ISSN 1044-2138

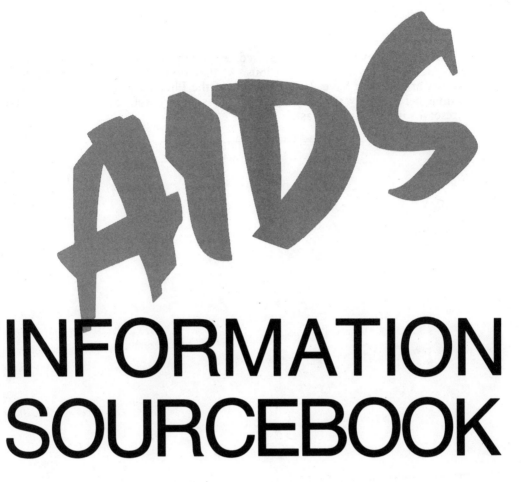

INFORMATION SOURCEBOOK

Second Edition 1989–90

Edited by H. Robert Malinowsky
and Gerald J. Perry

Foreword by James L. Holm
Acting Executive Director
National AIDS Network

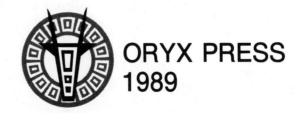

ORYX PRESS
1989

The rare Arabian Oryx is believed to have inspired the myth of the unicorn. This desert antelope became virtually extinct in the early 1960s. At that time several groups of international conservationists arranged to have 9 animals sent to the Phoenix Zoo to be the nucleus of a captive breeding herd. Today the Oryx population is nearly 800, and over 400 have been returned to reserves in the Middle East.

ISSN 1044-2138
ISBN 0-89774-544-2

CONTENTS

FOREWORD

As the 1990s approach, the face of AIDS continues to change, and it continues to spread with a seemingly unabated momentum. On one front, there are significant medical advances. Where once there were no therapies of proven efficacy, today AZT and other drugs are being recommended as possible interventions not only for the person with a full-blown AIDS diagnosis, but also for individuals at other points on the Human Immunodeficiency (HIV) infection continuum. Medical researchers are developing treatments which use advanced biomedical blocking techniques to disable the disease-causing virus. Prophylactic interventions such as the newly licensed aerosolized pentamidine are reducing the incidence of the opportunistic and often lethal infection, pneumocystis pneumonia. Persons with AIDS (PWAs) who have access to these new life-prolonging therapies are learning to *live* with AIDS.

This focus on living with AIDS does not minimize the lethal nature of the epidemic. AIDS has touched people from all walks of life including increasing numbers of Blacks, Hispanics, women, adolescents, and infants. IV drug use is now a primary transmission factor, and since IV drug use is frequently a concurrent phenomenon of poverty and unemployment, those most disproportionately affected by these social ills are now the target of HIV. Gay and bisexual men are still the majority population group infected with HIV despite the rising numbers of other population groups.

The 100,000th person diagnosed with AIDS is being reported as this book goes to press. Even more alarming is the fact that over a million infected people in the U.S. are living with the ambiguity of an unknown health future.

At the time it was identified, AIDS was known as Gay Related Immunodeficiency Complex (GRID) because it was prevalent among groups of gay men in New York, San Francisco, and Los Angeles. Today, AIDS is rapidly spreading to other population groups, although this does not need to continue to be true in the future.

The "vaccine" for AIDS is public information that promotes behavior change. HIV infection is clearly preventable. *The AIDS Information Sourcebook* contains what medical science cannot yet provide, information on how to keep others from being infected. Resources for education and prevention services and materials are clearly and thoroughly listed for cities in the United States and Canada.

Most of the facilities listed in the *Sourcebook* are a part of the community-based response to AIDS and are members of the National AIDS Network. They represent over 800 organizations that have provided opportunities for volunteerism by those moved by the epidemic to contribute their time and/or careers to stem the spread of AIDS and to care for those who are ill. This response is unprecedented in depth and effectiveness. We at the National AIDS Network urge you to join this response by utilizing and contributing to these organizations.

Take advantage of all available education resources. Follow the lead of outgoing U.S. Surgeon General C. Everett Koop who stresses the use of condoms as a safeguard against the spread of HIV. The leadership of this staunchly conservative physician in frankly and explicitly discussing sexual behavior as it relates to transmission of HIV and in concentrating on disease prevention over ideology has brought a greatly needed lucidity to the fight against this retrovirus. As he has shown us, informed, clear thinking and action is needed.

You *have* access to today's vaccine against AIDS: Information! You carry this preventive innoculation of information which you can use to stop the spread by helping those at risk to change their behavior.

Thank you to the publishers and editors of *The AIDS Information Sourcebook* for giving us all one more tool to help us be part of the solution.

James L. Holm
Acting Executive Director
National AIDS Network

PREFACE

In the past, the group at highest risk of contracting the AIDS-causing Human Immunodeficiency Virus (HIV) has been the homosexual population. In fact, many of the resources which exist today are based upon efforts established by and for the gay community to provide education in an attempt to control the spread of AIDS. Similarly, many of the organizations today providing services to persons with AIDS (PWAs) grew from the early efforts of the gay community to provide basic human necessities, from health care to support groups, from food and shelter to telephone counseling, for those stricken with the deadly virus. The toll has been overwhelming, both in terms of human life and in medical costs. However, the effort has paid off. Due to the education campaigns in the gay community, the incidence of new cases of AIDS among gay men in this country is at the lowest level in years and is steadily decreasing. However, other groups are now at a higher risk of contracting HIV than ever before, namely intravenous drug users and minorities. Efforts to provide education to these groups have been hampered by many barriers including illiteracy, religion, language, and cultural factors. As the shift in demographics of AIDS occurs, so must the resources for prevention and treatment of the disease change. Accordingly, a special emphasis has been made in this edition of the *Sourcebook* to include sources of information and services for these high-risk groups, especially the intravenous drug users.

The 1989/90 edition of *The AIDS Information Sourcebook* continues to be a guide to educational resources about the acquired immunodeficiency syndrome which are intended for the general public. First and foremost, it directs users to a wide variety of sources that help to answer questions about how AIDS is contracted, who is at risk, how to lessen one's chances of contracting AIDS, what is being done for people with AIDS, and what is being done to combat the AIDS-causing virus. It brings together a wide variety of information sources, providing a chronology of the history of the AIDS epidemic; alerting the user to the existence of agencies, facilities, and organizations established to handle questions about AIDS; and presenting a select, briefly annotated bibliography of literature on AIDS and AIDS-related topics.

ARRANGEMENT

The *Sourcebook* has been organized into three parts: Chronology, Directory of Organizations, and Bibliography. Appendices include information on drugs currently in development for diagnosis, treatment, and prevention of AIDS as well as a statistical analysis of the numbers of AIDS cases reported in the United States as of Spring 1989.

Chronology Section

The Chronology lists important milestones and events in the history of the AIDS epidemic from June 1981 to April 1989. Dates and events were selected that have a substantial impact on AIDS awareness and research. The events leading up to the original discovery of the syndrome were rather easy to identify, although there is considerable discussion as to whether AIDS is a new or old health problem. Until the development of a cure or vaccine, the history of AIDS must make mention of ongoing research, demographic trends, shifting public reactions, discussions of funding priorities, and news about major public personalities who have died of AIDS or related diseases. The Chronology has been continually updated with new milestones, and each new edition of the *Sourcebook* will reprint the Chronology with additions and corrections. A subject index to the Chronology has been added so that specific topics can be easily located.

Directory Section

The Directory of Organizations is arranged by state, then alphabetically by name of facility. Canadian facilities are listed alphabetically following facilities in the United States and Puerto Rico. Data for this section were compiled between August 1988 and April 1989 and were obtained through a questionnaire mailing to facilities listed in the first edition and others identified through the efforts of the authors and staff at The Oryx Press. Incomplete entries represent facilities from which no response was received.

Complete entries include the following information: complete name of organization, facility, or program, including any acronyms; previous name(s); address; telephone numbers including hotlines and toll-free numbers; key personnel with titles; organizational affiliation; type of organization, facility, or program; staff size; year founded; sources of funding support; outreach or educational services provided; network or consortia affiliations; names and dates of sponsored seminars, conferences, workshops, or symposia; areas of research interest; additional information, including descriptions of special services provided, history of the program, and other descriptive information; publications available, including newsletters, journals, books, audiovisuals, pamphlets, posters, buttons, and other promotional materials; and languages spoken other than English, including American Sign Language. A facility type index, new to this edition, as well as an alphabetical listing of facilities follow this section.

Over 800 facilities in the United States and Canada are listed in this edition. With this edition of the *Source-*

book, the coverage has been greatly expanded so that it includes not only facilities whose primary or only purpose is to deal with AIDS but also facilities such as clinics, hospices, hospitals, alternative health groups, counseling and testing sites, substance abuse counseling and treatment programs, and public aid organizations.

Users of this book should contact the facility in their area when seeking information about AIDS. Many have toll-free hotline telephone numbers. Volunteers frequently staff these hotlines, and hours of operation may be limited. If you cannot get through to your local hotline, try one in another region.

All listed organizations consider public education a primary goal and most either produce or distribute educational materials; all have expressed a willingness to widely distribute these materials either free or for a small handling fee. Be aware, however, that some may use sexually explicit language or illustrations presenting information in "street language" with a minimum of technical jargon. The primary purpose of these materials is to educate the public and therefore they include simple terminology and, in many cases, frank illustrations.

Bibliography Section

The last portion of this book is a bibliography of publications which have appeared over the past six years and which pertain to AIDS. This bibliography is divided into section by type of publication: periodical articles, bibliographies, books, brochures/pamphlets, curriculum/education programs, directories, fiction, film/video/audio resources, online databases, periodicals, plays, and posters. All but the articles are cumulated from the first edition. A subject index is provided.

Complete entries include the following information, where appropriate: title; author; publisher's name and address; year produced; pagination or running time; cost; ISBN; document number; an annotation; and for journal articles, periodical title, volume number, and date. Each entry is assigned an accession number for easy reference.

More educational materials are now being developed which target intravenous drug users, since they are now one of the higher risk groups. Educational materials for minorities are also more widely available with more and more materials in languages other than English, especially Spanish.

One unassailable fact is that AIDS may be transmitted through sexual contact. Therefore, a large portion of the available literature focuses on the prevention of AIDS through the practice of safer sex. The use of condoms is a recommended practice for prevention of AIDS and many of the posters are rather explicit in this promotion. Similarly, educational materials that discuss the connection between intravenous drug abuse and AIDS are often considered taboo. There are numerous brochures describing the hazards of needle-sharing; many give advice on how to clean needles and most encourage drug users to seek help in breaking their habit. This literature may be controversial, and as a result, may not find its way into the hand of the general public. The *Sourcebook* should help to make this information more available to those needing it.

Appendices

Two appendices, new to the 1989/90 edition, will be of importance to those interested in statistical representation of the incidence of AIDS in this country or to anyone interested in the current status of any of the drugs currently in development for prevention, diagnosis, or treatment of AIDS. The first appendix, reproduced with the permission of the United States Centers for Disease Control, is the monthly *HIV/AIDS Surveillance Report*, containing information on AIDS cases reported through April 1989. It is followed by information compiled by the Pharmaceutical Manufacturers Association giving the status of AIDS products in development, including anti-virals, immuno-modulators, anti-infectives, diagnostics, and vaccines.

ACKNOWLEDGMENTS

Compassion empowered with knowledge can achieve miracles. Short of a miracle, education is the only way to prevent the spread of AIDS and save lives. The authors hope this book will help in the educational process and that it does not have to go through too many editions before a cure or vaccine is developed.

The authors would like to thank their colleagues for alerting them to specific items to include, and facilities that answered the questionnaire. Special thanks to Rhonda Shapiro who located additional information to be included in the chronology and did most of the proofreading; to Michael Musheno of the Arizona State University School of Justice Studies who made suggestions as to the coverage of legal events and publications; to Peter Kelly of the Arizona AIDS Project, Inc., who made himself available for questions and consultation; to Linda Webster for her expertise in indexing the chronology; and especially to Susan Johnson of Oryx Press for her suggestions, support, consultations, and help in keeping deadlines.

The authors welcome comments and suggestions, as well as new information for inclusion in future editions. Please address communications to *The AIDS Information Sourcebook*: The Oryx Press, 2214 North Central at Encanto, Phoenix, AZ 85004-1483.

LIST OF ABBREVIATIONS

AIDS	Acquired immune deficiency syndrome (or Acquired immunodeficiency syndrome)
AMA	American Medical Association
AmFAR	American Foundation for AIDS Research
ARC	AIDS-related complex
AZT	Azidothymidine (now known as Retrovir)
CAIN	Computerized AIDS Information Network
CDC	Centers for Disease Control
DDC	Dideoxycytidine
FDA	Food and Drug Administration
HIV	Human immunodeficiency virus = HTLV-III = AIDS virus
HTLV-III	Human T-cell leukemia virus III
LAV	Lymphadenopathy virus
NAN	National AIDS Network
NCI	National Cancer Institute
NIAID	National Institute of Allergy and Infectious Diseases
NIDA	National Institute on Drug Abuse
NIH	National Institutes of Health
NIMH	National Institute of Mental Health
PWA	Person with AIDS
PWARC	Person with AIDS-related complex
STD	Sexually transmitted disease
WHO	United Nations World Health Organization

PART I

CHRONOLOGY

1981

June

2. **Pneumocystis pneumonia** CDC reports five unusual cases of pneumocystis pneumonia among homosexual men in Los Angeles

July

3. **Pneumocystis pneumonia and Kaposi's sarcoma** CDC reports cases of pneumocystis pneumonia and Kaposi's sarcoma among homosexual males in New York City

December

4. **Blood supply** CDC reports that infant who received blood transfusions developed serious immune deficiency disease that has principally afflicted homosexuals

1982

May

5. **Immune disorder** Serious disorder of immune system that has been known to doctors for less than one year and that appears to affect primarily male homosexuals, afflicts 335 people, killing 136

June

6. **Pneumocystis pneumonia and Kaposi's sarcoma** CDC reports clusters of pneumocystis pneumonia and Kaposi's sarcoma in Los Angeles and Orange counties of California

July

7. **Opportunistic infections** CDC reports the occurrence of opportunistic infections and Kaposi's sarcoma among Haitians in the US

8. **Pneumocystis pneumonia and hemophilia** CDC reports cases of pneumocystis pneumonia among persons with hemophilia

August

9. **New York City** Nearly one half of nation's cases of serious disease whose victims are primarily homosexual men have been reported in New York City. Disease has been recently termed Acquired Immune Deficiency Syndrome (AIDS)

November

10. **Occupational concerns** CDC issues precautions for clinical and laboratory staff working with blood and other laboratory samples

December

11. **Red Cross policy** American Red Cross says it will review policy for selecting blood donors, following reports that child developed often-fatal immune deficiency (AIDS) from donor

12. **Transfusions and AIDS** CDC reports a possible transfusion-linked case of AIDS

1983

January

13. **Women and AIDS** CDC reports immune deficiency among female partners of males with AIDS

March

14. **At-risk groups** American Red Cross says it will inform homosexual males, Haitian immigrants, drug users, and others considered at high risk of carrying AIDS that they should not donate blood

15. **First AIDS prevention guidelines** CDC reports on the Public Health Service inter-agency recommendations for the prevention of AIDS

16. **Transmission of AIDS** Report in *New England Journal of Medicine* cites study of seven female sexual partners of men with AIDS, which suggests that disease may be sexually transmitted between heterosexual men and women

May

17. **Detection of HTLV-III/LAV** American and French scientists report in the journal *Science*, the detection of a retrovirus, HTLV-III/LAV, among those either with, or at risk, for AIDS

18. **HTLV-III/LAV and AIDS** American scientists publish evidence of a direct relationship between HTLV-III/LAV infection and the subsequent development of AIDS

19. **Public health** Health and Human Services Asst Secretary Edward N Brandt says investigation of AIDS has become number one priority of US Public Health Service

June

20. **At-risk groups** AIDS, thought to be caused by a virus found in bodily secretions causing near-total collapse of body's immune system, is found in Haitian men and women, intravenous drug users and their female partners, and infants and children, in addition to homosexual men

August

21. **Universities** Recent trend on university campuses not to recognize gay/lesbian student organizations prompts opinion that spread of AIDS is encouraging fear and intolerance of homosexuals across the nation

September

22. **Occupational concerns** Medical study group at the Univ of California at San Francisco concludes that there is no scientific reason why health care personnel who are reluctant to treat PWAs should be excused from doing so

23. **Occupational precautions** Federal government urges dentists, morticians, and medical examiners to take special precautions against contracting AIDS. CDC issues precautions for health care workers and allied health professionals regarding exposure to AIDS

October

24. **US-Haitian link** Study of 61 Haitians suspected of having AIDS, published in *The New England Journal of Medicine*, finds many lived in Haitian prostitution center and had homosexual relations with Americans, providing possible link in spread of the disease

November

25. **Global concern** Laurence K Altman reports that AIDS is now seen as a worldwide problem with incidence doubling in Europe within one year

26. **Immune system abnormalities** Study by Mt Sinai School of Medicine shows that Haitian immigrants do not have any of immune system abnormalities discovered in homosexual men, another group susceptible to syndrome

27. **Multiple causes** Dr Joseph A Sonnabend, in report to international scientific meeting on AIDS in Manhattan, says there may be no single cause of AIDS even though many scientists are searching for proof that some single virus or other infectious agent is responsible

1984

January

28. **Transmission of AIDS** New evidence is reported that AIDS can be spread heterosexually and transmitted even before a person shows outward manifestations of disease

April

29. **Discovery of virus** Federal researchers announce they have found virus that is believed to be the cause of AIDS; call virus HTLV-III and say they have developed process to mass-produce it for purpose of developing tools needed to conquer AIDS, which now afflicts more than 4000 Americans

30. **Research controversy** Controversy regarding credit for discovery of virus believed to be the cause of AIDS is sorted out in article noting contributions of scientists at both Pasteur Institute in Paris and NCI (*New York Times*, Apr 29, 1987)

June

31. **STD decline** CDC reports declining rates of sexually transmitted diseases among males in New York City

August

32. **Animal research** Researchers from CDC and NIH succeed in infecting chimpanzees with AIDS, thus taking crucial step toward development of vaccine against disease; transmission of disease to primates strengthens case that virus causes AIDS

October

33. **Blood supply** Abbott Laboratories gets FDA approval for diagnostic to screen blood for antibodies to virus believed to be the cause of AIDS

34. **Genetic variations** NCI researcher Dr Robert Gallo says genetic variations have been found in samples of virus believed to cause AIDS which could pose significant problems for vaccine development

November

35. **AIDS in infants** NY Hospital/Cornell Medical Center researchers say six infants in New York City have contracted AIDS from healthy mothers, supporting theory that disease can exist in remissive state that can become deadly when passed on to infants

December

36. **Blood testing** Researchers at Univ of California say one of first blood tests to detect AIDS virus in humans will be used in as many as 10,000 samples next year; samples will be taken at random from blood donor centers

1985

January

37. **Blood supply** CDC reports provisional Public Health Service inter-agency recommendations for the screening of donated blood for antibodies to HTLV-III/LAV

38. **Transmission of AIDS** As epidemic of AIDS continues unabated, CDC experts fear that disease may now pose a threat to heterosexuals; warnings against promiscuity issued. (Based only on preliminary figures, mostly from Africa and Haiti, with scant US numbers)

February

39. **Experimental drugs** Pasteur Institute researcher Dr Jean Claude Chermann reports that new compound drug, HPA-23, appears for first time to have inhibited reproduction of virus believed to cause AIDS

40. **Religion and AIDS** Group of Protestant, Roman Catholic, and Jewish leaders issues joint statement calling on public "not to stand in judgement" of PWAs, but to show compassion for them

March

41. **Blood supply** Blood banks across nation begin issuing screening test designed to protect blood supplies from contamination by virus suspected of causing AIDS

April

42. **Haitians and AIDS** CDC drops recent Haitian immigrants from list of those considered at greatest risk of contracting AIDS

May

43. **AIDS symptoms** Report in *New England Journal of Medicine* indicates that AIDS virus may persist without symptoms in infected people for more than four years

44. **AIDS virus** AIDS is now known to be caused by virus LAV or HTLV-III and follows persistent pattern of contagion

45. **Occupational concerns** Dr David Henderson of NIH says study of hundreds of doctors, nurses, and others exposed at hospitals to AIDS shows that even such close contact is unlikely to spread the disease

June

46. **AIDS test** Method of detecting antibodies in blood samples that indicate presence of HTLV-III is patented for Dept of Health and Human Services by Drs Robert C Gallo, Mikulas Popovic, and M G Sarngadharan

47. **Gene discovery** Reports in journal *Science* indicate scientists have discovered previously unidentified gene in virus that causes AIDS; believed important key to understanding how virus produces some of its effects. Report also suggests that closer study may eventually lead to new ways to treat or prevent AIDS

July

48. **AZT** Burroughs Wellcome Co begins testing their drug AZT (azidothymidine) with 33 patients with AIDS

49. **Immune system breakdown** Government scientists identify critical defect in immune system of AIDS patients; report virus selectively destroys key set of blood cells, T-4 helper cells, that are supposed to detect invading viruses and set immune system into motion to destroy them

50. **Rock Hudson** French confirm that Rock Hudson has AIDS

August

51. **AIDS education** Los Angeles County Supervisors label the first safe sex materials pornographic; say it "attempts to subsidize deviant behavior"

52. **Blood supply** NIH reports that new test has apparently succeeded in screening AIDS-tainted blood from US supply of blood for transfusions

53. **Causes of AIDS** New findings suggest that other viruses in addition to LAV/HTLV-III may play role in causing AIDS

54. **Genetic variations** NCI researchers report AIDS virus has so many variations in its genetic structure that developing preventive vaccine may prove difficult

55. **Military and AIDS** Asst Defense Secretary William E Mayer announces that department will screen all prospective military recruits for possible exposure to AIDS virus

56. **Public opinion** CDC reports results from two Gallup polls on AIDS indicating that 95% of the US population has heard of AIDS

57. **Schools and AIDS** Western Middle School in Kokomo, IN bars Ryan White, 13-year-old who contracted AIDS while being treated for hemophilia, for fear he might pose a health threat to other pupils

58. **Schools and AIDS** Los Angeles officials report 3-year-old boy with AIDS has been barred from class for handicapped children and will receive private instruction at home if he is accepted into county special education program

59. **Schools and AIDS** CDC issues guidelines indicating school-aged children infected with the AIDS virus should be allowed to attend school, and school officials should do their best to protect pupils' privacy. However, the guidelines recommend that preschoolers and handicapped children be kept out of school until more is known about how the disease is transmitted. CDC also recommends that adoption and foster care agencies administer AIDS antibody tests to children whose parents are in high-risk groups, or whose parents' histories are not known

60. **State reactions to AIDS** Colorado Board of Health, over objections from the ACLU, tentatively agrees to start keeping list of people who have been exposed to AIDS virus

September

61. **AIDS benefit** Hollywood "Night of 1000 Stars" raises $1.3 mil for AIDS research

62. **At-risk groups** The FDA redefines gay-related high-risk group for AIDS to include "any male who has had sex with another male since 1977"

63. **Discrimination** Test developed to protect US blood supply from AIDS has sparked controversy regarding question of personal liberties vs public interests. Civil libertarians say personal trauma of individuals exposed to AIDS is intensified by fear that test results will be disclosed, leading to discriminatory practices

64. **Experimental drugs** FDA approves experimental use in US of HPA-23, which apparently prevents AIDS virus from reproducing, but does not eliminate immune system suppression that leaves victims vulnerable to disease

65. **Federal AIDS funding** A House appropriations subcommittee is told that $70 mil more is needed for AIDS research and treatment, twice what the Reagan administration had originally requested

66. **Insurance and AIDS** Insurance industry, fearing large claims by PWAs, is considering new ways to find out if applicants have disorder

67. **National AIDS Research Foundation** Elizabeth Taylor named national chairperson of the National AIDS Research Foundation

68. **Public opinion** New York Times/CBS News poll finds that about one-half of Americans believe that AIDS can be transmitted through casual contact, despite what federal scientists say is overwhelming evidence to the contrary

69. **Research** CDC reports results of *Acquired Immunodeficiency Syndrome in San Francisco Cohort Study, 1978-1985*. According to the report, 73.1% of those active in the study, about 6800 homosexual and bisexual men who sought treatment for STDs at a San Francisco city clinic, demonstrated antibodies to HTLV-III/LAV

70. **Schools and AIDS** Parents in two community school districts in Queens, NY organize boycott to protest city's decision to allow second-grader with AIDS to attend regular classes. 11,000 students stay home from school on the first day; 9000 do so on the second day

71. **Schools and AIDS** Orange County, FL, bars 5-year-old with AIDS from kindergarten; action comes despite recommendation by Florida Medical Assn that students and teachers who have AIDS should not be denied access to public schools

October

72. **Behavioral changes** CDC reports self-imposed behavioral changes among gay and bisexual males in San Francisco

73. **Control of AIDS** US Public Health Service unveils long-range plan to control spread of AIDS; plan sets two goals: Reduction in steady increase in transmission of AIDS virus by 1990, and elimination of spread of virus by year 2000

74. **Insurance and AIDS** Lincoln National Life Insurance Co instructs its underwriters to examine applicants' personal lives and use marital status, age, and residence in attempt to screen out possible PWAs. Company policy is that marital status is possible indicator of homosexuality. Underwriters told to flag applicants if "lifestyle, habits, or medical history suggest a person is in one of the AIDS risk groups." Company spokesman Al Parsons defends suggestions, noting high medical costs often incurred in treatment of AIDS (*Dallas Times-Herald*, 10/6/85)

75. **Military and AIDS** Defense Dept decides to screen all 2.1 million military personnel for AIDS virus; those who develop disease would be treated, counseled, and receive honorable medical discharges

76. **Public reaction** Two protestors chain themselves to the Federal Office Building in San Francisco until more federal money is allocated for AIDS research and ARC patients receive the same benefits as AIDS patients

77. **Rock Hudson** Rock Hudson's death creates a national swell of support for AIDS research

78. **Schools and AIDS** New York City Schools Chancellor Nathan Quinones reveals that three children had been removed from classes because their mothers' boyfriends were suspected of having AIDS

79. **Schools and AIDS** National Education Assn suggests schools test students or teachers for AIDS if there is reasonable cause to suspect that they have been infected; also urges that districts decide on case-by-case basis whether children with AIDS should attend regular classes

80. **Spread of AIDS** Newark, Miami, and Houston join the list of cities with increased AIDS cases. AIDS was first reported in large numbers in this country in Manhattan, San Francisco, and Los Angeles

81. **Transmission of AIDS** CDC says study indicates that risk of transmitting AIDS from daily contact in the home apparently is non-existent, even when sharing razors, toothbrushes, and other household items with PWAs

82. **Transmission of AIDS** Harvard School of Public Health warns that AIDS is spreading through sexual activity into general population

November

83. **AIDS and the media** NBC presents *An Early Frost*, the first made-for-TV family drama with an AIDS theme

84. **AIDS in Africa** Researchers in Africa report AIDS seems to be spreading by conventional sexual intercourse among heterosexuals in Africa, and striking women nearly as often as men; women with the disease are giving birth to infected babies

85. **AIDS in Africa** Controversial new research results that point both to and against Africa as origin of AIDS fuels international furor. Origin is regarded as key factor in search for cause and cure. Also at issue is whether disease is truly new, or merely newly recognized. Some American and European scientists say it is so widespread in Central Africa that they doubt it could have been introduced there recently

86. **AIDS in Africa** Scientists think risky blood transfusion practices throughout Africa may be one reason why so many African men and women suffer from AIDS. With rare exception, donor blood in Africa is not tested for evidence of the AIDS virus

87. **AIDS in China** China announces strategy against AIDS, including checks on foreigners and Chinese who work with them

88. **Blood supply** Statco Co president Dr Henry Tomizawa says company may soon make available for hospital and emergency use AIDS-free blood substitutes originally developed by US Army researchers

89. **Blood supply** Thousands of people in US store their own blood for use in elective surgery rather than risk getting AIDS from donated blood

90. **Discrimination** San Francisco Board of Supervisors votes unanimously to outlaw discrimination against AIDS/ARC patients

91. **Economic impact** Hospital administrators tell Congressional sub-committee that growing number of PWAs who are unable to pay their hospital bills threatens financial stability of nation's health care system

92. **International conference on AIDS** International conference on AIDS is held in Brussels

93. **Occupational concerns** US Public Health Service says there is generally no need to place special restrictions on food handlers and health care workers infected with AIDS. There is no evidence virus has spread through casual contact; urges instead adherence to sanitary precautions already in place to deal with wide variety of diseases

94. **Prostitutes and AIDS** Scientists say the fear that prostitutes will be the major conduit of AIDS spread into the heterosexual community at large is unjustified; spread of AIDS virus from women to men through sexual contact has rarely been documented

95. **Schools and AIDS** Indiana hearing officer rules teenager with AIDS, Ryan White, may return to classroom studies in Kokomo, where he had been barred by school officials

December

96. **AIDS and meningitis** *New England Journal of Medicine* reports effects of AIDS virus on brain may appear before there is evidence of destruction of immune system. This raises possibility that central nervous system may serve as sanctuary for virus, which, because of blood-brain barrier, might complicate task of developing effective drug treatment against virus

97. **AIDS in Africa** Cases of AIDS in Africa continue to mount and doctors, lacking manpower and money, have been unable to carry out surveys needed to measure severity and nature of epidemic

98. **AIDS in Africa** African countries start to become more open about AIDS. Some governments have, in the past, suppressed scientific reports for fear that publicity might threaten tourism and foreign exchange. WHO officials, in expression of mounting concern, say they plan new push to control global epidemic of usually fatal disease

99. **Condoms** Univ of California at San Francisco researchers show that the AIDS virus is blocked by the use of condoms

100. **Drugs and AIDS** New York State Health Commissioner David Axelrod warns Congressional committee hearing that there has been little progress in curbing spread of AIDS through addicts who inject drugs and doubts providing free single-use needles would work

101. **Federal AIDS funding** Office of Management and Budget proposes to cut spending on AIDS as part of Pres Reagan's budget for fiscal year 1987

102. **Federal AIDS funding** Pres Reagan signs appropriations bill that includes $234 mil for AIDS-related funding

103. **Insurance and AIDS** Increasingly, insurance companies are trying to pre-screen applicants for AIDS, either through blood tests or by making judgments based on applicants' personal and medical profiles

104. **LaRouche speaks out on AIDS** Lyndon H LaRouche, Jr says AIDS is caused by "the dirty sexual habits of gays and by elected officials who have traded away their morals" in support of gay civil rights

105. **Pregnancy and AIDS** CDC says pregnant women infected with AIDS may run risk as high as 65% of passing infection to unborn child; issues guidelines calling for testing of high-risk women who are or may become pregnant

106. **Premarital testing** AMA considers resolution calling for mandatory premarital testing of all couples for presence of AIDS virus

107. **Research controversy** Pasteur Institute director Raymond Dedonder contends that its research team headed by Dr Luc Montagnier found virus that causes AIDS and developed first test to detect antibodies to virus in 1983, a year before US team led by Dr Robert Gallo of NCI

108. **Schools and AIDS** School district in Hazelwood, MO drops training in cardiopulmonary resuscitation because of fear that high school students might be exposed to AIDS

109. **Transmission of AIDS** New report, published in *New England Journal of Medicine* indicates that AIDS virus was detected in saliva of only one of 71 homosexual men known to be infected with disease. Scientists say finding should help allay public fears that AIDS can be spread through casual social contact

1986

January

110. **AIDS education** CDC places 14 proposals for safe sex education materials "on hold" because of their sexually explicit content

111. **AIDS in Saudia Arabia** Saudi Arabia requires a negative AIDS test to obtain a visa to visit

112. **Charles Lee Morris** Charles Lee Morris, former San Francisco publisher, dies at age 42 of AIDS. He had been ill since 1978 and was one of the longest-surviving PWAs

113. **Economic impact** First published estimate of national impact of AIDS states that first 10,000 cases will total nearly $6.3 bil. $1.4 bil in hospital expenses and nearly $5 bil in earnings have been lost because of disability and premature death. Study finds hospital expenses have averaged $147,000 per AIDS patient

114. **Experimental drugs** Japanese researcher says new drug treatment for AIDS tested on 15 patients in US has proved effective in keeping virus from multiplying but cannot be considered cure

115. **Research** CDC scientists discover way AIDS virus zeroes in on its target in body's immune system. Dr Steven J McDougal says finding suggests new ways of stopping or preventing AIDS infection

116. **Transmission of AIDS** US government indicates that the spread of AIDS in the general population is not expected to be rapid as first thought, but AIDS is still one of the highest killers

117. **Tuberculosis and AIDS** CDC and New York City health officials investigate possible link between AIDS virus and increased number of tuberculosis cases in city. Scientists are finding that areas with the largest increase in tuberculosis are identical to those with the highest rates of AIDS

February

118. **AZT** Phase II testing of AZT with 300 patients begins. Placebo control used initially, but dropped quickly when 16 on placebo die as opposed to only one on AZT

119. **Experimental drugs** FDA challenges Newport Pharmaceuticals Inc's report that it had some success treating AIDS with isoprinosine

120. **Insurance and AIDS** Revised New York State legislation proposed by Gov Mario Cuomo would bar insurance companies from requiring policy applicants to take blood test for AIDS. Test could only be used to screen blood and organs for donations

121. **Reagan administration** Pres Reagan says that the administration is committed to finding cure for disease; asks Surgeon General C Everett Koop to prepare a "major report" on AIDS. Rep Henry A Waxman (D-CA) terms Reagan's pronouncement "outrageous," noting that Reagan's budget, made public Feb 6, includes reductions in spending for AIDS research (*New York Times*, Feb 6, 1986)

122. **Schools and AIDS** Howard County, IN Circuit Court Judge R Alan Brubaker bars 14-year-old PWA Ryan White from attending his seventh-grade classes after he returns to school for one day following 15-month absence

123. **Transmission of AIDS** A mother contracts AIDS as result of extensive contact with the blood and bodily fluids of a child with AIDS. The woman did not wear gloves and did not "often wash her hands" after blood or secretion contact

March

124. **Insurance donations** Insurance companies donate $1.1 mil towards AIDS education and research

125. **Religion and AIDS** Mormon Church excommunicates Clair Howard after he is diagnosed as having AIDS

126. **Research** Scientists at NCI have identified and produced in pure form enzyme that is key to ability of AIDS virus to infect human cells

127. **Research** Scientists at NCI, led by Dr Flossie Wong-Staal, and team at Harvard Univ's Dana Farber Cancer Institute, led by Dr William A Haseltine, find way to make AIDS virus harmless by inactivating one of its genes in laboratory experiments

128. **Women and AIDS** Scientists say that new evidence of AIDS virus in women could help explain how disease can be spread among heterosexuals

April

129. **AIDS testing** Researchers at Cincinnati Veterans Administration Medical Center and Cincinnati blood center report that people afflicted with both alcoholism and hepatitis B virus could incorrectly test positive for AIDS virus

130. **Drugs and AIDS** The number of reported cases of AIDS among drug users rises dramatically

131. **Experimental drugs** Federal program expected to get under way this summer to treat up to 2000 people with AIDS at 10 hospitals using an experimental drug therapy for AIDS. Dr Ian MacDonald of Dept of Health and Human Services says drugs to be tested will be selected from "most promising" ones being developed

132. **Experimental vaccine** Two research teams successfully use genetic engineering techniques to modify smallpox vaccine and plan to seek approval before end of 1986 to test it on humans as protection against AIDS

133. **Immigration regulations** American consular officers receive authority to require aliens who seek temporary visas to undergo test for AIDS. Public Health Service says new regulation would add AIDS to list of "dangerous contagious diseases" which prohibit entry into United States

134. **Public opinion** Two-thirds of people surveyed would permit their children to attend school with an AIDS patient

135. **Public reaction** Some people feel PWAs should be quarantined, tattooed, or identified in some way

136. **Research controversy** US Patent and Trademark Office reportedly decides to allow formal proceedings to determine whether French or American scientists were first to invent AIDS antibody test

137. **Schools and AIDS** Ryan White, 14-year-old PWA, returns to his seventh-grade classes in Kokomo, IN, less than two hours after judge throws out injunction barring him from school. Parents of 27 other children remove them from school, fearful they might develop disease. Parents of at least 15 students plan to enroll their children at makeshift school in nearby Russiaville, rather than expose them to Ryan White

May

138. **AIDS in Africa** Uganda acknowledges the AIDS epidemic and launches a mass education drive to prevent its spread

139. **Insurance and AIDS** Washington, DC City Council unanimously approves legislation requiring life insurance companies to provide coverage to people exposed to AIDS virus

140. **New York City** New York City Health Dept epidemiologist Dr Alan R Kristal reports that AIDS has become leading killer in New York City of men aged 30 to 44 and women aged 25 to 29

141. **Research** Researchers have for the first time grown the AIDS virus in animal tissues

142. **Research** Article in journal *Science* reports that researchers have prevented AIDS virus from invading and infecting human cells in test tube; laboratory techniques could become basis for immunization against AIDS

143. **Research** Discovery of a seventh gene makes the AIDS virus the most complex of any of the retroviruses

144. **Research funding** The American Foundation for AIDS Research (AmFAR) awards its first grants for AIDS research totaling more than $1 mil

145. **Spread of AIDS** New York and California now account for less than 50% of AIDS cases, compared with 75% in 1981 and 1982

146. **Transfusions and AIDS** CDC study finds that average time lag between infection with AIDS virus and onset of AIDS has been at least five years among people who developed disease after receiving contaminated blood transfusions

June

147. **AIDS and child visitation** Court orders divorced gay father in Chicago to take HTLV-III test before he can visit his children

148. **AIDS and the media** *AIDS Show* airs on San Francisco PBS-TV station and shows the sadness and humor in the AIDS crisis

149. **AIDS in Africa** WHO reports at least 50,000 Africans may have contracted AIDS since 1980, and estimated one to 2 million people on continent may be symptomless carriers of virus that causes disease

150. **AIDS in Haiti** AIDS spreads in Haiti now predominantly through heterosexual intercourse. Researchers report that since 1983 there has been a sharp rise in AIDS cases among heterosexuals and a decline in the number of cases among homosexual men and intravenous drug users

151. **Blood supply** Health researchers at the CDC report the first case of a patient becoming infected with the AIDS virus from a blood transfusion that had been tested and showed no signs of the deadly disease

152. **Civil rights** Lawyers in Justice Dept civil rights division say people with AIDS are entitled to protection under federal civil rights law because they meet statutory definition of "handicapped individuals," having physical impairment that limits one or more "major life activities"

153. **Civil rights** The US Justice Dept rules that federal civil rights laws do not prohibit the arbitrary firing of employees with AIDS or other contagious diseases. Ruling states in part that "An employer may not fire an AIDS victim on the basis of any disabling effect of AIDS, but may do so if concerned about contagious effects." Decision interprets legal rights of PWAs much more narrowly than department's civil rights lawyers had recommended

154. **Economic impact** Anne A Scitovsky, leading health economist, reports that per capita cost of providing hospital care to AIDS patients in 1984 ranged from $60,000 to $75,000 per patient, or about half the amount projected last year by CDC. Government's "astronomical projections" have frightened employers and insurers

155. **Federal AIDS funding** The US government announces contracts for $100 mil to speed up the search for an AIDS cure

156. **Hospital for AIDS** 150-bed Citizens General Hospital, Houston, TX, converts into nation's first hospital devoted solely to AIDS patient care and research under agreement reached by American Medical International Inc and Univ of Texas System

157. **International conference on AIDS** The second International Conference on AIDS is held in Paris

158. **Kaposi's sarcoma** Proportion of patients with Kaposi's sarcoma with AIDS drops to 14% through April from 34% in 1981. Some researchers say there may be unknown factor in addition to AIDS virus that puts homosexual men at risk for Kaposi's sarcoma, and that exposure to co-factor is declining, perhaps as result of safer sexual practices among homosexual and bisexual men

159. **Military and AIDS** Petty Officer Second Class Phillip J Nolan, who refused to take blood tests for antibodies to AIDS, is found guilty at court-martial of disobeying order. Military spokesman says he is first serviceman to challenge test for AIDS

160. **Proposition 64** Followers of the political extremist Lyndon H LaRouche Jr succeed in placing a referendum on the Nov 4 California ballot that could lead to the quarantine of PWAs. The initiative, which has been denounced by the California Medical Assn and public health officials, would redefine AIDS as an infectious disease, similar to measles and tuberculosis, and would authorize health officials to use a variety of controls, including quarantine, to restrict the activities of PWAs and carriers of the virus

161. **Recovery** Research team at NIAID in Bethesda, MD reports that for the first time a human immune system severely damaged by AIDS has been restored to apparently normal health. Team expresses caution and describes results as crucial early step toward long-term development of therapy for AIDS. Bone marrow transplant, obtained from healthy twin of patient, transfusions of lymphocytes, and antiviral drug were used as treatment

162. **Schools and AIDS** The AMA maintains public schools should be open to children with AIDS, except for pre-schoolers and handicapped

163. **Spread of AIDS** Federal health officials predict tenfold increase in number of AIDS cases and deaths in next five years. Virus spreads widely outside New York and San Francisco and infects larger segment of heterosexual population

July

164. **AIDS and child visitation** Court allows divorced gay father in Chicago to have daughters visit him without the HTLV-III test

165. **Blood supply** Greater New York Blood Program says that it is working to identify about 700 people who received transfusions since 1977 that might have been contaminated with AIDS virus

166. **Blood supply** Public anxiety about transfusions mounts. Blood supply is safer than it has ever been because of dramatic changes in nation's blood banks. Concern that increased precautions at blood banks may contribute to anxiety that could lead patients who need transfusions to refuse them

167. **Discrimination** AMA, in a legal brief filed with the Supreme Court, charges that Justice Dept decision permitting certain types of job discrimination against people with AIDS is legally incorrect and unjustified

168. **Federal AIDS funding** Five months after Pres Reagan asked Congress to cut federal spending for AIDS, Public Health Service proposes more than doubling federal budget for all activities related to AIDS

169. **Haitians and AIDS** CDC reports clusters of disease showing up in Florida do not match pattern elsewhere in nation. Haitians will become first group listed at risk by heterosexual transmission

170. **Murder by AIDS** Florida charges two prisoners with a conspiracy of murder when they placed AIDS-contaminated blood serum in the coffee of a corrections officer

171. **Research** Immunologists at Georgetown Univ Hospital will begin human clinical trials of treatment for AIDS aimed at revitalizing immune system of those afflicted

172. **Schools and AIDS** Group of parents in Kokomo, IN drops legal fight to bar Ryan White from classroom

173. **Swine fever** Researchers test blood of AIDS patients for the presence of African swine fever as well as blood serum collected from pigs in Belle Glade, FL for presence of human AIDS virus as a result of disputed report that antibodies to African swine fever were found in a single pig there. African swine fever, one of the world's most devastating livestock diseases, has never been found in North America

174. **Transmission of AIDS** Indiana Univ School of Medicine criticizes as "premature" New York study of families of PWAs that concluded they were highly unlikely to become infected with deadly disease through nonsexual contact

August

175. **AIDS in Africa** French scientists say that specimens of numerous insects from central Africa have been found to contain AIDS. Despite discovery, transmission of AIDS to humans by insects is considered extremely unlikely

176. **Airlines** AIDS patient Mark Sigers returns to San Francisco on Eastern Air Lines after Delta refused to carry him (*Los Angeles Times*, Aug 8, 1986)

177. **Blood supply** Growth of commercial blood banks that freeze and store supply of customer's own blood

178. **Discovery of virus** Dr Shyh-Ching Lo of Armed Forces Institute of Pathology discovers hitherto unknown virus among AIDS patients. Too soon to know what relationship, if any, microbe has to AIDS. Scientists are intrigued by unusual way Dr Lo isolated virus, which has never been found in any patient other than those with AIDS. Several possible ways in which new virus might contribute to AIDS infection noted

179. **Discrimination** Dept of Health and Human Services accuses the Charlotte Memorial Hospital in North Carolina of discrimination when a nurse was fired after he was discovered to have AIDS

180. **Discrimination** California State Assembly approves bill barring job and housing discrimination against PWAs

181. **Experimental drugs** Dr Mathilde Krim contends patients with other life-threatening diseases for which there are no established therapy can avail themselves of latest, most hopeful treatments, even if they are still experimental. Americans who have AIDS should be entitled to some measure of hope

182. **Gift of Peace** Nobel Prize winner Mother Teresa opens second home called Gift of Peace for PWAs in Washington, DC. The first home is located in New York City

183. **Organ transplants** Two patients have received transplanted organs that were later discovered to have been donated by a PWA who had received such large blood transfusions that the AIDS virus present in his blood was not detected. Transplanted organs, however, have not been found to transmit AIDS, according to CDC spokesperson Dr Betty Hooper

184. **Reporting categories** New knowledge surfaces about heterosexual transmission of disease; category in which heterosexual PWAs are listed now includes foreign-born people with disease. More than half of those now in revised category are Haitians. CDC reports new category lists 862 PWAs

185. **Research** NCI researchers report that they have created new form of AIDS virus that appears harmless to human cells in test tubes and could help development of AIDS vaccine

186. **Schools and AIDS** Ryan White is cleared for school by county health officials, provided certain precautions are taken. These precautions, called unnecessary by leading scientists, include giving Ryan a separate bathroom and disposable utensils

187. **Schools and AIDS** New York City officials say 6 of 13 children known to have AIDS, or less-severe disorder, AIDS-related complex, will be allowed to attend public schools. Identities of children and schools will not be disclosed

September

188. **Airlines** Mark Sigers wins apology from Delta for refusing to transport him (*Chicago Tribune*, Sep 2, 1986)

189. **Discrimination** Majority of states have adopted policies barring discrimination against AIDS patients, despite Justice Dept position that federal law does not prevent employers from refusing jobs to such people

190. **Drugs and AIDS** Fear of AIDS is cited as factor in shift from heroin to crack and powdered cocaine as drug of choice for young drug users in New York City

191. **Edward Lebowitz** Man posing as doctor prescribes change in medication of Edward Lebowitz, PWA, and Lebowitz subsequently dies. Police in Santa Monica, CA, theorize call could have been attempt at mercy killing. Hal Speers Rachman, a private-duty nurse is arrested on murder charges. He is also charged with stealing $10,000 from Lebowitz, for whom he cared at home before his hospitalization. Autopsy proves Lebowitz died of disease effects, not from the change of medication

192. **Experimental vaccine** University researchers in California say that vaccine, based on the polio vaccine, has protected monkeys from deadly AIDS-like monkey virus for over one year

193. **Religion and AIDS** California's 20 Roman Catholic Bishops criticize voter-initiated referendum that would impose control on PWAs

194. **State reactions to AIDS** Michigan Civil Rights Commission lists AIDS as a handicap

195. **Swine fever** CDC scientists say series of blood tests conducted indicate that African swine fever is not related to spread of AIDS, hoping to stop theory that swine fever somehow contributed to the spread of AIDS

October

196. **AIDS and child visitation** AIDS continues as subject of court battles between many divorced couples in cases where former husband is homosexual and seeks visiting rights with children. Ben Schatz, lawyer for National Gay Rights Advocates, expects increase in number of custody cases in which AIDS is a factor

197. **At-risk groups** Of more than 25,000 AIDS cases in US, 1133 were initially placed in "no identified risk" category because there was no clear indication about how they got disease

198. **AZT** Burroughs Wellcome applies to FDA for formal approval to market AZT. The company is producing small quantities of AZT in 100 mg capsule form

199. **Classification of AIDS** Researchers say government's definition of AIDS excludes many people who almost certainly have disease. Revised definition of AIDS would raise total number of recorded PWAs in US by 14%, to nearly 30,000

200. **Control of AIDS** US Surgeon General C Everett Koop issues the first major federal government statement on controlling the spread of AIDS by calling for education about AIDS in elementary schools and stresses "the best protection against infection right now, barring abstinence, is use of a condom." Urges parents to be frank in discussing sex and AIDS with their children

201. **Experimental drugs** CS-85, ST, and D-Penicillamine are being tested for their effect on AIDS

202. **Federal AIDS funding** National Academy of Sciences report charges that government's response to AIDS epidemic has been "dangerously inadequate" and calls for $2 bil-per-year educational and research effort to avert medical catastrophe

203. **Global concern** WHO reports sharp increase in number of cases of AIDS recorded worldwide in first 9 months of year. Spread of viral infection has reached pandemic proportions, affecting countries in all continents of world

204. **Insurance and AIDS** Senate passes amendment that would overturn law barring insurance companies from testing people applying for policies for exposure to AIDS virus. Several insurance companies have stopped writing policies in Washington since law was enacted

205. **Jerry Smith** First prominent athlete, Jerry Smith, formerly of the Washington Redskins, dies of AIDS-related complications

206. **Minorities** The CDC announces that Blacks account for 25% and Hispanics for 15% of the US AIDS cases. According to the same report, about 70% of the women with AIDS are Black or Hispanic

207. **Organ transplants** Unidentified Georgian who received kidney last August has tested positive for antibodies to AIDS. Antibodies were found in donor after transplant

208. **Transmission of AIDS** Evidence presented by Drs Brian R Saltzman and Thomas A Peterman suggests there is small chance that single heterosexual relations will spread AIDS infection, although heterosexual relations appear to play key role in transmission in Africa and Haiti

November

209. **AIDS in Africa** Research by Dr Luc Montagnier says new African AIDS virus discovered last year may be as deadly as original virus and could pose international health threat. New evidence suggests new virus has already spread from west Africa to several countries in western Europe

210. **AIDS in Africa** Some African nations, in dramatic reversal, are beginning to acknowledge impact of AIDS and allow international experts to visit so they can track spread of disease closely and give advice about preventive steps

211. **At-risk groups** Vast majority of PWAs continue to be male homosexuals and intravenous drug addicts. In African countries like Zaire and Uganda, disease spreads differently, affecting men and women alike. With homosexual community acting to educate and protect itself, prime target for preventive efforts remains intravenous drug addicts. There is no proof yet that general public is equally at risk

212. **Blood supply** New York City area blood program begins effort to find and notify estimated 500-700 former hospital patients who may have contracted AIDS virus through blood transfusions dating back to 1977, long before screening tests became available in early 1985

213. **Blood supply** FDA seeks to further reduce risk of AIDS; adds prostitutes and their recent heterosexual customers to its list of those who should not donate blood

214. **Condoms** Insure, Inc launches a new anti-AIDS condom product. Ten percent of the brand's profits will go to AIDS research

215. **Federal AIDS funding** Pres Reagan signs legislation that provides over $410 mil for AIDS research

216. **Global concern** WHO announces first coordinated global effort to combat AIDS, calling disease "a health disaster of pandemic proportions"

217. **Proposition 64** California voters reject LaRouche-backed proposition on quarantining PWAs by 71% to 29% margin

218. **Research** Scientists discover third virus causing AIDS, raising prospect that researchers will eventually need to refine current AIDS test that safeguards blood supplies against disease. Drs Robert C Gallo, Luc Montagnier, and Myron Essec win the Albert Lasker Research Award for their discovery

219. **Research** NCI researchers report that AIDS virus attacks different types of cells in brain and central nervous system than in rest of body. Finding may complicate treatment of AIDS

December

220. **AIDS in China** Beginning in 1987, all students wishing to study in China will be required to test negative for AIDS

221. **Clofazimine** FDA approves new drug, clofazimine, which Ciba-Geigy will market as Lamprene. The drug, primarily for treatment of lepromatous leprosy, has been used to treat infection related to AIDS

222. **Discrimination** $190,000 settlement that reinstated Todd Shuttleworth, Broward County, FL municipal worker, and paid his medical bills is considered "tremendous victory" for other PWAs

223. **Discrimination** A fingernail salon in West Hollywood becomes the first California business to be charged with discrimination under the new antidiscrimination law

224. **Experimental vaccine** NCI scientists take another step toward producing vaccine against AIDS by showing that only fragment of protein from AIDS virus is necessary for developing antibodies against it

225. **Insurance and AIDS** National Assn of Insurance Commissioners approves set of guidelines that would prevent insurance companies from discriminating against homosexuals

226. **Prostitutes and AIDS** AIDS virus infects thousands of prostitutes who work in bars that cluster around Subic Bay Naval Station and Clark Air Base in the Philippines, stirring concern about spread of AIDS through local population and American servicemen

227. **Religion and AIDS** Roman Catholic Archdiocese of Los Angeles withdraws support for program for Hispanic Americans that recommends use of condoms to prevent spread of AIDS. Archbishop Roger Maloney prohibits AIDS education seminars in churches because the use of condoms implies either heterosexual promiscuity or homosexual activity, both of which are condemned by the church

228. **Research** Scientists discover type of human white blood cell which inhibits duplication of AIDS virus in test tube, suggesting possible new approach to treatment

229. **Research** Scientists discover AIDS virus can infect cells from colon and rectum and may enter body by route other than directly into bloodstream

230. **Research** Scientists from Zaire and France report experiments on small number of people to stimulate body's immune system to produce huge army of special white blood cells known as killer lymphocytes. Experiments have astonished other AIDS experts who had believed that first human experiments of any form of immunization would not come for at least a year

231. **Research** Pasteur Institute researchers clone newly discovered virus that can cause AIDS in humans but is quite different from main AIDS virus and somewhat similar to third virus that causes disease in monkeys

232. **Research** NIAID researchers find dormant AIDS virus can be stimulated by DNA viruses into reproducing itself, which may explain why some people suddenly develop AIDS years after becoming infected

1987

January

233. **AIDS awareness** San Francisco survey finds that most students know what AIDS is but do not know how to prevent it

234. **AIDS in Africa** Government of Zaire gives its support to experimental immunization project against AIDS being conducted in that country by team of French and Zairian scientists

235. **AIDS in Great Britain** British Government begins large-scale campaign to teach country that AIDS is spreading in Britain and that is it is a fatal disease with no known cure. Campaign seeks to educate nation in a matter of weeks by using radio and TV and sending leaflets to country's 23 million households

236. **Condom ads** Radio and TV stations in Detroit and San Francisco are among the first to air condom ads

237. **Confidentiality** California health officials refuse to participate in federal study of AIDS on grounds that testing of blood specimens without patients' permission violates state confidentiality laws

238. **Drugs and AIDS** Edinburgh, Scotland experiences epidemic proportions of AIDS since crackdown on drug paraphernalia forced city's addicts to share dirty needles and syringes. Government has not acted on recommendation of Scottish health experts that free clean needles and syringes be provided to addicts to better contain AIDS. Glasgow, with no similar needle ban, has twice as many drug abusers but far fewer AIDS cases

239. **Experimental drugs** ICN Pharmaceuticals' product Ribavirin is not a cure for disease, although it is first time any drug has seemed to prevent AIDS from developing in patients with early signs of infection

240. **Experimental vaccine** Anthony S Fauci, Coordinator of AIDS Research at NIH tells Senate panel that testing on humans for some vaccine for AIDS could take place as early as end of 1987 or early 1988

241. **Federal AIDS treatment research center** Univ of Minnesota Hospital becomes the first midwestern hospital to be designated as a Federal AIDS treatment research center

242. **Insurance and AIDS** The National Assn of Insurance Commissioners adopts model rules barring insurers from asking applicants whether they are homosexual but the rules do not cover whether insurers can require AIDS tests

243. **Religion and AIDS** Msgr James F Rigney, rector of St Patrick's Cathedral, New York City, reverses decision of priest at cathedral and refuses to perform marriage there for David Hefner, man dying with AIDS who wanted to renew civil marriage vows with his wife

244. **Research** Study published in *New England Journal of Medicine* indicates men infected with AIDS virus have been identified with five traits associated with development of disorder

245. **Research** Researchers find blood plasma of some persons infected with AIDS virus to have large quantities of antibodies that inactivate virus in test tube

246. **Spread of AIDS** Federal officials, in effort to learn where and how fast AIDS virus is spreading, begin screening anonymous blood samples drawn in hospitals for other purposes

247. **Spread of AIDS** Health and Human Services Secretary Otis R Bowen tells National Press Club that worldwide AIDS epidemic will become so serious that it will dwarf earlier medical disasters such as Black Plague, smallpox and typhoid

February

248. **AIDS benefit** The annual Grammy Awards names "That's What Friends Are For," written by songwriters Burt Bacharach and Carol Bayer Sager, song of the year. The song has raised $750,000 for AIDS research

249. **AIDS benefit** "The Night of a Thousand Gowns," the largest drag ball of the year at New York's Waldorf Astoria Hotel, raises nearly $500,000

250. **AIDS education** Pres Reagan decides to support federal campaign to educate public about dangers of AIDS, but only if campaign stresses "responsible sexual behavior" within marriage and teaches children to avoid sex, according to internal White House memorandum made available by Congressional sources

251. **AIDS in Bavaria** Conservative Bavarian government announces tight restrictions on some groups believed to be at high risk of exposure to AIDS, including compulsory testing for prostitutes and prison inmates as well as for certain foreigners wishing to reside in state

252. **AIDS in Japan** Japanese go to clinics for blood tests and prod government to start special programs to keep disease in check. Health officials report 26 cases, including 18 deaths. Experts estimate that 7000 to 10,000 people carry AIDS virus

253. **AIDS in Japan** Japan adopts anti-AIDS program that includes plans to keep out foreigners found to be carriers of AIDS

254. **AIDS in the Soviet Union** Soviet weekly *Literaturnaya Gazetta* reports Soviet Union has developed and is mass-producing test for AIDS virus infection that has already been used on tens of thousands of people; includes interview with Georgi N Khlyabich, country's chief public health inspector, which offered most detailed information to date on AIDS prevention and treatment programs under way in the Soviet Union

255. **AIDS testing** Participants in federally-sponsored conference on control of AIDS reach broad agreement on need for wider testing for infection with AIDS virus, provided testing is voluntary and accompanied by adequate counseling and safeguards to keep results confidential; call for more systematic offering of blood test to detect infection with virus that causes AIDS

256. **Condom ads** Surgeon General C Everett Koop calls for advertising condoms on TV, reiterating position that condoms offer best protection from deadly AIDS virus for those who "will not practice abstinence or monogamy." Says he is particularly concerned about rise in AIDS cases among Blacks and Hispanics

257. **Condom ads** WMCA Radio in New York City agrees to accept condom advertisements, and will run them for free for 6 months. New York City affiliates of CBS and NBC TV networks announce that effective immediately they will accept condom advertising as long as it is related to combating AIDS. ABC-TV, although still refusing to broadcast such commercials, has agreed to run public service spot supplied by American Foundation for AIDS research. WCBS and WNBC will not run the ads before 11 pm

258. **Condoms** New York City to offer free condoms to fight AIDS

259. **Confidentiality** Rep Henry A Waxman (D-CA) argues that neither voluntary nor mandatory testing policies can succeed unless there is a guarantee that test results will be confidential and there will not be discrimination against those who test positive. Justice Dept position is if test is positive, any subsequent discrimination is legal and is not government's concern

260. **Drugs and AIDS** Pres Reagan rejects proposal to combine warnings about AIDS with his anti-narcotics campaign

261. **Hospital for AIDS** The only AIDS hospital in the US (Houston) stops accepting PWAs who cannot pay due to over $2 mil in losses

262. **Liberace** Noted entertainer Liberace dies, and controversy arises over whether AIDS was the cause of death. Liberace's physician, Dr Ronald Daniels, says there is enough doubt as to whether Liberace had AIDS to justify his decision to report heart failure as cause of death. He obeyed law by informing officials that AIDS tests prior to death did not disclose whether entertainer had disease. Denies cover-up

263. **Military and AIDS** Sources report that Pentagon, more than halfway through its screening of military personnel on active duty for infection with AIDS virus, has identified about 2100 men and women who were infected; Defense Dept is reportedly now debating whether testing should be extended to civilian employees

264. **Occupational concerns** Some funeral directors have refused to embalm bodies of AIDS victims or insist on costly extra equipment

265. **Occupational concerns** Cook County, IL, hospital debates whether or not a physician with AIDS can continue to see patients

266. **Religion and AIDS** Dallas Conference of Roman Catholic Bishops concludes that abstinence and marital fidelity are better weapons to fight AIDS than condoms, because condoms create a false sense of security

267. **Religion and AIDS** Maria and David Hefner renew wedding vows at St Patrick's Cathedral more than a month after rector refused to allow ceremony. Mr Hefner is dying of AIDS. John Cardinal O'Connor, who arranged compromise that allowed ceremony to be performed, attends

268. **Research** Researchers at Univ of California Davis have discovered virus that caused disease in domestic cats and is similar to one that caused AIDS in humans. Development can make cat useful animal model for research on AIDS. There is no indication that cat virus can infect human beings

269. **Spread of AIDS** In Nuremburg, officials arrest former US Army sergeant with AIDS on suspicion of knowingly spreading disease to his sexual partners. Arrest is first ordered under crackdown on spread of disease in Bavaria ordered by Premier Franz Josef Strauss

March

270. **AIDS education** Reagan Administration issues AIDS education plan that calls for specific information to be made available to Americans on how to prevent spread of disease, including use of condoms for sexually active people

271. **AIDS education** California approves AIDS education in high school

272. **AIDS in Brazil** Brazil ranks third after United States and France in total number of official reported cases of AIDS; alarm at disease's rapid spread has turned problem into public issue; Health Ministry is sponsoring radio and television spots recommending precautions, with more explicit spots to be aired in late evenings; gradual change in sexual behavior patterns is seen

273. **AIDS in Europe** The AIDS epidemic, which once seemed to affect Africa and the US far more severely than the rest of world, hits hard in Western Europe in the last year or so

274. **AIDS in the Soviet Union** Soviet newspaper for young people, in rare public disclosure, reports that homosexuality is increasing in Soviet Union and should continue to be treated as crime to prevent spread of AIDS

275. **AZT** Burroughs Wellcome receives FDA approval to market their product, AZT. The name of the drug is changed to Retrovir (zidovudine) so that it could be trademarked throughout the world. A total of 4000 clinical trial patients received the drug at a cost of $10 mil to the developer/manufacturer. The plan at the time of approval was to provide Retrovir to the most seriously ill and to trial patients already using it

276. **AZT** Britain approves experimental drug AZT for treatment of AIDS, saying it appears to prolong lives of people suffering from disease, although it is not a cure

277. **Discrimination** Supreme Court rules 7 to 2 that recipients of federal money may not discriminate against people who are physically or mentally impaired by contagious diseases; although decision involves Gene H Arline, Florida school teacher suffering from tuberculosis, it could benefit many PWAs

278. **Experimental drugs** Reagan Administration announces that it will soon propose new regulations to make promising experimental drugs available more rapidly to patients suffering from AIDS and other life-threatening diseases

279. **Experimental vaccine** Severe practical and ethical dilemmas plague researchers working to develop AIDS vaccine, especially as they move to next phase of process: Experimenting with potential vaccines on humans and eventually bringing to market any that prove effective; experts feel government must now play more assertive role in defining framework within which a vaccine can be developed and marketed

280. **Experimental vaccine** French researcher, Daniel Zagury, injects himself with an experimental AIDS vaccine

281. **Immigration regulations** Federal health officials say that Reagan Administration intends to proceed with plan to bar PWAs from immigrating to US, despite objections raised when proposal was announced in 1986

282. **Mandatory testing** Rep Dan Burton (R-IN) proposes a bill requiring annual AIDS testing for every US citizen

283. **Occupational concerns** Many US employers treat AIDS as any other major illness and urge employees to stay on the job as long as possible

284. **Public opinion** Survey for American Assn of Blood Banks finds AIDS has replaced heart disease in public mind as second most serious health problem in US, ranking behind cancer

285. **Research** Study by San Francisco Health Dept and CDC indicates that risk of developing AIDS increases yearly after infection with virus, dampening hopes that rates of illness might plateau or even drop five years or so after infection. Study fails to identify any factor other than time that triggers onset of disease. Research is based on analysis of blood and data collected in San Francisco since 1978

286. **Research** AIDS virus reveals surprising complexity as research continues; is shown to have far more genes than expected, to be capable of attacking more different human cells than was thought, and to have more complex means of destroying immune system defenses. It is expected to prove difficult vaccine target

287. **Research** Dr Robert C Gallo and Dr Mikulas Popovic of NCI patent method of producing virus that causes AIDS; process creates large quantities of virus for use in research

288. **Schools and AIDS** Throughout New York metropolitan region, many schools begin to teach students about AIDS, its transmission, and methods of prevention

289. **Women and AIDS** Surgeon General C Everett Koop recommends that all women be tested for AIDS virus, on voluntary basis, before becoming pregnant and says he does not understand controversy over proposed mandatory AIDS testing for couples seeking marriage licenses

April

290. **AIDS benefit** The Duchess of Windsor's jewelry collection was auctioned in Geneva by Sotheby's, netting $50,281,887 for the Pasteur Institute in Paris

291. **Bobby Reynolds** Longest surviving AIDS patient, first diagnosed in 1978, dies in San Francisco

292. **Condom ads** FDA approves condom ads as an AIDS preventive

293. **Discrimination** Judge rules that the nail salon in West Hollywood does not have to provide pedicures to PWAs

294. **Insurance and AIDS** New York State regulation prevents insurance companies from testing for AIDS

295. **Research** French scientists say that the AIDS virus may have been present in humans long before its current outbreak

296. **Research controversy** Pres Reagan and French Premier Jacques Chirac announce the settlement of a dispute over who discovered the AIDS-causing virus. French scientists have been credited with its initial discovery and isolation

297. **State reactions to AIDS** Anti-pornography crusaders in California want AIDS materials removed from schools because they consider the materials obscene

298. **Women and AIDS** *Journal of the American Medical Association* reports the percentage of women who contracted AIDS from men more than doubled between 1982 and 1986 with Black women 13 times more likely to get AIDS than White women

May

299. **Condom ads** New Haven, CT displays ads for condoms in its public buses

300. **Condom ads** Consumer Data Bureau reports that 65% of American women polled support condom advertising on television. All respondents were over 28 years old and 70% over 45

301. **Immigration regulations** Public Health Service recommends the testing of all aliens for AIDS before they can become US citizens

302. **Presidential commission** Pres Reagan forms a special commission on AIDS

June

303. **AIDS conference** The third International Conference on AIDS is held in Washington, DC

304. **Experimental drugs** Early tests indicate that Hoffmann-La Roche's product DDC (dideoxycytidine) is an effective drug against AIDS with less side effects than Retrovir (formerly AZT). It has been shown to possibly be just as effective but less toxic than Retrovir, only causing skin rashes and temporary loss of platelets. A rise in beneficial T-4 helper cells was also reported, without causing bone marrow suppression or weight loss.

305. **Insurance and AIDS** Several of the nation's largest insurance companies limit amounts of insurance coverage if applicant refuses a blood test for AIDS

306. **Presidential commission** Dr W Eugene Mayberry of the Mayo Clinic in Rochester, MN is named chair of the Presidential advisory commission on AIDS

307. **Presidential speech on AIDS** Pres Reagan makes first speech on AIDS, stressing the need for compassion, education, and commitment to treatment. Calls for mandatory AIDS testing within 2 years

308. **Public reaction** US Gay and Lesbian Pride Week celebrations focus on AIDS

309. **Research funding** Sotheby's Art Against AIDS nets $400,000 for AmFAR

310. **Ribavirin** Ribavirin fails to receive FDA marketing approval for treatment of AIDS

July

311. **AIDS benefit** Art Against AIDS raises $1.25 mil for AIDS research

312. **Airlines** An American tourist, Brent Anderson, becomes stranded in China when asked to leave because he had AIDS. Commerical airlines refused to transport him; US Air Force flies him home

313. **Hospital for AIDS** Due to limited funding, the Houston hospital devoted entirely to AIDS patients reports it is in danger of closing

314. **New York City** Report cites that 2650 people died from AIDS in New York City during 1986, up 59% over 1985 figures

315. **Presidential AIDS commission** Pres Reagan appoints 12 members to his advisory commission

316. **Pro Football AIDS testing** Many professional football teams offer voluntary AIDS testing

August

317. **At-risk groups** Chicago provides bleach to drug addicts for cleaning needles; also furnishes condoms to prostitutes to help prevent the spread of AIDS

318. **Experimental vaccine** MicroGeneSys, Inc receives FDA approval to undertake phase I human clinical trials of VaxSyn, its AIDS vaccine

319. **Public opinion** SRI Gallup Poll reports that 32% of Americans say AIDS is now their most serious health problem

320. **Public reaction** A Florida family leaves their home town because their children have AIDS and cannot attend school. Their home was destroyed by a fire termed "suspicious" by the local sheriff. Authorities added that "blaze capped a week of bomb and death threats" and a school boycott

September

321. **AIDS testing** Illinois governor Jim Thompson signs bill requiring premarital testing for AIDS

322. **Discrimination** The Reagan Administration opposes a bill which would ban discrimination against PWAs. Dr Otis R Bowen, Secretary of Health and Human Services says states should be free to adopt or reject civil rights laws protecting such people according to local conditions

323. **Military and AIDS** Costa Rica demands that the US Navy certify that all crew members test negative for AIDS before they can visit the country. Navy cancels visit

324. **Religion and AIDS** Pope John Paul II faces protestors but visits over 60 AIDS patients and "proclaims a message of divine and unconditional love"

325. **Retrovir (AZT)** Burroughs Wellcome announces Retrovir now available to all PWAs, not just the critically ill. Company now able to supply drug to as many as 50,000 patients per year

326. **Women and AIDS** New Jersey State Dept of Health study shows that inner-city women at high risk of AIDS infection are well-informed of the risk, but few are changing their behavior as a result

October

327. **AIDS education** *AIDS and the Education of Our Children: A Guide for Parents and Children* contains advice written primarily by Education Secretary William J Bennett, urging all parents and teachers to stress "appropriate moral and social conduct" as the first line of defense against the spread of the AIDS virus

328. **At-risk groups** New York City health officials report AIDS has killed more IV drug users in city than homosexuals, contrasting sharply with official statistics. According to Health Commissioner Stephen C Joseph, "Homosexual men are no longer the major group at risk in the city"

329. **Confidentiality** New York City Health Commissioner Stephen C Joseph says that physicians and public health officials should warn sex partners of AIDS patients of substantial risk of infection

330. **Control of AIDS** Dr Jonathan Mann, director of WHO Special Program on AIDS warns that expelling PWAs from society would only force the problem underground and "wreak havoc with health authorities' efforts to keep track of the disease." Currently there are 62,438 active cases of AIDS in 126 countries, projecting up to 3 million new cases in 5 years

331. **Drugs and AIDS** A shortage of drug treatment facilities creates waiting lists of up to a year long in certain cities, contributing to the failure to contain the spread of the AIDS virus among IV drug users and their sexual partners

332. **Early AIDS infection** A Saint Louis teenager who died of mysterious causes in 1969 was found to have had AIDS

333. **Experimental drugs** Pharmacy press announces FDA created new category, 1-AA, for AIDS products to mark them for top priority review

334. **Experimental drugs** NIAID expresses hopes that Hoffmann-La Roche's AIDS drug, DDC (dideoxycytidine) will be less toxic than Retrovir (formerly AZT)

335. **Experimental drugs** Federal health officials report the focus of AIDS drug therapy is shifting away from vaccines to drugs which may control the syndrome, treat the illness, and prolong life

336. **Experimental drugs** California passes legislation allowing drugs produced in California for AIDS to be tested before the FDA tests the same drug

337. **Gay Rights** AIDS has energized but complicated the battle for gay rights. Gay groups have more money and more supporters, but their resources are now concentrated on the disease, rather than on basic rights

338. **Organ transplants** Transplanting livers or kidneys into AIDS patients raises ethical questions because of the scarcity of such organs

339. **Presidential commission** Adm James D Watkins (retired), appointed to head the Presidential AIDS Commission after the resignation of W Eugene Mayberry, says, "We frankly haven't done the job that we were tasked to do." Commission has been criticized as incompetent and ideologically biased

340. **Public reaction** Over 250,000 gays, lesbians, and friends march on Washington, DC for human rights and recognition

341. **Public reaction** A Longmeadow, MA teenager dies of AIDS, but during the entire time after diagnosis, the town supported him and his family and allowed him to attend school without incident

342. **Research** A Finnish study reports AIDS antibodies take longer to form in some infected people than most experts had believed; indicates negative results on commonly-used AIDS tests which detect antibodies may be premature

343. **Transmission of AIDS** An airline steward from Montreal who died of AIDS in 1984 was found to have had sexual relations with 4 of the first 19 cases of AIDS reported in Los Angeles, and 4 others had sexual relations with one of his sexual partners, suggesting that this man played a key role in the early spread of AIDS in North America

344. **Women and AIDS** Researchers indicate that women with AIDS become sicker and die more quickly than men. Trend may be rooted in hormonal differences

November

345. **Experimental drugs** There are now at least 40 products being researched by various companies hoping to find vaccines or therapeutics for AIDS

346. **Immigration testing** US Government implements testing for AIDS of all persons wishing to immigrate

347. **Jerry Carlson** Conductor of Gay Men's Chorus of Los Angeles dies of AIDS at 31 years old. He was the founder of the Windy City Chorus and charter member of the Chicago Gay Pride Band

348. **Schools and AIDS** Vincent Chalk of Irvine, CA, instructor for the hearing-impaired, returns to classroom after 9th US Circuit Court of Appeals grants an injunction against Orange County Dept of Education ruling it has no grounds to keep Chalk at desk job; he was reassigned after he informed the school he had AIDS

December

349. **Religion and AIDS** In a 30-page statement entitled *The Many Faces of AIDS: A Gospel Response*, US Roman Catholic bishops acknowledge that some people do not adhere to the church's teachings on sexuality and indicate that they would tolerate educational programs that describe how condoms may prevent the spread of AIDS

1988

January

350. **AIDS awareness** Federal health officials announce they will boost their attack on AIDS by expanding mass advertising and by mailing a government-produced AIDS education pamphlet to every American household by the end of June

351. **AIDS in infants** According to a New York State study, one in every 117 babies born during November 1987 throughout the state has tested positive for the presence of antibodies to HIV, the AIDS-causing virus. New York City reported the greatest rate of antibody prevalence. State officials now consider AIDS a major threat to infant health in New York City

352. **Antibody testing** US Surgeon General C Everett Koop suggested that blood samples be drawn from the entire student body of a major, urban university and be tested for antibodies to the AIDS-causing virus during an all-day AIDS prevention "gala." The effort was recommended as a method of determining the spread of HIV infection

353. **Australia** A variety of AIDS-prevention measures were adopted by the Queensland (Australia) cabinet, in an effort to stem the spread of AIDS. The measures include a comprehensive AIDS and sex education program for schools, an hypodermic needle exchange program for drug abusers and funding for azidothymidine (AZT) therapy, a costly drug used in the treatment of AIDS

354. **Canada** According to a survey conducted by the *Toronto Globe and Mail*, about 10,000 people in Canada have been infected with the AIDS-causing virus. The survey was based on nation-wide voluntary AIDS testing results, and though not conclusive, was an indication that the syndrome has spread outside recognized high-risk groups

355. **HIV-2** A second AIDS virus that was discovered in West Africa during the summer of 1985 and later spread to Europe has now been discovered for the first time in a patient in the US, according to researchers at the Univ of Medicine and Dentistry of New Jersey. According to Dr Myron Essex, a Harvard Univ researcher, HIV-2 does not cause illness as severe or in the same frequency as the HIV-1, a view disputed by French and American researchers

356. **HTLV-I** Cancer researchers reported in New York the discovery of HTLV-I, a leukemia-causing virus similar to the virus responsible for AIDS, in the blood of six patients who had received blood transfusions. Public officials called for the screening of blood supplies for the HTLV-I virus

357. **London conference** The World AIDS Summit, jointly sponsored by the World Health Organization and the British government, was held in London and was attended by delegates from nearly 150 countries. Attendees drafted the "London Declaration," calling on all governments and people to act to stem the spread of AIDS

358. **Mosquitos and AIDS** A study reported in the journal *Science*, found no evidence that AIDS may be spread by mosquitos. The study attempted to explain a disproportionate number of AIDS cases in Belle Glade, FL. The study found no AIDS cases in people under age 10 or over age 60, as would be expected if mosquitos were responsible for the syndrome's spread

359. **New Jersey** Gov Thomas Kean announced the establishment of a new state agency to deal with AIDS

360. **New York City** New York City health officials were given permission by state authorities to distribute free hypodermic syringes to drug addicts in an effort to combat the spread of AIDS through the sharing of needles

361. **Occupational exposure** According to an article in the journal *Science*, a laboratory worker handling AIDS-contaminated materials reportedly has become infected with the AIDS-causing virus through no apparent means of exposure, such as by a needle or break in the skin. According to the study, the risk of occupational exposure in the laboratory is "very low"

362. **Research** A medical research team led by Dr James L Matthews successfully uses a laser to cleanse a sexually transmitted disease from donated blood and is confident the method will prove effective against the AIDS virus. The research, carried out by a team from Baylor Univ Medical Center and the Baylor Research Foundation, was financed in part by the Pentagon's "Star Wars" anti-missile program

363. **Research** In an interview published in *SPIN* Magazine's monthly AIDS column, Dr Peter Duesberg states that HIV cannot be the cause of AIDS because of its relative inactivity. In fact, Duesberg cites that HIV is found in far more healthy humans than sick humans

364. **Research** The United States and Soviet Union sign a scientific accord in Moscow Jan 12 which includes pledges of cooperation in AIDS research

365. **Tuberculosis and AIDS** The CDC reports a substantial increase in reported cases of tuberculosis, and link the increase to the spread of AIDS where the tuberculosis occurs as a secondary infection in AIDS patients.

366. **World Summit on AIDS** 600 health officials from more than 150 nations attend the first world summit on AIDS, sponsored by the World Health Organization and the British government. The 3-day conference, held in London, was formally opened by Britain's Princess Anne, who urged attendees, including 120 national health ministers, to push their anti-AIDS efforts

February

367. **AIDS Advisory Commission** Adm James D Watkins, Chair of Pres Reagan's AIDS Advisory Commission, issued a report calling for an increase in spending for substance abuse rehabilitation and health care programs to fight the spread of AIDS. According to the report, the focus on drug users and their sexual partners is due to the concern that these groups pose the greatest threat for spreading the AIDS-causing virus. Additionally, the report called for: federally-funded health care for uninsured people with AIDS, group homes for children with AIDS awaiting foster-home placement, and the training of nurses and doctors to work in poor communities where AIDS is prevalent

368. **AIDS and politics** The House of Representatives approves a $1.2 trillion budget plan for fiscal year 1989, including $1.47 billion for AIDS research, up $100 million over the amount suggested by Pres Reagan in his budget proposal

369. **AIDS and the military** The Defense Dept announces that 5890 of almost 4 million active-duty military personnel and recruits have tested positive for exposure to the AIDS-causing virus, for an infection rate of 0.3%. The tests were conducted from October 1985 through September 1987

370. **AIDS in Australia** According to a report issued by Australia's National Advisory Committee on AIDS, between 50,000 and 100,000 people in Australia have been exposed to the AIDS-causing virus

371. **AIDS in the workplace** The Wall Street Journal reported that several major American corporations have adopted a set of "AIDS Workplace Principles" developed to protect people with AIDS from bias. The principles prohibit discrimination against people with AIDS and testing of job applicants for exposure to the AIDS-causing virus

372. **AIDS quilt** The national tour of the AIDS quilt, promoted by the NAMES Project, began its tour of several American cities, culminating in October in a rally presentation in Washington, DC. The quilt bears the names of those who have died, and is constructed of panels made by their friends, families and lovers

373. **AIDS screening** US Surgeon General C Everett Koop discloses a plan to screen every student of a major American university to help determine the incidence of AIDS among young adults. The details of the plan, on which the US government had not yet reached a decision, were unveiled during a 3-day international summit on AIDS held in London

374. **AIDS vaccine** Final testing of any AIDS vaccine may have to be done in Africa rather than in the US, because the US AIDS infection rate is not high enough to determine whether a vaccine is working, according to NIAID director Dr Anthony Fauci

375. **Blood supply** Dr Condon Hughes hopes to open LifeBlood, a Christian blood bank that will not accept "promiscuous" donors. Blood donors will be asked to sign a statement confirming that they have abstained from sex or been faithful to a spouse since 1977, a move which could dangerously limit the pool of potential donors

376. **Drugs and AIDS** District of Columbia health officials will begin giving drug addicts vials of bleach to clean hypodermic needles in an effort to slow the spread of AIDS

377. **Drugs and AIDS** James Watkins, chairman of Pres Reagan's AIDS commission, recommends a 10-year, $15 bil expansion of rehabilitative treatment for IV drug abuse, including establishment of 3300 new drug abuse clinics, and hiring 32,000 specialists to staff them in an effort to help control the spread of AIDS. There is a growing scientific consensus that IV drug users are now the main source of new AIDS infections

378. **Drugs and AIDS** Drug addicts accounted for 53% of all deaths due to AIDS in New York City from 1978 to 1986, according to an article published in the journal *Science*, Feb 12

379. **Federal AIDS funding** President Reagan's proposed budget for fiscal year 1989 includes $1.3 bil for AIDS research, a 38% increase

380. **Haiti** Deposed Haitian President Duvalier claimed in a *Paris Match* interview that the spread of AIDS was the cause of his ouster. According to Duvalier, the AIDS epidemic and reports linking it with Haiti had caused a drop in tourism, resulting in economic problems that forced him out of office

381. **Home AIDS test** The FDA acts to stop the development of home-administered tests for determining exposure to the AIDS-causing virus. The action was taken due to concern over test accuracy and the need for psychological counseling for persons testing positive

382. **Insurance and AIDS** According to a survey issued by the Office of Technology Assessment, most health insurance companies now screen applicants for exposure to the AIDS-causing virus. The survey of commercial insurers found that 86% screened insurance candidates using AIDS-related questions on application forms and medical histories supplied by the applicants' physicians

383. **Origin of the AIDS virus** A report in the journal, *Science* indicates that a Harvard research team, apparently working with contaminated samples, was studying a virus which came from rhesus monkeys, not from humans, as had been originally thought. The findings could weaken the link thought to exist between AIDS-like viruses in monkeys and those in humans

384. **Politics and AIDS** The *Baltimore Sun* discloses an internal Justice department memorandum calling for the "polarization" of debate over a number of important social issues, including AIDS. According to the memo, department officials were called on to argue the point that, in jurisprudence, AIDS should not be considered a civil rights or privacy issue

385. **Premarital testing** A bill requiring AIDS tests before couples could marry in Arizona narrowly clears a House panel amid charges that Gov Evan Mecham ordered state officials not to criticize the measure. A similar measure was defeated in 1987, but has been resurrected by Rep Brenda Burns, a Mecham supporter

386. **Research** Dr Peter Duesberg, a respected virus researcher at UC Berkeley, has been invited to appear before the Presidential Commission on the HIV epidemmic at a hearing Feb 20 in New York. Duesberg claims that federal researchers are wrong in their conclusion that HIV is the cause of AIDS, and are embarrassed to admit their mistake

387. **Research** Reports of unsatisfactory test results involving traditional approaches to AIDS vaccine development, which target HIV envelope proteins, such as gp120 and gp160, create a great deal of pessimism among scientists once committed to these approaches. As evidence mounts suggesting that AIDS vaccines based on isolated viral envelope proteins may be very limited in their effectiveness, many AIDS researchers are turning their attention to core proteins like p17

388. **Research** Pres Reagan's budget for fiscal year 1989 includes nearly $2 billion for AIDS programs, including research, education and prevention measures. The appropriation represents a 38% increase in spending for AIDS over the previous year. Of the $2 bil, $900 mil would go for research, $600 mil for Medicaid for PWAs and $400 mil for education

389. **Surgeon with AIDS** A coroner's investigation reveals that a Canadian surgeon performed at least 700 operations over five years while he was suffering from AIDS. The College of Physicians and Surgeons of Ontario has been asked to examine whether surgeons with AIDS have an ethical or moral obligation to tell patients about their illness. A spokesman for the college said there are currently no guidelines about physicians performing surgery when they have a transmissible disease

390. **Tranfusion risk** The CDC reports a low risk of AIDS transmission through blood transfusion. However, there remains a one in 40,000 chance of contracting AIDS through blood transfusion

March

391. **AIDS in adolescents** Three independent studies indicate teens may be more resistant to AIDS than infants or adults. According to the studies, there seemed to be an unusually long lag-time before onset of the syndrome in teens as opposed to adults and infants

392. **AIDS in heterosexuals** According to a study by sex therapists Dr William H Masters, Virginia E Johnson and colaborator Dr Robert C Kolody, "the AIDS virus is now running rampant in the heterosexual community." Their findings, reported in the book, *Crisis: Heterosexual Behavior in the Age of AIDS*, were met with criticism from other AIDS researchers and public health offcials. Excerpts from the book were published in *Newsweek*. Defending their work, Masters said, "What we have done is identify another group at high risk," being "sexually active heterosexuals with many partners." In their study, the authors call for mandatory testing for exposure to HIV

393. **AIDS in heterosexuals** Dr Matilda Krim of the American Federation for AIDS Research (AmFAR) criticized the Masters, Johnson and Kolodny study of AIDS in heterosexuals, saying it "...will serve no purpose except to fuel senseless hysteria."

394. **Discrimination** Congress overrides Pres Reagan's veto of the Civil Rights Restoration Act, a law barring institutions receiving federal assistance from practicing discrimination based on sex, race, age, or physical handicap. Under the law, persons with AIDS (and other contagious diseases) will be considered as handicapped and will be protected

395. **Homeless** Reports indicate that hundreds of homeless people with AIDS are living in shelters in New York City, despite city policy providing alternative housing for those with the syndrome

396. **Joseph E Markowski** Joseph E Markowski, 29, is acquitted by a Los Angeles jury of attempted poisoning when he reportedly sold his blood to a blood bank after being informed that he was tested positive for exposure to the AIDS-causing virus

397. **Pulitzer Prize** Jacqui Banaszynski of the *St Paul Pioneer Press Dispatch* receives a Pulitzer Prize in journalism for her series of articles about two rural Minnesotan farmers diagnosed with AIDS

April

398. **AIDS in heterosexuals** According to a report in the *Journal of the American Medical Association (JAMA)*, the risk of exposure to AIDS through heterosexual intercourse is low. The degree of risk, according to the study, is determined by whether one's sexual partner is from a high-risk group (bisexual males, prostitutes or IV drug abusers), whether condoms are used, and abstinence from high-risk sexual behaviors

399. **Epidemiology** According to New York City Health Commissioner Stephen C Joseph, the number of new AIDS cases in intravenous drug abusers has now surpassed the number of cases seen in homosexual or bisexual men

400. **Ford Foundation** The Ford Foundation, along with other major corporate philanthropies, announces the establishment of the National Community AIDS Partnership, a program for financing the care of AIDS patients and providing assistance to their families

401. **HTLV-I** The American Red Cross reports it will soon begin testing blood donations for HTLV-I, a virus similar to the AIDS-causing virus HIV (HTLV-III), that causes a form of leukemia

402. **Infection rates** The CDC reports that according to a study of 12,000 patients at four Midwest hospitals, 0.3% demonstrated exposure to the AIDS-causing virus, HIV

403. **Insurance** New York State Supreme Court Justice Daniel H Prior Jr invalidates a state regulation barring insurers from giving applicants blood tests for HIV, the AIDS-causing virus

404. **Needles** During April and May, the District of Columbia distributes over 2000 vials of bleach in a move to get intravenous drug users to clean their needles, a move to help stem the transmission of AIDS

405. Origin of AIDS University of California biologist Peter Duesberg reports in the March issue of the journal *Cancer Research* his belief that exposure to the human immunodeficiency virus (HIV) is not the precipitating factor for contracting AIDS. Rather, he contends that a lifestyle of substance abuse and sexual promiscuity brought about the syndrome. Duesberg debated his position at a forum sponsored by the American Foundation for AIDS Research (AmFAR) held at George Washington University in Washington, DC

406. Premarital testing Several bills are introduced in the State of Illinois legislature to repeal a law mandating prenuptual AIDS tests, which went into effect Jan 1, 1988. According to the law's opponents, those most in need of testing were unlikely candidates for marriage licenses. Additionally, perhaps due to the new law, applications for marriage licenses decreased in Chicago by 42%, while neighboring states were reporting dramatic increases in license applications by Illinois residents

407. Quarantine Florida Governor Bob Martinez calls for the quarantine of people with AIDS who refuse to limit their sexual contacts

408. Research Dr Anthony S Fauci of the National Institute of Allergy and Infectious Diseases reported that human clinical trials of experimental AIDS drugs have been delayed due to insufficient staffing to direct the drugs through the clinical testing process

409. Research The Office of AIDS Research is created by the National Institutes of Health (NIH), in an effort to centralize and coordinate national AIDS research activities. Dr Anthony Fauci, NIH coordinator for AIDS research, is named head of the office which will report directly to Dr James Wyngaarden, NIH Director

May

410. AIDS and politics Presidential candidate Jesse Jackson announces a 5-year budget plan which would shift substantial federal spending priorities from defense to education, housing and AIDS research

411. AIDS in Africa The Organization of African Unity (OAU) at its 24th annual meeting held in Addis Ababa issues a resolution calling for the promotion of "research by African scientists" on AIDS

412. AZT AZT manufacturer Burroughs Wellcome Co reports to the FDA that in human clinical trials of 144 persons with AIDS or ARC, nearly 85% are still alive after one year of treatment. All patients in the trials given placebo are now dead

413. Canada The Canadian Human Rights Commission issues regulations prohibiting most employers from requiring employees and job applicants to undergo mandatory AIDS antibody testing. The commission's regulations also prohibit discrimination against groups at high risk for AIDS and those with the syndrome

414. Economics A study by Fred Hellinger of the Dept of Health and Human Services and published in the journal *Public Health Reports* predicts that the medical cost of treating AIDS patients will reach $4.5 billion by the year 1991

415. Hemophiliacs Nearly 7500 American hemophiliacs are now believed to be infected with HIV, the AIDS-causing virus, due to blood transfusions given prior to screening for the virus

416. Prisons The Johns Hopkins School of Public Health reportedly will test the blood of 10,000 new prisoners across the country in an effort to measure the spread of AIDS in prisons. The study will be funded by the CDC

417. Prostitution The Newark, NJ City Council drafts an ordinance requiring those convicted of prostitution be tested for exposure to the AIDS-causing virus both at the time of conviction and six months later. Newark Mayor Sharpe James opposes the new ordinance on the grounds that it is unconstitutional

418. Public health The US government begins distribution to all American homes an 8-page pamphlet about AIDS, produced under the direction of Surgeon General C Everett Koop. The pamphlet directly addresses the routes of AIDS transmission: sexual contact with infected partners or sharing contaminated needles. The brochure discusses the use of condoms for preventing the spread of AIDS

419. Veterans and AIDS Pres Reagan signs into law an order providing confidentiality of medical records for veterans with AIDS

June

420. AIDS and politics Presidential candidate George Bush announces his support for the AIDS Advisory Commission's recommendation banning discrimination of people with AIDS or those who test positive for HIV infection

421. AIDS and politics The National Academy of Sciences issues a report criticizing the Reagan administration for failing to provide "strong federal leadership" in the fight against AIDS. The report also calls on the Congress to act to protect the civil rights of people with AIDS

422. AIDS and the Catholic Church Roman Catholic bishops in the US vote to rewrite a policy statement regarding AIDS, in which the bishops give qualified support to an AIDS education program that discusses the use of condoms to prevent the tranmission of AIDS. The policy was attacked by some church leaders, fearing the statement may be read as condoning artificial birth control

423. AIDS in infants According to a report presented at the Fourth International Conference on AIDS, 40% of infants born exposed to HIV develop AIDS within 10 months

424. AIDS lethality The CDC predicts in the journal *Science* that it is likely all persons infected with the AIDS-causing virus will eventually die of the syndrome. It had been hoped that if some people didn't develop the syndrome within a few years of infection, they would never go on to develop AIDS. The findings were based on a long-term San Francisco study of 6000 gay and bisexual men

425. AIDS play opens in New York Playwright Harry Kondoleon's absurdist drama *Zero Positive,* a play about a playwright who tests positive for exposure to HIV, opens in New York

426. AL-721 The FDA reverses an earlier decision and will continue to allow the sale of AL-721, a drug as yet clinically untested as an AIDS treatment though frequently used as such by people with AIDS

427. Antibody testing AIDS experts Drs Robert Gallo (US) and Luc Montaigner (France) report at the Fourth International Conference on AIDS that an undetermined number of cases of infection with HIV will go undetected by conventional HIV antibody-detecting tests. According to the doctors, in some cases people may be infected and yet not test positive

428. CD4 Reviews of CD4 therapy for AIDS surfaced and were mixed. The therapy entails injecting into patients the synthetic white blood cell protein CD4 onto which the AIDS-causing virus HIV attaches and begins its corruption of the immune system. Theoretically, it is expected that the virus will attach itself to the synthetic CD4, leaving the patients' own white blood cells alone. Dr William Haseltine of Harvard has suggested the therapy might cause in some patients an immune reaction against the synthetic CD4, and that this may cause those patients to develop an immunologic response to their own CD4

429. Confidentiality The president's AIDS Advisory Commission, in its final report to Pres Reagan, proposes that health care professionals be required to report to state officials—in confidence—the names of all people who test positive for exposure to the AIDS-causing virus. Furthermore, the commission proposes that state health officials then report this information to the sex partners of those infected

430. Discrimination Adm James D Watkins, Chair of Pres Reagan's AIDS Advisory Commission, calls on the president to issue an executive order prohibiting AIDS discrimination, saying that bias against people with AIDS was the "foremost obstacle" to combating the syndrome. The commission approved the proposal by a narrow margin, with opponents preferring that individual states be allowed to adopt legislative remedies

431. Drugs and AIDS A Portland, OR community clinic announces it will begin distributing clean hypodermic needles to intravenous drug abusers in an effort to stem the spread of AIDS

432. Herpes and AIDS US scientists report at the Fourth International Conference on AIDS that herpes virus infection may increase susceptibility to infection by HIV, the AIDS-causing virus. According to the researchers, both viruses attack the same blood cell, with the herpes virus apparently activating the HIV. Genital herpes in one of the most commonly-reported venereal diseases in the US, affecting nearly 40 million people

433. India An Indian health officer proposes making sex between Indians and foreigners illegal, in a step to curb the spread of AIDS

434. Mass screening A private children's hospital in Rockland, DE announces plans to test all incoming patients for exposure to HIV and refer all those testing positive to other health care facilities

435. Mexico Mexican researchers announce at the Fourth International Conference on AIDS that there was a decrease from 1987 to 1988 in the percentage of gay men in Mexico City infected with the AIDS-causing virus. The decrease was attributed to educational efforts to limit the spread of the syndrome

436. Monkeys Japanese researchers report in the journal *Nature* that after analyzing the genetic structure of the AIDS-causing virus, they believe the virus did not cross from African green monkeys to humans, as has been proposed. This "monkey connection" has been considered a possible source of the AIDS epidemic in humans

437. Quarantine Californians vote down in primary elections a proposal sponsored by Lyndon H LaRouche, Jr to quarantine people with AIDS

438. Vaccine Pharmaceutical manufacturer Ciba-Geigy Corp announces it will soon begin human tests on a vaccine against HIV

439. Vaccine NIH AIDS researchers announce at the Fourth International Conference on AIDS results of their tests with a genetically-engineered vaccine developed from the AIDS-causing virus HIV. According to the researchers, none of a small human test group had become infected with HIV through the administration of the vaccine, though some did develop antibodies to it

440. Vaccine Dr Jonas Salk, known for his work on the polio vaccine, suggests that whole, dead HIV cells be used as a vaccine, rather than genetically-engineered portions of the virus

441. World conference on AIDS The Fourth International Conference on AIDS is held June 12-16 in Stockholm, Sweden. Over 6,000 experts from 125 countries attend. In his opening remarks, Dr Jonathan Mann, director of the World Health Organization's AIDS program, reports that at least 5 million people from 130 countries have been exposed to the AIDS-causing virus

July

442. AIDS and politics The Democratic Party adopts a platform emphasizing "...that the HIV/AIDS epidemic is an unprecedented public health emergency requiring increased support for accelerated research on, and the expedited approval of, treatments and vaccines, comprehensive education and prevention, compassionate patient care, adoption of the public health community consensus on voluntary and confidential testing and counseling, and protection of the civil rights of those suffering from AIDS or AIDS-related complex or testing positive for the HIV antibody..."

443. AIDS and the military Adrian G Morris, Jr, a US Army private infected with the AIDS-causing virus, is acquitted of aggravated assault charges for reportedly having unprotected sex with three other soldiers. Pvt Morris was found guilty of two lesser charges

444. Biomaterial dumping Central Diagnostic Laboratories of Perth Amboy, NJ, is accused of dumping vials of blood, some containing the AIDS-causing virus, in vacant lots in Woodbridge, Old Bridge and Perth Amboy, NJ

445. Confidentiality The AMA's policy-making body issues a statement suggesting physicians breach confidentiality and warn the sexual partners of patients testing positive for exposure to HIV. The warning is recommended if there is concern the partners would not find out about their own personal risk by any other means

446. Dextran sulfate Federally-sponsored human clinical trials of the anti-AIDS drug dextran sulfate begin. The drug has been used for some time by people with AIDS, who have been getting it from foreign sources

447. Foreign drugs FDA Commissioner Dr Frank E Young announces his agency will permit the import of FDA-unapproved anti-AIDS drugs in small quantities and for personal use. The announcement is made at the Lesbian and Gay Health Conference and AIDS Forum, held in Washington, DC

448. Handicap A federal court rules that the Federal Rehabilitation Act of 1973, which bars discrimination of the handicapped, protects healthy persons carrying HIV, as well as those who have gone on to develop AIDS

449. Minorities The New York State Health Dept releases statistics based on 141,000 anonymous tests for exposure to the AIDS-causing virus showing infection was greater among males, Blacks, Latinos, people in their 30s and residents of New York City than any other demographic group. The statistics also indicate that Black mothers and their babies are 13 times more likely to have been exposed to HIV than White women giving birth

450. New York City New York City health officials release revised projections for the number of New Yorkers believed exposed to HIV, setting the figure at 240,000. Three years ago, officials projected the number at 400,000

451. Treatments FDA Commissioner Dr Frank E Young testifies that he expects only one or two new anti-AIDS drugs would be available by 1991

August

452. AIDS Advisory Commission Pres Reagan issues an "action plan" for combatting AIDS, minus several recommendations made by his AIDS Advisory Commission, including the commission's central recommendation that he support federal legislation barring discrimination against people with AIDS and those infected with the AIDS-causing virus. Rather, Reagan called on federal agencies to implement voluntary antibias workplace regulations

453. AIDS and politics The Republican Party platform adopted at the national convention in New Orleans states that "Those who suffer from AIDS, their families, and the men and women of medicine who care for the afflicted deserve our compassion and help...We will vigorously fight against AIDS, recognizing that the enemy is one of the deadliest diseases to challenge medical research...We must not only marshall our scientific resources against AIDS, but must also protect those who do not have the disease. In this regard, education plays a critical role. AIDS education should emphasize that abstinence from drug abuse and sexual activity outside of marriage is the safest way to avoid infection with the AIDS virus..."

454. AIDS education According to results of a Gallup Poll published in the education journal *Phi Delta Kappan*, 90% of the general public believes instruction about AIDS belongs in the classroom. However, almost 25% felt children exposed to the AIDS-causing virus should not be allowed to attend school with other healthy children

455. Antibody testing A study by Oregon state public health officials reported in the journal *Lancet* suggests that anonymous testing for exposure to the AIDS-causing virus may result in greater numbers of high-risk people submitting to the test

456. Artificial insemination According to a study conducted for Congress, nearly 44% of the nation's physicians performing artificial insemination procedures test the donated sperm for HIV

457. Epidemiology According to analysts for the Hudson Institute, nearly 1.9 million Americans may be infected with HIV, twice the number suggested by the federal government

458. Jean-Paul Y Aron, writer, dies French social philosopher and author Jean-Paul Y Aron dies from AIDS at the age of 60. Aron taught philosophy at Tourcoing and Lille Universities, contributed to the newspapers *Le Matin* and *Le Monde,* and authored both plays and novels

459. Needles New York City Health Commissioner Stephen Joseph announces testing will begin of a program to distribute free needles to 200 intravenous drug users. The program, aimed at stopping the spread of AIDS among needle-sharers, has met significant resistance from opponents contending that the giveaway promotes the abuse of drugs

September

460. AZT The British pharmaceutical corporation Wellcome PLC offered a grant of $5 million to the US Congress for the provision of the anti-AIDS drug AZT to the medically-indigent, provided Congress extend a program supplying the life-prolonging drug to low-income AIDS patients. The program extension is expected to cost $10 million. A year's treatment with AZT costs approximately $10,000. The original congressional program, set to expire Sept 30, was sponsored by Sen Lowell Weicker (R-CT) in response to protests from advocates for AIDS patients over the high cost of AZT treatments

461. **AZT** The Senate approves a six-month extension of a program providing AZT to medically-indigent AIDS patients

462. **Hotline** A toll-free AIDS hotline run by teens is established in Kansas City, MO, for other teenagers to call with questions about the syndrome

463. **Legislation** New York State Governor Mario Cuomo signs a bill allowing physicians to warn needle-sharing or sex partners of people infected with HIV that they may be in danger of contracting the virus

464. **Proposition 102** A California initiative prepared by US Rep William Dannemeyer and by radiologist Lawrence McNamee promotes passage of a law requiring that doctors report patients or blood donors with positive AIDS test results to state health officials or be fined $250. The proposed law would also require that anyone known or "reasonably believed" by doctors or health authorities to be infected with AIDS must divulge a list of intimate partners to the state or be charged with a misdemeanor and would permit use of the AIDS antibody test by insurers and employees. The measure would allow doctors to use the same test on a patient's blood without the patient's written consent and make willful transmission of the virus a crime, stiffening sentences for rape or assault by HIV carriers. The measure, if passed and upheld in court, would make the nation's most populous state a leader in the legal countertrend toward favoring alleged public interests and insurers over patients' rights. No states have passed laws as sweepingly restrictive as the California proposal

465. **School district settlement** The Florida DeSoto County School District agrees in an out-of-court settlement to pay $1.1 million to the family of Clifford and Louise Ray, whose three sons have been exposed to the AIDS-causing virus. The Rays had moved to Sarasota from Arcadia, FL, after community residents attempted to prevent the three boys from attending local schools. In addition, their home was burned by a an unknown arsonist. The suit filed by the Rays charged school district officials with abuse of power, depriving their sons of their rights, and promoting community hatred against the boys

October

466. **Ad campaign** CDC officials unveil a series of new television and print AIDS awareness advertisements. Unlike a similar 1987 AIDS information campaign, the new ads avoid mentioning the word "condom." The 1987 ads that directly addressed the use of condoms to prevent HIV transmission met resistance from local television stations and were rarely broadcast

467. **AIDS bill passes congress** Congress approves an AIDS bill providing for $1 billion to support research, counseling, testing, and home health care. The original bill included funding to insure the confidentiality of test results. Opposition to confidentiality funding, particularly from North Carolina Republican Sen Jesse Helms, lead to a Congressional compromise, and this provision was dropped

468. **AZT** A study published in the *New England Journal of Medicine* indicates that children with AIDS can benefit from the drug AZT just as adults do. Most strikingly, children with AIDS-related brain disease and developmental abnormalities improved while on the drug, as shown by IQ test scores. However, children, like adults, suffer AZT's side effects—mainly bone marrow suppression and a drop in certain white blood cells, which requires transfusions. This limitation is leading doctors to explore reduced dosages and combination therapies to try to evade AZT's toxicity

469. **Condoms** The three major television broadcasting networks, ABC, CBS and NBC, agree to run public service ads promoting condom use in the prevention of AIDS

470. **Discrimination** The Justice Dept issues a report supporting federal policies barring bias against people with AIDS who are employees of the government or of organizations receiving Federal funding

471. **Epidemiology** Federal health officials announce Allegheny County, PA, will be the first test site of a controversial door-to-door AIDS survey to include blood sampling and interviews with questions regarding sexual orientation, race, education and in-

come level. The pilot study is considered a precursor to a proposed similar national survey. Federal health officials contend the national survey is necessary to accurately determine the extent of infection with the AIDS-causing virus

472. **FDA speeds drug approval process** The FDA announces adoption of a new policy providing for quicker access by patients to experimental drugs for life-threatening illness, including AIDS

473. **Long-term care** The US government awards $7 million in grants for the construction of nineteen health care facilities specifically geared to provide long-term and intermediate care for AIDS patients. The facilities will be located in nine states

474. **New York City** Mayor Edward Koch designates 8 sites throughout New York City for housing homeless people with AIDS. The plan, which has met stiff opposition in the designated neighborhoods, will create nearly 850 beds

475. **Pneumonia** The CDC reports AIDS may be responsible for an increase in deaths due to pneumonia among young adults in New York City

476. **Research** Dr Bernard Poiesz and his colleagues at the State Univ of New York in Syracuse discover that the HIV virus does not lurk in sperm cells but instead is found only in the cells of the seminal fluid in which sperm cells are suspended. The discovery may mean that it will be possible for men infected with the AIDS virus to safely father children through a form of artificial insemination

477. **Schools and AIDS** Ground-breaking is held in Newark, NJ for the nation's first Head Start facility for children with AIDS

478. **Transplant guidelines** Federal health officials release guidelines for the collection and storage of tissues and organs following the discovery that a bone marrow transplant recipient was recently diagnosed with AIDS

479. **USSR** Dr Valentin I Pokrovsky, leading Soviet AIDS expert, visits the AIDS unit of the Montefiore Medical Center. According to Dr. Pokrovsky, AIDS is not yet a crisis in the Soviet Union, but is a major concern

November

480. **AIDS bill signed** President Reagan signs into law a bill creating a $1 billion AIDS program providing for testing, counseling, home care, and research

481. **Author Ernest Matthew Mickler dies** Ernest Matthew Mickler, author of the 1986 bestseller *White Trash Cooking*, dies of AIDS at the age of 48

482. **California voters reject mandatory test result reporting** California voters, by a two-to-one margin, reject a proposal requiring doctors to report to state officials all individuals who test positive for exposure to HIV, the AIDS-causing virus. The same proposal would have also lifted a ban on employers and insurers from testing for HIV exposure

483. **Colleges** Preliminary results from a study conducted jointly by the CDC and the American College Health Association suggests three of every 10,000 students now carry the AIDS-causing virus. The study was conducted at 20 college campuses across the country

484. **Condoms** The November issue of *Spin,* a popular culture magazine for young adult readers, features a free condom with explicit instructions for its use and the notice that for sexually active people condoms are the only protection against AIDS. Many newsstands, drugstores, retail outlets and magazine distributors refuse to sell the issue. The magazine's cover featured the message, "Free condom inside." The notice was found objectionable by some vendors

485. **Drugs and AIDS** According to unpublished research studies conducted in San Francisco and New York City, transmission of HIV, the AIDS-causing virus, may be spreading faster among people who inject cocaine than those injecting heroin. The higher infection rate apparently is due to the practice of injecting cocaine more often than one would heroin, sometimes several times a day. Data from the studies is due to be published in the *Journal of the American Medical Association*

486. **FDA approves alpha-Interferon** The Food and Drug Administration (FDA) announces its approval of alpha-Interferon as a treatment for Kaposi's sarcoma, a form of skin cancer seen in some people with AIDS. Alpha-Interferon is a substance produced by the body to fight disease, and its use as a commercial pharmaceutical has been made possible by the application of gene-splicing technologies

487. **Homeless** According to a study conducted by Covenant House, nearly 1500 of an estimated 20,000 homeless adolescents in New York City have been exposed to the AIDS-causing virus

488. **Mandatory testing** The New York State Supreme Court rejects a move by several New York state physicians' groups to force the state's health commissioner to declare AIDS a sexually transmitted disease (STD). Had the groups prevailed, measures including mandatory testing as well as partner tracing and notification could have been put into effect

489. **New York City needle exchange** The New York City Health Dept begins distributing sterile needles to drug abusers in an program designed to combat the spread of AIDS via needle-sharing by intravenous drug users

490. **Surgeon General Koop** According to Surgeon General C Everett Koop, discrimination, language problems and poverty are as much to blame for the AIDS epidemic as shared needle use and sexual promiscuity

December

491. **AIDS in children** As of December 1988, 1,291 cases of AIDS in children had been reported to the CDC. Of that number, 717 have died. Federal health experts estimate that by 1991, between 10,000 and 20,000 children in the US will be infected with HIV, the AIDS-causing virus

492. **AIDS in children** According to a study presented to Dept of Health and Human Services (HHS) Secretary Otis Bowen, AIDS is now the ninth-leading cause of death for American children ages 1 to 4

493. **Blood banks** A San Francisco blood bank is successfully sued for negligence after a five-year-old child contracted AIDS from blood supplied by the bank. The child received the blood during open-heart surgery Feb 24, 1983. The Irwin Memorial Blood Bank will pay $750,000 in damages and medical costs as awarded by a state Supreme Court jury. According to the child's family's lawyer, "The date Feb 24, 1983 now provides a baseline. Beyond that date, blood banks are vulnerable to jury verdicts"

494. **Hemophilia** A federal judge in Atlanta overturns a jury award of $1.6 million to a man who claimed he contracted AIDS from a drug used to treat his hemophilia. The judge ruled there was insufficient evidence to prove negligence on the part of the drug's manufacturer, Miles Inc

495. **Newscaster Max Robinson dies** Max Robinson, the first Black to anchor a television newscasting, dies of complications from AIDS. Robinson worked for the American Broadcast Company (ABC) from 1978 to 1983 and was co-anchor of the *World News Tonight* program. Robinson was 49

496. **Syphilis** According to a study conducted by the CDC, the incidence of syphilis appears to be on the rise in America's urban centers, particularly among prostitutes, intravenous drug users and their sexual partners. The study suggests that with the rise in syphilis there may also be a rise in infection with the AIDS-causing virus among those same groups

497. **Treatments** According to a report published in the journal, *Proceedings of the National Academy of Sciences,* serum from healthy carriers of HIV has been shown to remove the virus from the blood of patients with AIDS

1989

January

498. **CD4** According a report in the journal *Nature,* the experimental protein CD4 has been found effective in preventing the infection of cells with the AIDS-causing virus in monkeys. CD4 is currently being tested on humans for potential negative side effects

February

499. **AIDS in infants** According to a *New York Times* report, intravenous drug abusers, their sexual partners and infants born to HIV-infected mothers now constitute over one-fourth of diagnosed cases of AIDS. The statistics support evidence that AIDS is quickly becoming a serious health problem for poor, urban, minority-group heterosexuals

500. **AIDS survey** Findings of a survey conducted by *American Demographics* magazine indicate that most Americans are aware that AIDS can be transmitted by sex or sharing needles for intravenous drug use and that pregnant women can pass the virus to their babies, although ignorance about other means of transmission persists. Over half of Americans believe that AIDS may be contracted by kissing and 24% erroneously believe that the virus may be transmitted by mosquitos and other insects. Twenty-nine percent have the impression that AIDS can be contracted by being coughed on or sneezed on by someone with the virus. Of those surveyed, 82% say that there is no chance that they are carrying the virus and 75% believe that there is no chance that they will ever contract it. Only 4% say they don't know what their chances are of getting AIDS

501. **AZT** According to a report in *The New York Times,* over the past three years the average time from diagnosis with AIDS to death has expanded from 10 to 15 months. Experts credit AZT, an anti-viral drug used to combat HIV, as a possible explanation. The report was based on an analysis of data drawn from studies of gay men with AIDS in San Francisco

502. **Economics** According to a report published in *The New York Times,* the average lifetime cost per patient of AIDS is $60,000, with regional variations. According to the same report, estimated national expenditures for AIDS care for 1989 will be $3 billion

503. **Gangcyclovir** The FDA announces it is reappraising its decision not to allow sales of gangcyclovir, an anti-viral drug used to treat cytomegalovirus infections in AIDS patients that can cause blindness. The announcement came after protests from advocates for people with AIDS and physicians decrying the decision

504. **Health care delivery** *The New York Times* reports that, according to Dr Jo Ivy Boufford, President of New York City's Health and Hospitals Corp, "AIDS highlights all the flaws in American health care: the lack of preventive medicine, primary physician care, long-term facilities, home care, universal insurance and drug treatment"

505. **Pentamidine** The FDA allows expanded access to an experimental, aerosol version of pentamidine, a drug used to treat AIDS patients stricken with Pneumocystis carinii pneumonia. The aerosol drug is manufactured by the pharmaceutical firm, Lyphomed, and one year's supply of the medication is expected to cost $1200

506. **Public awareness** Workers who receive only brochures about AIDS from their employers are more likely to have negative feelings toward AIDS-infected colleagues than employees who receive no information, according to Georgia Tech researcher David Herold. Only comprehensive education lessens fears, he says

507. **Substance abuse** The FDA and the National Institute on Drug Abuse (NIDA) propose that expanded access to methadone would be effective in helping to curb the spread of AIDS by reducing the use of needles among intravenous drug abusers. Heroin addicts frequently share needles and thus infect one another with the AIDS virus. They, in turn, can infect their sexual partners and unborn children. Methadone, which relieves an addict's craving for heroin, is taken orally. As part of the Interim Care proposal, clinics dispensing methadone would be required to counsel addicts on how to avoid AIDS infection

508. **USSR** Soviet health officials investige the exposure of 27 babies and five mothers to AIDS in the city of Elista, located on the Caspian Sea, 750 miles south of Moscow. The use of unsterilized syringes at a children's hospital appeared to be the source of transmission

March

509. **Imreg-I** Imreg Inc is awarded a patent for Imreg-I, the first specifically anti-AIDS and ARC treatment to receive patent protection. Reports of ongoing clinical trials presented at the Fourth International Conference on AIDS in Stockholm indicate that fewer patients with ARC receiving Imreg-I went on to develop AIDS than those receiving a placebo

510. **Patients develop viruses resistant to AZT** Researchers discover drug-resistant strains of HIV appear to be cropping up in patients undergoing long-term treatment with the antiviral drug AZT, causing AIDS patients and advocates to increase pressure on the FDA to speed up testing and approval of alternative therapies

CHRONOLOGY – SUBJECT INDEX

PART II

DIRECTORY OF ORGANIZATIONS

ALABAMA

1. AIDS Control Program, Mobile County Health Dept
251 N Bayou St
Mobile, AL 36603
(204) 690-8810
KEY PERSONNEL: Virginia B Midgette; Director
AFFILIATION: Mobile County Government
FACILITY TYPE: Educational; Clinic; HIV counseling and testing; Health department
STAFF: Paid professional 5
YEAR FOUNDED: 1985
FUNDING: Federal government; State government
OUTREACH: Speakers bureau
NETWORKS: Mobile AIDS Coalition; Alabama AIDS Prevention Network
ADDITIONAL INFO: This agency became an alternate test site in 1987. Provides educational activities
LANGUAGES: Spanish, Vietnamese

2. Birmingham AIDS Outreach
PO Box 73062
Birmingham, AL 35253
(205) 930-0440; (800) 445-3741
KEY PERSONNEL: Rick Adams

3. Mobile AIDS Support Services (MASS)
PO Box 16341
Mobile, AL 36616
(205) 342-5092
KEY PERSONNEL: Robb Sanborn; Coordinator
AFFILIATION: Unitarian Universalist Fellowship of Mobile, AL
FACILITY TYPE: Educational; Hospital; Support group; HIV counseling and testing; Client services/case management; Visitation
STAFF: Volunteers 5
YEAR FOUNDED: 1987
FUNDING: Private; Fund-raisers
OUTREACH: Program training, informal community training
NETWORKS: National AIDS Network (NAN)
SEMINARS: "AIDS—What You Need to Know;" "AIDS—A Religious Response"

4. Montgomery AIDS Outreach, Inc
PO Box 5213
Montgomery, AL 36103
(205) 284-2273; Hotline: (205) 284-CARE
KEY PERSONNEL: Sandra Langston; President, Board of Directors
FACILITY TYPE: Educational; Support group; Fund-raising
STAFF: Volunteers 30
YEAR FOUNDED: 1987
FUNDING: Private; Fund-raisers
OUTREACH: Speakers bureau, educational presentations in drug rehabilitation centers, public educational forums on AIDS-related issues
NETWORKS: National AIDS Network (NAN)
AVAILABLE LITERATURE: *We Choose to Care*, an educational pamphlet; *In Sight*, a quarterly newsletter

ALASKA

5. AIDS Program
PO Box 240249, 3601 C St, Ste 540
Anchorage, AK 99524-0249
(907) 561-4406
KEY PERSONNEL: Marvin Bailey; Contract Health Education/Risk Reduction Program Coordinator
AFFILIATION: Alaska State Dept of Health and Social Services, Division of Public Health, Section of Epidemiology
FACILITY TYPE: Research; Educational; Task force; HIV counseling and testing
YEAR FOUNDED: 1985
FUNDING: State government
ADDITIONAL INFO: Provides surveillance and counseling/testing and health education/risk reduction education to all communities in Alaska
AVAILABLE LITERATURE: *AIDS Program*, informational brochure

6. Alaskan AIDS Assistance Association (4A's)
417 W 8th Ave
Anchorage, AK 99501
(907) 276-1400; Hotline: (907) 276-4880; Toll-free: (800) 478-AIDS (AK only)
KEY PERSONNEL: Alison King; Program Director
FACILITY TYPE: Educational; Support group; Client services/case management; HIV counseling and testing
STAFF: Paid professional 1; Paid nonprofessional 2; Volunteers 14
YEAR FOUNDED: 1985
FUNDING: State government; Local government; Private; Fund-raisers
NETWORKS: Computerized AIDS Information Network (CAIN); Interior AIDS Assistance Association; Shanti of Juneau; Stop AIDS Project
SEMINARS: May 1988—"Ministers' Conference;" Aug 1988—"Lovie Nassaney Workshop;" Apr 1989—"Empowering Our Lives"
AVAILABLE LITERATURE: Newsletter; agency description pamphlets; distributes materials from other agencies

7. American Red Cross, Tanana Valley Chapter
626 2nd St
Fairbanks, AK 99708
(907) 456-5937
FACILITY TYPE: Educational
ADDITIONAL INFO: Source of AIDS information. Also, check other local chapters of the American Red Cross

8. Arctic Gay and Lesbian Association
PO Box 82290
Fairbanks, AK 99708
FACILITY TYPE: Educational; Support group
ADDITIONAL INFO: Source of AIDS information

9. Fairbanks Health Center
800 Airport Way
Fairbanks, AK 99701
(907) 452-1776
KEY PERSONNEL: Elaine McKenzie; Nursing Manager
AFFILIATION: Alaska State Division of Public Health
FACILITY TYPE: Clinic; HIV counseling and testing
FUNDING: Federal government; State government
AVAILABLE LITERATURE: Distributes materials from other agencies

10. Identity, Inc
PO Box 2000070
Anchorage, AK 99520-0070
(907) 276-3918
FACILITY TYPE: Educational
ADDITIONAL INFO: Source of AIDS information

11. Municipality of Anchorage, Dept of Health and Human Services
PO Box 196650, 825 L St
Anchorage, AK 99511-6650
(907) 343-4611
KEY PERSONNEL: Micki Boling; AIDS Coordinator
AFFILIATION: Anchorage Dept of Health and Human Services
FACILITY TYPE: Educational; Clinic; HIV counseling and testing
STAFF: Paid professional 5; Volunteers 20
FUNDING: Federal government; State government
OUTREACH: Speakers bureau provided for schools, civic groups, and workshops; provides workshops for AIDS network members, health care workers, schools, and the gay community
NETWORKS: AIDS Network
ADDITIONAL INFO: Provides sexually transmitted disease services, family planning and general clinic services. Clinic provides confidential HIV counseling and testing

12. Northern Region AIDS/STD Program
212A Arctic Health Research Bldg, UAF
Fairbanks, AK 99775
(907) 474-6001
KEY PERSONNEL: Cheryl Kilgore; Public Health Representative
AFFILIATION: Alaska State Division of Public Health, Section of Epidemiology
FACILITY TYPE: Educational; Task force; HIV counseling and testing
FUNDING: Federal government; State government
OUTREACH: Educational services and staff training to the general public, health care providers, and teachers; speakers bureau
ADDITIONAL INFO: Arranges for and/or conducts numerous community educational presentations. Provides HIV antibody pre-and post-test counseling, epidemiology, community networking, AIDS Task Force, and a speakers bureau
AVAILABLE LITERATURE: Distributes materials from various agencies

13. Sexually Transmitted Disease Program, Municipality of Anchorage
PO Box 196650
Anchorage, AK 99519-6650
(907) 343-4611
KEY PERSONNEL: Jan Nichols; Program Coordinator
AFFILIATION: Anchorage Dept of Health and Human Services
FACILITY TYPE: Educational; Clinic; HIV counseling and testing
STAFF: Paid professional 6; Paid nonprofessional 2
FUNDING: State government; Local government; Fees for services or products
OUTREACH: Public speaking to schools and other community groups, visits bars and other places where at-risk people gather to distribute condoms and educational materials
NETWORKS: National AIDS Network (NAN); Alaska Public Health Association; Alaskan AIDS Assistance Association; AIDS Speakers Bureau
ADDITIONAL INFO: Provides HIV testing, counseling, and referral service
AVAILABLE LITERATURE: *Have You Got It Together*, brochure about STDs; *Let's Stand Together and Fence Off AIDS*, sticker and poster on the use of condoms; *Confidential Sexually Transmitted Disease Services*, matchbook; *Erase AIDS*, pencil; *Sex, Drugs, and AIDS*, pocket ruler
LANGUAGES: Spanish

14. Sitka Health Center
210 Moller St
Sitka, AK 99835
(907) 747-3255
KEY PERSONNEL: Nancy McMonagle; Public Health Nurse
AFFILIATION: Alaska State Division of Public Health Nursing
FACILITY TYPE: HIV counseling and testing; Health department
STAFF: Paid professional 2; Paid nonprofessional 1
FUNDING: State government; Local government
OUTREACH: STD clinic, alternative testing site for AIDS screening with counseling
SEMINARS: 1988—"AIDS Workshop"
ADDITIONAL INFO: An alternative site for HIV testing. Provides other adult and child services such as immunizations, health assessments, cancer screening, and resource referral

ARIZONA

15. Arizona AIDS Information Line
PO Box 16423
Phoenix, AZ 85011
(602) 234-2753; Hotline: (602) 234-2752
KEY PERSONNEL: Ron Barnes; Co-Director
AFFILIATION: Lesbian and Gay Community Switchboard
FACILITY TYPE: Educational; Switchboard
STAFF: Paid professional 2; Volunteers 30
YEAR FOUNDED: 1979
FUNDING: Fund-raisers
NETWORKS: National Gay and Lesbian Task Force (NGLTF)
ADDITIONAL INFO: This is an information and referral service for the gay and lesbian community. Provides information and referral to the greater Phoenix area

16. Arizona AIDS Project, Inc (AAP)
FORMER NAME: Arizona Stop AIDS Project
736 E Flynn Lane
Phoenix, AZ 85014
(602) 277-1929; Hotline: (602) 277-1929
KEY PERSONNEL: Marilyn R Lanza; Operations Manager
FACILITY TYPE: Educational; Support group; Fund-raising; Client services/case management
STAFF: Paid professional 3; Paid nonprofessional 1; Volunteers 150
YEAR FOUNDED: 1984
FUNDING: Federal government; Local government; Private; Fund-raisers
OUTREACH: Provides educational information in the workplace, schools, and community
SEMINARS: Sep 30, 1988—"AIDS: Challenges for Caregivers;" Oct 18, 1988—"Inter-Faith Conference on AIDS"
ADDITIONAL INFO: "The services AAP provides to people with AIDS and AIDS-Related Complex, as well as their families and friends, include practical and emotional support, and coordination with medical, legal, and social service resources, both public and private."
AVAILABLE LITERATURE: *Arizona AIDS Project*, brochure describing the organization; Newsletter
LANGUAGES: Spanish, American Sign Language

17. CODAMA Services Connection to Care
2025 N Central
Phoenix, AZ 85004
(602) 234-0053
KEY PERSONNEL: Sam Spradlin; Physician Assistant
FACILITY TYPE: HIV counseling and testing; Substance abuse treatment

18. Community AIDS Council (CAC)
PO Box 32903
Phoenix, AZ 85064
(602) 890-1776
KEY PERSONNEL: Robert M Aronin; Chairperson
FACILITY TYPE: Educational; Support group; Fund-raising; Client services/case management
STAFF: Volunteers 751
YEAR FOUNDED: 1987
FUNDING: Local government; Private; Fund-raisers
OUTREACH: Risk prevention education
NETWORKS: Computerized AIDS Information Network (CAIN); National AIDS Network (NAN)
SEMINARS: 1989—"AIDS Treatment Seminars for Physicians"
ADDITIONAL INFO: CAC is the primary source of direct financial assistance for people with AIDS in Maricopa County. Approximately 85% of CAC's income is distributed to PWAs for emergency medical care, housing, and food
AVAILABLE LITERATURE: *AIDS in Phoenix Newsletter*
LANGUAGES: Spanish

19. Cristo AIDS Ministry
1029 E Turney
Phoenix, AZ 85014
KEY PERSONNEL: Rev Fred L Pattison
AFFILIATION: Casa de Cristo Evangelical Church
FACILITY TYPE: Educational; Religious; Client services/case management; Food bank

STAFF: Volunteers 15
YEAR FOUNDED: 1986
FUNDING: Private
NETWORKS: Food bank for PWAs, PWARCs and others; weekly hot lunch program (free to PWAs); delivery of monthly food baskets through foodshare; spiritual outreach with healing ministry
SEMINARS: T-E-N: The Evangelical Network of AIDS Ministry Groups

20. Maricopa County Dept of Health Services
1825 E Roosevelt
Phoenix, AZ 85006
(602) 258-6381 ext 261
KEY PERSONNEL: Charles Juels; Director, Disease Control Services
FACILITY TYPE: Educational; HIV counseling and testing
STAFF: Paid professional 5; Paid nonprofessional 3
FUNDING: Federal government; State government; Local government
OUTREACH: Speakers bureau, inservice training
SEMINARS: 1988—"How I Do AIDS Counseling and Testing;" Sep 30, 1988—"Care for the Care Giver"
LANGUAGES: Spanish

21. The People With AIDS Coalition of Tucson (PACT)
PO Box 2488
Tucson, AZ 85702
(602) 792-3775
KEY PERSONNEL: James Fisher; Director
AFFILIATION: National Association of People With AIDS (NAPWA)
FACILITY TYPE: Research; Educational; Support group
STAFF: Volunteers 20
YEAR FOUNDED: 1987
FUNDING: Private; Fund-raisers
OUTREACH: Speakers bureau provides PWAs to speak about the experience of living with AIDS to various organizations and groups
ADDITIONAL INFO: PACT is an information and referral organization comprised of HIV positive members and concerned others. Maintains an HIV wellness clinic once a week
AVAILABLE LITERATURE: *Living with AIDS*, newsletter; *AIDS Resource List*, a brochure of resources

22. Phoenix Shanti Group
PO Box 17618
Phoenix, AZ 85011
(602) 265-3884
KEY PERSONNEL: Randall Gorbette; Executive Director
FACILITY TYPE: Educational; Support group; HIV counseling and testing
STAFF: Paid professional 2; Volunteers 175
YEAR FOUNDED: 1986
FUNDING: State government; Local government; Private; Fund-raisers
OUTREACH: Volunteer training program, weekly support groups, monthly open forum workshops, PWA library, community and professional inservices
RESEARCH: Alternative therapies
ADDITIONAL INFO: Shanti is a Sanskrit word meaning "inner peace" which reflects the approach of the services that the group provides. The Phoenix Shanti Group is a volunteer organization providing one-to-one nondirective peer support, advocacy, and companionship, as well as other psychosocial services to people with AIDS and their family, friends, and loved ones. Holds six volunteer training programs a year
AVAILABLE LITERATURE: *Rudy's Rocket: For and from PWAs with a Little Help from Their Friends*, newsletter; *Love and Light: Phoenix Shanti Group*, brochure describing the group
LANGUAGES: Spanish

23. Shanti Foundation of Tucson, Inc
602 N 4th Ave
Tucson, AZ 85705
(602) 622-7107
KEY PERSONNEL: Natalie Perry; Executive Director
FACILITY TYPE: Educational; Support group
STAFF: Volunteers 60
YEAR FOUNDED: 1985
FUNDING: Local government; Private; Fund-raisers
OUTREACH: Safer sex workshops, "Living Through Death" grief support group, HIV "Letting Go of Fear" support group

AVAILABLE LITERATURE: Distributes safer sex brochures, buttons, posters, coasters, and stickers
LANGUAGES: Spanish, American Sign Language

24. Tucson AIDS Project, Inc (TAP)
151 S Tucson Blvd, Ste 252
Tucson, AZ 85716
(602) 322-6226; Hotline: (602) 326-AIDS
KEY PERSONNEL: Craig Bradford Snow; Executive Director
FACILITY TYPE: Educational; Support group; Fund-raising; Client services/case management
STAFF: Paid professional 14; Volunteers 200
YEAR FOUNDED: 1985
FUNDING: Federal government; State government; Local government; Private; Fund-raisers; Fees for services or products
OUTREACH: Outreach to IV drug users and their sex partners and to gays and lesbians
NETWORKS: National AIDS Network (NAN); AIDS Action Council
ADDITIONAL INFO: This agency provides local forums on legal and policy issues of AIDS, pediatrics and AIDS, and workplace policies for human service agenicies
AVAILABLE LITERATURE: *On Tap*, monthly newsletter; *One Strike You're Out*, matchbook with information for drug users; *If You're an I.V. Drug User, You May be at Double Risk for Getting the AIDS Virus*, a pocket card with information for IV drug users; *Don't Get AIDS, Clean Your Works*, a pocket card in English and Spanish; *Si Usted usa Drogas Intravenosas, es Posible que Corra Doble Riesgo de Contraer el Virus de SIDS*, a Spanish-language pocket card for IV drug users; *Tucson is Taking Loving Care*, a package with condom and instructions
LANGUAGES: Spanish, American Sign Language

ARKANSAS

25. AIDS Support Group
210 Pulaski
Little Rock, AR 72201
(501) 374-3605
KEY PERSONNEL: Ralph A Hyman; Administrator
AFFILIATION: The Psychotherapy Center
FACILITY TYPE: Support group
STAFF: Volunteers 4
YEAR FOUNDED: 1983
FUNDING: Donations
OUTREACH: Support for PWAs
NETWORKS: Arkansas AIDS Foundation

26. Arkansas A.I.D.S. Foundation
PO Box 5007
Little Rock, AR 72225
(501) 663-7833; Hotline: (501) 666-3340
KEY PERSONNEL: Chip Montgomery; Executive Director
FACILITY TYPE: Educational; Support group; Fund-raising; HIV counseling and testing
STAFF: Paid professional 1; Paid nonprofessional 2; Volunteers 40
YEAR FOUNDED: 1985
FUNDING: State government; Private; Fund-raisers; Fees for services or products
OUTREACH: Speakers bureau, hotline, AIDS educational resource center, consultation to employers, support groups, buddy programs, transitional residence for PWAs, statewide educational seminars for health and lay professionals
NETWORKS: Arkansas Coalition for the Handicapped; American Civil Liberties Union; Planned Parenthood; Disabilities Network Council
SEMINARS: Provides educational programs
ADDITIONAL INFO: "The Arkansas AIDS Foundation is a community-based organization founded in 1985 to educate the people of Arkansas about AIDS, to prevent the spread of the disease, and to provide urgently needed patient services."
AVAILABLE LITERATURE: *AIDS in Arkansas: You Can Make a Difference*, a brochure about the organization; *Services in Arkansas for People with AIDS-Related Concerns*, brochure describing the organization with application form; *AIDS: Lecture Material for the Helping Professional Including AIDS Fantasy, History, Statistics, Stages, Psychosocial Aspects, and AIPS*, a booklet by Ralph A Hyman, a licensed psychologist

27. Arkansas Dept of Health AIDS Prevention Program (APP)
4815 W Markham
Little Rock, AR 72205-3867
(501) 661-2408; Hotline: (800) 445-7720 AR only
KEY PERSONNEL: Robin Bailey; AIDS Program Training Coordinator
AFFILIATION: Arkansas State Government
FACILITY TYPE: Research; Educational; Clinic; Task force; HIV counseling and testing
YEAR FOUNDED: 1985
FUNDING: Federal government
OUTREACH: Speakers bureau, technical assistance in policy development, HIV counseling
NETWORKS: Arkansas Medical Society; Arkansas AIDS Foundation; Arkansas Dept of Education
SEMINARS: Nov, 1987—"Statewide AIDS Symposium;" Apr, Oct, 1988—"Minority AIDS in Arkansas;" Dec, 1988—"Ministerial AIDS Workshop;" 1989—"Statewide Speakers Bureau Network Meeting"
RESEARCH: Knowledge, attitude, behavior, and belief surveys
AVAILABLE LITERATURE: *HIV Antibody Test*, a brochure describing the test; *Surveillance Update, November 1, 1988: AIDS*, a 22-page booklet of graphical statistics

28. Washington County AIDS Task Force
PO Box 4224
Fayetteville, AR 72702
Hotline: (501) 443-AIDS
KEY PERSONNEL: Diane Lyddon; President
FACILITY TYPE: Educational; Support group; Fund-raising; Task force; Client services/case management; Emergency fund
STAFF: Volunteers 13
YEAR FOUNDED: 1987
FUNDING: Private; Fund-raisers
OUTREACH: Speakers bureau
SEMINARS: Nov 1987—"NW Arkansas AIDS Conference"
ADDITIONAL INFO: This agency is widening its service area to include all of northwest Arkansas
LANGUAGES: American Sign Language

CALIFORNIA

29. Adult Immunodeficiencies Clinic/San Francisco
400 Parnassus, Rm 555A
San Francisco, CA 94143-0324
(415) 476-3226
KEY PERSONNEL: Harry Hollander, Director; Susan Stringaki, Head Nurse
AFFILIATION: Univ of California San Francisco
FACILITY TYPE: Research; Educational; Clinic
FUNDING: State government
LIBRARY: Information on all aspects of AIDS for staff, public and students
NETWORKS: Social Work AIDS Network (SWAN)
SEMINARS: "AIDS/ARC Update '86;" "AIDS/ARC Update '87"
RESEARCH: AZT clinical trial center
ADDITIONAL INFO: Founded in 1984 as a research, educational, and clinical facility for AIDS patients

30. Aid For AIDS, Inc
8235 Santa Monica Blvd, Ste 200
West Hollywood, CA 90046
(213) 656-1107
KEY PERSONNEL: Phil Sciaroni; Client Services Director
FACILITY TYPE: Support group; Client services/case management; Financial support
STAFF: Paid professional 2; Volunteers 20
YEAR FOUNDED: 1983
FUNDING: Local government; Fund-raisers
ADDITIONAL INFO: This agency is dedicated to greater awareness of and providing for the needs, comfort and dignity of persons with AIDS or ARC
AVAILABLE LITERATURE: *Agency Profile*, information about the agency; *Aid for AIDS*, an informational brochure
LANGUAGES: Spanish

31. AIDS Advisory Committee of San Bernardino County
351 N Mountain View Ave
San Bernardino, CA 92415-0010
(714) 387-6230
KEY PERSONNEL: Samuel Johnson; Chief of Preventive Medical Services
AFFILIATION: San Bernardino County Government
FACILITY TYPE: Advisory
STAFF: Paid professional 4
YEAR FOUNDED: 1987
FUNDING: Local government

32. AIDS and Employment Protection
1663 Mission St, Ste 400
San Francisco, CA 94103
(415) 864-8848
KEY PERSONNEL: Robert Barnes; Acting Director
AFFILIATION: Legal Aid Society of San Francisco
FACILITY TYPE: Legal
STAFF: Paid professional 10; Paid nonprofessional 9
YEAR FOUNDED: 1986
FUNDING: Private; Fund-raisers; Fees for services or products
SEMINARS: Nov 11, 1988—"AIDSlaw Conference," San Francisco
AVAILABLE LITERATURE: Pamphlets on state and federal laws protecting PWAs from employment discrimination
LANGUAGES: Spanish

33. AIDS/ARC Clothing Depot
1715 Castro St, Ste 3
San Francisco, CA 94131
(415) 282-6493; Hotline: (415) 282-6493
KEY PERSONNEL: J Rolph; Director
AFFILIATION: New Friends of San Francisco, CA
FACILITY TYPE: Support group; Client services/case management; Clothing distribution
STAFF: Volunteers 6
YEAR FOUNDED: 1984
FUNDING: Fund-raisers; Donations
OUTREACH: Clothing distribution
NETWORKS: New Friends of San Francisco, CA; People With AIDS, San Francisco (PWASF); Lambda Institute
ADDITIONAL INFO: The purpose of this group is to connect the PWA/ARC with the right resources without government help. Assists in obtaining housing, clothing, appliances, and financial aid. Provides clean, new/used clothing and appliances to PWA/PWARCs.

34. AIDS/ARC Services Division of the Catholic Charities, San Francisco
FORMER NAME: AIDS/ARC Program, Saint Joseph's Fund
1049 Market St, Ste 200
San Francisco, CA 94103
(415) 864-7400
KEY PERSONNEL: Bob Nelson; Coordinator of Direct Services
AFFILIATION: Catholic Charities, Archdiocese of San Francisco
FACILITY TYPE: Educational; Fund-raising; Residential facility (adults); Religious
STAFF: Paid professional 12; Volunteers 15
YEAR FOUNDED: 1986
FUNDING: Federal government; State government; Local government; Private; Fund-raisers; Fees for services or products
OUTREACH: Educational outreach to congregations and church related agencies and schools
NETWORKS: BAYCARE; Homeless Coalition; Women's AIDS Network; Latino AIDS Task Force; Third World AIDS Advisory Task Force; Interfaith Coalition on AIDS
SEMINARS: Mar, 1987—"Interfaith Conference on AIDS"
AVAILABLE LITERATURE: *Catholic Charities Effective Philanthropy*, a booklet describing the agency; *Peter Claver Community*, a brochure describing the home for homeless PWAs/PWARCs *Peter Claver Community Opening Ceremony*, a program booklet about the community; *Emergency Health Fund: AIDS/ARC Division*, a brochure describing funds available; *Catholic Charities: AIDS/ARC Division*, newsletter; *Archdiocese of San Francisco: AIDS and ARC Programs Information and Pastoral Kit*, a kit for pastors *A Day in the Life of an AIDS Minister*, *AIDS and ARC Program Services Offered*, *When a Member Has AIDS*, *AIDS: A Serious and Special Opportunity for Ministry*, *AIDS: A Challenge to the Church*, *Talking to Your Family About AIDS*
LANGUAGES: Spanish, Ameslan, German, Italian

35. AIDS Clinic, County/University of Southern California Medical Center
1175 N Cummings, 5P21 Outpatient Bldg
Los Angeles, CA 90033
(213) 226-5028
KEY PERSONNEL: Michael Shubert; Nurse Manager
AFFILIATION: AIDS Clinical Trials Group
FACILITY TYPE: Research; Educational; Clinic
YEAR FOUNDED: 1985
FUNDING: Federal government; State government; Local government
OUTREACH: Education
ADDITIONAL INFO: Provides comprehensive care including ambulatory services, in-patient follow-up, and home care coordination
LANGUAGES: Spanish

36. AIDS: Counseling and Assistance Program (AIDS:CAP), Gay and Lesbian Resource Center (GLRC)
417 Santa Barbara St, Ste A18
Santa Barbara, CA 93101
(805) 963-3636; Hotline: (805) 965-2925
KEY PERSONNEL: Geni Cowan; Executive Director
AFFILIATION: Western Addiction Services Program, Inc
FACILITY TYPE: Educational; Support group
STAFF: Paid professional 5; Paid nonprofessional 3; Volunteers 40
YEAR FOUNDED: 1976
FUNDING: State government; Local government; Private; Fund-raisers; Fees for services or products
OUTREACH: AIDS education for IV drug users, general public, HIV antibody testing
NETWORKS: Santa Barbara County AIDS Task Force
SEMINARS: Provides direct patient assistance, professional training, consultation and program development
AVAILABLE LITERATURE: Monthly newsletter; brochures about the program

37. AIDS Education Project/Division of Northern California Coalition for Rural Health, Inc
2850A West Center St
Anderson, CA 96007
(916) 365-2559; Hotline: (916) 365-2304
KEY PERSONNEL: Jan McAdams; Project Director
AFFILIATION: Northern California Coalition for Rural Health, Inc (NCCRH, Inc)
FACILITY TYPE: Educational; Support group; Fund-raising
STAFF: Paid professional 1.25; Paid nonprofessional 1.75; Volunteers 14
YEAR FOUNDED: 1987
FUNDING: Federal government; State government; Private; Fund-raisers; Fees for services or products
OUTREACH: Home parties for women, AIDS prevention displays and outreach for workers at Women, Infants and Children (WIC) nutritional clinics in six counties, outreach to women in jail
NETWORKS: Rural AIDS Network; California Association of AIDS Agencies (CAAA); Shasta County Drug Abuse Network
SEMINARS: Aug 1988—"Youth and AIDS Seminar;" Nov 1988—"Physicians AIDS Diagnosis and Treatment Seminar;" Apr 1989—"Funding Community AIDS Projects—A Teleconference"
RESEARCH: Funding, grants, and contracts for services; condom sales and distribution
ADDITIONAL INFO: The first California AIDS project to combine Women, Infants and Children nutritional information and AIDS education. Provides on-going efforts on behalf of women including home parties, AIDS confidence barometer quiz, and outreach efforts to curtail the spread of AIDS in rural northern California
AVAILABLE LITERATURE: Publish a monthly newsletter; *AIDS Prevention Confidence Barometer for Women*, a brochure
LANGUAGES: Spanish, French, Sign Language

38. AIDS Emergency Fund (AEF)
FORMER NAME: San Francisco AIDS Fund
1550 California St, Ste 7L
San Francisco, CA 94109
(415) 441-6407
KEY PERSONNEL: Hank Cook; President
FACILITY TYPE: Support group
STAFF: Paid nonprofessional 2; Volunteers 20
YEAR FOUNDED: 1982
FUNDING: Private; Fund-raisers
ADDITIONAL INFO: Provides financial grants to PWAs and PWARCs living within the greater Bay Area

39. The AIDS Health Project
1855 Folsom St, Ste 506, Box 0884
San Francisco, CA 94143-0884
(415) 476-6430
KEY PERSONNEL: Paul Causey; Public Relations Associate
AFFILIATION: University of California, San Francisco
FACILITY TYPE: Research; Educational; Support group
STAFF: Paid professional 60; Paid nonprofessional 10; Volunteers 125
YEAR FOUNDED: 1984
FUNDING: Federal government; State government; Local government; Private; Fund-raisers; Fees for services or products
OUTREACH: Outreach to high risk populations for prevention and risk reduction services, support groups for PWAs, PWARCs, and HIV positive individuals, education for health care professionals and educators
NETWORKS: Computerized AIDS Information Network (CAIN)
SEMINARS: "Beyond the Basics: AIDS and Mental Health," "Alternate Antibody Test Site Trainings," "Volunteer Therapist Training"
RESEARCH: Substance abuse and AIDS/ARC/HIV Positive, neuropsychiatry and AIDS, AIDS and mental health, care for the AIDS caregiver
ADDITIONAL INFO: The AIDS Health Project is an AIDS prevention and mental health promotion program serving people at risk for AIDS, those with HIV infection, and their health care providers. Facilitates risk reduction and health promotion through individual and group activities and trains health professionals about the psychological and social impact of the epidemic. Founded by a group of mental health professionals from UCSF and the private practice community. The program has trained over 70,000 professionals, disclosed over 30,000 HIV antibody test results and helped over 25,000 high-risk individuals in various activities
AVAILABLE LITERATURE: *Focus: A Guide to AIDS Research*, a newsletter; *AIDS Effects on the Brain*, an informational brochure; *El SIDA (AIDS) y sus Efectros en el Cerebro*, an informational brochure; *Stress Management Leader's Guide*, a facilitator's manual on stress management for people at risk for AIDS; *AIDS and Substance Abuse*, a training manual for health care professionals; *Working With AIDS*, a resource guide for mental health professionals; *Guidelines for Disclosing AIDS Antibody Test Results*, a protocol for health professionals; *The Other Crisis: AIDS and Mental Health*, a video; *What's Next? After the Test*, a training video; *Relaxation and Visualization*, a stress management video
LANGUAGES: Spanish

40. AIDS Minority Health Initiative (AMHI)
FORMER NAME: Bay Area Black Health Consortium
1440 Broadway, Ste 403
Oakland, CA 94618
(415) 763-1872
KEY PERSONNEL: Mabel W. Hazard; Director
AFFILIATION: Black Area Black Consortium for Quality Health Care, Inc.
FACILITY TYPE: Task force; Social service agency
STAFF: Paid professional 6; Paid nonprofessional 2; Volunteers 30
FUNDING: State government; Local government; Private
OUTREACH: Case mangement coordination, psychological counseling, crisis intervention and support groups
NETWORKS: Bay Area Black Health Professionals Network; Statewide Black Health Conferences
SEMINARS: Apr, 1989—"California State Health Conference"
ADDITIONAL INFO: "The AMHI was created to increase the availability of medical, treatment, counseling, and coordination services through case mangement to minority people with Acquired Immune Deficiency Syndrome (AIDS) and AIDS Related Conditions (ARC)."
AVAILABLE LITERATURE: *AIDS Minority Health Initiative*, flyer describing the agency

41. AIDS Positive Action League (APAL)
1154 N Lake Ave
Pasadena, CA 91104
(213) 684-8411
KEY PERSONNEL: Sonny King, Director; Richard Esquer, Director
FACILITY TYPE: Educational
FUNDING: Donations
NETWORKS: Los Angeles County Health Dept, AIDS Consortium
ADDITIONAL INFO: Founded in 1983 to provide preventative and alternative educational material as it pertains to safe sex and AIDS

AVAILABLE LITERATURE: *Guidelines for Health Risk Reduction*, a 2-fold brochure giving guidelines for safe sex including risk reduction, "What happens to people with AIDS?," "But what are the symptoms or signs of AIDS?," "Sexual practices," and other factors; *The Art of Loving You*, a sexually explicit booklet for gay and bisexual adult males, not for distribution to the general public or to minors under 18. It covers penile and anal masturbation as safe sex alternatives. Also available are several memos discussing AIDS facts, terms, sex, blood test, and sexually transmitted diseases
LANGUAGES: Spanish

42. AIDS Project Los Angeles (APLA)
3670 Wilshire Blvd, Ste 300
Los Angeles, CA 90010
(213) 380-2000; Hotline: (800) 922-AIDS southern CA only; Spanish Hotline: (800) 222-SIDA southern CA only; TDD Hotline: (800) 553-AIDS southern CA only
KEY PERSONNEL: Janet Martinez; Media Relations Assistant
FACILITY TYPE: Educational; Support group; Fund-raising
YEAR FOUNDED: 1982
FUNDING: Federal government; State government; Local government; Private; Fund-raisers
OUTREACH: Comprehensive case management, mental health counseling, no-charge food program, buddy program, religious resources, chemical dependency and addictive behaviors program, residential care, no-charge dental clinic, hotlines, community education, speakers bureau, AIDS in the workplace outreach, professional training programs for health care providers and emergency service workers, and government affairs office
ADDITIONAL INFO: "AIDS Project Los Angeles (APLA), a non-profit organization, provides support services for people with AIDS and ARC and their loved ones throughout Los Angeles County. APLA is committed to increasing compassion for people with AIDS and ARC and reducing the incidence of AIDS through risk-reduction education."
AVAILABLE LITERATURE: *Issues: An AIDS Forum*, informational brochure for the general public; *AIDS: A Self-Care Manual*, for PWAs, PWARCs, family members, training programs, and the general public; various brochures

43. AIDS Project of the East Bay (APEB)
400 40th St, Ste 204
Oakland, CA 94609
(415) 420-8181; Information and Referral: (415) 420-8181
FACILITY TYPE: Educational; Support group; Client services/case management
STAFF: Paid professional 17; Volunteers 150
YEAR FOUNDED: 1983
FUNDING: State government; Private; Fund-raisers
OUTREACH: Direct services for PWAs, PWARCs, HIV positive individuals, friends, family and lovers, educational outreach for health care providers, mental health professionals, high risk groups, and general population
NETWORKS: Computerized AIDS Information Network (CAIN); National AIDS Network (NAN); California Association of AIDS Agencies (CAAC)
SEMINARS: Nov, Dec 1987, Apr, Jun 1988—"AIDS Education Training for Health Care Workers and Emergency Service Workers;" May 1988—"The Changing Epidemic: A Media Symposium;" Sep 1988—"AIDS Action Alameda;" Mar 1988—"A Working Conference;" Jul, 1988—"Update on California AIDS Legislation;" Feb, Sep 1988—"Emotional Support Volunteer Training"
LANGUAGES: Spanish, American Sign Language

44. AIDS Provider Education Experience (APEX)
995 Potrero Ave, Ward 95, Bldg 90
San Francisco, CA 94110
(415) 550-6890
KEY PERSONNEL: Sam Broyles; Program Assistant
AFFILIATION: San Francisco General Hospital
FACILITY TYPE: Educational
STAFF: Paid professional 2
YEAR FOUNDED: 1986
FUNDING: Private; Fees for services or products
NETWORKS: Infectious Disease Society of America
SEMINARS: Oct 31; Nov 18, 1988—"Program IV;" Feb 6; Feb 24, 1989—"Program V"

ADDITIONAL INFO: "APEX is a hospital-based, patient-oriented, 3-4 week educational program headquartered at San Francisco General Hospital. Experience has indicated that the program is best suited to individuals who have had at least some direct experience in the care of patients with AIDS because the program delves heavily into specific management of all of the opportunistic infections, malignancies, and virology of HIV infection."
AVAILABLE LITERATURE: *A.P.E.X—AIDS Provider Education Experience*, informational flyer about the program

45. AIDS Response Program of Orange County (ARP)
12832 Garden Grove Blvd, Ste B
Garden Grove, CA 92643
(714) 534-0961
KEY PERSONNEL: Nancy Radclyffe; Director
AFFILIATION: Gay and Lesbian Community Services Center of Orange County
FACILITY TYPE: Educational; Support group
STAFF: Paid professional 3; Paid nonprofessional 4; Volunteers 50
YEAR FOUNDED: 1983
FUNDING: State government; Private; Fund-raisers
OUTREACH: Speakers bureau, support groups
NETWORKS: National AIDS Network (NAN); California Association of AIDS Agencies (CAAA)
AVAILABLE LITERATURE: *AIDS Digest*, a bimonthly newsletter; *Teens and AIDS*, a brochure for teens; *Face It: Safe Sex Is a Decision You Can Live With*, a safer sex brochure; *Common Sense About Condoms*, a brochure on condom use

46. AIDS Services, County Health Care Services
FORMER NAME: Tri-Counties AIDS Project
300 N San Antonio Rd
Santa Barbara, CA 93110
(805) 681-5120
KEY PERSONNEL: Valwyn Hooper; Administrator
AFFILIATION: Santa Barbara County Health Care Services
FACILITY TYPE: Educational; Clinic; Task force; HIV counseling and testing; Mental health agency
STAFF: Paid professional 5; Paid nonprofessional 3; Volunteers 5
YEAR FOUNDED: 1983
FUNDING: Federal government; State government; Local government; Private; Fees for services or products
OUTREACH: Provides outreach to gay community, IVDUs, health care workers, schools, emergency service workers, general public, social service providers, jail inmates, substance abusers
NETWORKS: California Association of AIDS Agencies (CAAA)
SEMINARS: Jan 20-22, 1989—"Caring for the Caring"
ADDITIONAL INFO: This agency is an infectious disease clinic for all HIV-infected persons. Facilitates cooperation between public and private agencies to provide a complete range of AIDS-related services.
AVAILABLE LITERATURE: *AIDS Update*, a quarterly bulletin for physicians; physician resource manual on AIDS
LANGUAGES: Spanish, Portuguese, Italian

47. AIDS Services Foundation for Orange County (ASF)
1685-A Babcock St
Costa Mesa, CA 92627
(714) 646-0411; Toll-free: (714) 458-2000 (South Orange County)
KEY PERSONNEL: Randy L Pesqueira; Director of Volunteer Services
AFFILIATION: Orange County Government
FACILITY TYPE: Educational; Support group; Hospice; Fund-raising; Client services/case management; Food bank
STAFF: Paid professional 11; Volunteers 115
YEAR FOUNDED: 1985
FUNDING: Federal government; State government; Local government; Private; Fund-raisers
OUTREACH: Speakers bureau, psychosocial educational forums
NETWORKS: California Association of AIDS Agencies (CAAA); California Association of Non-Profits; National AIDS Network (NAN); Life Lobby, California
ADDITIONAL INFO: The foundation is dedicated to the mission of providing and developing quality direct services to PWAs and those affected by AIDS in and around Orange County. Maintains a Persons Living with AIDS Coalition (PLWA) that provides psychosocial educational forums
AVAILABLE LITERATURE: *ASF Newsletter*

48. AIDS Support Group/West Hollywood
7377 Santa Monica Blvd
West Hollywood, CA 90038
FACILITY TYPE: Support group
ADDITIONAL INFO: Source of additional AIDS information

49. AIDS Treatment News
PO Box 411256
San Francisco, CA 94141
(415) 255-0588
KEY PERSONNEL: Denny Smith; Office Manager
FACILITY TYPE: Educational
STAFF: Paid professional 3; Paid nonprofessional 3
YEAR FOUNDED: 1986
FUNDING: Fees for services or products
NETWORKS: Community Research Alliance; Community Health Coalition
ADDITIONAL INFO: Interested in all promising therapies for HIV infection and related opportunistic infections
AVAILABLE LITERATURE: *AIDS Treatment News*, a biweekly newsletter reporting on new and experimental treatments for HIV, AIDS positive, and ARC and discusses new developments in public policy

50. American Association of Physicians for Human Rights (AAPHR)
PO Box 14366
San Francisco, CA 94114
(415) 558-9353
KEY PERSONNEL: David Ostrow, President; Pierre R Ludington, Executive Director
FACILITY TYPE: Educational
FUNDING: Dues
OUTREACH: Referral panel of doctors
ADDITIONAL INFO: A source of additional information on AIDS, especially for physicians
AVAILABLE LITERATURE: *AIDS and Healthful Gay Sexual Activity*, a 2-fold brochure discussing safe sex and AIDS; *AAPHR Letter*, a quarterly newsletter with information\of interest to members about seminars, resources, and position statements

51. American Foundation for AIDS Research (AmFAR)
FORMER NAME: AIDS Medical Foundation
9601 Wilshire Blvd
Beverly Hills, CA 90210-5294
(213) 273-5547
KEY PERSONNEL: Elizabeth Taylor, National Chairperson; Mervyn F Silverman, President; Mathilde Krim, Co-Chair; Michael S Gottlieb, Co-Chair
FACILITY TYPE: Research; Educational; Granting agency
FUNDING: Donations
LIBRARY: Contains information on AIDS and drug development and is open to qualified health professionals
OUTREACH: Developing a youth education pilot project in cooperation with the American Social Health Association
ADDITIONAL INFO: A California not-for-profit public benefit corporation created in 1985 primarily to meet an urgent need for biomedical research on AIDS and the conditions related to it. Promotes the development of AIDS treatments, vaccines, and an improved understanding of the natural history and causes of AIDS. The foundation awards grants for laboratory and clinical investigations. There is also a New York office: 40 W 57th St, New York, NY 10019 (212) 333-3118
AVAILABLE LITERATURE: *The Facts About AIDS*, a pamphlet of general AIDS facts; *The AmFAR Periodical Index of Experimental Treatments for AIDS and ARC*; *AIDS Targeted Information Newsletter*

52. The Aquarian Effort Heroin Detox Unit
1550 Juliesse Ave
Sacramento, CA 95815
(916) 920-3588
KEY PERSONNEL: H Scott Strain; Program Director
FACILITY TYPE: HIV counseling and testing; Substance abuse treatment

53. Aris Project
595 Millich Dr, Ste 104
Campbell, CA 95008
(408) 370-3272

KEY PERSONNEL: Robert A Sorenson, Executive Director; F Julian di Ciurcio, Coordinator of Volunteer Services
FACILITY TYPE: Educational; Support group
FUNDING: Donations; County government; Grants
LIBRARY: A resource library for volunteers
OUTREACH: Provides speakers who stress the experiences of people with AIDS and the service needs demonstrated in these situations, encouraging members of the community to respond and assist
ADDITIONAL INFO: Founded in 1986 as an educational facility providing support groups
AVAILABLE LITERATURE: Agency brochure, monthly volunteer bulletin, and a quarterly community newsletter
LANGUAGES: Spanish

54. Asian AIDS Project
1596 Post St
San Francisco, CA 94106
(415) 929-1304
KEY PERSONNEL: Darryl Ng; Interim Program Coordinator
FACILITY TYPE: Research; Educational; Task force
STAFF: Paid professional 7; Volunteers 2
YEAR FOUNDED: 1987
FUNDING: State government; Local government; Private; Fund-raisers
OUTREACH: Presentations to Asian groups in their native languages
NETWORKS: Asian AIDS Task Force
ADDITIONAL INFO: The project's ultimate goal is "to reduce and halt the incidence of AIDS in the Asian population."
AVAILABLE LITERATURE: *Asian AIDS Task Force*, a brochure describing the task force; *The Asian AIDS Project*, a brochure describing the services of the project. Also provides brochures and posters in the Asian languages
LANGUAGES: Chinese, Tagolog, Japanese, Vietnamese, Korean

55. Association for Women's AIDS Research and Education (Project AWARE)
995 Potrero Ave, Bldg 90, Ward 95, Rm 513
San Francisco, CA 94110
(415) 476-4091
KEY PERSONNEL: Judith B Cohen; Program Director
AFFILIATION: University of California, San Francisco
FACILITY TYPE: Research; Educational; Clinic
STAFF: Paid professional 2; Paid nonprofessional 11
YEAR FOUNDED: 1985
FUNDING: Federal government; State government
OUTREACH: Research and education, counseling, medical diagnostic services to high risk and HIV positive women
NETWORKS: Women's AIDS Network
RESEARCH: Transmission of the virus in prostitutes
ADDITIONAL INFO: Educates prostitutes to reduce the risk of AIDS transmission
LANGUAGES: Spanish

56. Bay Area Physicians for Human Rights (BAPHR)
2940 16th St, Ste 309
San Francisco, CA 94103
(415) 558-9353
KEY PERSONNEL: Arthur J. McDermott; Executive Coordinator
FACILITY TYPE: Educational
STAFF: Paid professional 1; Volunteers 20
YEAR FOUNDED: 1977
FUNDING: Private; Dues
OUTREACH: Monthly educational seminars and frequent social events, including annual retreat and awards banquet for professional members; BAPHR physician referral line; consultation with other AIDS-related boards, commissions, and AIDS service organizations
SEMINARS: Jun, 1989—"Physician Burn-Out," BAPHR retreat; Aug, 1989—"AAPHR/BAPHR Symposium," San Francisco
ADDITIONAL INFO: This agency was founded in 1977 to promote human rights and quality medical care for the gay and lesbian community. BAPHR was the first to publish "safe sex" guidelines, setting a standard and format on which all others are based.
AVAILABLE LITERATURE: *The BAPHRON*, a newsletter; *Medical Evaluation of Persons at Risk for HIV Infection*, a booklet
LANGUAGES: American Sign Language

57. Bayview-Hunter's Point Foundation, AIDS Education Unit
FORMER NAME: Multicultural Alliance for the Prevention of AIDS
6025 3rd St
San Francisco, CA 94124

(415) 822-7500
KEY PERSONNEL: Tanis Dasher; Project Director
FACILITY TYPE: Educational; Hospital; Support group
STAFF: Paid professional 2; Paid nonprofessional 5; Volunteers 15
YEAR FOUNDED: 1974
FUNDING: State government; Local government

58. Being Alive/People with AIDS Action Coalition, Inc, Los Angeles
4222 Santa Monica Blvd, Ste 105
Los Angeles, CA 90029
(213) 667-3262
KEY PERSONNEL: Ron Rose, Chairman; Rick Ewing, Vice-Chair
FACILITY TYPE: Educational; Support group
FUNDING: Donations; Grants
OUTREACH: Speakers bureau, referrals for services for people with AIDS, Spanish support group, veterans' support group
NETWORKS: National Association of People with AIDS
ADDITIONAL INFO: Founded in Dec 1986 focusing on self-empowerment, social activities, and speaking out on issues concerning people with AIDS
AVAILABLE LITERATURE: *Body Positive*, a newsletter for people with AIDS

59. California Association of AIDS Agencies (CAAA)
1900 K St, Ste 200
Sacramento, CA 95814
(916) 447-7199
KEY PERSONNEL: Arthur J. McDermott; Executive Director
FACILITY TYPE: Educational; Coalition
STAFF: Paid professional 2; Volunteers 8
YEAR FOUNDED: 1986
FUNDING: Private; Dues
OUTREACH: Statewide networking and technical assistance among AIDS service providers, annual conference, regional meetings, and topical institutes, association committees and public policy advocacy
NETWORKS: Computerized AIDS Information Network (CAIN)
SEMINARS: Jan, 1989—"Annual Conference;" Sep, 1989—"Regional Conference"
ADDITIONAL INFO: CAAA serves as a strong, unified voice before the state legislature on issues affecting AIDS education and direct services. CAAA promotes organizational development and resource sharing among member agencies as well as local public policy surveillance.
AVAILABLE LITERATURE: *CAAA Reports*, newsletter

60. California Dept of Health Services, Office of AIDS
PO Box 942732, 714/744 P St
Sacramento, CA 94234-7320
(916) 445-0553; Hotline, Northern CA: (800) 367-AIDS; Hotline, Southern CA: (800) 922-AIDS
KEY PERSONNEL: Thelma Fraziear; Chief
AFFILIATION: California State Government
FACILITY TYPE: Educational
STAFF: Paid professional 154
YEAR FOUNDED: 1983
FUNDING: Federal government; State government
OUTREACH: Provides educational support at all levels through speakers and published information
NETWORKS: Computerized AIDS Information Network (CAIN)
SEMINARS: Mar 1989—"Bi-Coastal National Conference on AIDS," Los Angeles
RESEARCH: Basic and clinical AIDS statewide research and statewide seroprevalence studies
ADDITIONAL INFO: This is the lead agency for dealing with AIDS in California with a 1988-89 fiscal year budget of $48.5 million. Operates 4 major programs. The AIDS Prevention and Education Program contracts with community-based organizations and agencies to carry out educational efforts. The Alternative Test Site Program contracts with counties to carry out free, anonymous HIV antibody counseling and testing. The Pilot Care Projects Program contracts with various health care and health support organizations to implement certain services. The Epidemiology and Research Program monitors the AIDS epidemic in California through the study of AIDS case data, AIDS case follow-up, and serologic testing studies. Administers funding support for AIDS vaccine development and clinical trials of new AIDS vaccines, and supports AIDS research at the University of California

AVAILABLE LITERATURE: *Black People Do Get AIDS*, a safer sex brochure; *DHS Issues Guidelines on HIV Testing*, a flyer outlining the guidelines for testing; *Information for People of Color*, a brochure of general AIDS information for Asians, Blacks, Latinos, and Native Americans; *Teens and AIDS*, a brochure of general AIDS information for 15- to 19-year-olds and their parents and teachers; *People of Color "Because We Care" Let's Talk*, a brochure for Blacks covering general AIDS information and safer sex guidelines; *AIDS: Facts for Californians*, a general brochure of AIDS facts for California; *Catalogue of Education and Prevention Projects, 1983-1987*, a 57-page book giving agency information about projects and educational materials available; *Acquired Immune Deficiency Syndrome in California: A Prescription for Meeting the Needs of 1990*, a 53-page report published in March 1986 with long-range plans for California

61. Center for Interdisciplinary Research in Immunology and Disease (CIRID) at UCLA
12-248 Factor Bldg, Dept of Microbiology and Immunology
Los Angeles, CA 90024-1747
(213) 825-1510
KEY PERSONNEL: John L Fahey; Director
AFFILIATION: University of California at Los Angeles School of Medicine
FACILITY TYPE: Research; Educational
STAFF: Paid professional 90
YEAR FOUNDED: 1978
FUNDING: Federal government
OUTREACH: Educational conferences and training programs for physicians, fellows/trainees, nurses, and other medical professionals, publication distribution, postdoctoral fellowships
NETWORKS: AIDS Clinical Treatment Group of the National Institute of Allergy and Infectious Diseases
SEMINARS: Nov 1-2, 1988—"A State-of-the-Art Symposium on Immunodeficiency Disorder;" Nov 12, 1988—"AIDS: Risks and Issues for the Dental Professional;" Dec 2, 1988—"AIDS: Risks and Issues for the Practicing Nurse"
RESEARCH: AIDS research related to diagnosis and pathogenesis, treatment, epidemiology, prevention, and education
AVAILABLE LITERATURE: *AIDS/HIV Reference Guide for Medical Professionals, 3rd ed.*; *AIDS/HIV Reference Guide for Nursing Professionals*; *AIDS Medical Update*, a newsletter; *AIDS Nursing Update*, a newsletter
LANGUAGES: French, Italian, Spanish, Japanese, Chinese

62. Central Valley AIDS Team (CVAT)
PO Box 4640, 606 E Blemont
Fresno, CA 93744
(209) 264-2436; Hotline: (209) 264-2437
KEY PERSONNEL: Catherine Calkins; Project Director
AFFILIATION: Gay United Services, Inc.
FACILITY TYPE: Educational; Support group; Fund-raising; Task force
YEAR FOUNDED: 1984
FUNDING: State government; Fund-raisers
OUTREACH: Provides printed educational materials, speakers bureau, library and access to Computerized AIDS Information Network (CAIN), disseminates brochures and other materials through several locations, and provides a street outreach service
NETWORKS: California Association of AIDS Agencies (CAAA); National AIDS Network (NAN); Computerized AIDS Information Network (CAIN); Area AIDS Task Force
ADDITIONAL INFO: CVAT provides direct support services to those diagnosed with AIDS in Fresno and surrounding counties, as well as many others affected by the AIDS epidemic. In addition to the outreach educational services, it provides peers who are volunteers trained to work one-to-one with PWAs, social service agency advocacy, support groups, the Fairy Godmother Fund, which is a community-supported fund to provide PWAs with essentials for living, and referrals for medical, dental, legal, financial, mental, hospice, insurance, religious/spiritual, and funeral/mortuary needs.
AVAILABLE LITERATURE: *Children and AIDS*, a brochure with facts for parents; *CVAT Newsletter*, a monthly newsletter; *I'm Positive*, a brochure with information for those who test positive; *When a Friend has AIDS*, a brochure with suggestions on what to say and do when a friend has AIDS; *What is AIDS*, a brochure with questions and answers about AIDS, its causes, diagnosis, treatment, and preventive measures; *Women and AIDS*, a brochure with questions and answers on AIDS and women; *HTLV III Testing:*

What You Need to Know, a brochure answering questions about the test with recommendations; *Play Safe—Stay Safe,* a calling card with safe sex suggestions; *Stay Alive,* a brochure of safe sex information; *Mantangas Vivo,* a Spanish-language brochure on AIDS
LANGUAGES: Spanish

63. Ciaccio Memorial Clinic of the Beach Area Community Health Center
FORMER NAME: Well Gay Male Screening Program of the BACHC
3705 Mission Blvd
San Diego, CA 92109
(619) 488-2841
KEY PERSONNEL: Rick Siordian; Program Assistant
FACILITY TYPE: Educational; Clinic; Fund-raising
STAFF: Paid professional 5; Paid nonprofessional 25; Volunteers 12
YEAR FOUNDED: 1971
FUNDING: State government; Local government; Private; Fund-raisers; Fees for services or products
OUTREACH: Outreach education through an AIDS prevention education grant
RESEARCH: Risk behavior change documentation
ADDITIONAL INFO: Provides peer educator/trainer project programs and psychological counseling
LANGUAGES: Spanish, French, American Sign Language

64. Clinic for AIDS and Related Disorders (C.A.R.D.)
FORMER NAME: AIDS Clinic/Sacramento
2035 Stockton Blvd, Rancho Grande Annex
Sacramento, CA 95817
(916) 453-3282
KEY PERSONNEL: Richard Rennie; Administrative Assistant
AFFILIATION: University of California, Davis, Medical Center
FACILITY TYPE: Research; Educational; Hospital; Clinic
STAFF: Paid professional 7; Paid nonprofessional 3; Volunteers 15
YEAR FOUNDED: 1983
FUNDING: State government; Local government; Fees for services or products
OUTREACH: Speakers for community programs for in-service education with talks varying from basic AIDS information to treatment modalities, prevention aspects, intravenous drug use, and minority issues
NETWORKS: Sacramento AIDS Foundation; Bi-Valley Medical Clinic; The Aquarian Effort
SEMINARS: Sep 16, 1988—"AIDS: A Practical Program for Community Based Physicians," Feb 4-5, 1989—"Surviving AIDS: 1989," first international major AIDS symposium to discuss new techniques for surviving AIDS
RESEARCH: Investigational drug research, epidemiological data research, education/prevention programs for intravenous drug users
ADDITIONAL INFO: The AIDS Clinic at UCDMC provides health care to people who are HIV positive, have ARC or AIDS. The clinic also provides mental health workers, social services and referrals for home health care and supportive services. There is provision for referral to agencies such as Hand to Hand Project.

65. Coming Home/Coming Home Support Services
One Sansome St, Ste 2000
San Francisco, CA 94104
(415) 951-4652
KEY PERSONNEL: Donald J Catalano; President
FACILITY TYPE: Fund-raising; Client services/case management
STAFF: Paid professional 2; Volunteers 25
YEAR FOUNDED: 1981
FUNDING: Private; Fund-raisers; Fees for services or products
NETWORKS: Coming Home Hospice
ADDITIONAL INFO: The Coming Home organization administers the Coming Home Hospice Endowment Fund. It also administers the support services program which provides daily money managment, legal support, and protective services to people with AIDS, ARC, other debilitating conditions and/or advanced age
AVAILABLE LITERATURE: *Support Services,* flyer describing the services

66. Community Outreach Risk/Reduction Education Program (CORE Program)
FORMER NAME: AID for AIDS CORE Program
6570 Santa Monica Blvd
Los Angeles, CA 90038
(213) 460-4444
KEY PERSONNEL: William M Green; Director
FACILITY TYPE: Educational
STAFF: Paid professional 2; Paid nonprofessional 2; Volunteers varies
YEAR FOUNDED: 1985
FUNDING: Local government; Fund-raisers
OUTREACH: Bar presentations and street outreach to specific segments of the gay community
AVAILABLE LITERATURE: Safe sex posters; *Are You Man Enough?,* leather and condom poster; *Are You Man Enough?,* safe sex brochure; *Que Tan Hombre es Usted?,* safe sex brochure; *Chicos Modernos, vol 1,* comic book in Spanish
LANGUAGES: Spanish

67. Computerized AIDS Information Network (CAIN)
1213 N Highland Ave
Los Angeles, CA 90038
(213) 464-7400 ext 277
KEY PERSONNEL: Torie Osborn; Executive Director
AFFILIATION: Gay and Lesbian Community Services Center, Los Angeles
FACILITY TYPE: Educational
STAFF: Paid professional 3; Paid nonprofessional 45; Volunteers varies
YEAR FOUNDED: 1983
FUNDING: State government
AVAILABLE LITERATURE: Online computer database specifically designed for AIDS information and education; *CAIN,* an informational brochure; as part of the Gay and Lesbian Community Services Center the following brochures are available: *STD and AIDS; Safer Sex,* a guide for everyone concerned about AIDS; *Las Mujeres y SIDA,* a Spanish brochure for women; *Women and AIDS,* a brochure for women; *Referral Guide; AIDS Related Complex,* a brochure about ARC; *Together We Can Prevent AIDS,* an informational brochure; *Juntos Podemos Prevenir el SIDA,* a Spanish informational brochure; *Informational Guide,* a brochure on the HIV antibody test; *Guia de Informacion,* a Spanish-language brochure on the HIV antibody test; *The Center,* a packet of information about the center

68. Desert AIDS Project
750 S Vella Rd
Palm Springs, CA 92264
(619) 323-2118
KEY PERSONNEL: Bill Smith; Executive Director
FACILITY TYPE: Educational; Clinic; Support group; Fund-raising; Task force; HIV counseling and testing
STAFF: Paid professional 7; Paid nonprofessional 3; Volunteers 125
YEAR FOUNDED: 1985
FUNDING: Federal government; State government; Local government; Private; Fund-raisers
OUTREACH: Street outreach, IV Drug users and prostitutes, native American Indian tribe outreach, general community, teens and AIDS, minorities
NETWORKS: Coachella Valley Consortium; Southern California Multi-Cultural AIDS Council
SEMINARS: Presents numerous seminars and workshops on AIDS legal issues, nutrition, self-care, social security system, AIDS update, and AIDS and drugs
ADDITIONAL INFO: This agency is making a concerned effort to reach the rural areas where the rate of infection is increasing.
AVAILABLE LITERATURE: *Desert AIDS Project Forum Newsletter; Desert AIDS Project Volunteers Resource Manual; I Support the Desert AIDS Project,* buttons
LANGUAGES: Spanish

69. Division of AIDS Activities/San Francisco
995 Potrero, SFGH, Ward 84
San Francisco, CA 94110
(415) 321-5531
KEY PERSONNEL: Paul A Volberding, Chief
AFFILIATION: San Francisco General Hospital
FACILITY TYPE: Research; Educational; Hospital; Clinic
FUNDING: Federal government; State government; Local government; Private; County government
LIBRARY: A collection of AIDS materials for use in-house
OUTREACH: Physician AIDS training program; San Francisco General Hospital visitors program
SEMINARS: Sep 1986 and May 1987—"Comprehensive Care of the AIDS Patient: A Workshop"
RESEARCH: AIDS clinical research

ADDITIONAL INFO: Founded in 1983 as a division of the San Francisco General Hospital providing clinical research programs for AIDS care in the public sector of San Francisco
LANGUAGES: Spanish

70. Documentation of AIDS Issues and Research Foundation, Inc (DAIR)
2336 Market St, no 33
San Francisco, CA 94114
(415) 552-1665
KEY PERSONNEL: Michael Flanagan; Presdent of Board of Directors
FACILITY TYPE: Research; Educational
STAFF: Volunteers 10
YEAR FOUNDED: 1985
FUNDING: Private
OUTREACH: DAIR prepares dossiers of information from their collection (copies of articles, research papers, clippings, and pamphlets) in response to requests for information on particular topics
ADDITIONAL INFO: DAIR collects printed media on medical, scientific, civil rights, funding, education, patient service, management, international, legislative, direct action, and public opinion issues. Besides acting as a source of printed information on AIDS it acts as a repository for individuals and organizations wishing to donate printed information. DAIR acted as a sponsor to Project Inform until April 1988, at which time it became an independent organization.
AVAILABLE LITERATURE: *DAIR Update*, a quarterly newsletter which discusses current reports and issues involved in AIDS treatment, management, social, political, and information issues; *DAIR Archive Classification System*, a schedule for the classification of articles contained in the DAIR collection of over 60,000 articles

71. East Bay AIDS Center (EBAC)
FORMER NAME: ACCESS
2640 Telegraph Ave
Berkeley, CA 94704
(415) 540-1870
KEY PERSONNEL: Grace Farinacci; Administrative Director
AFFILIATION: Alta Bates-Herrick Hospital
FACILITY TYPE: Educational; Hospital; Clinic; HIV counseling and testing
STAFF: Paid professional 8; Volunteers 20
YEAR FOUNDED: 1987
FUNDING: Private; Fund-raisers; Fees for services or products
OUTREACH: Educational outreach
SEMINARS: 1987, 1988—"AIDS Symposium for Medical Care Providers"
ADDITIONAL INFO: The East Bay AIDS Center offers comprehensive services educating about and dealing with AIDS and ARC. One location offers testing, counseling and treatment
AVAILABLE LITERATURE: *East Bay AIDS Center*, an informational brochure
LANGUAGES: Spanish

72. El Centro Human Services Organizations, Milagros AIDS Project
741 S Atlantic Blvd
Los Angeles, CA 90022
(213) 261-2722
KEY PERSONNEL: David R Marquez; Project Coordinator
FACILITY TYPE: Educational; Support group; Client services/case management
STAFF: Paid professional 6; Paid nonprofessional 6
YEAR FOUNDED: 1986
FUNDING: State government; Local government; National AIDS Network
OUTREACH: Presentations to the general public, substance abusers, youth, health care professionals, multiple sex partners, women, and union workers
NETWORKS: National AIDS Network (NAN); California Association of AIDS Agencies (CAAA)
RESEARCH: Cost effectiveness of care provision in the home versus hospitalization
ADDITIONAL INFO: A comprehensive AIDS agency which provides bilingual and bicultural services to the Latino community. Services include community education and prevention seminars, case management services, mental health counseling, support groups, pilot in-home health care project
LANGUAGES: Spanish

73. Face To Face, Sonoma County AIDS Network (SCAN)
FORMER NAME: River AIDS Support Group
PO Box 1599
Guerneville, CA 95446
(707) 887-1581
KEY PERSONNEL: Jacquie Robb; Office Manager
FACILITY TYPE: Support group; Fund-raising; Client services/case management
STAFF: Paid professional 8; Volunteers 80
YEAR FOUNDED: 1985
FUNDING: Local government; Private; Fund-raisers
OUTREACH: Referral service, advocate training, in-home care and practical support training, support groups
NETWORKS: Santa Rosa AIDS Awareness Group
ADDITIONAL INFO: The purpose of this agency is to provide emotional, informational and practical assistance to persons living with AIDS and persons living with ARC residing in Sonoma County
AVAILABLE LITERATURE: *Face to Face: The Sonoma County AIDS Network*, a brochure describing the agency
LANGUAGES: Spanish

74. Families Who Care (FWC)
3900 E Pacific Coast Hwy
Long Beach, CA 90804
(213) 498-6366
KEY PERSONNEL: Gena Wilson; Program Director
FACILITY TYPE: Educational; Support group; Fund-raising
STAFF: Paid professional 1.5; Paid nonprofessional 1.25; Volunteers 35
YEAR FOUNDED: 1986
FUNDING: Fund-raisers; Donations
OUTREACH: Follow-up with persons who contact the agency for support; speakers bureau; developing a family caregiver training program to be made available to interested caregivers
NETWORKS: National AIDS Network (NAN); Long Beach AIDS Network
SEMINARS: 1989—"Family Caregiver Training Workshops"
ADDITIONAL INFO: "FWC was formed by and for families of people with AIDS" and is intended "to help people cope with the pain and stress of caring for a relative with AIDS." Includes a support group, volunteer friends of the family, telephone reassurance, referrals, family care guide, family caregiver training program, and speakers
AVAILABLE LITERATURE: *Families Who Care*, a pamphlet describing the services of FWC; a caregivers packet with information on community resources for new families and caregivers of PWAs
LANGUAGES: Spanish, Vietnamese

75. The Family Link
PO Box 42007
San Francisco, CA 94142-2007
(415) 346-0770
KEY PERSONNEL: Ruth Cope; Resident Manager
AFFILIATION: National AIDS Network (NAN)
FACILITY TYPE: Residential facility (adults)
STAFF: Paid professional 2; Volunteers 10
YEAR FOUNDED: 1985
FUNDING: Private; Fund-raisers; Fees for services or products
ADDITIONAL INFO: The Family Link has provided accommodations for 280 guest families from 34 different states, the Philippines, England, Puerto Rico, and Canada
AVAILABLE LITERATURE: *The Family Link*, a newsletter published three times a year

76. The Gay and Lesbian Community Services Center
1213 N Highland Ave
Los Angeles, CA 90038
(213) 464-7400 x251; TDD (213) 464-0029
FACILITY TYPE: Educational; Clinic; Support group; Fund-raising; Task force
STAFF: Paid nonprofessional 70; Volunteers 700
YEAR FOUNDED: 1971
FUNDING: State government; Local government; Donations
ADDITIONAL INFO: This agency currently has nine programs—Counseling Services, Health Services, Lesbian Central, Alcohol Abuse Program, Legal Services, Vocational Services, Dept of Education, Information and Referral, and Youth Services. The Health Services includes a sexually transmitted disease clinic, the Philip Mandelker AIDS Prevention Clinic, HIV/HTLV-III Antibody Alternative Test Site, and mobile outreach

AVAILABLE LITERATURE: *The Center*, a packet of information about the center

77. Gay and Lesbian Resource Center/Santa Barbara
232 E Montecito St
Santa Barbara, CA 93101
(805) 963-3636
AFFILIATION: Western Addiction Services
FACILITY TYPE: Educational
ADDITIONAL INFO: Source of additional AIDS information

78. Gay Men's Health Collective/Berkeley
2339 Durant Ave
Berkeley, CA 94704
(415) 644-0425
KEY PERSONNEL: John Day, Co-Director; Jerry Thornhill, Co-Director
FACILITY TYPE: Clinic
ADDITIONAL INFO: Founded in 1978 as a gay clinic within the Berkeley Free Clinic

79. Haight-Ashbury Free Clinics
FORMER NAME: Haight-Ashbury Free Medical Clinic
1696 Haight St
San Francisco, CA 94117
(415) 864-6090, 621-2016
KEY PERSONNEL: John Newmeyer; Epidemiologist
FACILITY TYPE: Research; Educational; Clinic
STAFF: Paid professional 45; Paid nonprofessional 27; Volunteers 70
YEAR FOUNDED: 1967
FUNDING: Federal government; State government; Local government; Private; Fund-raisers
OUTREACH: Outreach to individuals at high risk of AIDS, education
SEMINARS: Nov 1987—"AIDS and Chemical Dependency;" Nov 1988—"Cocaine, Alcohol, and Prescription Drugs: Recent Advances in Treatment"
RESEARCH: AIDS epidemiology, treatment of the cocaine or methamphetamine abuser, drug abuse epidemiology
AVAILABLE LITERATURE: *Journal of Psychoactive Drugs*; *MidCity Numbers*, a monthly bulletin of AIDS-related statistics; *"Your Turn, Man"*, a comic strip on using clean needles to prevent AIDS
LANGUAGES: Spanish, Cantonese, Mandarin, Tagalog

80. Harbor/UCLA Medical Center
1000 W Carson St
Torrance, CA 90509
(213) 533-2365
FACILITY TYPE: Clinic
ADDITIONAL INFO: A part of the Dept of Medicine, Immunology, and Allergy that provides AIDS medical evaluation. By appointment only

81. Louise L Hay AIDS Support Group (HAYRIDE)
FORMER NAME: Wednesday Night AIDS Support Group
PO Box 2212
Santa Monica, CA 90406
(213) 828-3666
KEY PERSONNEL: Louise L Hay, Counselor/Teacher; Warren Bayless, Hay House Vice President; Joseph Vattimo, Assistant; Ron Tillinghast, Assistant
FACILITY TYPE: Educational
FUNDING: Donations; Grants
LIBRARY: Contains health practice, spiritual and mind growth studies and materials. Open by appointment
OUTREACH: Workshops and lectures
SEMINARS: Sep 26, 1987—"Annual Hay Foundation Symposium on Health and Social Awareness Practices," 1987 symposium
ADDITIONAL INFO: Founded in 1985 to provide educational workshops and lectures, information concerning re-established life practices, nutrition, alternative health therapies, and other programs
LANGUAGES: French, German, Swedish, Dutch, Spanish

82. Hemophilia Council of California (HCC)
1507 21st St, Ste 300
Sacramento, CA 95814
(916) 448-7444
KEY PERSONNEL: George Lobdell; Programs Director
FACILITY TYPE: Educational; Hospital; Clinic; Support group; Task force

STAFF: Paid professional 9; Paid nonprofessional 3
YEAR FOUNDED: 1982
FUNDING: State government
OUTREACH: Provides AIDS education to people with hemophilia, blood transfusion recipients, their spouses/sexual partners, youth, parents, health care providers, nurses, dental hygienists. A psychosocial services program provides counseling to individuals and families
SEMINARS: Several educational seminars and workshops are sponsored throughout the year to target groups
RESEARCH: Cure for hemophila, cure for AIDS
ADDITIONAL INFO: This agency has regional offices in Oakland, San Diego, and Los Angeles. It also represents consumer based hemophilia organizations throughout the state.
AVAILABLE LITERATURE: Distributes publications from the National Hemophilia Foundation

83. Homosexual Information Center/Hollywood
PO Box 8252
Universal City, CA 91608
(213) 464-8431
FACILITY TYPE: Research
ADDITIONAL INFO: Source of additional information on AIDS

84. Hope and Help Center/San Francisco
PO Box 14286
San Francisco, CA 94114
(415) 861-HOPE; Hotline: (800) AID-TALK
KEY PERSONNEL: Alba Barreto-Jelinek, Director
FACILITY TYPE: Educational; Support group
FUNDING: Donations; Grants
LIBRARY: Contains videos, brochures, magazine articles, pastoral publications, and prevention education materials. Open to interested persons to use in-house
OUTREACH: Speakers bureau, workshops, and educational materials
SEMINARS: Mar 4-7, 1986—"National Episcopal Conference on AIDS/ SF;" Nov 8, 1986—"Diocesan Mini Convention on AIDS"
ADDITIONAL INFO: Founded in 1986 as an advocacy and resource entity within the Episcopal Church for AIDS prevention educators, persons with AIDS/ARC, and their loved ones
AVAILABLE LITERATURE: *Hope and Help Center Newsletter*, a bimonthly newsletter with information about the center's activities. Also provides a resource packet for parishes in the Episcopal Diocese of California

85. Human Health Organization (HHO)
PO Box 4569
Berkeley, CA 94704
KEY PERSONNEL: Dominic Cappello; Director
FACILITY TYPE: Educational
STAFF: Paid professional 3; Volunteers 12
YEAR FOUNDED: 1985
FUNDING: Private; Fund-raisers; Fees for services or products
OUTREACH: Educational materials development, outreach education on AIDS, safe sex, AIDS and the workplace, and AIDS media development
SEMINARS: 1989—"Health and Creativity Workshop Series"
ADDITIONAL INFO: HHO is an educational agency with an interest in program and materials development and Native American STD education projects
AVAILABLE LITERATURE: *We Owe It to Ourselves and Our Children*, book; slideshows on AIDS and sexually transmitted diseases

86. Humboldt County Dept of Public Welfare
929 Koster St
Eureka, CA 95501
(707) 445-6023
KEY PERSONNEL: John Frank; Director
AFFILIATION: Humboldt County Government
FACILITY TYPE: Research; Educational; Task force
STAFF: Paid professional 227
YEAR FOUNDED: 1936
FUNDING: Federal government; State government; Local government
OUTREACH: Education to schools, churches, foster parents, and community at-large
RESEARCH: Information about AIDS; who, when, how and why to test for AIDS; usage to develop protocol for testing foster children

ADDITIONAL INFO: This agency is a child protective service and adult protective service

AVAILABLE LITERATURE: Publishes a monthly newsletter

87. Imperial AIDS Foundation
1906 Orlando Dr
San Jose, CA 95122
FACILITY TYPE: Educational
ADDITIONAL INFO: Source of additional AIDS information

88. Inland AIDS Project
3638 University Ave
Riverside, CA 92501
(213) 784-2437; Toll-free: (800) 451-4133
KEY PERSONNEL: John E Sailey; Executive Director
FACILITY TYPE: Educational; Support group
STAFF: Paid professional 7; Paid nonprofessional 2; Volunteers 85
YEAR FOUNDED: 1984
FUNDING: Federal government; State government; Private; Fund-raisers
OUTREACH: Speakers bureau, peer outreach prevention
NETWORKS: Computerized AIDS Information Network (CAIN); Stop AIDS
SEMINARS: May 1988—"Interfaith AIDS Council Workshop;" Jun 1988—"Putting a Face on AIDS;" Jun 1988—"Caregivers Workshop"
LANGUAGES: American Sign Language, Spanish

89. Institute for Advanced Study of Human Sexuality (IASHS)
1523 Franklin St
San Francisco, CA 94109
(415) 928-1133
KEY PERSONNEL: Ted McIlvenna, President
FACILITY TYPE: Research; Educational
RESEARCH: Research into all areas of sexology
ADDITIONAL INFO: Founded in 1976 as a research organization on sexology

90. International Gay and Lesbian Archives
PO Box 38100
Los Angeles, CA 90038-0100
FACILITY TYPE: Educational
ADDITIONAL INFO: Source of additional AIDS information

91. Isla Vista Medical Clinic
970-C Embarcadero Del Mar
Isla Vista, CA 93117
(805) 968-1511
KEY PERSONNEL: Dennis Feeley; County Director
FACILITY TYPE: HIV counseling and testing; Substance abuse treatment

92. Kern County AIDS Task Force
PO Box 10961
Bakersfield, CA 93389
(805) 397-8588, 328-0729
KEY PERSONNEL: Norman Prigge; Nancy Bailey

93. KS Research and Education Foundation/San Francisco
54 10th St
San Francisco, CA 94103
FACILITY TYPE: Research; Educational
ADDITIONAL INFO: Source of additional AIDS information

94. Lesbian and Gay Rights Chapter/Los Angeles
633 Shatto Pl
Los Angeles, CA 90005
FACILITY TYPE: Educational
ADDITIONAL INFO: Source of additional AIDS information

95. Los Angeles County Dept of Health Services, AIDS Program Office
313 N Figueroa St
Los Angeles, CA 90012
(213) 974-7803
KEY PERSONNEL: Robert E Frangenberg; Program Diirector
AFFILIATION: Los Angeles County Government

FACILITY TYPE: Contract agency
YEAR FOUNDED: 1984
FUNDING: Local government
OUTREACH: AIDS education to health educators, community outreach
RESEARCH: AIDS epidemiology
ADDITIONAL INFO: The AIDS program provides services in three main areas—policy and planning, contracts and grants, and AIDS education. Holds numerous conferences covering AIDS education or risk reduction
AVAILABLE LITERATURE: *Los Angeles County Monthly AIDS Report*, newsletter
LANGUAGES: Several languages

96. Los Angeles Sex Information Helpline (LASIH)
8489 W 3rd St, Ste 1080
Los Angeles, CA 90048
(213) 653-1123; 655-2165
KEY PERSONNEL: Lynda Smith, Administrator
AFFILIATION: Los Angeles Free Clinic
FACILITY TYPE: Educational
FUNDING: Los Angeles Free Clinic
OUTREACH: Speakers bureau
ADDITIONAL INFO: Established in 1975 as a helpline for accurate, non-judgmental information and referrals concerning all aspects of human sexuality

97. Los Angeles Shanti Foundation
9060 Santa Monica Blvd, Ste 301
West Hollywood, CA 90069
(213) 273-7591; TDD: (213) 273-7217
KEY PERSONNEL: Paul D Zak; Executive Director
FACILITY TYPE: Educational; Support group
STAFF: Paid professional 9; Paid nonprofessional 1; Volunteers 100
YEAR FOUNDED: 1983
FUNDING: Federal government; State government; Local government; Private; Fund-raisers
OUTREACH: Speakers bureau, Special Health Education Program (SHE) aimed at risk reduction behavior modification through seminars and follow-up
NETWORKS: United AIDS Coalition of Los Angeles County; AIDS Programs Together (APT) California Association of AIDS Agencies (CAAA); AIDS Community Educators of Los Angeles
SEMINARS: 1987-1988—"Emotional Support Volunteer Trainings" and "SHEP Group Co-Facilitator Trainings;" 1988, 1989—"Emotional Support Volunteer Training," "SHEP Trainings," and "Volunteer Workshops"
ADDITIONAL INFO: Founded in 1983 as a volunteer support and educational service for individuals and their loved ones facing AIDS and related issues
AVAILABLE LITERATURE: *Heartspace*, a quarterly newsletter for donors and the general public; *Newsletter*, a newsletter for volunteers; *Shanti*, a brochure about the foundation; *Shanti SHEP*, a brochure describing the Special Health Education Program of the foundation; other miscellaneous brochures, buttons, and T-shirts
LANGUAGES: Spanish

98. Mayor's Task Force on AIDS/San Diego
1700 Pacific Hwy
San Diego, CA 92101
FACILITY TYPE: Task force
ADDITIONAL INFO: Source of additional AIDS information

99. Minority AIDS Project/Los Angeles
5882 W Pico Blvd, Ste 210
Los Angeles, CA 90019
(213) 936-4949
FACILITY TYPE: Educational; Support group
ADDITIONAL INFO: Provides direct service to persons with AIDS and their loved ones through support groups and educational outreach

100. Mission Crisis Service
111 Potrero Ave
San Francisco, CA 94103
(415) 558-2071
KEY PERSONNEL: Tom Gallagher; Director
FACILITY TYPE: Clinic
STAFF: Paid professional 15; Paid nonprofessional 3; Volunteers 1
FUNDING: Local government

OUTREACH: Psychiatric evaluation in clients' homes, long-term outpatient psychotherapy services in clients' homes if they have AIDS and are too ill to come to the office
NETWORKS: Latino Consortium of San Francisco; Bay Area Crisis Directors Association
ADDITIONAL INFO: Mission Crisis has been designated as the AIDS psychiatric crisis service for San Francisco residents. Lesbian, gay, and gay sensitive staff are available and all staff are AIDS sensitive
LANGUAGES: Spanish, French, Russian, American Sign Language, Arabic

101. Mothers of AIDS Patients (MAP)
PO Box 3132
San Diego, CA 92103-0040
(619) 293-3985
KEY PERSONNEL: Barbara Peabody, Coordinator
FACILITY TYPE: Support group
ADDITIONAL INFO: A national support group for mothers of AIDS patients

102. Multi-Focus, Inc
FORMER NAME: Multi Media Resource Center
1525 Franklin St
San Francisco, CA 94109
(415) 673-5100; Toll-free: (800) 821-0514
KEY PERSONNEL: Renee Jones; Film Booking and Distribution Coordinator
FACILITY TYPE: Educational
STAFF: Paid professional 4
YEAR FOUNDED: 1976
FUNDING: Fees for services or products
ADDITIONAL INFO: Provides videos, films, slides, and filmstrips on all topics including introduction to sexuality, youth and teenage sexuality, childbirth, vasectomy, abortion, AIDS and STDs, women's issues, incest, prostitution, sex roles, humor and satire, erotica, touch and massage, masturbation, heterosexuality, sex and pregnancy, sex and later life, sex and disability, multiple partners, bisexuality, homosexuality, anatomy, physiology, and sex therapy
AVAILABLE LITERATURE: A 35-page media and audiovisual catalog plus supplement describing videos, films, slides, and filmstrips on human sexuality is available

103. The Names Project, sponsors of the AIDS Memorial Quilt
2362 Market St
San Francisco, CA 94114
(415) 863-1966; Toll-free: (800) USA-NAME
KEY PERSONNEL: Sue Baelen; Director of Communications
FACILITY TYPE: Educational; Fund-raising
STAFF: Paid professional 18; Volunteers 200-2000
YEAR FOUNDED: 1987
FUNDING: Private; Fund-raisers; Fees for services or products
OUTREACH: Quilt displays are arranged throughout the country, educational and outreach programs focusing on the quilt
SEMINARS: In 1988 there were more than 100 displays of the Quilt, ranging from small displays with 12 panels, to the Washington, DC, display in October, 1988, with 8,288 panels. There will be another tour across the US in 1989 and through Canada
ADDITIONAL INFO: The Names Project, organized in June of 1987, works to illustrate the impact and human toll of the AIDS epidemic, to provide a positive and creative means of expression for those whose lives have been touched by the epidemic, and to raise vital funds and encourage support for people with AIDS and their loved ones.
AVAILABLE LITERATURE: *The Quilt: Stories from the Names Project*, a hardcover book that chronicles the creation of the Names Project Quilt; note cards; *The Names Project*, etched logo pin; 1988 DC commemorative poster; *The Inaugural Display of the Names Project Quilt*, a 15-minute video commemorating the dawn unfolding ceremony of the Quilt on October 11, 1987; *The Names Project: A National AIDS Memorial*, a full-color poster; *We Bring a Quilt*, a 30-minute video; *Quilt Visitor*, reproduction of a painting to Thomas Rohnacher; Names Project t-shirts
LANGUAGES: Spanish, German, Finnish, French

104. National Association for Lesbian and Gay Gerontology (NALGG)
1853 Market St
San Francisco, CA 94103
(415) 626-7000
KEY PERSONNEL: Elaine Porter; President

FACILITY TYPE: Research; Educational
STAFF: Volunteers 4
YEAR FOUNDED: 1980
FUNDING: Fees for services or products; Dues
OUTREACH: Participates in annual conferences
NETWORKS: American Society on Aging
SEMINARS: Nov 20, 1988—"1988 Meeting of the Gerontological Society of America," San Francisco (a session on AIDS and Aging); Mar 18-21, 1989—"1989 Meeting of the Gerontological Society of America," Washington, DC (a session on AIDS and Aging)
ADDITIONAL INFO: While the primary focus of the organization is on lesbian and gay aging, several members lead discussions at national forums and in local communities to talk about the research, psychological and social service parallels experienced among people with AIDS/ARC and older persons
AVAILABLE LITERATURE: *Bibliography on Lesbian and Gay Aging*

105. National Gay Rights Advocates (NGR)
540 Castro St
San Francisco, CA 94114
(415) 863-3624
KEY PERSONNEL: Benjamin Schatz; Director, AIDS Civil Rights Project
FACILITY TYPE: Legal
STAFF: Paid professional 11; Volunteers 40
YEAR FOUNDED: 1977
FUNDING: Private; Fund-raisers; Fees for services or products
ADDITIONAL INFO: NGRA is the nation's leading law firm promoting equality for gay men and women. Founded in 1978 as a non-profit, membership-supported organization, NGRA focuses on impact litigation coordinated by a professional staff and supported by pro bono assistance from the country's most prestigious law firms and attorneys
AVAILABLE LITERATURE: *Wills Give You Power*, a guide for gay men and women; *AIDS and Your Legal Rights*, a pamphlet of facts that you should know; *Security Clearances for Gay Men and Women*, an informational brochure; *AIDS Practice Manual*; *AIDS and Handicap Discrimination*, a brochure outlining the rights of PWAs; *Pros and Cons of the HIV Antibody Test*; *Tax Strategies for Lesbians and Gay Men*; *The AIDS Insurance Crisis*, a brochure about AIDS and how it has affected the insurance industry; *AIDS, Civil Rights and the Public*, an informational brochure about your civil rights; *American Corporate Policy—AIDS and Employment*, a brochure about your rights
LANGUAGES: Japanese

106. National Lawyers Guild AIDS Network
211 Gough St, 3rd Fl
San Francisco, CA 94102
(415) 861-8886
KEY PERSONNEL: Paul Albert; Director
AFFILIATION: National Lawyers Guild
FACILITY TYPE: Educational; Legal; Network
STAFF: Paid professional 1; Paid nonprofessional 1; Volunteers 300
YEAR FOUNDED: 1985
FUNDING: Private; Fund-raisers; Fees for services or products
AVAILABLE LITERATURE: *The Exchange*, a bimonthly periodical covering the legal and political analysis of AIDS issues; *AIDS Practice Manual*, a legal and educational guide

107. National Mobilization Against AIDS
2120 Market St
San Francisco, CA 94114
FACILITY TYPE: Educational
ADDITIONAL INFO: Source of additional AIDS information

108. National Native American AIDS Prevention Center (NNAAPC)
6239 College Ave, Ste 201
Oakland, CA 94618
(415) 658-2051
KEY PERSONNEL: Ron Rowell; Executive Director
FACILITY TYPE: Research; Educational
STAFF: Paid professional 4; Paid nonprofessional 1; Volunteers 12
YEAR FOUNDED: 1988
FUNDING: Federal government
OUTREACH: Outreach to Native American organizations and local Native American communities, national clearinghouse for Native American AIDS education materials, national online bulletin board for Indian physicians working with AIDS

NETWORKS: National Minority AIDS Council
RESEARCH: Research on health status of Native Americans, infectious diseases and substance abuse as they relate to AIDS
AVAILABLE LITERATURE: Will be publishing a quarterly newsletter focusing on AIDS for Native Americans
LANGUAGES: Tiwa

109. North State AIDS Project (NSAP)
PO Box 4542
Redding, CA 96099
(916) 225-5252; Hotline: (916) 225-5252; Toll-free: (800) 821-5252
Eastern Shasta County
KEY PERSONNEL: Marilyn Traugott; President of Board of Directors
FACILITY TYPE: Educational; Support group; Task force
STAFF: Volunteers varies
YEAR FOUNDED: 1986
FUNDING: Private; Fund-raisers
OUTREACH: Educational presentations
SEMINARS: Feb 18, 1988—"Symposium on AIDS," sponsored by Superior, CA Medical Education Council; projecting seminars for clergy and dentists, education/inservice for physicians and nurses
ADDITIONAL INFO: Founded as a community-based task force working to cultivate and coordinate local resources for PWAs. Provides personal and professional education, support, and referral for those infected with HIV and their caregivers. Residents of Shasta, Siskiyou, Trinity, and Tehama counties are eligible for services

110. Office for Civil Rights
50 United Nations Plaza, Rm 322
San Francisco, CA 94102
(415) 556-8586; Hotline: (800) 368-1019
KEY PERSONNEL: Virginia P Apodaca; Regional Manager
AFFILIATION: US Dept of Health and Human Services
FACILITY TYPE: Educational
STAFF: Paid professional 30; Paid nonprofessional 8
FUNDING: Federal government
OUTREACH: Outreach to minority communities, handicapped groups, senior citizens, and low-income persons; technical assistance to health care and social service providers; conducts workshops; gives presentations; staff exhibit booths
SEMINARS: Jul 1988—"National AIDS/ARC Update," San Francisco
ADDITIONAL INFO: Founded as part of the federal government's effort to eliminate discrimination in health, education and welfare programs funded by federal dollars. Since the passage of the Civil Rights Act of 1964, additional statutes have been added to increase the protection of the federal government against discrimination. The agency receives complaints of discrimination and reaches a resolution in each case. Undertakes to review cases where unlawful discrimination may be present
AVAILABLE LITERATURE: Your Rights as a Person With AIDS or Related Conditions, a fact sheet available in English, Spanish, Tagalog, Japanese, and Portuguese
LANGUAGES: Spanish, Tagalog, American Sign Language, Japanese, Portuguese

111. Orange County Health Care Agency
511 N Sycamore
Santa Ana, CA 92701
(714) 834-2015; Hotline: (714) 834-8700
KEY PERSONNEL: Penny C Weismuller; AIDS Coordinator
AFFILIATION: Orange County Government
FACILITY TYPE: Research; Educational; Clinic; Support group; Task force; Health department
YEAR FOUNDED: 1987 (AIDS Coordination)
FUNDING: Federal government; State government; Local government
OUTREACH: Grand Rounds monthly professional education at UCIMC hospital, AIDS education, AIDS outreach, speakers bureau, juvenile/criminal justice for incarcerated minors at juvenile hall
NETWORKS: California Association of AIDS Agencies (CAAA)
SEMINARS: Feb 25, 1988—"AIDS on the Front Line;" Feb 1, 1989—"Second Annual AIDS Conference," Anaheim; Sep 12-13, 1988, Oct 31, 1988, Nov 1, 1988, Feb 6-7, 1989, Apr 24-25, 1989—"Emergency Service Worker Training"
ADDITIONAL INFO: Provides AIDS education to health professionals, supports development of AIDS residential and in-home supportive services, provides case management services to PWAs and PWARCs

AVAILABLE LITERATURE: When You Buy Sex: You May Get More Than You Paid For, a brochure about prostitutes; AIDS: Protect Your Family, Your Friends, Yourself: Learn the Facts, a brochure of AIDS facts; AIDS: What Your HIV Antibody Test Tells You, a brochure describing the test; AIDS/SIDA: Que Significa la Prueba de Anticuerpos VIH (HIV), a Spanish-language brochure about the HIV test; Physicians' Bulletin, a newsletter; Resultados e Indicaciones, a Spanish-language AIDS informational flyer; What Do You Know About AIDS?, a test about your knowledge of AIDS; Que Sabe Usted Acerca del S.I.D.A., a test in Spanish about your knowledge of AIDS; AIDS Monthly Report, an HIV monthly monitoring report for Orange County
LANGUAGES: Spanish, Vietnamese

112. People with AIDS/ARC of San Francisco
FORMER NAME: People with AIDS/SF
333 Valencia St, 4th Fl
San Francisco, CA 94103-3597
(415) 861-6703; 864-4376
KEY PERSONNEL: Jack Townsend, Coordinator
FACILITY TYPE: Educational; Support group
FUNDING: Grants
LIBRARY: Contains various medical books, journals, and other materials pertaining to AIDS and ARC for in-house use by anyone
NETWORKS: PWA International; San Francisco AIDS Foundation
ADDITIONAL INFO: Founded in 1983 as a support and educational agency for PWAs and PWARCs
AVAILABLE LITERATURE: Distributes publications from the San Francisco AIDS Foundation including the following: Hot 'n Healthy Times, an irregularly published newspaper that covers safe sex; Resource Manual for Persons With AIDS, a 52-page book in its 3rd edition outlining the resources available in the San Francisco area including financial, medical, counseling, and social services; Shooting Up and Your Health, a 2-fold brochure on IV drugs and your health; AIDS in the Workplace, a 3-fold brochure discussing AIDS in the workplace; AIDS Lifeline, a 2-fold brochure with general information about AIDS; Can We Talk?, a 5-fold brochure on safe sex; Fact vs. Fiction: Ten Things You Should Know About AIDS, a 1-fold brochure of AIDS facts; Information for People of Color, a 2-fold brochure of AIDS information for Asians, Blacks, Latinos, and Native Americans; Lesbians and AIDS: What's the Connection?, a 2-fold brochure of AIDS information for lesbians; Poppers: Your Health and AIDS: Can You Afford the Risk?, a 3-fold brochure discussing poppers and the possible AIDS connection; Straight Talk About Sex and AIDS, a 2-fold brochure of AIDS information for the general public; Women and AIDS; Coping with AIDS, an 8-page booklet for PWAs; Coping with ARC, an 18-page booklet for PWARCs; AIDS and Safe Sex, a pocket card of safe sex guidelines
LANGUAGES: Spanish, Tagalog, Chinese

113. Placer County Health Dept
11484 B Ave
Auburn, CA 95603
(916) 823-4541
KEY PERSONNEL: Sandra Medlin; Coordinator
AFFILIATION: Placer County Government
FACILITY TYPE: Educational; Clinic; Task force; Health department
STAFF: Paid professional 2
YEAR FOUNDED: 1900
FUNDING: State government; Local government
OUTREACH: AIDS education and prevention presentations to businesses, schools, churches, organizations, and agencies; public health nurse visitations to PWAs; coordinate and help lead the Placer County AIDS Task Force
SEMINARS: Apr 1988—"Teaching AIDS," for persons teaching AIDS in Placer County high schools
RESEARCH: Follow-up on changes in sexual behaviors after an individual has been to an antibody test site and tested both positive and negative
ADDITIONAL INFO: Provides programs for substance abusers in both in-patient recovery wards and residential treatment programs. In some recovery homes, antibody testing is offered at the home following AIDS information programs
AVAILABLE LITERATURE: Safer Sex Guidelines to Prevent Transmission of AIDS, a card with safer sex information; AIDS: Don't Risk It, a folded card with safer sex information and information for IV drug users; Welcome to HAT, a brochure describing the HIV Antibody Test
LANGUAGES: Spanish

114. Project AHEAD (AIDS Health Education and Assistance Delivery)
2017 E 4th St
Long Beach, CA 90814
(213) 439-3948
KEY PERSONNEL: Avery L Loschen; Administrative Director
AFFILIATION: One In Long Beach, Inc
FACILITY TYPE: Educational; Support group; Fund-raising; Client services/case management
STAFF: Paid professional 2; Paid nonprofessional 1; Volunteers 350
YEAR FOUNDED: 1983
FUNDING: Private; Fund-raisers

115. Riverside County Office of AIDS Coordination (COAC)
PO Box 1370
Riverside, CA 92502
(714) 787-1608
KEY PERSONNEL: Barry L. Kaplan; Administrator
AFFILIATION: Riverside County Health Dept
FACILITY TYPE: Educational; Clinic; Task force; HIV counseling and testing
STAFF: Paid professional 7; Paid nonprofessional 1
YEAR FOUNDED: 1986
FUNDING: State government; Local government
OUTREACH: Outreach and education in the county jails, drug rehabilitation centers and law enforcement agencies, coordinate educational programs with local AIDS projects
NETWORKS: Computerized AIDS Information Network (CAIN); National AIDS Network (NAN); California Association of AIDS Agencies (CAAA)
SEMINARS: Feb, 1988—"AIDS Information for Educators and Mental Health Professionals," with California State University in San Bernadino; Apr, 1989—"Current Perspectives on AIDS," Mirage
ADDITIONAL INFO: This agency provides HIV antibody testing both anonymous and confidential, education and training of county workers, including emergency and public safety staff
AVAILABLE LITERATURE: *Facts About AIDS*, brochure of AIDS facts; *My Plan to Better Health*, a brochure of safer sex information; *Referral Sources*, a 5-page pamphlet
LANGUAGES: Spanish

116. Sacramento AIDS Foundation (SAF)
FORMER NAME: Sacramento AIDS/KS Foundation
1900 K St, Ste 201
Sacramento, CA 95814
(916) 448-2437; Hotline: (916) 448-2437
KEY PERSONNEL: Nurk Franklin; Office Supervisor
FACILITY TYPE: Educational; Support group; Client services/case management
STAFF: Paid professional 20; Volunteers 300
YEAR FOUNDED: 1983
FUNDING: State government; Local government; Private; Fund-raisers
OUTREACH: Speakers bureau, speakers training, inservices for health care providers and social service providers, outreach to gay and bisexual men, wellness and risk reduction workshops, women's workshops, AIDS in the workplace programs
NETWORKS: California Association of AIDS Agencies (CAAA)
SEMINARS: Various programs held throughout the year including "Hot, Horny and Healthy," "You and Your Health," "Legal Planning for Gays and Lesbians," "Transforming Our Approach to AIDS—a Holistic Perspective," "Achieving Intimacy in Relationships," "Nutrition and Your Health," "Relationship Building: Making Good Contact," "Breathing for Health"
ADDITIONAL INFO: Provides counseling, case management, referral for medical and psychosocial services, home health programs, and emotional and practical support volunteers
AVAILABLE LITERATURE: *Healthy Living*, a calendar of events for gay and bisexual men; *Black People Get AIDS Too*, an informational brochure; *Women and Children Have Special Needs*, an informational brochure
LANGUAGES: Spanish, French, Hindi, American Sign Language

117. Sacramento County Health Dept, AIDS Unit
3701 Branch Center Rd
Sacramento, CA 95827
(916) 366-2922
KEY PERSONNEL: Dennis Webb; Program Coordinator
AFFILIATION: Sacramento County Government
FACILITY TYPE: Educational; HIV counseling and testing; Health department

STAFF: Paid professional 7; Paid nonprofessional 1; Volunteers 3
YEAR FOUNDED: 1988
FUNDING: Federal government; State government; Local government
OUTREACH: Minority outreach, presentations at the worksite and for the general public
NETWORKS: Sacramento County AIDS Advisory Board; Computerized AIDS Information Network (CAIN)
SEMINARS: Jun 2, 1988—"AIDS and Substance Abuse;" Sep 1988— "Grant-Writing Workshop for People of Color"
ADDITIONAL INFO: Provides HIV counseling, testing and referrals and distributes educational materials to agencies upon request. Presents various community workshops and presentations on AIDS targeting high risk groups and people of color
AVAILABLE LITERATURE: *SCAN*, a newsletter; *AIDS: Don't Risk It*, a brochure of general preventive measures
LANGUAGES: Spanish

118. San Diego AIDS Project
3777 4th Ave
San Diego, CA 92103
(619) 543-0300; Hotline: (619) 543-0300; Spanish Line: (619) 548-0604
KEY PERSONNEL: Kristie Mills; Director
FACILITY TYPE: Educational; Support group; Fund-raising
STAFF: Paid professional 19; Volunteers 350
YEAR FOUNDED: 1983
FUNDING: Federal government; State government; Local government; Private; Fund-raisers
OUTREACH: Information and referral, community health education, client services
AVAILABLE LITERATURE: *Support Groups*, a flyer with times of meetings; *Services of San Diego AIDS Project*, a flyer describing the facility; *On a Positive Note*, a newsletter for PWAs and PWARCs; *Project Times*, a newsletter for the project
LANGUAGES: Spanish, Russian, American Sign Language

119. San Francisco AIDS Foundation
PO Box 6182, 25 Van Ness
San Francisco, CA 94101-6182
(415) 864-4376; Hotline: (415) 863-AIDS in English and Spanish; TDD: (415) 864-6606; Toll-free: (800) FOR-AIDS in English and Spanish
KEY PERSONNEL: Anne Goddard; Director of Communications
FACILITY TYPE: Educational; Support group; Client services/case management; Consulting
STAFF: Paid professional 58; Paid nonprofessional 25; Volunteers 700
YEAR FOUNDED: 1982
FUNDING: State government; Local government; Private; Fund-raisers; Fees for services or products
OUTREACH: Educational materials, speakers bureau, hotline, client services including food bank, emergency housing, social workers, advocacy, outreach to all communities, safer sex programs, fear reduction
NETWORKS: National AIDS Network (NAN); AIDS Action Council; California Association of AIDS Agencies (CAAA)
SEMINARS: Participates in most national public health, human resource, and AIDS events in the US
ADDITIONAL INFO: Provides a variety of programs that educate the public and provide direct services to those affected by the HIV virus
AVAILABLE LITERATURE: *Impetus*, a newsletter; *The Speakers Bureau Talks About AIDS*, an informational brochure about the service; *AIDS in the Workplace*, a brochure describing a comprehensive policy development and education program designed for business by business; *AIDS in the Workplace: A Guide for Employees*, an informational brochure; *SIDA en el Sitio de Trabajo: Una Guia para Empleados*, a Spanish-language informational brochure; *AIDS Care Beyond the Hospital*, a videotape program; *AIDS and the Healthcare Worker*, a brochure about AIDS in the healthcare field; *Condoms for Couples*, an informational brochure for heterosexuals; *Consulting Programs from the San Francisco AIDS Foundation*, an informational brochure; *The Adventures of BleachMan*, a comic strip format aimed at the IV drug user; *Poppers: Your Health and AIDS*, a brochure about AIDS and poppers; *AIDS Safe-Sex Guidelines*, a card of safe sex tips for the wallet; *Practicas Sexuales Sanas*, a safe sex card for the wallet in Spanish; *Sharing Needles Can Give You AIDS/Tu Puedes Contraer el SIDA, al Compartir Agujas*, a wallet card for IV drug users about keeping needles clean; *Inyectandos y su Salud*, an informational brochure in Spanish; *Coping with AIDS*, an informational brochure with AIDS facts;

When a Friend Has AIDS, a brochure of tips on what to say and what to do; *Lesbians and AIDS: What's the Connection?*, a brochure for lesbians; *Alcohol Drugs and AIDS*, a brochure discussing the connections between the three; *Information for People of Color*, an informational brochure; *Fact vs. Fiction: Ten Things You Should Know About AIDS*, an informational brochure; *Play Safe*, a condom; *Your Child and AIDS*, a simple guide for parents with children in daycare and public schools; *El Embarazo y el SIDA*, a brochure about AIDS and pregnancy in Spanish; *Pregnancy and AIDS*, a brochure about AIDS and pregnancy; *AIDS Kills Women and Babies*, informational brochure for women; *AIDS (SIDA) Mata a las Mujeres y a los Ninos*, an informational brochure for women in Spanish; *Women and AIDS*, a brochure for women; *Las Mujeres y el SIDA*, a brochure for women; *Informacion a las parejas sobre AIDS/SIDA*, a brochure of AIDS facts and safe sex information in Spanish; *Straight Talk About Sex and AIDS*, a brochure of AIDS facts and safe sex information; *AIDS Lifeline: The Best Defense Against AIDS is Information*, an informational brochure available in English, Spanish, and Chinese; *Strengthen Your Community, Strengthen Yourself, Volunteer at the S.F. AIDS Foundation*, an informational brochure about the foundation; *Talking With Your Teen About AIDS*, a guide for parents; *Hablando con sus Hijos Sobre el SIDA (o AIDS)*, a guide for parents in Spanish; *AIDS Antibody Testing at Alternative Test Sites*, a pamphlet describing the test; *La Prueba del Anticuerpo de AIDS*, a pamphlet in Spanish about the test; *Women, Children and AIDS*, a pamphlet of information on educational resources that are available; *Can We Talk?*, a safe sex guide; *Talk About AIDS*, an AIDS in the workplace videotape; *An Important Message for Gay and Bisexual Men*, a pamphlet/poster about safe sex; *BETA*, a bulletin of experimental treatments for AIDS; *San Francisco AIDS Foundation*, an informational brochure; *Annual Report*; *Onward*, a newsletter for volunteers; *San Francisco AIDS Foundation Catalog*
LANGUAGES: American Sign Language, all other languages

120. San Francisco Dept of Public Health, The AIDS Office
1111 Market St, 3rd Fl
San Francisco, CA 94103
(415) 864-5571
KEY PERSONNEL: Linda Udall; Assistant to the Medical Director
AFFILIATION: San Francisco Dept of Public Health
FACILITY TYPE: Research; Educational; Support group; Hospice
STAFF: Paid professional 58
YEAR FOUNDED: 1983
FUNDING: Federal government; State government; Local government
OUTREACH: Contracts with community-based organizations to provide education and outreach to the general public, minority communities, gay and bisexual communities, substance abusers, etc.; host provider education seminars aimed at offering the most current AIDS information to community physicians and other health care professionals
NETWORKS: University of California, Berkeley; University of California, San Francisco; State of California Health Dept; Centers for Disease Control; Federal Health, Resources and Services Administration
SEMINARS: Sep 29-Oct 1, 1988—"2nd National Conference on AIDS," San Francisco Dept of Public Health
RESEARCH: Evaluation of the effectiveness of various educational strategies, natural history of HIV infection, clinical trials, behavioral issues related to prevention of HIV transmission, etc
AVAILABLE LITERATURE: Publishes many research papers each year; *AIDS in San Francisco: 1987-88 Status Report and Projections for Services, Demands and Costs 1988-1993*, a 280-page document
LANGUAGES: Spanish, Tagalog, Mandarin

121. San Joaquin AIDS Foundation
PO Box 8277, 4410 N Pershing Ste C-5
Stockton, CA 95208-8277
(209) 476-8533
KEY PERSONNEL: Al Krumrey; Executive Director
FACILITY TYPE: Educational; Support group; Fund-raising; Task force
STAFF: Paid professional 4; Volunteers 50
YEAR FOUNDED: 1986
FUNDING: State government; Local government; Private; Fund-raisers; Donations
OUTREACH: Hand-to-hand support groups, emotional support groups, practical support groups, alternative test site training
AVAILABLE LITERATURE: Distributes materials from other agencies
LANGUAGES: Spanish, Indo-Chinese, American Sign Language

122. San Luis Obispo County AIDS Education and Prevention Project
FORMER NAME: San Luis Obispo County AIDS Task Force
PO Box 1489, 12191 Johnson Ave
San Luis Obispo, CA 93406
(805) 549-5540
KEY PERSONNEL: Wendy Holaday-Giggy; AIDS Program Coordinator
AFFILIATION: San Luis Obispo County Health Dept
FACILITY TYPE: Educational; Clinic; Task force; HIV counseling and testing; Health department
STAFF: Paid professional 3
FUNDING: State government
OUTREACH: Speakers bureau for high risk groups, health care workers, and emergency service workers plus general public, HIV counseling and testing, medical care of HIV infected individuals, resource distribution
LANGUAGES: Spanish

123. Santa Clara County Health Dept AIDS Program
2220 Moorpark
San Jose, CA 95128
(408) 299-4151
FACILITY TYPE: Educational; Clinic; Support group; HIV counseling and testing
ADDITIONAL INFO: Source of additional information on AIDS and an alternative HIV test site and evaluation/screening clinic. The test site is free, confidential, and anonymous

124. Santa Cruz AIDS Project (SCAP)
PO Box 5142, 1606 Soquel Ave
Santa Cruz, CA 95062
(408) 427-3900; Hotline: (408) 458-4999
KEY PERSONNEL: Jo Kenny; Executive Director
FACILITY TYPE: Educational; Support group; HIV counseling and testing
STAFF: Paid professional 3; Paid nonprofessional 4; Volunteers 250
YEAR FOUNDED: 1985
FUNDING: State government; Local government; Private; Fund-raisers
OUTREACH: Community-wide education, outreach services to IV drug users, gay and bisexual men, service providers, and migrant farm workers
NETWORKS: National AIDS Network (NAN); California Association of AIDS Agencies (CAAA); Computerized AIDS Information Network (CAIN)
ADDITIONAL INFO: Provides educational programs and direct emotional and practical support services to PWAs and their loved ones
AVAILABLE LITERATURE: *Volunteer Newsletter*
LANGUAGES: Spanish

125. Shanti Project
525 Howard St
San Francisco, CA 94105
(415) 777-CARE
KEY PERSONNEL: Chris Sandoval; Assistant Director
FACILITY TYPE: Support group
STAFF: Paid professional 67; Volunteers 700
YEAR FOUNDED: 1974
FUNDING: Local government; Private; Fund-raisers
OUTREACH: Provides 22-hour training programs for practical support volunteers, 44-hour training programs for emotional support volunteers, weekly orientation sessions for the public, 22-hour community participant training and trainings out of San Francisco for organizations desiring our one-on-one peer counseling model
SEMINARS: 1988—"National AIDS Conference," San Francisco, as a co-sponsor
ADDITIONAL INFO: This is the parent organization of all other Shanti projects in the United States. Shanti was formed to deal with the psychosocial aspects of persons facing life-threatening illnesses with its current focus on those affected with AIDS.
AVAILABLE LITERATURE: *Shanti Project*, informational brochure and membership application; *Eclipse: The Shanti Project Newsletter*, quarterly newsletter; 22 training videotapes available for practical and emotional support volunteers
LANGUAGES: Spanish, American Sign Language

126. Shasta County Public Health (SCPH)
2650 Hospital Lane
Redding, CA 96001
(916) 225-5591
KEY PERSONNEL: Judith Townley, RN

FACILITY TYPE: Educational; Clinic; Health department
STAFF: Paid professional 18; Paid nonprofessional 8
FUNDING: Federal government; State government; Local government; Fees for services or products
OUTREACH: Educational programs throughout the community, support groups for HIV positive, PWAs, PWARCs, and their family and friends
NETWORKS: North State AIDS Project (NSAP)
ADDITIONAL INFO: Serves as an alternative test site and acts as a resource for community education by providing educational programs for schools, hospitals, service organizations, juvenile hall, substance abuse programs, parent organization, and other interested groups. They have gone into the community for those at-risk persons who are unable to come into the site because of lack of transportation, fear of lack or anonymity, etc
LANGUAGES: Spanish, Vietnamese

127. Solano County Health Dept, AIDS Program
355 Tuolumne St
Vallejo, CA 94590
(707) 553-5401; Hotline: (707) 553-5552
KEY PERSONNEL: Alice Gandelman; AIDS Program Coordinator
AFFILIATION: Solano County Government
FACILITY TYPE: Educational; Clinic; Task force; HIV counseling and testing; Health department; Client services/case management
STAFF: Paid professional 6; Paid nonprofessional 4; Volunteers 4
YEAR FOUNDED: 1985
FUNDING: Federal government; State government
OUTREACH: Educational trainings and inservices to all specified target populations and others on request, street outreach, anonymous and confidential HIV antibody testing and counseling, surveillance, home care, case management
NETWORKS: Solano AIDS Task Force; AIDS Community Forum; Planned Parenthood; Computerized AIDS Information Network (CAIN)
RESEARCH: Behavior changes among individuals pertaining to needle cleaning practices and safe sex practices
ADDITIONAL INFO: This agency has four AIDS-related branches: AIDS Community Education Project, AIDS Surveillance Program, AIDS Clinic for HIV testing, and AIDS Home Care Project
AVAILABLE LITERATURE: *AIDS Related Services in Solano County*, a pocket card with services provided and telephone number; *About AIDS...Why Everyone Must Care*, a brochure of AIDS facts; *AIDS Resource Directory*, a 33-page booklet of resources
LANGUAGES: Spanish

128. Southern California Mobilization Against AIDS
1428 N McCadden Pl
Los Angeles, CA 90028
FACILITY TYPE: Educational
ADDITIONAL INFO: Source of additional AIDS information

129. Southern California Physicians for Human Rights (SCPHR)
PO Box 931507
Los Angeles, CA 90093-1507
(213) 464-7666
KEY PERSONNEL: Steven L Harris, President
FACILITY TYPE: Educational; Support group
FUNDING: Dues
OUTREACH: Speakers bureau, physicians referral service
SEMINARS: Annual continuing medical education conference held each Oct; monthly educational meetings
ADDITIONAL INFO: Founded in 1978 as an organization to provide physicians with educational support and social activities. Primary concern is human rights
AVAILABLE LITERATURE: Publishes brochures and a newsletter

130. Spanish Language AIDS Hotline
5350 E Beverly Blvd
Los Angeles, CA 90022
(213) 726-2201; Hotline: (800) 222-7432
KEY PERSONNEL: Elena Alvarado; Executive Director
AFFILIATION: East Los Angeles Rape Hotline, Inc.
FACILITY TYPE: Educational
STAFF: Paid professional 10; Paid nonprofessional 20; Volunteers 30
YEAR FOUNDED: 1974
FUNDING: State government; Local government; Fund-raisers

OUTREACH: Teen Teatro AIDS Prevention Program for youths, Teatro AIDS Prevention Program for adults, information and referral services on the SIDA Hotline
SEMINARS: 1988—"Symposium on Los Angeles Youth and AIDS"
RESEARCH: Knowledge and attitudes assessment research project of Latino and Black families in Los Angeles
ADDITIONAL INFO: Provides a 24-hour crisis line for sexual assault and child sexual abuse, long- and short-term therapy for sexual assault survivors, and child abuse prevention training
AVAILABLE LITERATURE: Currently producing a video on AIDS prevention which will be bilingual and culturally relevant to the Latino community
LANGUAGES: Spanish

131. Stanislaus Community AIDS Project (SCAP)
820 Scenic Dr
Modesto, CA 95350
(209) 572-2437; Hotline: (209) 572-2437
KEY PERSONNEL: Kris Owens; Education Director
FACILITY TYPE: Educational; Support group; Fund-raising; Client services/case management; Lobbying
STAFF: Paid professional 6; Paid nonprofessional 1; Volunteers 70
YEAR FOUNDED: 1985
FUNDING: State government; Fund-raisers
OUTREACH: Safer sex workshops for gay and bisexual men, HCW training, IV drug use outreach and education, school presentations, phoneline, jail outreach, literature distribution, HIV positive support groups
SEMINARS: The goals of SCAP are the prevention of AIDS through education, the assurance of quality medical and psychological care for people with AIDS and the promotion of understanding and sensitivity among the general public. Provides medical and counseling referrals, speakers bureau, counseling, special education programs and supportive services. Provides a "Hand-To-Hand" service of volunteers who offer emotional and practical support to people with AIDS and their families or care partners in the Stanislaus area
AVAILABLE LITERATURE: *SCAP: Stanislaus Community AIDS Project*, a brochure outlining the services of the agency
LANGUAGES: Spanish

132. Stop AIDS/Los Angeles
8512 Santa Monica Blvd
West Hollywood, CA 90069
(213) 659-4778; TDD: (213) 659-4779
KEY PERSONNEL: Jeff Campbell; Director of Education
FACILITY TYPE: Educational
STAFF: Paid professional 5; Volunteers 250
YEAR FOUNDED: 1986
FUNDING: State government; Local government
OUTREACH: Discussion groups for gay and bisexual men and women dealing with AIDS, safe sex, testing, and commitment to halting the spread of AIDS
NETWORKS: National AIDS Network (NAN); AIDS Community Educators of Los Angeles (ACE-LA); Los Angeles AIDS Consortium
LANGUAGES: Spanish, American Sign Language

133. Stop AIDS Project—California
1931 L St
Sacramento, CA 95814
(916) 442-5801
KEY PERSONNEL: Tim Warford; Executive Director
AFFILIATION: Lambda Community Fund
FACILITY TYPE: Educational .25; Hospital 50; Support group; Task force
STAFF: Paid professional 4
YEAR FOUNDED: 1978
FUNDING: State government; Private; Fund-raisers
OUTREACH: Works with gay men and heterosexual college students
NETWORKS: Sacramento County AIDS Network; Stop AIDS Resource Center
LANGUAGES: Spanish

134. Suicide Prevention Center Methadone Maintenance
1041 S Menlo Ave
Los Angeles, CA 90006
(213) 306-5111
KEY PERSONNEL: Dianne Graham; Manager
FACILITY TYPE: HIV counseling and testing; Substance abuse treatment

135. UCLA Medical Center, Immunology Clinic
10833 Le Conte Ave
Los Angeles, CA 90024
(213) 825-3718
FACILITY TYPE: Clinic
ADDITIONAL INFO: Provides AIDS medical evaluations by appointment only

136. UCSF AIDS Clinical Research Center
VA Medical Center, 4150 Clement St, Rm 141
San Francisco, CA 94121
(415) 750-2048
KEY PERSONNEL: John L Ziegler, Director
AFFILIATION: Univ of California San Francisco
FACILITY TYPE: Research; Educational; Hospital; Clinic
FUNDING: State government
RESEARCH: Clinical trials in AIDS
ADDITIONAL INFO: Founded in 1983 to do research and education on AIDS

137. UCSF AIDS Health Project
PO Box 0884, 1855 Folsom St, Ste 506
San Francisco, CA 94143-0884
(415) 476-6430
KEY PERSONNEL: James W Dilley, Director
AFFILIATION: Univ of California San Francisco
FACILITY TYPE: Educational
FUNDING: Federal government; State government; Local government
LIBRARY: AIDS information for in-house use
OUTREACH: Various educational and training services for the San Francisco Bay Area
ADDITIONAL INFO: Founded in 1984 as a provider of information on AIDS and educational materials that can be used in the classroom and work areas. It offers five programs: AIDS Prevention, AIDS Mental Health, AIDS and Substance Abuse, AIDS Antibody Counseling, and AIDS Health Professional Training
AVAILABLE LITERATURE: *Focus: A Review of AIDS Research*, a monthly newsletter reporting on AIDS research. Feature articles published to date include "AIDS antibody testing," "AIDS and substance abuse," "Impact of AIDS on women," "AIDS and ethnic communities," "AIDS-related suicide," "AIDS and children." Subscription: $24.00 per year (California), $30.00 per year (US), and $42.00 per year (foreign); *AIDS Substance Abuse Program*, a pamphlet presenting facts about AIDS and drugs; *Leaders Guides for Educational Support Groups*, consists of 3 educational guides on wellness-integrated health behaviors, stress management, and safe sex; *Teaching Curriculum for High School Teachers*, basic AIDS information for high school teachers; *Stress Management Tape*, a 20-minute stress tape; *What's Next?: After the Test*, a 15-minute videotape summarizing what the AIDS antibody test means and how individuals can cope with the results. Produced by Adair Films with AIDS Health Project as the Executive Producer

138. University of California at Los Angeles AIDS Clinical Research Center (UCLA AIDS Clinical Research Center)
Room 60-051 CHS, UCLA
Los Angeles, CA 91423
(213) 206-6414, 206-6415
KEY PERSONNEL: Virginia Campen; Program Director, Outreach and Education
AFFILIATION: University of California at Los Angeles (UCLA)
FACILITY TYPE: Research; Educational; Clinic
YEAR FOUNDED: 1983
FUNDING: Federal government; State government; Private
OUTREACH: Speakers bureau, CME courses, publication distribution
NETWORKS: Computerized AIDS Information Network (CAIN)
SEMINARS: Oct 26, 1987—"2nd UCLA AIDS Researchers Symposium;" Sep 17, 1988—"Primary Care of the HIV Infected Patient;" Oct 28, 1988—"3rd UCLA AIDS Researchers Symposium;" Oct 28, 1988—"Primary Care Course"
RESEARCH: Therapeutics and diagnostics
ADDITIONAL INFO: The UCLA AIDS Clinical Research Center conducts clinical trials of drugs and treatments for HIV infection, AIDS-related opportunistic infections and milignancies
AVAILABLE LITERATURE: *AIDS Medical Update*, monthly newsletter that reviews important medical journal articles with editorial comments; *AIDS Nursing Update*, quarterly newsletter of articles on AIDS issues of importance to nursing professionals
LANGUAGES: Interpreters available

139. Visiting Nurses and Hospice of San Francisco (VNH)
FORMER NAME: Hospice of San Francisco; AIDS Home Care and Hospice Program
1390 Market St, Ste 510
San Francisco, CA 94102
(415) 861-8705
KEY PERSONNEL: Jeannee Parker Martin; Director, Hospice Programs
AFFILIATION: Pacific Presbyterian Medical Center
FACILITY TYPE: Hospice; Home care
STAFF: Paid professional 40; Paid nonprofessional 80; Volunteers 210
YEAR FOUNDED: 1979
FUNDING: Federal government; State government; Local government; Fund-raisers; Fees for services or products
OUTREACH: Training sessions, bereavement support groups and referrals to support groups
NETWORKS: National Hospice Organization
ADDITIONAL INFO: Serves persons with AIDS/ARC and their families and loved ones who reside in the city and county of San Francisco. Through a grant given by the Gannett Foundation, VNH has organized two-day training sessions given throughout northern California
AVAILABLE LITERATURE: *AIDS Home Care and Hospice Manual*, a brochure describing the forthcoming manual; *AIDS Home Care and Hospice Training*, a brochure describing the various courses and workshops that are available; *Hospice Programs Fact Sheet*, various sheets that provide information about the services of the hospice with statistics; *Developing AIDS Residential Settings: A Manual*
LANGUAGES: Interpreters available for most languages

140. Women's AIDS Network (WAN)
333 Valencia St, 4th Fl
San Francisco, CA 94103
(415) 864-4376 ext 2030; TDD: (415) 864-6606
KEY PERSONNEL: Ruth Schwartz; Acting Coordinator
FACILITY TYPE: Educational; Task force; Advocacy
STAFF: Volunteers 60
YEAR FOUNDED: 1983
FUNDING: Fees for services or products; Dues
OUTREACH: Educational materials, educational events, centralized resources on women and AIDS
NETWORKS: California Association of AIDS Agencies (CAAA); Lobby for Individual Freedom and Equality (LIFE)
SEMINARS: Mar 1987—"Bay Area Researchers Conference on Women, Children and AIDS"
RESEARCH: Educational, psychosocial, service, and medical needs of women, particularly underserved women—teens, IV drug users, women of color, incarcerated women
ADDITIONAL INFO: Founded to provide support, assistance, and a forum for information exchange among members; to develop support strategies, educational materials, and events and to provide liaison with other community groups and services relating to AIDS
AVAILABLE LITERATURE: *San Francisco Resources for HIV-Affected Women*, a brochure of resource information for women; *Women and AIDS*, a brochure of AIDS and how it relates to women; *Mujeres y el SIDA*, a Spanish-language brochure for women; *Lesbians and AIDS: What's the Connection*, an informational brochure
LANGUAGES: Spanish

141. Women's AIDS Project
8235 Santa Monica Blvd
West Hollywood, CA 90046
KEY PERSONNEL: Suzann Gage; Administrator
FACILITY TYPE: Educational; Clinic; Support group; HIV counseling and testing
YEAR FOUNDED: 1986
FUNDING: Donations

142. World Hemophilia AIDS Center (WHAC)
2400 S Flower St
Los Angeles, CA 90007-2697
(213) 742-1357
KEY PERSONNEL: Shelby L Dietrich, Director
AFFILIATION: World Federation of Hemophilia
FACILITY TYPE: Educational
FUNDING: Donations; Grants
RESEARCH: Conducts an annual case survey for epidemiological purposes to determine the numbers of AIDS and AIDS-related conditions in hemophilia. Survey is conducted external to USA with respondents from 55 countries

ADDITIONAL INFO: Founded in 1983 to collect and disseminate data pertaining to AIDS and hemophilia
AVAILABLE LITERATURE: *Hemophilia World*, a quarterly newsletter with research reviews of AIDS drugs and tests. Former title *AIDS Center News*

COLORADO

143. Colorado AIDS Project
PO Box 18529
Denver, CO 80218
(303) 837-0166
KEY PERSONNEL: Julian Rush, Executive Director
FACILITY TYPE: Educational; Support group
FUNDING: Donations; Grants
LIBRARY: Contains brochures, posters, information sheets, and other materials pertaining to AIDS. Open to interested persons
OUTREACH: Speakers bureau, safer sex seminars, educational information
NETWORKS: Metro Area AIDS Education Group; Directors of Volunteers in Agencies; Southwest AIDS Project Directors; National AIDS Network; AIDS Action Council; Fund for Human Dignity
ADDITIONAL INFO: Founded in 1984 to assist those Coloradans who have developed AIDS, to educate those who are at risk for AIDS, and to educate the public about AIDS. Provides an AIDS information hotline, support group for persons with AIDS, support group for partners and friends of PWAs, support for parents of PWAs, volunteer services for PWAs, network and advocacy service for PWAs, emergency funding for PWAs, training programs for volunteers, educational outreach to high-risk groups, educational outreach to the general population, advocacy networking for risk groups, support for the worried well, and support for women
AVAILABLE LITERATURE: *AIDS: The Colorado AIDS Project*, a 1-fold brochure describing the project; *AIDS: What Gay Men Need to Know*, a 2-fold brochure with general information on AIDS and safe sex; *AIDS: The Contents of this Package Could Save Your Life*, a 1-fold brochure on how to use a condom; *AIDS: What You Need to Know About the AIDS Virus and Antibody Testing*, a 2-fold brochure with general information on AIDS and the antibody test; *AIDS: What Everyone Needs to Know*, a 1-fold brochure about AIDS for the general public; *AIDS: What Women Need to Know*, a 2-fold brochure with information for women; *Wellspring*, a bi-monthly newsletter with news of the project, national AIDS news, calendar of events, and statistics

144. Colorado Dept of Health, STD/AIDS Control
4210 E 11th St
Denver, CO 80220
(303) 331-8320; Hotline: (303) 333-4336; Toll-free: (800) 252-AIDS
KEY PERSONNEL: Jean Finn; Program Manager, Education/Training
AFFILIATION: Colorado State Government
FACILITY TYPE: Research; Educational; Support group; Health department
STAFF: Paid professional 60
FUNDING: Federal government; State government
OUTREACH: Targeted risk reduction projects, minority education, school and workplace education, public information campaigns, STD/AIDS training courses, partner notification
NETWORKS: AIDS Coalition for Education
SEMINARS: "4th Annual Rocky Mountain Regional Conference;" six regularly scheduled courses on HIV/AIDS
RESEARCH: Epidemiology
AVAILABLE LITERATURE: *Your Choice About AIDS*, a secondary school curriculum
LANGUAGES: Spanish, French

145. Denver AIDS Prevention Program
605 Bannock St
Denver, CO 80204-4507
(303) 893-6300; Hotline: (303) 893-6300
KEY PERSONNEL: Peter Ralin; Director, AIDS Information Services
AFFILIATION: Denver Dept of Health and Hospitals
FACILITY TYPE: Research; Educational; Hospital; Clinic
STAFF: Paid professional 22
FUNDING: Federal government; Local government
OUTREACH: Education for the workplace, health care workers, and schools, speakers bureau outreach to minorities and gays

SEMINARS: Feb 1987—"2nd Annual Rocky Mountain Regional Conference on AIDS;" Jan 1988—"3rd Annual Rocky Mountain Regional Conference on AIDS;" Jan 1989—"4th Annual Rocky Mountain Regional Conference on AIDS"
RESEARCH: AZT in early HIV infection, aerosolized pentamidine for PCP prophlaxis, CRC funded community-based AIDS demonstration project, HIV natural history study, high-risk study
AVAILABLE LITERATURE: *AIDS Questions and Answers*, a brochure of AIDS information in the form of questions and answers; *SIDA Parael Heterosexual*, a Spanish-language brochure for heterosexuals; *AIDS: The Sexually Active Heterosexual*, a brochure of general AIDS information for the heterosexual; *AIDS: Why Should I Take the AIDS Virus (HIV) Antibody Test?*, a brochure describing the test; *AIDS: Safer Sex*, a brochure of safe sex tips; *AIDS: Information for the Individual with a Positive AIDS Virus (HIV) Antibody Test*, a brochure of general information for the HIV positive individual; *AIDS: Information for the Individual with a Negative AIDS Virus (HIV) Antibody Test*, a brochure of information on what it means to be negative and the precautions one must take
LANGUAGES: Spanish

146. Eastside Neighborhood Health Center
501 28th St
Denver, CO 80206
(303) 297-1241
KEY PERSONNEL: Richard E Poole; Administrator
FACILITY TYPE: Clinic
YEAR FOUNDED: 1966
FUNDING: Federal government; State government; Local government; Fees for services or products
NETWORKS: Denver Disease Control, Infectious Disease Clinic
LANGUAGES: Spanish

147. Gay and Lesbian Community Center of Colorado, Inc (GLCCC)
PO Drawer E
Denver, CO 80218
(303) 831-6168; Hotline: (303) 837-1598
KEY PERSONNEL: B Galasso; Director
FACILITY TYPE: Support group; Fund-raising; Referral
STAFF: Paid professional 1; Paid nonprofessional 1; Volunteers 140
YEAR FOUNDED: 1976
FUNDING: Private; Fund-raisers; Dues
AVAILABLE LITERATURE: Bi-monthly newsletter

148. Hospice of Saint John
1320 Everett Court
Lakewood, CO 80215
(303) 232-7900
KEY PERSONNEL: Linda S Barley; Administrator
FACILITY TYPE: Hospice
STAFF: Paid professional 50; Paid nonprofessional 25; Volunteers 110
YEAR FOUNDED: 1984
FUNDING: Federal government; State government; Fund-raisers; Fees for services or products
OUTREACH: Terminal care of PWAs
NETWORKS: Colorado AIDS Project; AIDS Coalition for Education
ADDITIONAL INFO: This is an inpatient hospice with 38 beds
LANGUAGES: Spanish, Yiddish

149. Larimer County Health Dept
363 Jefferson St
Fort Collins, CO 80524
(303) 221-7460
KEY PERSONNEL: Ann Watson; Health Educator
FACILITY TYPE: HIV counseling and testing; Health department
STAFF: Paid professional 2.5; Paid nonprofessional .5
YEAR FOUNDED: 1968
FUNDING: Federal government; State government; Local government
OUTREACH: Speakers bureau, education and consultation on staff training for worksites, programs for the general public, clubs, organizations, curriculum development and staff training for schools, education of high-risk groups
NETWORKS: Northern Colorado AIDS Project; ACE-AIDS Coalition for Education; Larimer County AIDS Education Committee
SEMINARS: Mar 1988—"AIDS in the Workplace," luncheon and breakfast seminar for business people
ADDITIONAL INFO: The department has been an HIV antibody counseling and testing site since July 1985

AVAILABLE LITERATURE: *Larimer County Health Department: Keeping You Healthy*, a brochure describing the services of the department
LANGUAGES: Spanish

150. Southern Colorado AIDS Project (S-CAP)
PO Box 311
Colorado Springs, CO 80901
(719) 578-9092; Hotline: (719) 578-9092
KEY PERSONNEL: James Williams; Administrator
FACILITY TYPE: Educational; Support group; Fund-raising
STAFF: Volunteers 50
FUNDING: Private; Fund-raisers
OUTREACH: HIV positive support group, PWA support group, PWA family and friends support group, speakers bureau
ADDITIONAL INFO: The Southern Colorado AIDS Project (S-CAP) is a non-profit organization serving El Paso and Pueblo counties. It was created to coordinate resources and referral services for people with HIV infection, ARC, and AIDS; to educate the public about HIV infection; to train and support volunteers; and to raise funds for people coping with this disease, their families, and loved ones
AVAILABLE LITERATURE: *Southern Colorado AIDS Project (S-CAP)*, a brochure describing the project; *Volunteer Newsletter*

151. Weld County AIDS Coalition
1516 Hospital Rd
Greeley, CO 80631
(303) 353-0639
KEY PERSONNEL: Glenda Schneider; Chairperson
AFFILIATION: Weld County Health Dept
FACILITY TYPE: Educational; Support group; Task force
STAFF: Volunteers 30
YEAR FOUNDED: 1987
FUNDING: Fund-raisers; Fees for services or products
OUTREACH: Speakers bureau, technical assistance for businesses and organizations
NETWORKS: AIDS Coalition for Education; Northern Colorado AIDS Project
LANGUAGES: Spanish, American Sign Language

CONNECTICUT

152. AIDS Ministries Program
1335 Asylum Ave
Hartford, CT 06105
(203) 233-4481; Toll-free: (800) 842-0126 (CT only)
KEY PERSONNEL: Thaddeus Bennett; Director
FACILITY TYPE: Educational; Support group; Task force; Religious
STAFF: Paid professional 1; Paid nonprofessional 1.5; Volunteers 4
YEAR FOUNDED: 1987
FUNDING: Private; Fund-raisers; Donations; Church contributions
OUTREACH: Educational programs, preaching, consultation on residences for PWAs, referral services, regional resource guides
NETWORKS: Connecticut AIDS Residence Coalition; National Episcopal AIDS Coalition; AIDS National Interfaith Network
SEMINARS: 1988—"Educational Workshop for Religious Educators;" 1988—"Workshop on Residences for PWAs;" 1989—"Training Pastoral Caregivers;" 1989—"Retreats for PWAs and for Caregivers"
ADDITIONAL INFO: The purpose of this program is to involve the religious communities in Connecticut in the AIDS crisis with the goals to train pastoral caregivers and to develop educational programs, model residences for PWAs, and regional care teams
AVAILABLE LITERATURE: *Resources for Healing Services*, a 1987 directory of resources; *AIDS Educational Program for Christian Community*, a 1988 informational brochure

153. AIDS Project Greater Danbury
PO Box 91
Bethel, CT 06801
(203) 426-5626; Hotline: (203) 797-7900
KEY PERSONNEL: Donald Evans; Administrator
FACILITY TYPE: Educational; Support group
STAFF: Volunteers 30
YEAR FOUNDED: 1985
FUNDING: Private; Fund-raisers
AVAILABLE LITERATURE: Distributes various pamphlets
LANGUAGES: Spanish

154. AIDS Project/Greater New Britain (AP/GNB)
PO Box 1214, 147 W Main St
New Britain, CT 06050-1214
(203) 225-7634; Hotline: (203) 225-6789
KEY PERSONNEL: Ellen Lang; Coordinator
AFFILIATION: Connecticut AIDS Action Council
FACILITY TYPE: Educational; Support group; Task force
STAFF: Paid professional 1; Volunteers 56
YEAR FOUNDED: 1987
FUNDING: Private; Grants
OUTREACH: Educational presentations
NETWORKS: Connecticut AIDS Action Council; National AIDS Network (NAN)
SEMINARS: Nov 17, 1988—"AIDS Workshop," New Britain
AVAILABLE LITERATURE: *The AIDS Project—Greater New Britain, Inc.*, a flyer about the organization with membership form
LANGUAGES: Spanish

155. AIDS Project/Hartford (AP/H)
30 Arbor St
Hartford, CT 06106
(203) 523-7699; Hotline: (203) 247-AIDS
KEY PERSONNEL: Patricia C Ruot; Executive Director
FACILITY TYPE: Educational; Support group
STAFF: Paid professional 2; Volunteers 80
YEAR FOUNDED: 1985
FUNDING: State government; Local government; Fund-raisers
OUTREACH: Speakers bureau, educational outreach to Hispanic community, support groups for HIV positive individuals, PWAs, PWARCs, women and children, and caregivers
NETWORKS: National AIDS Network (NAN); Connecticut AIDS Action Council (CARC); Greater Hartford AIDS Residence Coalition; Hartford AIDS Collaborative
ADDITIONAL INFO: Provides outreach and education to the community through information tables, speakers, and workshops. Individual and group support is provided to HIV positive individuals, PWAs, PWARCs, women and children, and caregivers. Provides counseling and information referrals to the Hispanic community with Spanish-speaking counselors
AVAILABLE LITERATURE: Distributes brochures and information from other agencies

156. AIDS Project: Middlesex County
Middletown Dept of Health
Middletown, CT 06457
(203) 344-3482; Hotline: (203) 344-9998
KEY PERSONNEL: Louis Carta; Health Educator
AFFILIATION: Middletown Dept of Health
FACILITY TYPE: Educational; Hospital; Support group; Task force; HIV counseling and testing
STAFF: Paid professional 7
YEAR FOUNDED: 1987
FUNDING: Federal government; State government
OUTREACH: Support groups, educational materials, audiovisual loans, presentations, workshops, inservice training, press releases to print and electronic media
NETWORKS: AIDS Grant Committee; AIDS Consortium
SEMINARS: Feb 14-20, 1988—"AIDS Awareness Week," Middlesex; Jun 23, 30, 1988—"AIDS Buddy Training Symposium," Middlesex
ADDITIONAL INFO: Provides a hotline, HIV counseling and testing, and AIDS education. Networks with other agencies and private industries
AVAILABLE LITERATURE: *AIDS Project Middlesex County*, a brochure describing the services
LANGUAGES: Spanish

157. AIDS Project New Haven (APNH)
PO Box 636
New Haven, CT 06503
(203) 624-0947; Hotline: (203) 624-2437
KEY PERSONNEL: Jean Hess; Executive Director
FACILITY TYPE: Educational; Support group
STAFF: Paid professional 3; Volunteers 250
YEAR FOUNDED: 1983
FUNDING: Federal government; State government; Private; Fund-raisers
OUTREACH: Hotline, speakers bureau, outreach, support groups, PWAs coalition, Meals on wheels, buddies, interfaith network

NETWORKS: National AIDS Network (NAN); Connecticut AIDS Council

AVAILABLE LITERATURE: *AIDS is Deadly: Don't Pass the Spike*, a brochure for IV drug users; newsletter

158. AIDS Project/Norwalk
137 East Ave
Norwalk, CT 06851
(203) 854-7976
AFFILIATION: Norwalk Health Dept
FACILITY TYPE: Educational; Clinic; HIV counseling and testing
ADDITIONAL INFO: An anonymous AIDS testing facility maintained by the Norwalk Health Dept and source of additional information on AIDS

159. Bridgeport AIDS Advisory Committee
2710 North Ave
Bridgeport, CT 06604
(203) 336-AIDS, 7-9 pm, M,W,F
KEY PERSONNEL: Jay Ferrori, Coordinator
FACILITY TYPE: Educational
ADDITIONAL INFO: Source of additional AIDS information

160. Connecticut AIDS Action Council (CAAC)
254 College St
New Haven, CT 06510
(203) 624-0947
KEY PERSONNEL: Sher Herasko; Coordinator
FACILITY TYPE: Task force; Advocacy
STAFF: Volunteers 20
YEAR FOUNDED: 1987
FUNDING: Private
ADDITIONAL INFO: CAAC is an advocacy and coordination agency for the coalition of leadership of all AIDS projects in Connecticut
LANGUAGES: Spanish

161. Connecticut Counseling Centers, Inc
951 Chase Pkwy
Waterbury, CT 06708
(203) 755-8874
KEY PERSONNEL: Helen Kotler; Program Director
FACILITY TYPE: HIV counseling and testing; Substance abuse treatment

162. Connecticut Dept of Health Services, AIDS Section
150 Washington St
Hartford, CT 06106
(203) 566-1157
KEY PERSONNEL: Ann McLendon; AIDS Education Director
AFFILIATION: Connecticut State Government
FACILITY TYPE: Educational
YEAR FOUNDED: 1985
FUNDING: Federal government; State government
OUTREACH: Speakers bureau
ADDITIONAL INFO: Coordinates AIDS prevention and HIV counseling and testing services in the state
AVAILABLE LITERATURE: *AIDS and IV Drug Users*, a brochure of information for drug users; *What You Should Know about HIV Antibody Testing*, a brochure describing the test; *AIDS: How to Avoid It*, a brochure of general AIDS information; *Connecticut Responds to AIDS*, a 20-page pamphlet describing the statewide AIDS prevention programs

163. Danbury Health Dept AIDS Program
20 West St
Danbury, CT 06810
(203) 796-1613; Hotline: (203) 797-7900
KEY PERSONNEL: Gingee Zazueta; AIDS Education Coordinator
FACILITY TYPE: Educational; Hospital; Clinic; Support group; Task force
STAFF: Paid professional 4; Paid nonprofessional 3
FUNDING: Federal government; State government
OUTREACH: Speakers bureau, outreach to IV drug abusers
NETWORKS: Danbury Task Force on AIDS; Danbury Alcohol and Drug Abuse Program; AIDS Project Greater Danbury

ADDITIONAL INFO: Works with community support programs and trains staff and others interested in educating PWAs
AVAILABLE LITERATURE: Eleven posters are in the process of being developed pinpointing various ages and target groups in the community

164. Greenwich AIDS Task Force
101 Field Point Rd
Greenwich, CT 06836-2540
(203) 622-6460
KEY PERSONNEL: John Wiesman; Co-Chairperson
AFFILIATION: Greenwich Dept of Health
FACILITY TYPE: Educational; Support group; Task force
STAFF: Volunteers 20
YEAR FOUNDED: 1986
FUNDING: Private; Coalition funding
OUTREACH: Speakers bureau, HIV positive support group, buddy system
NETWORKS: Southern Fairfield County AIDS Coalition; HIV Legislative Network—CT
ADDITIONAL INFO: The task force's 60 members include service providers, concerned citizens and a growing number of volunteers. The group's purpose is to plan, coordinate and monitor existing services and advocate for future needs and to provide services that would not otherwise be offered

165. Greenwich Dept of Health, Office of HIV Information and Services
FORMER NAME: Office of AIDS Information and Services
101 Field Point Rd
Greenwich, CT 06836-2540
(203) 622-6460; Hotline: (203) 622-6460
KEY PERSONNEL: John Wiesman; Directory
AFFILIATION: Greenwich Dept of Health
FACILITY TYPE: Educational; Clinic; HIV counseling and testing; Health department
STAFF: Paid professional 2
YEAR FOUNDED: 1987
FUNDING: Federal government; State government; Local government
OUTREACH: Community education, professional and corporate education, hotline
NETWORKS: Southern Fairfield County AIDS Coalition, Greenwich AIDS Task Force
SEMINARS: 1988—"AIDS and Early Childhood Programs: Are You Prepared?," "HIV Seminar for Dentists," "HIV Seminar for Funeral Directors/Morticians"
ADDITIONAL INFO: Administers the HIV antibody test with counseling. The primary purpose is to prevent additional cases of HIV infection, act as the local HIV resource, and provide referrals to those with HIV infection. The main focus is on education for school children, professionals, and adults, community coordination and facilitation of services, and anonymous HIV counseling and testing

166. Hartford Gay and Lesbian Health Collective, Inc
PO Box 2094
Hartford, CT 06145-2094
(203) 236-4431
KEY PERSONNEL: Ken Griffin; Executive Director
FACILITY TYPE: Educational; Clinic; HIV counseling and testing
STAFF: Paid professional 2; Volunteers 30
YEAR FOUNDED: 1983
FUNDING: State government; Fund-raisers; Donations
OUTREACH: Telephone counseling for HIV positive, STD screening and treatment, Hepatitis screening, HIV counseling and testing
NETWORKS: National Coalition of Gay Sexually Transmitted Disease Services (NCGSTDS)
SEMINARS: Sep 18, 1988—"AIDS: Women to Women"
ADDITIONAL INFO: This collective is committed to fostering healthful lifestyles for lesbians and gay men. The group supports the essential psychological health of a variety of alternative lesbian, gay and bisexual lifestyles, and seeks counseling and support strategies to aid all potential clients in improving their life quality.
AVAILABLE LITERATURE: *Gay Health in Gay Hands*, an informational brochure about the clinic; *Salud Homosexual en Manos Homosexuales*, a Spanish-language brochure about the clinic
LANGUAGES: American Sign Language, Spanish

167. Hispanos Unidos Contra El SIDA/AIDS, Inc
263 Grand Ave
New Haven, CT 06513
(203) 772-1777
KEY PERSONNEL: Carlos E. Allende-Ramos; Executive Director
FACILITY TYPE: Educational; Support group
YEAR FOUNDED: 1987
FUNDING: Federal government; State government; Fund-raisers
OUTREACH: Conferences in Spanish, brochure distribution, counseling, workshops on AIDS
NETWORKS: Northeast Hispanic AIDS Consortium; National Latino/Hispanic AIDS Committee
ADDITIONAL INFO: The twofold mission of this group is to curb the spread of infection by providing AIDS education to Hispanic people and to care for the infected and their families by identifying or providing support services. Provides outreach to the schools and churches in the Hispanic communities and psychosocial training for health care workers so they can address the problems of AIDS in the Hispanic community.
AVAILABLE LITERATURE: *Cuida Tu Salud*, Spanish-language informational brochure; *AIDS*, brochure on AIDS in Spanish and English
LANGUAGES: Spanish

168. Liberation Programs, Inc
119 Main St
Stamford, CT 06901
(203) 359-3134
KEY PERSONNEL: Doris De Huff; Executive Director
FACILITY TYPE: HIV counseling and testing; Substance abuse treatment

169. Mayor's Task Force on AIDS
1 State St
New Haven, CT 06511
(203) 686-6957
KEY PERSONNEL: Sher Horosko; Coordinator
AFFILIATION: New Haven Mayor's Office
FACILITY TYPE: Task force
STAFF: Paid professional 1; Paid nonprofessional 1
YEAR FOUNDED: 1986
FUNDING: Local government
NETWORKS: National AIDS Network (NAN); Connecticut AIDS Action Council
ADDITIONAL INFO: Works in co-creating other community groups to fight AIDS. Helped form the New Haven Women's AIDS Coalition of the Task Force, Hispanics United Against AIDS, and Project AIM, a Black outreach effort. The task force is a policy-recommending body of 25 community-based individuals and AIDS professionals. Meets monthly to work through various policy questions like needle exchange, anti-discrimination, confidentiality, etc., and then advocates for these positions at city- and state-wide levels
AVAILABLE LITERATURE: Distributes the following posters produced by the Women's AIDS Coalition—*I Care About Myself, I Use Condoms*; *Love as if Your Life Depended on It, It Does, Insist on Condoms*; *You Care About Your Kids, You Care About Him, Care About Yourself, Insist on Condoms*; *AIDS is a Fact, When You Teach Them the Facts of Life, Remember the Most Important One Today, Condoms Make Sex Safer!*; *I'm Serious About Love, I Use Condoms*; *Tomo, en Serio el Amor, Uso Condones*; *AIDS Doesn't Discriminate*; *Cuidas de los Hijos, Cuidas de el, Cuidate a ti misma, Insiste en Condones*; all posters depict women and children of all ages, both sexes, and different nationalities
LANGUAGES: Spanish

170. Mid-Fairfield AIDS Project, Inc
FORMER NAME: Mid-Fairfield AIDS Task Force
30 France St
Norwalk, CT 06851
(203) 854-7979
KEY PERSONNEL: Jan Boardman; AIDS Coordinator
FACILITY TYPE: Educational; Support group; Fund-raising; Task force
STAFF: Volunteers 75
YEAR FOUNDED: 1986
FUNDING: Fund-raisers; Donations
OUTREACH: Speakers bureau, educational programs, AIDS support groups for HIV positive men and women and their families, volunteer buddy group, support for PWAs
NETWORKS: Norwalk Health Dept; Southern Fairfield County AIDS Coalition
SEMINARS: Apr, May 1987—"Volunteer Buddy Training Program"

171. New London AIDS Educational, Counseling and Testing Service
120 Broad St, Health Dept
New London, CT 06320
Hotline: (203) 447-AIDS
KEY PERSONNEL: Lizabeth Love Ryan; Coordinator
AFFILIATION: New London Health Dept
FACILITY TYPE: Educational; HIV counseling and testing; Health department
STAFF: Paid professional 4; Paid nonprofessional 1; Volunteers 15
YEAR FOUNDED: 1987
FUNDING: Federal government; State government
OUTREACH: Provides outreach to those out of the mainstream of education
LANGUAGES: Spanish

172. Northwest Connecticut AIDS Project
PO Box 985
Torrington, CT 06790
(203) 567-4111

173. Norwalk Health Dept, AIDS Program
137 East Ave
Norwalk, CT 06851
(203) 854-7979; Hotline: (203) 854-7979
KEY PERSONNEL: Jan Boardman; AIDS Coordinator
AFFILIATION: Norwalk City Government
FACILITY TYPE: Educational; Clinic; Support group; Hospice; HIV counseling and testing; Health department
STAFF: Paid professional 4; Paid nonprofessional 1
YEAR FOUNDED: 1986
FUNDING: Federal government; State government; Local government; Fees for services or products
OUTREACH: Educational programs for community organizations, outreach programs directed to IV drug users and minorities
NETWORKS: Mid-Fairfield AIDS Project, Inc.; Southern Fairfield County AIDS Coalition
ADDITIONAL INFO: Provides anonymous counseling and testing, support groups for HIV positive men and women, education and information services, home care, and hospice services
LANGUAGES: Spanish

174. Southern Fairfield County AIDS Coalition
137 East Ave
Norwalk, CT 06851
(203) 866-9123
KEY PERSONNEL: Deborah L May; Regional AIDS Coordinator
FACILITY TYPE: Educational; Support group; Fund-raising; Task force; Coordination
STAFF: Paid professional 1; Paid nonprofessional 1; Volunteers 200
YEAR FOUNDED: 1987
FUNDING: Private; Fund-raisers; Fees for services or products
OUTREACH: Coordination of all regional educational and outreach services
NETWORKS: National AIDS Network (NAN); HIV Legislative Network; Connecticut AIDS Action Council (CAAC); Greater Bridgeport AIDS Project; Mid-Fairfield AIDS Project; Stamford AIDS Task Force; Greenwich AIDS Task Force
ADDITIONAL INFO: The coalition was created to provide a forum and mechanism for the cooperation and coordination of the Greater Bridgeport AIDS Project, Mid-Fairfield AIDS Project, Stamford AIDS Task Force, and Greenwich AIDS Task Force
AVAILABLE LITERATURE: *Southern Fairfield County AIDS Coalition Newsletter*, a bimonthly newsletter; *Southern Fairfield County AIDS Coalition*, a brochure describing the coalition; *Resource Guide for People Affected by AIDS in Southern Fairfield County*, a 23-page resource directory with addresses and telephone numbers

175. Stamford Health Dept: AIDS Program
888 Washington Blvd, 8th Fl
Stamford, CT 06904
(203) 967-2437; Hotline (203) 967-3356
KEY PERSONNEL: Debra Katz; Education Coordinator
AFFILIATION: Stamford Health Dept
FACILITY TYPE: Educational; Fund-raising; Task force; HIV counseling and testing
STAFF: Paid professional 2; Paid nonprofessional 5
YEAR FOUNDED: 1986
FUNDING: Federal government; State government

OUTREACH: Outreach education to IV drug users, minorities, women, and youth
NETWORKS: Stamford AIDS Taskforce
LANGUAGES: Haitian French, Spanish

176. Waterbury Dept of Public Health, AIDS Program
402 E Main St
Waterbury, CT 06702
(203) 574-6883
KEY PERSONNEL: Laura Minor; AIDS Education Coordinator
AFFILIATION: Waterbury Government
FACILITY TYPE: Educational; Clinic; HIV counseling and testing
STAFF: Paid professional 3; Paid nonprofessional 2
YEAR FOUNDED: 1986
FUNDING: Federal government; State government; Fees for services or products
OUTREACH: Educational programs for police, nursing home staffs, drug treatment facilities, and high schools, outreach to Black and Hispanic communities, IV drug users and prostitutes
NETWORKS: AIDS Project Waterbury; Connecticut AIDS Action Council
SEMINARS: Oct 1988—"Seminar on AIDS and Ethics"
ADDITIONAL INFO: Provides anonymous counseling and testing for HIV. Co-sponsors support groups for HIV positive individuals, their friends, and families
AVAILABLE LITERATURE: Pamphlets describing the services of the agency
LANGUAGES: Spanish

177. Yale University Health Services
17 Hillhouse Ave
New Haven, CT 06520
(203) 432-0123
KEY PERSONNEL: Daniel S Rowe, Director; Sally Rinaldi, Assistant
FACILITY TYPE: Clinic
FUNDING: State government; Insurance premiums
LIBRARY: Contains medical books, general books, periodicals, pamphlets, brochures, audio visuals, and other materials for professional staff, faculty, employees, and students
OUTREACH: Speakers bureau
NETWORKS: Mayor's Task Force on AIDS; AIDS Task Force at Yale; AIDS Project New Haven; Shirley Frank Foundation; Yale-New Haven Hospital; Yale School of Medicine
ADDITIONAL INFO: Founded in 1971 as an HMO for Yale students providing general information on AIDS
AVAILABLE LITERATURE: *AIDS Prevention; Stop AIDS; Safe Sex is for Everyone*, a 2-fold brochure with general information on safe sex and the control of AIDS

DELAWARE

178. AIDS Program Office (APO)
3000 Newport Gap Pike, Bldg G
Wilmington, DE 19808
(302) 995-8422; Hotline: (800) 422-0429 (DE only)
KEY PERSONNEL: James C Welch; Director
AFFILIATION: Delaware State Division of Public Health
FACILITY TYPE: Educational; Support group; Task force; HIV counseling and testing; Client services/case management
STAFF: Paid professional 7
YEAR FOUNDED: 1985
FUNDING: Federal government; State government
OUTREACH: Outreach and educational services to ethnic, minority communities, IV drug users, public and private sectors, schools, community and civic organizations
NETWORKS: AIDS Committee of the Delaware Lesbian and Gay Health Advocates (DLGHA); Gay and Lesbian Alliance of Delaware (GLAD); The Alliance of Black and Hispanic Communities Against AIDS; AIDS Advisory Task Force; Delaware Council on Crime and Justice
SEMINARS: Sep 28-29, 1987—"The Impact of AIDS on the Family and Society;" Oct 20-21, 1988—"AIDS: Beyond the Basics"
ADDITIONAL INFO: Provides anonymous counseling and testing services to 5 alternate test sites throughout Delaware and educational programming to public and private sectors throughout Delaware. Provides case management services and support groups to PWAs and PWARCs, family members and significant others
AVAILABLE LITERATURE: *AIDS: It's Everybody's Problem*, an informational brochure; *AIDS Program Office*, a flyer

179. Delaware Lesbian and Gay Health Advocates, Inc (DLGHA)
214 N Market St
Wilmington, DE 19801
(302) 652-6776; Hotline: (800) 422-0429 (DE only)
KEY PERSONNEL: Ivo Dominguez, Jr; Executive Director
FACILITY TYPE: Research; Educational; Support group; HIV counseling and testing; Residential facility (adults)
STAFF: Paid professional 4; Paid nonprofessional 1; Volunteers 87
YEAR FOUNDED: 1984
FUNDING: Federal government; Private; Fund-raisers
OUTREACH: Health education, HIV counseling and testing, buddy system, housing, library, financial assistance, pastoral care, meditation, and alternative therapies
NETWORKS: Computerized AIDS Information Network (CAIN); National AIDS Network (NAN)
SEMINARS: "AIDS: Beyond the Basics"
RESEARCH: Homophobia and health care
ADDITIONAL INFO: Provides support services and education on AIDS and related health issues and concerns. Committed to work with substance abuse and mental health issues, especially as they relate to sexual minorities
AVAILABLE LITERATURE: *AIDS Update*, a monthly newsletter; *When a Friend Has AIDS*, a brochure of what to say and what to do; *Safer Sex*, a brochure of safer sex tips; *AIDS and Kids*, information for parents; *If Your HIV Antibody Test is Positive*, a brochure for those who test positive; *AIDS: Definition, Cause, Transmission, and Prevention*, an informational brochure; *Working for Health in the Human Family*, an informational brochure about DLGHA; *AIDS and Minorities*, an informational brochure; *Cleaning Your Works*, a brochure for IV drug users
LANGUAGES: Spanish, American Sign Language

DISTRICT OF COLUMBIA

180. AIDS Action Council/Washington
FORMER NAME: FARO—AIDS Action Council
729 8th St SE, Ste 200
Washington, DC 20003
(202) 547-3101
KEY PERSONNEL: Ann E McFarren, Executive Director
FACILITY TYPE: Lobbying
FUNDING: Donations; Dues
NETWORKS: National AIDS Network
SEMINARS: Presents a symposium the first Monday of each month
ADDITIONAL INFO: Founded as a non-profit lobbying organization representing the interests of community-based AIDS agencies to Congress, the federal administration, and the public health service
AVAILABLE LITERATURE: *AIDS Action Update*, a newsletter with AIDS lobbying effort news

181. AIDS Campaign Trust/Washington
PO Box 1396
Washington, DC 20013
FACILITY TYPE: Educational
ADDITIONAL INFO: Source of additional AIDS information

182. AIDS Clinical Trials Unit (ACTU)
2300 Eye St, Ste 202
Washington, DC 20037
(202) 994-2417
KEY PERSONNEL: Jane Courtless, RN
AFFILIATION: George Washington Univ Medical Center AIDS Research
FACILITY TYPE: Research
FUNDING: Federal government
NETWORKS: Whitman-Walker Clinic
AVAILABLE LITERATURE: *reSEARCH*, a newsletter to inform patients and health professionals of current medical research which may prevent or delay the progression of AIDS
LANGUAGES: Spanish

183. American Association of Sex Educators, Counselors and Therapists (AASECT)
11 Dupont NW, Ste 220
Washington, DC 20036
(202) 462-1171
KEY PERSONNEL: Ann McFarren; Interim Executive Director
FACILITY TYPE: Educational

STAFF: Paid professional 3; Paid nonprofessional 2
YEAR FOUNDED: 1967
FUNDING: Fees for services or products
OUTREACH: Professional training programs
NETWORKS: National Organizations Responding to AIDS (NORA)
SEMINARS: Provides regional workshops and conferences
ADDITIONAL INFO: "The American Association of Sex Educators, Counselors and Therapists links thousands of professionals in sex education, counseling and therapy. AASECT is the professional body which certifies the qualifications of sexual health practitioners."
AVAILABLE LITERATURE: *AASECT: Professionals on the Move*, brochure describing the association; *Journal of Sex Education and Therapy*, a quarterly reporting clinical studies and research; *AASECT Newsletter*, a general newsletter; *Membership Directory*

184. American College of Obstetricians and Gynecologists (ACOG)
409 12th St SW
Washington, DC 20024
(202) 638-5577
FACILITY TYPE: Educational; Professional
STAFF: Paid professional 150
YEAR FOUNDED: 1951
FUNDING: Federal government; Private; Fund-raisers; Fees for services or products; Dues
OUTREACH: Patient education
RESEARCH: Women's health
AVAILABLE LITERATURE: *Prevention of Human Immune Deficiency Virus Infection and Acquired Immune Deficiency Syndrome*, a pamphlet on prevention of HIV infection and AIDS; a card with all future meetings of ACOG; *ACOG 1988 Publications and Educational Materials Catalog*; *ACOG 1989 Continuing Medical Education Catalog*

185. American Red Cross, AIDS Education Program
1730 E St NW
Washington, DC 20006
(202) 639-3223
KEY PERSONNEL: Carole Kauffman; Manager
FACILITY TYPE: Research; Educational
STAFF: Paid professional 931; Paid nonprofessional 300; Volunteers 150
YEAR FOUNDED: 1881
FUNDING: Federal government; State government; Local government; Private; Fund-raisers; Fees for services or products
OUTREACH: AIDS prevention program for the workplace, AIDS prevention programs for Black and Hispanic youth and their families
RESEARCH: Education—market effectiveness, program effectiveness, educational effectiveness
ADDITIONAL INFO: The program's goal is to provide reliable, factual information to help prevent the spread of the disease.
AVAILABLE LITERATURE: *AIDS: The Facts*, an informational brochure covering the basic facts about AIDS; *Surgeon General's Report on Acquired Immune Deficiency Syndrome*; *AIDS and Children*, an informational brochure for parents of school-age children; *AIDS and Children*, an informational brochure for teachers and school officials; *Gay and Bisexual Men and AIDS*, an informational brochure of AIDS facts; *Facts About AIDS and Drug Abuse*, a brochure for IV drug users; *AIDS, Sex, and You*, a brochure of brief facts about AIDS transmission; *Caring for the AIDS Patient at Home*, an informational brochure giving some guidelines; *AIDS and the Safety of the Nation's Blood Supply*, an informational brochure; *AIDS and Your Job—Are There Risks?*, a brochure discussing AIDS in the workplace; *Informate de lo que es el SIDA*, a Spanish-language brochure of AIDS facts; *If Your Test for Antibody to the AIDS Virus is Positive*, a brochure describing what the test means and what HIV positive means; *American Red Cross AIDS Public Education Program*, a flyer describing the program; *AIDS Prevention Program for Youth*, a flyer covering the basics of the youth program; *Don't Forget Sherrie*, video; *Printed/Audio Visual Materials*, a catalog of materials available from the American Red Cross; *See Beyond Fear: You Can't Get AIDS...*, a poster of how you cannot get AIDS; *AIDS: Beyond Fear*, video
LANGUAGES: Wide range of languages

186. Damien Ministries
PO Box 10202
Washington, DC 20018
(202) 387-2926
KEY PERSONNEL: Louis J Tesconi; Executive Director
FACILITY TYPE: Educational; Support group; Hospice; Fund-raising; Task force
STAFF: Paid professional 4; Volunteers 150
YEAR FOUNDED: 1987
FUNDING: Local government; Private
OUTREACH: Speakers bureau
SEMINARS: May 4-7, 1988—"AIDS: Religions Respond," a national conference for Roman Catholic clergy to address AIDS both as a ministry and an illness among clergy
ADDITIONAL INFO: Provides retreats for PWAs and conducts jail ministry. Operates three homes in the DC area for PWAs
AVAILABLE LITERATURE: *Damienews*, a newsletter
LANGUAGES: Spanish, Italian, Dutch

187. Dupont West Medical Center
2032 P St NW
Washington, DC 20036
(202) 775-8500
FACILITY TYPE: Educational
ADDITIONAL INFO: Source of additional AIDS informaton

188. Everyday Theater Youth Ensemble
1st and Eye St SW, Randall Bldg
Washington, DC 20024
(202) 727-5930 ext 65, 38
KEY PERSONNEL: Thom Workman; Associate Director
AFFILIATION: Youth Awareness Group
FACILITY TYPE: Educational; Theater
STAFF: Paid professional 7
YEAR FOUNDED: 1978
FUNDING: Local government; Fund-raisers; Fees for services or products
OUTREACH: Touring productions, videotapes, workshops, discussions
NETWORKS: Washington DC Commission of Public Health; Washington DC Dept of Human Services; Regional Organization of Theaters South (ROOTS)
SEMINARS: Mar 31, 1988—"National Red Cross Conference," performed; Aug 15, 1988—"National CDC Conference," performed; May 20, 1988—"Africare Conference," performed
RESEARCH: Minorities
ADDITIONAL INFO: This group works primarily with inner city youth at risk. Educates through the theater
AVAILABLE LITERATURE: *Til Death Do Us Part*, a videotape on AIDS awareness and prevention; *The Lost Prize*, a live theater production on AIDS awareness and prevention

189. Family Research Institute, Inc
PO Box 2091
Washington, DC 20013
(301) 963-7463
KEY PERSONNEL: Paul Cameron; Chairperson
FACILITY TYPE: Research; Educational
STAFF: Paid professional 3; Volunteers 5
YEAR FOUNDED: 1982
FUNDING: Private; Fees for services or products
OUTREACH: Distribution of publications
RESEARCH: Control the spread of AIDS through traditional public health measures
AVAILABLE LITERATURE: *Family Research*, newsletter; also publishes pamphlets and articles in medical and psychological journals

190. Gay Men's Venereal Disease Clinic/Washington
1407 S St NW
Washington, DC 20009
FACILITY TYPE: Clinic
ADDITIONAL INFO: Source of additional AIDS information

191. Gay Rights National Lobby/AIDS Project
PO Box 1892
Washington, DC 20013
(202) 783-1828
FACILITY TYPE: Lobbying
ADDITIONAL INFO: Source of additional AIDS information

192. Human Rights Campaign Fund (HRCF)
1012 14th St NW, 6th Fl
Washington, DC 20005
(202) 628-4160

KEY PERSONNEL: Vic Basile, Executive Director; Philip Dufour, Press
FACILITY TYPE: Lobbying
FUNDING: Donations
ADDITIONAL INFO: Founded in 1981 to provide financial support on behalf of the gay and lesbian community to candidates for the US Senate and the House of Representatives who pledge to support gay civil rights legislation and responsible AIDS policy
AVAILABLE LITERATURE: *The Campaign Fund Report*, a newsletter reporting the activities of the Human Rights Campaign Fund; *Human Rights Campaign Fund: An Introduction*, a 2-fold brochure describing the activities of the HRC

193. LifeLink, PWA Coalition of Washington, DC
2025 Eye St NW, Ste 417
Washington, DC 20006
(202) 833-3070
KEY PERSONNEL: Robert Thewes; Service Coordinator
AFFILIATION: National Association of People with AIDS (NAPWA)
FACILITY TYPE: Educational; Fund-raising; Client services/case management; Advocacy
STAFF: Paid professional; Volunteers 50
YEAR FOUNDED: 1987
FUNDING: Local government; Private; Fund-raisers
OUTREACH: Personal perspectives provided to enhance existing educational programs throughout the DC area
NETWORKS: National Association of People with AIDS (NAPWA)
ADDITIONAL INFO: LifeLink is a nonprofit community-based organization of PWAs working for PWAs—men, women and children, regardless of color, sexual preference, or risk behavior. The organization is primarily for fostering the self-empowerment of people with AIDS
AVAILABLE LITERATURE: *LifeLink*, a brochure describing the organization; *NAPWA: National Association of People with AIDS*, a brochure describing the national association; *Background History*, an informational sheet about LifeLink; *LifeLink NewsLink*, a monthly newsletter

194. National AIDS Network (NAN)
2033 M St NW, Ste 800
Washington, DC 20036
(202) 293-2437
KEY PERSONNEL: James L Holm, Acting Executive Director
FACILITY TYPE: Network
STAFF: Paid professional 20; Paid nonprofessional 5; Volunteers 10
YEAR FOUNDED: 1986
FUNDING: Federal government; Private; Fund-raisers; Fees for services or products; Dues
OUTREACH: Public service announcements on TV, radio and in print with Advertising Council and with Warner Records Clearinghouse
SEMINARS: Oct, 1988, 1989—"NAN Skills Building Conference"
ADDITIONAL INFO: NAN serves as a national organization responding to the community-based efforts on AIDS.
AVAILABLE LITERATURE: *NAN Monitor*, quarterly newsletter; *Network News*, bi-weekly newsletter; *NAN Multicultural Notes*, monthly newsletter; Technical assistance series: *2176 Medicaid Waivers, Buddy Programs, Volunteer Management*; *History of the National AIDS Network*
LANGUAGES: Spanish

195. National AIDS Vigil Commission
2335 18th St NW
Washington, DC 20009
FACILITY TYPE: Educational; Support group
ADDITIONAL INFO: Source of additional AIDS information

196. National Association of People with AIDS (NAPWA)
2025 Eye St NW, Ste 415
Washington, DC 20006
(202) 429-2856
KEY PERSONNEL: Mike Merdian; Executive Director
FACILITY TYPE: Educational; Support group; Fund-raising; Task force
FUNDING: Private; Donations; Grants
OUTREACH: Education, support, advocacy
ADDITIONAL INFO: Assists all people with AIDS and people with ARC regardless of race, color, creed, ethnicity, gender, age, disability, sexual orientation or affectional preference. NAPWA has more than 70 locally-based PWA organizations across the United States, each serving their own community

AVAILABLE LITERATURE: *NAPWA News*, a newsletter produced by and for people with AIDS
LANGUAGES: Spanish

197. National Association of Public Hospitals (NAPH)
1001 Pennsylvania Ave NW, Ste 6355
Washington, DC 20004
(202) 347-1136
KEY PERSONNEL: Dennis P Andrulis; Vice President
FACILITY TYPE: Research; Educational
STAFF: Paid professional 6
YEAR FOUNDED: 1980
FUNDING: Dues
AVAILABLE LITERATURE: *Safety Net*, a quarterly magazine

198. National Gay and Lesbian Task Force (NGLTF)
FORMER NAME: National Gay Task Force (NGTF)
1517 U St NW
Washington, DC 20009
(202) 332-6483
KEY PERSONNEL: Jeffrey Levi; Executive Director
FACILITY TYPE: Lobbying
STAFF: Paid professional 10; Volunteers 50
YEAR FOUNDED: 1973
FUNDING: Fund-raisers; Dues
AVAILABLE LITERATURE: *Task Force Report*, a newsletter; *It Takes Time*, a brochure with chronology of lobbying efforts throughout the United States; *AIDS-Related Issues and Insurance*, a position paper; *Dealing with Violence*, a guide for gay and lesbian people; *Anti-Gay Violence: Causes, Consequences, Responses*, a 30-page report; *Anti-Gay/Lesbian Victimization*, results of a survey; *Anti-Gay Violence and Victimization in 1985 and 1986*, reports; *Information on Police Entrapment and Abuse*, an informational brochure; *Hate Crime Statistics Packet*; *Eight Good Reasons to Decriminalize Sexuality*, a handout; *Youth Support Packet*, comprehensive resources for young lesbians and gay men

199. National Leadership Coalition on AIDS
1150 17th St NW, Ste 202
Washington, DC 20036
(202) 429-0930
KEY PERSONNEL: B J Stiles; President
FACILITY TYPE: Educational; Task force
STAFF: Paid professional 3; Volunteers 1
YEAR FOUNDED: 1987
FUNDING: Federal government; Private; Fees for services or products
OUTREACH: Disseminates of AIDS in the workplace information and resources among members and interested parties, provides consultation to those developing AIDS workplace policies, stimulates private sector involvement with efforts to meet the demands posed by the epidemic
NETWORKS: Univ of Maryland at Baltimore; American National Red Cross; National Association of Manufacturers; National Coalition of Hispanic Health and Human Services Organizations; Gay Men's Health Crisis; United Board for Homeland Ministries; American Medical Association; Joseph E Seagram and Sons, Inc; AFL-CIO; US Conference of Mayors; Center for Corporate Public Involvement; National AIDS Network (NAN); International Business Machines Corp; Wells Fargo Bank; Indiana State Board of Health; Transamerica Occidental Life Insurance; National Urban League; American Pharmaceutical Institute; Addiction Research Treatment Corp; American Foundation for AIDS Research (AmFAR); Episcopal Diocese of California; Allstate Insurance Co
SEMINARS: Oct 1987, Jan 1988—"AIDS: Corporate America Responds," co-sponsored with Allstate Insurance Co; Sep 16, 1988—"Private Sector Leadership Conference on AIDS"
ADDITIONAL INFO: The goal of this agency is to bring together the collective resources of the private sector—corporate, non-profit and charitable—to respond to the AIDS crisis. Supports improved education and services and promotes the policies and strategies required to cope with the awesome challenges of AIDS
AVAILABLE LITERATURE: *AIDS: Risk Prevention Understanding*, a brochure describing the facts about AIDS to be used in workplace education; *A Private Sector Leadership Response to the Challenges of AIDS: National Leadership Coalition on AIDS*, a brochure describing the coalition

200. National Lesbian and Gay Health Foundation (NLGHF)

1638 R St NW Ste 2
Washington, DC 20009
(202) 797-7104, 797-3708
KEY PERSONNEL: Bea Roman; Executive Director
FACILITY TYPE: Educational; Support group; Fund-raising; Task force
STAFF: Paid professional 3; Paid nonprofessional 1; Volunteers 74
YEAR FOUNDED: 1983
FUNDING: Federal government; Private; Fees for services or products
OUTREACH: Organizes national and international conferences
SEMINARS: 1987—"9th National Lesbian/Gay Health Conference and 5th AIDS Forum," Los Angeles; 1988—"10th National Lesbian/Gay Health Conference and 6th AIDS Forum," Boston; 1989—"11th National Lesbian/Gay Health Conference and 7th AIDS Forum," San Francisco
ADDITIONAL INFO: Provides training for psychosocial and medical support for PWAs, networks for youth, prisons, and organizes international conferences
AVAILABLE LITERATURE: *Lesbian Health Survey*; *Sourcebook on Lesbian/Gay Health Care*; *Sexual Health Report*
LANGUAGES: Spanish, German, American Sign Language

201. Saint Francis Center

5417 Sherier Pl, NW
Washington, DC 20016
(202) 363-8500
KEY PERSONNEL: Judy Pollatsek; Associate Executive Director of Programs
FACILITY TYPE: Educational; Support group; HIV counseling and testing Training
STAFF: Paid professional 6; Paid nonprofessional 2; Volunteers 40
YEAR FOUNDED: 1975
FUNDING: Private; Fund-raisers; Fees for services or products
OUTREACH: AIDS training program; Friends program, AIDS-related service support group for those affected by AIDS in the family
SEMINARS: May 1988—"Children and Death," conference; Oct 1988—lecture by Dr Bernie Siegel; Oct 1989—lecture by Harold Kushner; Nov 1988—"Counseling and Understanding Persons with AIDS," workshop; 4 times per year—"Thanatology and AIDS," workshops
RESEARCH: Psychosocial issues facing PWAs and their families; stress and burn-out for care givers working with AIDS patients; AIDS education for community groups
ADDITIONAL INFO: Provides professional counseling, agancy training, and volunteer support for PWAs, family members, and care givers since 1983
AVAILABLE LITERATURE: *Centering*, newsletter; pamphlets describing the center

202. United States Conference of Local Health Officers (USCLHO)

FORMER NAME: United States Conference of City Health Officers
1620 Eye St NW
Washington, DC 20006
(202) 293-7330
KEY PERSONNEL: Richard D Johnson; Deputy Executive Director
AFFILIATION: United States Conference of Mayors
FACILITY TYPE: Health department
STAFF: Paid professional 13; Volunteers 1
YEAR FOUNDED: 1960
FUNDING: Federal government; Private; Fees for services or products
SEMINARS: Nov 14, 1988, Oct 23, 1989—"Annual Meeting," held in conjunction with the American Public Health Association, 1988 in Boston, 1989 in Chicago; two regional meetings are to be held in the spring of 1989
RESEARCH: Federal policies on AIDS, development of national preventive health objectives, federal family planning clinic regulations, smoking on airlines, childhood nutrition
ADDITIONAL INFO: USCLHO is the national organization representing the interests of local health department officials. It is an affiliate of the U.S. Conference of Mayors and promotes the local perspective on national public health policy before Congress, the Administration, and various federal agencies. Represents over 1,500 health departments nationwide
AVAILABLE LITERATURE: *Local Health Department Directory, March 1988*, a directory of health departments; *Local Health Officers News*, a bimonthly newsletter; *AIDS Information Exchange*, a bimonthly newsletter; *Local AIDS Policies, June 1988*, a directory of

policies pertaining to AIDS at the local level; *Local AIDS Services Directory, May 1988*, a directory of local AIDS services; *United States Conference of Local Health Officers*, a brochure describing the agency

203. The United States Conference of Mayors (USCM)

1620 Eye St NW
Washington, DC 20006
(202) 293-7330
KEY PERSONNEL: Richard D Johnson; Assistant Executive Director
FACILITY TYPE: Educational; Public interest group
YEAR FOUNDED: 1933
FUNDING: Federal government; Local government; Private; Fees for services or products
OUTREACH: Information exchange among local governments, grants to community-based organizations for AIDS education
SEMINARS: Every June —"UCSM Annual Conference;" Feb 1988—"4th Annual Conference on AIDS," for local health dept staff and community-based organizations
ADDITIONAL INFO: The AIDS program of this agency was founded in 1983. Provides publications, including a directory of local AIDS services
AVAILABLE LITERATURE: *Local AIDS Policies*, a June 1988, 79-page book of various policies throughout the United States; *Local AIDS Services: The National Directory*, a May 1988 directory; *AIDS Information Exchange Newsletter*, a bimonthly newsletter

204. US Public Health Service, Public Affairs Office

200 Independence Ave SW
Washington, DC 20201
(202) 245-6867
FACILITY TYPE: Educational
ADDITIONAL INFO: Source of additional information on AIDS

205. Washington Area Council on Alcohol and Drug Abuse

1232 M St NW
Washington, DC 20005
(202) 682-1700
FACILITY TYPE: Substance abuse treatment
ADDITIONAL INFO: Source of additional information on AIDS and drug abuse

206. Whitman-Walker Clinic, Inc

1407 S St NW
Washington, DC 20009
(202) 797-3500; Hotline: (202) 332-2437; Spanish Line: (202) 328-0697
KEY PERSONNEL: Jim Graham; Administrator
AFFILIATION: National Leadership Coalition on AIDS
FACILITY TYPE: Research; Educational; Clinic; Support group; Fund-raising; HIV counseling and testing
STAFF: Paid professional 50; Volunteers 1000
YEAR FOUNDED: 1973
FUNDING: Local government; Private; Fund-raisers
OUTREACH: Outreach to IV drug users, male and female prostitutes, education outreach project to gay and bisexual men, outreach to prisons
NETWORKS: National AIDS Network (NAN); NOVA Cares
SEMINARS: Gives numerous presentations and workshops throughout the year
RESEARCH: Laboratory development of HIV associated measurements, AIDS-related health care delivery, AIDS drug evaluation
ADDITIONAL INFO: Provides medical evaluation and AIDS counseling and antibody testing. Support services are provided in the form of emotional, legal and financial. The Robert N Schwartz, MD, Housing Services provides low-cost, permanent housing for displaced persons with AIDS. Three projects are part of the Sunnye Sherman AIDS Education Project and include Operation H.E.A.R.T (Health Education and Risk Reduction Training), home meeting discussion groups where gay/bisexual men discuss lifestyle issues in the context of AIDS; Project A.O.R.T.A. (AIDS Education Outreach to the Alienated), operates outreach teams who discuss the issues of AIDS with male prostitutes, escorts, transvestite prostitutes, and the homeless; IV Drug Abuse/Prostitute Project, Outreach workers for street encounters. The clinic also provides STD services and alcoholism services

AVAILABLE LITERATURE: *Fight the Fear With the Facts 332-AIDS*, an informational card; *Alcohol, Drugs and Your Health*, a brochure discussing the relationships among the three; *AIDS Program*, an informational brochure about the clinic; *Staying Healthy: AIDS Information for Gay Men*; *Safer Sex: You Don't Have To Do It Alone*, a brochure of safer sex tips; *When a Friend Has AIDS*, a brochure of what to say and what to do; *AIDS: The More We Know, the Less We Have to Fear*, an informational brochure; *AIDS in the Black Community: The Facts*, a brochure for Blacks; *Whitman Walker Clinic News*, a newsletter; *What Are the Symptoms of AIDS?*, a flyer outlining the symptoms; *A Fighting Chance*, an annual report of the clinic; *Health—Mental Health Trainings*, a chronology of presentations for February-April 1987; *Speaker's Bureau*, a monthly list of where the various speakers have given presentations
LANGUAGES: Spanish, American Sign Language

FLORIDA

207. AID Jacksonville
PO Box 19-0488
Miami Beach, FL 33119-0488
(904) 399-4589
ADDITIONAL INFO: Source of additional AIDS information

208. AIDS Action Committee/Key West
PO Box 4073
Key West, FL 33041
AFFILIATION: Florida Keys Memorial Hospital
FACILITY TYPE: Educational
ADDITIONAL INFO: Source of additional AIDS information

209. AIDS Education Programs/Jacksonville
5900 Junior College Rd
Key West, FL 33040
FACILITY TYPE: Educational
ADDITIONAL INFO: Source of additional AIDS information

210. AIDS Help, Inc
PO Box 4374
Key West, FL 33041
(305) 296-6196
KEY PERSONNEL: Edward Seebol; Executive Director
FACILITY TYPE: Support group; Fund-raising
STAFF: Paid professional 2; Paid nonprofessional 2; Volunteers 30
YEAR FOUNDED: 1986
FUNDING: State government; Local government; Private; Fund-raisers; Grants
OUTREACH: Support groups for PWAs, their friends and lovers
NETWORKS: South Florida AIDS Network; Health Advisory Board of Key West; South Florida Health Council's AIDS Advisory Committee
ADDITIONAL INFO: This is a community-based service organization serving as an interim financial agency to assist needy PWAs and providing general support for all PWAs
AVAILABLE LITERATURE: *PWA Newsletter*

211. AIDS Project, Duval County Public Health Unit
515 W 6th St, Rm 2A
Jacksonville, FL 32206
(904) 630-3237; Hotline: (800) FLA-AIDS
KEY PERSONNEL: Ken Hunt; Director
AFFILIATION: Florida State Dept of Health and Rehabilitative Services
FACILITY TYPE: Educational; Clinic; HIV counseling and testing; Client services/case management
STAFF: Paid professional 9; Volunteers 20
YEAR FOUNDED: 1985
FUNDING: Federal government; State government; Local government; Fees for services or products
OUTREACH: Community education programs, staff training
NETWORKS: Duval County Case Management Network; State of Florida AIDS Program
ADDITIONAL INFO: Provides comprehensive outpatient clinic services for HIV infected individuals, PWARCs, and PWAs. The staff includes a physician, nurse, case managers, education specialists, and education counselors
LANGUAGES: Spanish, Vietnamese

212. AIDS Resource, Education and Assistance (AREA)
PO Box 160224
Altamonte Springs, FL 32716
(407) 843-4368; Hotline: (407) 843-4368
KEY PERSONNEL: Shari Ranger; Program Director
FACILITY TYPE: Educational; Support group; Fund-raising
STAFF: Volunteers 20
YEAR FOUNDED: 1987
FUNDING: Private; Fund-raisers
OUTREACH: Crisis intervention/suicide prevention training held every 6 weeks for the public and volunteers, speakers at various seminars and conferences held for professionals
NETWORKS: AIDS Network of Central Florida; Florida AIDS Coalition for Education and Support (FACES)
SEMINARS: Nov 21-22, 1987, Feb 6-7, 1988, Apr 16-17, 1988, Jun 11-12, 1988, Jul 23-24, 1988, Aug 20-21, 1988, Oct 1-2, 1988—"AIDS Awareness Weekend Seminar;" Apr 30-May 1, 1988—"FACES Quarterly Conference"
ADDITIONAL INFO: Formed to respond to the needs of people affected by AIDS. Provides area information, resources, education, and assistance
AVAILABLE LITERATURE: *Community Resources Directory for Orange, Osceola, Seminole Counties, State of Florida*, a 1987 directory; *AIDS Resource Education and Assistance*, newsletter; *AIDS Resources Education and Assistance: Meeting the Needs of the Community*, a brochure describing the agency; *What to do if You are AIDS Antibody Positive*, a brochure of information for those who test positive; *AIDS Nursing: Care and Safety Procedures for Medical Care Professionals*, a brochure
LANGUAGES: American Sign Language, Spanish, Creole

213. AIDS Support Group/Miami
23rd St and NE 2nd St
Miami, FL 33139
AFFILIATION: MCC/Miami
FACILITY TYPE: Educational
ADDITIONAL INFO: Source of additional AIDS information and support

214. Bay CPHU
FORMER NAME: Bay County Health Dept
605 N MacArthur Ave
Panama City, FL 32401-3680
(904) 785-4384
KEY PERSONNEL: John J Benton, Director
AFFILIATION: Florida Dept of Health and Rehabilitative Services
FACILITY TYPE: Educational; Clinic
FUNDING: Federal government; State government; County government
OUTREACH: Speakers bureau
ADDITIONAL INFO: Founded as a clinic and educational agency
AVAILABLE LITERATURE: Distributes publications of the State of Florida
LANGUAGES: Spanish

215. Betterway Inc 12-Step Halfway House
229 NE 24 St
Miami, FL 33137
(305) 573-6279
KEY PERSONNEL: Scott Bernard; Assistant Director
FACILITY TYPE: HIV counseling and testing; Substance abuse treatment

216. Center One, Anyone in Distress, Inc
FORMER NAME: AIDS Center One
PO Box 8152
Fort Lauderdale, FL 33310
(305) 561-0807; Hotline: (305) 561-0316
KEY PERSONNEL: Joe Repice; Executive Director
FACILITY TYPE: Educational; Support group; Fund-raising; Task force; Client services/case management; Residential facility (adults)
STAFF: Paid professional 9; Paid nonprofessional 3; Volunteers 240
YEAR FOUNDED: 1984
FUNDING: Federal government; Local government; Private; Fund-raisers
OUTREACH: Community education and outreach
NETWORKS: South Florida AIDS Network; National AIDS Network (NAN)
RESEARCH: Clients services

ADDITIONAL INFO: Center One provides referrals, support groups, buddy system, advocacy, spiritual counseling, direct financial aid, and information and education for the total community. Sponsors "Our House," a residence in Fort Lauderdale for people with ARC and PWAs who are homeless and need custodial care

AVAILABLE LITERATURE: *Heartbeat*, bimonthly newsletter; *Center One/Anyone in Distress*, a brochure describing the agency; *What is the Center One Volunteer Program*, a pamphlet describing the program; *AIDS Information Booklet: Family Edition*, a booklet of facts about AIDS

LANGUAGES: Spanish

217. Central Florida AIDS Unified Resources, Inc (CENTAUR)
PO Box 3725
Orlando, FL 32802
(407) 849-1453; Hotline: (407) 849-1452
KEY PERSONNEL: James Stucky; Executive Director
FACILITY TYPE: Educational; Support group
STAFF: Volunteers 50
YEAR FOUNDED: 1985
FUNDING: Private; Fund-raisers
AVAILABLE LITERATURE: *Centaur*, a monthly newsletter

218. Charlotte County AIDS Task Force
514 E Grace St
Punta Gorda, FL 33950
(813) 639-1181
KEY PERSONNEL: John J Piacitelli; Acting Chairman
AFFILIATION: Southwest Florida AIDS Task Force
FACILITY TYPE: Task force
STAFF: Volunteers 20
YEAR FOUNDED: 1988
FUNDING: Donations
OUTREACH: Educational materials made available to local libraries, agencies, and individuals
NETWORKS: Southwest Florida AIDS Task Force

219. Collier County AIDS Task Force
PO Box 428
Naples, FL 33939
(813) 774-8200
KEY PERSONNEL: Jane Polkowski; Director
AFFILIATION: Collier City Public Health Unit
FACILITY TYPE: Educational; Clinic; Support group; Task force
STAFF: Volunteers 100
YEAR FOUNDED: 1986
FUNDING: Federal government; State government; Private
OUTREACH: Court-ordered AIDS education program for people convicted of prostitution or drug-related offenses, door-to-door Creole outreach program
NETWORKS: South West Florida AIDS Task Force
SEMINARS: Apr 1989—"AIDS Update," Naples
ADDITIONAL INFO: Sponsors support groups and educational programs for the high risk populations of the inland migrant town of Immokalee in Spanish and Creole as well as programs for populations in the coastal resort city of Naples
LANGUAGES: Spanish, Creole

220. Comprehensive AIDS Program of Palm Beach County, Inc (CAP)
FORMER NAME: Inforum
PO Box 3084
Lantana, FL 33465-3084
(407) 582-HELP
FACILITY TYPE: Educational; Support group; Fund-raising; Home care
STAFF: Paid professional 15; Volunteers 35
YEAR FOUNDED: 1986
FUNDING: Federal government; State government; Local government; Private; Fund-raisers
ADDITIONAL INFO: CAP is an organization of professionals dedicated to providing care to those who are ill and support for those who need it, encouraging prevention for everyone, making maximum use of available community resources through a network of service providers who are members of the CAP coalition
AVAILABLE LITERATURE: *CAP of Palm Beach County, Inc*, an informational brochure about the agency
LANGUAGES: Spanish

221. The Fight For Life Committee, Inc
6231 SW 10th Court
North Lauderdale, FL 33068
(305) 972-0393
KEY PERSONNEL: Lenny Kaplan; Chairperson
FACILITY TYPE: Educational; Fund-raising
STAFF: Volunteers 12
YEAR FOUNDED: 1988
FUNDING: Private; Fund-raisers
OUTREACH: Speakers bureau, information on new drugs and testing
NETWORKS: Broward Act Now; Act Up; National Association of People with AIDS (NAPWA); PWA Coalition
ADDITIONAL INFO: Lobbies for new drugs through letter writing, news releases, and speaking
AVAILABLE LITERATURE: *You Don't Have to Stop Getting Down to Avoid Getting AIDS*, a safe sex brochure; tee shirts and buttons

222. Florida AIDS Hotline
PO Box 20169
Tallahassee, FL 32316
Hotline: (800) FLA-AIDS (FL only)
KEY PERSONNEL: Maryalice Thomas; Clinical Coordinator
AFFILIATION: Telephone Counseling and Referral Service, Inc.
FACILITY TYPE: Educational; Hotline
STAFF: Paid professional 4; Paid nonprofessional 10; Volunteers 40
YEAR FOUNDED: 1985
FUNDING: Federal government; State government
OUTREACH: Limited local community training

223. Health Crisis Network, Inc (HCN)
PO Box 42-1280, 1351 NW 20th St
Miami, FL 33242-1280
(305) 326-8833; Hotline: (305) 634-4636; Spanish Hotline: (305) 324-5148; Toll-free: (800) 443-5046
KEY PERSONNEL: Sally Dodds; Executive Director
FACILITY TYPE: Research; Educational; Support group; HIV counseling and testing
STAFF: Paid professional 22; Paid nonprofessional 4; Volunteers 150
YEAR FOUNDED: 1983
FUNDING: Federal government; State government; Fund-raisers; Fees for services or products
OUTREACH: Prevention education for gay men, IV drug users, women, migrant workers
NETWORKS: South Florida AIDS Network (SFAN); Biopsychosocial Research Center of AIDS
RESEARCH: Psychosocial stressors, exercise and immune system, education and prevention strategies
AVAILABLE LITERATURE: *Healthnotes*, a newsletter; *Health Sources*, a Dade County AIDS resource directory
LANGUAGES: Spanish

224. Hope House of the Palm Beaches, Inc
PO Box 812
Lake Worth, FL 33460
(407) 655-8949
KEY PERSONNEL: PG Ciotti; Executive Director
FACILITY TYPE: Residential facility (adults)
STAFF: Paid professional 1; Volunteers 50
YEAR FOUNDED: 1984
FUNDING: Private; Fund-raisers; Fees for services or products
NETWORKS: PWA Coalition of Palm Beach County; The Homeless Coalition; The Comprehensive AIDS Program; National AIDS Network (NAN)
ADDITIONAL INFO: Formed in 1984 when the congregation of the Metropolitan Community Church realized the need for a residential facility for PWAs who had become indigent and homeless as a result of their illness

225. HRS/Hillsbourough County Health Dept/AIDS Program
1112B E Kennedy Blvd
Tampa, FL 33675-5135
(813) 272-6155
KEY PERSONNEL: Mickey Tagliarini; Program Supervisor
AFFILIATION: Hillsbourough County Government
FACILITY TYPE: Educational; Clinic; Health department
STAFF: Paid professional 8; Paid nonprofessional 2
YEAR FOUNDED: 1889
FUNDING: Federal government; State government; Fees for services or products

OUTREACH: Informational talks to facilities addressing AIDS in jails and rehabilitative services
AVAILABLE LITERATURE: *HIV Antibody Testing*, *AIDS Patient Care Program*, a flyer explaining the purpose of the program

226. International Health Research Foundation
1780 NE 168th St
North Miami Beach, FL 33162
FACILITY TYPE: Educational; Research
ADDITIONAL INFO: Source of additional AIDS information

227. Jackson Memorial Hospital AIDS Center
1611 NW 12th Ave
Miami, FL 33136
FACILITY TYPE: Hospital
ADDITIONAL INFO: Source of additional AIDS information

228. Lee County AIDS Task Force (Volunteer Committee)
2231 McGregor Blvd
Fort Myers, FL 33901
(813) 337-2391; Hotline: (813) 332-AIDS
KEY PERSONNEL: Hans Cox; Coordinator
AFFILIATION: Southwest Florida AIDS Task Force
FACILITY TYPE: Educational; Support group; Fund-raising; Task force
STAFF: Volunteers 80
YEAR FOUNDED: 1988
FUNDING: Private; Fund-raisers
OUTREACH: Referrals for support groups for HIV positive individuals, PWAs, families and friends, referrals for free private counseling for newly diagnosed persons, assistance with Medicaid and Social Security applications, coordinates the buddy program, hotline, educational seminars for the public, information about local AIDS resources for PWAs, home for PWAs

229. Lee County Public Health Unit, Immunology Clinic
3920 Michigan Ave
Fort Myers, FL 33916
(813) 332-9614
KEY PERSONNEL: Adrian L Pollock; Senior Physician
AFFILIATION: Lee County Government
FACILITY TYPE: Educational; Clinic; HIV counseling and testing
STAFF: Paid professional 6; Paid nonprofessional 1
FUNDING: Federal government; State government; Local government; Fees for services or products
OUTREACH: AIDS/HIV educational seminars for health care professionals and the general public
ADDITIONAL INFO: This agency is an immunology clinic for HIV positive individuals, PWARCs, and PWAs. Part-time HIV counselor is available at the local soup kitchen to educate, counsel and test prostitutes and IV drug users

230. Leon County Public Health Unit
2965 Municipal Way
Tallahassee, FL 32304
(904) 487-3186
KEY PERSONNEL: Mary P Wegmann; Senior Community Health Nursing Director
AFFILIATION: Florida State Dept of Health and Rehabilitative Services
FACILITY TYPE: Clinic; HIV counseling and testing
STAFF: Paid professional 26; Paid nonprofessional 10
YEAR FOUNDED: 1931
FUNDING: Federal government; State government; Local government; Fees for services or products
OUTREACH: Educational sessions and information on AIDS to individuals and groups in Leon County
NETWORKS: Florida Dept of Health and Rehabilitative Services, AIDS Program, Disease Control
SEMINARS: Feb 24, 1988—"The Impact of AIDS on Leon County, AIDS Update 1988;" Feb 26, 1988—"AIDS Community Leadership Symposium"
ADDITIONAL INFO: Provides anonymous and confidential HIV counseling and testing with referrals. AIDS cases are reported to this agency for completion of the CDC Case Report. Provides trained professionals who conduct programs on AIDS

231. Monroe County Health Dept, AIDS Education Project (MCPHU, AEP)
513 Whitehead St.
Key West, FL 33040
(305) 294-8302
KEY PERSONNEL: Dan Geshrick, Director
FACILITY TYPE: Educational; Clinic
FUNDING: County government
LIBRARY: Contains videos and various printed literature on AIDS. Open to the general public
OUTREACH: Advocacy and public education
ADDITIONAL INFO: Founded in 1985 as an educational agency for the Key West area
AVAILABLE LITERATURE: *AIDS Newsletter*, a bimonthly newsletter with information about AIDS in the Key West area
LANGUAGES: Spanish

232. North Central Florida AIDS Network (NCFAN)
FORMER NAME: Gainesville AIDS Community Network
1005-I SE 4th Ave
Gainesville, FL 32601
(904) 372-4370; Hotline: (904) 372-4370
KEY PERSONNEL: Stephen C. Braswell; Office Manager
AFFILIATION: Florida AIDS Coalition for Education and Support Services (FACES)
FACILITY TYPE: Educational; Support group; Fund-raising; Task force
STAFF: Paid professional 1; Volunteers 150
YEAR FOUNDED: 1985
FUNDING: Private; Fund-raisers; Fees for services or products
OUTREACH: Speakers bureau; AIDS-101, a general overview of HIV and how to stop the spread of HIV; outreach to the workplace, teenagers, drug users, and the community
NETWORKS: Univ of Florida Task Force on AIDS
SEMINARS: Monthly, 1987-1989—"AIDS-101," a general overview of HIV and how to stop the spread of HIV; 1989—"Buddy Training," three times a year
ADDITIONAL INFO: NCFAN is a private, nonprofit organization providing services and support to the public and PWAs in 17 counties in north central Florida. "NCFAN's major goals are to provide professional and community education to help stop the spread of AIDS and to provide needed service and support to persons with AIDS or at risk for AIDS."
AVAILABLE LITERATURE: *North Central Florida AIDS Network Support Services*, brochure describing the organization; *AIDS in the Workplace*, brochure of facts about AIDS and the workplace; *AIDS in the Black Community: The Facts*, brochure about AIDS and Blacks; *AIDS and Drugs*, brochure of information about AIDS and drugs; *AIDS: What Everyone Needs to Know*, brochure of brief facts about AIDS; *Women and AIDS*, brochure of information for women about AIDS; *NCFAN Newsletter*
LANGUAGES: Spanish, French, American Sign Language

233. Okaloosa County Public Health Unit
221 Hospital Dr NE
Fort Walton Beach, FL 32548
(904) 244-5175
KEY PERSONNEL: Peggy A Collins; Nursing Director
AFFILIATION: Florida Dept of Health and Rehabilitative Services
FACILITY TYPE: Health department
STAFF: Paid professional 56
FUNDING: State government; Local government
OUTREACH: Community programs on request
LANGUAGES: French, Spanish

234. Planned Parenthood Association of Southwest Florida, Naples Chapter
900 5th Ave N
Naples, FL 33940
(813) 262-8441
KEY PERSONNEL: Nancy Bearss; Chapter Director
AFFILIATION: Planned Parenthood Federation of America (PPFA)
FACILITY TYPE: Educational; Clinic; Fund-raising
STAFF: Paid professional 14; Volunteers 4
YEAR FOUNDED: 1975
FUNDING: Federal government; Private; Fund-raisers; Fees for services or products
OUTREACH: Educational outreach program includes going door-to-door in minority communities with brochures and condoms
NETWORKS: Southwest Florida AIDS Task Force; Collier County AIDS Task Force

SEMINARS: Sep 1, 1987—"AIDS and Adolescents;" Oct 1, 1987—"AIDS and You;" Sep 15, 1988—"AIDS and Adolescents"
ADDITIONAL INFO: Provides reproductive health care and family planning which includes pregnancy testing and counseling, pelvic exams, pap smears, screening and treatment for STDs, birth control information and supplies
AVAILABLE LITERATURE: *I'm Glad I Found Them: It Makes Sense,* a brochure about the agency; *Planned Parenthood of Southwest Florida/Naples Chapter,* a quarterly newsletter
LANGUAGES: Spanish, Creole

235. Saint Lucie County Public Health Unit (SLCPHU)
714 Ave C
Fort Pierce, FL 34954
(407) 468-3945
KEY PERSONNEL: Carl Blair; STD Supervisor
AFFILIATION: Florida State Dept of Health and Rehabilitative Services
FACILITY TYPE: Clinic; Support group; HIV counseling and testing
STAFF: Paid professional 35; Paid nonprofessional 12
YEAR FOUNDED: 1947
FUNDING: Federal government; State government; Local government; Fees for services or products
OUTREACH: Literature to community centers, bars, and other locations, educational programs for worksites, schools, and community groups
NETWORKS: Saint Lucie School Board; AIDS Task Force
RESEARCH: Follow-up of heterosexual HIV positives for behavior modification
ADDITIONAL INFO: Provides anonymous and confidential HIV counseling and testing. The agency's main objective is educating schools, county workers, teachers, health aides, administrators, and counselors
LANGUAGES: Creole, Spanish

236. State of Florida Dept of Health and Rehabilitative Services, AIDS Program Office, District II
401 NW 2nd Ave, Ste S-811
Miami, FL 33128
(305) 252-AIDS; Anonymous Testing: (305) 325-1234; Case Reporting: (305) 324-2491
KEY PERSONNEL: Jeanne Easton; Senior Human Services Program Manager/AIDS
AFFILIATION: Florida Dept of Health and Rehabilitative Services
FACILITY TYPE: Research; Educational; Clinic; Support group; HIV counseling and testing
STAFF: Paid professional 14; Paid nonprofessional 5
FUNDING: Federal government; State government; Fees for services or products
OUTREACH: Educational seminars for all groups with an emphasis on Haitians, Blacks, and Latinos, and to high schools and health departments
NETWORKS: South Florida AIDS Network
RESEARCH: Seroprevalence in clinic populations/women and children
AVAILABLE LITERATURE: *Prevention Views,* a newsletter; buttons and bumper stickers; Creole posters; distributes materials from other agencies
LANGUAGES: Spanish, French, Creole

237. Tallahassee AIDS Support Services (TASS)
PO Box 14365
Tallahassee, FL 32317
(904) 656-AIDS
KEY PERSONNEL: Ginny Robson; Executive Director
AFFILIATION: Florida AIDS Coalition for Education and Support (FACES)
FACILITY TYPE: Educational; Support group; Fund-raising
STAFF: Paid professional 1; Volunteers 70
YEAR FOUNDED: 1985
FUNDING: State government; Local government; Fund-raisers
OUTREACH: Speakers bureau, education for health care professionals, students, churches, businesses, civic groups, minorities, and any other requesting group
ADDITIONAL INFO: Provides a support group for immunosuppressed persons and one for family, friends and health care workers. The major goal of TASS is to provide services and support to persons with AIDS or to anyone with AIDS-related concerns. Provides buddies for PWAs

AVAILABLE LITERATURE: *Tallahassee AIDS Support Services, Inc.,* a brochure describing the agency; publishes a monthly volunteer newsletter

238. Tampa AIDS Network (TAN)
PO Box 8333
Tampa, FL 33674-8333
(813) 221-6420
KEY PERSONNEL: Chuck Kuehn; President
AFFILIATION: National AIDS Network (NAN)
FACILITY TYPE: Educational; Support group
STAFF: Paid professional 2.5; Volunteers 100
YEAR FOUNDED: 1985
FUNDING: State government; Private; Fund-raisers
OUTREACH: Speakers bureau, outreach to Black and Hispanic communities, minority information and referral line
NETWORKS: Bay Area Community AIDS Response (BACAR); National AIDS Network (NAN)
ADDITIONAL INFO: This agency also provides a buddy program, food bank, limited financial assistance, and support groups.
AVAILABLE LITERATURE: Internal newsletter
LANGUAGES: Spanish

239. University of Miami, AIDS Clinical Research Unit (ACRU)
FORMER NAME: AIDS Project, University of Miami Medical School
1776 NW 10th Ave
Miami, FL 33136
(305) 549-7538
KEY PERSONNEL: Janie Reese; Director of Nursing, Protocol Coordinator
AFFILIATION: University of Miami Dept of Medicine
FACILITY TYPE: Research; Educational; Clinic; HIV counseling and testing
STAFF: Paid professional 27; Paid nonprofessional 26
YEAR FOUNDED: 1983
FUNDING: Federal government; State government; Fund-raisers; Donations
OUTREACH: AIDS education and information to concerned groups of people, social agencies, hospitals, therapeutic communities, and schools
NETWORKS: Comprehensive AIDS Program, University of Miami
SEMINARS: Feb 1989—"Comprehensive AIDS Update for Health Care Workers;" Sep 1989—"5th Annual AIDS Symposium"
RESEARCH: Heterosexual and household transmission study
ADDITIONAL INFO: Conducts research at various levels, maintains an HIV screening clinic, a drug protocol screening clinic, and an AZT clinic.
AVAILABLE LITERATURE: Currently preparing pamphlets, posters, and buttons
LANGUAGES: Spanish, Creole, French, German

GEORGIA

240. AID Atlanta
1132 W Peachtree St NW
Atlanta, GA 30309
(404) 872-0600; Infoline: (404) 876-9944; Toll-free: (800) 551-2728
KEY PERSONNEL: Buren W Batson, Jr; Executive Director
FACILITY TYPE: Educational; Support group; Fund-raising; Client services/case management
STAFF: Paid professional 25; Volunteers 525
YEAR FOUNDED: 1982
FUNDING: Federal government; State government; Local government; Fund-raisers
OUTREACH: Intake and needs assessment, buddies, practical support, transportation, support groups, meals on wheels, housing, AIDS health services, referral, info-line, speakers bureau, outreach to minorities and IV drug users, educational materials, AIDS awareness and action weekends, pastoral services
NETWORKS: Metropolitan Atlanta AIDS Educators Network; National AIDS Network (NAN); Coalition to Prevent Drug Abuse and AIDS; Atlanta AIDS Health Service Program; AIDS Action Council; Statewide Minority Advocacy Group for Drug and Alcohol Prevention (SMAGDAP)
SEMINARS: Jan 30-31, Mar 12-13, Jun 11-12, Aug 13-14, Oct 16-17, Nov 26-27, 1988—"AIDS Awareness Action Weekends"

ADDITIONAL INFO: AID Atlanta has one purpose: To respond to the AIDS epidemic with services to people with AIDS, their family and friends, and to educate everyone about this disease and its prevention. AID Atlanta's services are available to all who need them without regard to age, race, national origin, sex, sexual orientation, economic class or physical limitations

AVAILABLE LITERATURE: *AID Atlanta,* an informational brochure; *What is "The Test"?,* an informational brochure about the HIV antibody test; *Women and AIDS,* a brochure for women; *AIDS, Your Child and You,* a brochure of answers about children and AIDS; *Fight the Fear with Facts,* a flyer with telephone numbers to contact for additional information; *Journal of AID Atlanta,* a quarterly newsletter

LANGUAGES: Spanish

241. AIDS Coastal Empire (ACE) Foundation
PO Box 2442, c/o First City Network, Inc
Savannah, GA 31401
(912) 236-2489
KEY PERSONNEL: Mark Krueger; President
FACILITY TYPE: Educational; Support group; Fund-raising; Task force
STAFF: Volunteers 30
YEAR FOUNDED: 1985
FUNDING: Private; Fund-raisers
OUTREACH: Bi-monthly PWA/HIV positive support group, speakers bureau, disbursement of AIDS-related literature at gay/lesbian businesses
SEMINARS: 1987 and 1988—"AIDS 101," a 4-hour seminar for local health care providers
ADDITIONAL INFO: ACE is an all-volunteer organization that is devoted to supporting the best possible quality of life for persons in the Coastal Empire with AIDS
AVAILABLE LITERATURE: *ACE News: A Monthly Publication of the AIDS Coastal Empire Foundation,* a newsletter; *Health Crisis: Information for the Coastal Empire and Low Country—Acquired Immune Deficiency Syndrome (AIDS),* a brochure of AIDS information; *ACE Foundation,* a brochure describing the foundation; *Network News,* a newsletter of the First City Network, Inc

242. AIDS Program, Center for Infectious Diseases, Centers for Disease Control (CDC)
FORMER NAME: AIDS Activity
1600 Clifton Rd
Atlanta, GA 30333
Toll-free: (800) 342-AIDS
KEY PERSONNEL: Peter Drotman; Administrator
AFFILIATION: US Public Health Service
FACILITY TYPE: Research; Educational
STAFF: Paid professional 130
YEAR FOUNDED: 1981
FUNDING: Federal government
RESEARCH: Epidemiology, prevention, and laboratory diagnosis
AVAILABLE LITERATURE: *Morbidity and Mortality Weekly Report*

243. The Atlanta Gay Center, Inc
63 12th St NE
Atlanta, GA 30309
(404) 876-5372; Helpline: (404) 892-0661
KEY PERSONNEL: William S. Gripp; Chairperson of Board of Directors
FACILITY TYPE: Research; Educational; Clinic; Support group; Fundraising; Advocacy
STAFF: Paid professional 1; Volunteers 100
YEAR FOUNDED: 1976
FUNDING: State government; Local government; Private; Fund-raisers; Fees for services or products
ADDITIONAL INFO: This is a gay and lesbian facility that provides services for all gays and lesbians and information to the general public.
AVAILABLE LITERATURE: *Volunteer Opportunities and Community Resources at the Atlanta Gay Center,* a pamphlet describing the organization; *What Do Those Gay People Want, Anyway?,* an informational brochure about gays; *Homophobia and Anti-Gay/Lesbian Violence,* a brochure describing anti-gay/lesbian violence; *I Took the Text, It Was Positive, What Do I Do Now?,* a brochure for those who test positive; *The News,* a biweekly newspaper serving the lesbian and gay communities of Atlanta

244. Central City Network/Macon
PO Box 6452
Macon, GA 31211
(912) 742-2437
KEY PERSONNEL: Kathy Dillard

245. Clayton County Substance Abuse Program
853 Battlecreek Rd
Jonesboro, GA 30236
(404) 991-0111
KEY PERSONNEL: Thomas D Earles; Physician
FACILITY TYPE: HIV counseling and testing; Substance abuse treatment

246. Coastal Area Support Team, Inc (CAST)
PO Box 2356
Brunswick, GA 31521-2111
(912) 264-2111
KEY PERSONNEL: Andrea Humphries; Vice Chairperson
FACILITY TYPE: Educational; Support group
STAFF: Volunteers 42
YEAR FOUNDED: 1988
FUNDING: State government; Fund-raisers
OUTREACH: Speakers for schools, churches, and community organizations
ADDITIONAL INFO: CAST was founded in response to increasing incidence of AIDS in coastal Georgia. As the agency grows it will develop telephone crisis lines, speakers bureau, education and prevention, and treatment
AVAILABLE LITERATURE: Newsletter, buttons, and pamphlets in preparation
LANGUAGES: Spanish, American Sign Language

247. DeKalb County Board of Health
440 Winn Way
Decatur, GA 30030
(404) 294-3796
KEY PERSONNEL: Alan J Sievert; Director of the Division of Physical Health
AFFILIATION: Georgia Dept of Human Resources
FACILITY TYPE: Clinic; HIV counseling and testing
FUNDING: State government; Local government; Fees for services or products
OUTREACH: Provides counseling, HIV testing, and health education services for clinic patients, schools, and community organizations
RESEARCH: Sexually transmitted diseases
AVAILABLE LITERATURE: Newsletter for employees; pamphlets for patient use

248. Georgia Dept of Human Resources, Division of Public Health, Office of Infectious Disease, AIDS Project
878 Peachtree St NE, Rm 109
Atlanta, GA 30309
(404) 894-5304; Toll-free: (800) 551-2728
KEY PERSONNEL: Jane C Carr; Acting Director
FACILITY TYPE: Health department
OUTREACH: Counseling and testing, health education and training, laboratory, planning, seroprevalence, special studies, surveillance

249. Laurens County Health Department/South Central Health District
2121 Bellevue Rd
Dublin, GA 31021
(912) 272-2051; Hotline: (912) 275-AIDS
KEY PERSONNEL: George W Patterson; District Health Director
AFFILIATION: Georgia State Government
FACILITY TYPE: Educational; Clinic; Task force
STAFF: Paid professional 100
FUNDING: State government; Local government
OUTREACH: AIDS education in schools, civic organizations, colleges, private business, governmental offices, and general public

250. National Association of People With AIDS Atlanta Chapter (NAPWA Atlanta)
1132 W Peachtree St NW, Ste 106
Atlanta, GA 30309
(404) 874-7926
KEY PERSONNEL: Kurt Rahn; Executive Director

AFFILIATION: National Association of People With AIDS (NAPWA)
FACILITY TYPE: Educational; Support group; Fund-raising; HIV counseling and testing; Client services/case management
STAFF: Paid nonprofessional 3; Volunteers 25
YEAR FOUNDED: 1987
FUNDING: Private; Fund-raisers; Fees for services or products
OUTREACH: Legal issues clinic, research and drug information library, insurance issues, peer counseling
NETWORKS: National Association of People With AIDS (NAPWA); Southeastern Arts, Media and Education Project (SAME)
ADDITIONAL INFO: Holds regular weekly meetings to provide information of interest to PWAs, PWARCs and HIV positive individuals and their friends. Co-sponsors the local PWA play project "Higher Ground" with SAME and Rebekah Ransom
AVAILABLE LITERATURE: *Alive and Aware*, a newsletter
LANGUAGES: Spanish

251. New Start Residential Substance Abuse Treatment Program
138 Douglas St SE
Atlanta, GA 30317
(404) 527-3994
KEY PERSONNEL: Razikiwe Adisa; Director
FACILITY TYPE: HIV counseling and testing; Substance abuse treatment

252. Social Security AIDS Regional Office IV
PO Box 1684, 101 Marietta Tower, Ste 2001
Atlanta, GA 30301
(404) 331-2475
KEY PERSONNEL: Bruce Garner, Field Services Specialist
FACILITY TYPE: Educational
ADDITIONAL INFO: Fast-track system assures priority handling of cases involving AIDS
AVAILABLE LITERATURE: Newsletter

253. Spalding County Health Dept
PO Box 129, Magnolia Dr
Griffin, GA 30224
(404) 227-5588
KEY PERSONNEL: Jim Morgan, RN
AFFILIATION: Georgia State Dept of Human Resources
FACILITY TYPE: Clinic; HIV counseling and testing; Health department
STAFF: Paid professional 7
YEAR FOUNDED: 1930
FUNDING: State government; Local government; Fees for services or products
OUTREACH: STD clinic, AIDS information, general public health information
ADDITIONAL INFO: Provides AIDS counseling and HIV testing along with other STD services
AVAILABLE LITERATURE: Educational materials and pamphlets

HAWAII

254. Big Island AIDS Project
FORMER NAME: AIDS Helpline
75-5766 Kuakini Hwy, Ste 101
Kailua-Kona, HI 96740
(808) 969-6626
FACILITY TYPE: Support group; HIV counseling and testing; Information line; Alternative therapies
STAFF: Volunteers
ADDITIONAL INFO: Recorded message gives telephone numbers of various confidential testing facilities around the island and information on experimental drugs for treatment of AIDS. Also provides telephone numbers of several local support groups for PWAs, PWARCs, and HIV-positive asymptomatic individuals

255. Gay Community Center (GCC)
FORMER NAME: Sexual Identity Center
PO Box 3224, 1154 Fort Street Mall, Ste 415
Honolulu, HI 96801
(808) 536-6000; Gay Information Service: (808) 926-1000
KEY PERSONNEL: William E Woods; Executive Director
FACILITY TYPE: Educational; Support group; Fund-raising; Task force; HIV counseling and testing
STAFF: Volunteers 86

YEAR FOUNDED: 1973
FUNDING: Fund-raisers; Donations
OUTREACH: Education to public and private schools on sexual orientation and AIDS
NETWORKS: AIDS Task Group; AIDS Task Force; ACCT-AIDS Community Care Team
SEMINARS: Aug 1988—"Burnout Workshop for AIDS Care Givers;" Oct 1988—"Statewide AIDS Conference"
ADDITIONAL INFO: Interested in working with representatives of public policy making units to educate them on AIDS and the appropriate use of the various resources that are available. Conducts AIDS education programs
AVAILABLE LITERATURE: *Gay Community News*, a newsletter

256. Hawaii AIDS Task Group (HATG)
FORMER NAME: AIDS Task Group
1951 East-West Rd
Honolulu, HI 96822
(808) 948-7400
KEY PERSONNEL: Milton Diamond; Director
AFFILIATION: Pacific Center for Sex and Society
FACILITY TYPE: Research; Educational; Task force
STAFF: Paid professional 1; Volunteers 10
YEAR FOUNDED: 1985
FUNDING: Federal government; Private
SEMINARS: Aug 26, 1988—"1st Annual AIDS Care Giving Retreat;" Nov 16, 1988—"AIDS Practical Applications for Health Care Providers"

257. Kauai District Health Office
3040 Umi St
Lihue, HI 96766
(808) 245-4495
KEY PERSONNEL: Art Tani; Health Educator
AFFILIATION: Hawaii State Dept of Health
FACILITY TYPE: HIV counseling and testing; Health department
STAFF: Paid professional 109
YEAR FOUNDED: 1959
FUNDING: Federal government; State government
OUTREACH: AIDS education to community groups and organizations, free and anonymous HIV counseling, testing, and education
LANGUAGES: Hawaiian, Filipino, Ilocano, Tagalog

258. Life Foundation/Honolulu
PO Box 88980
Honolulu, HI 96830-8980
(808) 924-AIDS
KEY PERSONNEL: Sue Slavish, President; Michael Bridge, Client Services Director; Paul Landers, Educational Director
AFFILIATION: AIDS Foundation of Hawaii
FACILITY TYPE: Educational; Clinic
FUNDING: State government; Donations
OUTREACH: AIDS information line, speakers bureau, health care workers education, safer sex education, computerized AIDS information network
SEMINARS: Apr 4, 1986—"AIDS: Learning Together;" conducts an AIDS Awareness Month in Nov of each year
ADDITIONAL INFO: Founded in 1983 as an educational agency about AIDS and also maintains clinic services
AVAILABLE LITERATURE: Publishes a lifeline newsletter and provides a comprehensive educational packet

259. Malama Pono/Kauai AIDS Project
FORMER NAME: Kauai Shanti Project
PO Box 1500
Kapaa, HI 96746
(808) 822-0878 24 hours
KEY PERSONNEL: Dick Castilow; Executive Director
FACILITY TYPE: Educational; Client services/case management; Referral
STAFF: Paid professional 1; Volunteers 12
YEAR FOUNDED: 1986
FUNDING: Private
OUTREACH: Speakers bureau, panels for church groups, in-house presentation for residential recovery facilities, outreach efforts to IV drug users, media presentations, 24-hour hotline

ADDITIONAL INFO: Sponsors R&R program for primary care givers of AIDS patients. Arranges housing, transportation while on the island, and information on local resources. To date, over 40 people have taken advantage of this program, all of whom have been from the mainland. Application for program is available upon written request
LANGUAGES: Filipino dialects, Spanish, Hawaiian

260. Maui District Health Office, Hawaii State Dept of Health
54 High St
Wailuku, HI 92793
(808) 244-0336
KEY PERSONNEL: Joy Bridges; Epidemiology Specialist
AFFILIATION: Hawaii State Dept of Health
FACILITY TYPE: HIV counseling and testing; Health department
STAFF: Paid professional 1
FUNDING: Federal government
OUTREACH: Health educator available to speak to community groups, HIV antibody counseling and testing
AVAILABLE LITERATURE: Audiovisuals available for loan

261. Waikiki Health Center (WHC)
FORMER NAME: Waikiki Drug Clinic
277 Ohua Ave
Honolulu, HI 96815
(808) 922-4787; STD and AIDS Hotline: (808) 922-1313; Toll-free: (800) 321-1555
FACILITY TYPE: Educational; Clinic; HIV counseling and testing
STAFF: Paid professional 15; Paid nonprofessional 5; Volunteers 4
YEAR FOUNDED: 1967
FUNDING: State government; Local government; Private; Fees for services or products; Grants
OUTREACH: STD/AIDS educational talks at intermediate school, high school, and college, adult high risk, and general public, one-on-one education in medical clinic and HIV antibody clinic
ADDITIONAL INFO: WHC is an educational and medical clinic facility for drug users. Provides AIDS information and HIV antibody counseling and testing

IDAHO

262. Central District Health Dept
1455 N Orchard
Boise, ID 83706
(208) 375-5211; Hotline: (800) 833-AIDS ID only
KEY PERSONNEL: Linda Poulsen; Epidemiologist
AFFILIATION: Boise City Government
FACILITY TYPE: HIV counseling and testing; Health department
STAFF: Paid professional 103; Volunteers 1,004
YEAR FOUNDED: 1959
FUNDING: Federal government; State government; Local government; Fees for services or products
OUTREACH: Public information, educational or informational presentations for individuals, groups, or organizations
NETWORKS: Idaho AIDS Foundation; State of Idaho Bureau of Preventive Medicine
ADDITIONAL INFO: Provides testing, counseling, epidemiological and contact follow-up for HIV positive persons and persons with AIDS or ARC, medical and social service referral for individuals and families, educational and informational presentations, consultation with individuals, groups or organizations on AIDS-related issues, screening physicals on HIV positive individuals upon request
LANGUAGES: Spanish

263. Idaho AIDS Foundation
PO Box 421
Boise, ID 83701-0421
(208) 345-2277
KEY PERSONNEL: Robert C. Cross; Interim Executive Director
FACILITY TYPE: Educational; Support group; Fund-raising; Task force
STAFF: Paid professional 0.5; Volunteers 35
YEAR FOUNDED: 1985
FUNDING: Federal government; Private; Fund-raisers
OUTREACH: Speakers bureau, counseling, materials, buddy program, support groups for HIV positive, families, friends, and caregivers, financial support for PWAs
NETWORKS: WAMI AIDS Project; Hispanic AIDS Project; Idaho AIDS Program

SEMINARS: Jan, 1988—"AIDS and Children;" Oct, 1988—"AIDS Awareness Month;" Jul, 1988—"AIDS and Public Education;" May, 1989—"AIDS Information for Health Care Providers"
ADDITIONAL INFO: This foundation was established by members of gay and non-gay communities to provide education and social services to PWAs, PWARCs, HIV-positive and their loved ones.

264. Idaho AIDS Program, Dept of Health and Welfare
450 W State St, Bureau of Preventive Medicine
Boise, ID 83720
(208) 334-5937; Toll-free: (800) 833-AIDS
KEY PERSONNEL: Laurie Fitzpatrick: Health Education Specialist
AFFILIATION: Idaho State Government
FACILITY TYPE: Educational
STAFF: Paid professional 1
FUNDING: Federal government
OUTREACH: Educational resources, speakers bureau, training workshops
SEMINARS: Mar 1989—"AIDS in the Workplace;" Oct 1989—"AIDS Counseling and Training"
AVAILABLE LITERATURE: *AIDS: the Facts*, a brochure; *Learn About AIDS, You Can Help Stop It*, a poster; *Idaho Women and AIDS*, a brochure for women; *Should I be Tested Prior to Marriage*, a brochure describing the HIV test; *No One Can Afford to Ignore AIDS*, a poster

265. Southwest District Health Dept (SWDHD)
PO Box 489, 920 Main
Caldwell, ID 83606
(208) 459-0744
KEY PERSONNEL: Mary Murphy, RN
AFFILIATION: Idaho State Government
FACILITY TYPE: Educational; Clinic; HIV counseling and testing; Health department
STAFF: Paid professional 8; Paid nonprofessional 6
FUNDING: Federal government; State government; Local government; Fees for services or products
OUTREACH: Speakers bureau, support services to school education programs, aid in developing curricula for AIDS education in public schools
NETWORKS: National Family Planning
ADDITIONAL INFO: Serves the counties of Payette, Washington, Adams, Gem, Canyon, and Owyhee. SWDHD's main service is HIV counseling and testing and AIDS/HIV epidemiology. Gives presentations to schools, groups, and treatment centers
AVAILABLE LITERATURE: Distributes information produced by other agencies

ILLINOIS

266. AIDS Care Network
FORMER NAME: Rockford Area AIDS Task Force
401 Division St
Rockford, IL 61104
(815) 962-5092
KEY PERSONNEL: Jim Bailey; AIDS Program Coordinator
AFFILIATION: Winnebago County Dept of Public Health
FACILITY TYPE: Educational; Support group; Fund-raising; Task force; HIV counseling and testing
STAFF: Volunteers 12
YEAR FOUNDED: 1988
FUNDING: Fund-raisers
OUTREACH: Counseling, advocacy, buddy system
ADDITIONAL INFO: The health department provides other informational, counseling and testing services
LANGUAGES: Spanish

267. AIDS Foundation of Chicago (AFC)
2035 N Lincoln, Ste 619
Chicago, IL 60614
(312) 525-9466
KEY PERSONNEL: Marcia Lipetz; Executive Director
FACILITY TYPE: Fund-raising; Task force
STAFF: Paid professional 4; Paid nonprofessional 2
YEAR FOUNDED: 1985
FUNDING: Federal government; Private; Fund-raisers
OUTREACH: Professional education for service providing agencies
NETWORKS: National AIDS Network (NAN); AIDS Action Council

SEMINARS: Jan 1988—"Compliance Seminar on Illinois AIDS Laws;" Dec 1988—"Community Leaders' Conference for Staff and Volunteers of Non-AIDS Groups"
RESEARCH: Fund needs assessments as they are required to determine level of service, population served, access level
ADDITIONAL INFO: AFC is both a funding consortium, raising funds in the private sector for competitive distribution among agencies and acting as the lead agency for governmental collaborative programs, as well as an association of service providing agencies. There are now 48 organizations and institutions in the consortium.
AVAILABLE LITERATURE: *AIDS Foundation of Chicago*, a brochure describing the organization; *Action Bulletin*, a monthly newsletter for member agencies; *Frontiers*, a newsletter for press and contributors

268. American Medical Association (AMA)

535 N Dearborn
Chicago, IL 60610
(312) 645-5000
KEY PERSONNEL: John Henning; HIV/AIDS Coordinator
FACILITY TYPE: Educational; Professional
STAFF: Paid professional 750; Paid nonprofessional 350
YEAR FOUNDED: 1847
FUNDING: Dues
OUTREACH: Speakers bureau, publication of research
SEMINARS: All medically-related conferences are reported in the various journals published by the association
RESEARCH: All issues related to HIV/AIDS
ADDITIONAL INFO: Provides AIDS education to the public. AMA's journals provide information on all aspects of medicine
AVAILABLE LITERATURE: *AIDS: AIDS Action Plan and Activities*, a February 15, 1988 update; *American Medical News*, the news periodical of the association; *Journal of the American Medical Association*, the official journal of the association; publishes several other research journals in all areas of medical research
LANGUAGES: French, German, Spanish, Polish, Greek, Italian

269. Howard Brown Memorial Clinic (HBMC)

945 W George St
Chicago, IL 60657
(312) 871-5777
KEY PERSONNEL: Judith Johns; Executive Director
FACILITY TYPE: Research; Educational; Clinic; Support group; Fund-raising; HIV counseling and testing
STAFF: Paid professional 55; Volunteers 500
YEAR FOUNDED: 1974
FUNDING: Federal government; State government; Local government; Private; Fund-raisers; Fees for services or products; Donations; Grants
OUTREACH: Speakers bureau, risk reduction/safer sex meetings, advertising, distribution of AIDS-related posters and brochures, public forums
NETWORKS: AIDS Foundation of Chicago (AFC)
SEMINARS: Presents quarterly public forums on AIDS-related issues
RESEARCH: Research site for National Institutes of Health-funded Multi-center AIDS Cohort Study (MACS), CDC-funded Hepatitis B Prevalance Study, CDC-funded AIDS Epidemiological Study
ADDITIONAL INFO: Provides support services for PWAs, peer counselors, support groups for various individuals, buddies, case management, financial aid, legal aid, drop-in center, job bank, HIV counseling and testing, and STD testing and treatment.
AVAILABLE LITERATURE: *Support*, a quarterly newsletter for PWAs and support volunteers; *Wellspring*, a quarterly general circulation newsletter; *Diagnosis: Life*, a video tape featuring PWAs discussing the quality of their lives; distributes materials from other organizations
LANGUAGES: Spanish

270. Chicago Coalition of Black Lesbians and Gays (CCBLG)

5633 N Winthrop Ave, No 512
Chicago, IL 60660
(312) 878-7839
KEY PERSONNEL: Max Smith; Administrator
AFFILIATION: National Coalition of Black Lesbians and Gays (NCBLG)
FACILITY TYPE: Educational; Support group; Task force
STAFF: Volunteers 20
YEAR FOUNDED: 1979
FUNDING: Fund-raisers; Dues

OUTREACH: In-home rap groups, supports the safer sex club— Black Jack
SEMINARS: Nov 1987—"DuSable Museum Book Reading;" Oct 1 987—"National March on Washington;" Sep 1987—"NCBLG Conference," co-sponsor; Feb 1988—"Conference in Los Angeles"
RESEARCH: Some members are participants in the National Institutes of Health study at the Howard Brown Clinic
ADDITIONAL INFO: CCBLG organized the United Faith Affinitas Church of Chicago, which is similar to MCC, the AIDS information panels in Black gay bars which led to the formation of Kupona network and Black Jack, a Black safer sex club
AVAILABLE LITERATURE: *The Letter From Home*, a newsletter; *Black/Out*, a newsmagazine from the national office; *This Brochure Contains One Good Answer for Black Men Who Think Safe Sex Is Boring*, a brochure describing the activities of the Black Jack Club
LANGUAGES: Spanish

271. Chicago House and Social Service Agency, Inc

PO Box 14728
Chicago, IL 60614-0728
(312) 248-5200
KEY PERSONNEL: Thom Dombkowski; Executive Director
FACILITY TYPE: Support group; Residential facility (adults)
STAFF: Paid professional 8; Paid nonprofessional 2; Volunteers 150
YEAR FOUNDED: 1985
FUNDING: State government; Local government; Private; Fund-raisers; Fees for services or products
NETWORKS: AIDS Foundation of Chicago; National AIDS Network (NAN)
ADDITIONAL INFO: Owns and operates 3 housing sites with a total of 29 beds for PWAs and PWARCs. Provides linkage to support programs within the city
AVAILABLE LITERATURE: *Chicago House and Social Service Agency*, a newsletter; *Chicago House and Social Service Agency, Inc: A Special Place to Call Home in a Time of Need*, a brochure describing the facility; *Annual Report and Financial Statement*; *Chicago House: Making the Difference*, an informational packet
LANGUAGES: Spanish

272. Cook County Dept of Public Health (CCDPH)

1500 S Maybrook Dr
Maywood, IL 60153
(312) 865-6100
KEY PERSONNEL: Nancy Frank; AIDS Education Coordinator
FACILITY TYPE: Educational; Clinic; Task force; HIV counseling and testing; Health department
FUNDING: Federal government; State government
OUTREACH: AIDS information line, distribution of pamphlets and posters, testing and counseling, epidemiological follow-up, AIDS presentations, school curriculum, AIDS area network, education on AIDS in the workplace, professional education
SEMINARS: Mar 1988—"AIDS—Working with You;" May 1988—"Real Issues and Fears Concerning Health Care Workers;" Sep 1988—"Support Groups for PWAs and Their Families: Issues and Models"
AVAILABLE LITERATURE: *AIDS Prevention Programs and Services*, a flyer outlining the services of the department; *AIDS: Answers to Your Questions on AIDS*, a 1987 brochure of general AIDS information; *AIDS: Information on AIDS for Parents of School Age Children*, general AIDS information for parents; *AIDS: Importante Informacion Para Familias Latinas*, AIDS information for Latino families; *AIDS: Facts You Need for the 80s*, a brochure of AIDS information for young adults; *AIDS: Hechos que Usted Necesita Para los 80s*, a brochure of AIDS information for young adults; *How to Use a Rubber (Condom)*, a pocket card with a condom and instructions on how to use the condom; *Women...Is the AIDS Virus in Your Body?*, a flyer with information on AIDS for women; *Men...Is the AIDS Virus in Your Body?*, a flyer with information on AIDS for men; *IV Drug Users...Is the AIDS Virus in Your Body?*, a flyer of facts for IV drug users; *AIDS Virus Antibody Blood Test*, a flyer describing the test; *Testing: Who Should Be Tested?*, a poster; *Teaching About AIDS: Suggested Curriculum Content for Elementary and Intermediate Students*, a booklet of curriculum information; *Sexually Transmitted Diseases Including AIDS*, curriculum materials taken from the *Revised Sex Education Curriculum* for junior and senior high school students
LANGUAGES: Spanish

273. Cook County Hospital AIDS Service
FORMER NAME: Sable/Sherer Clinic
1835 W Harrison St
Chicago, IL 60612
(312) 633-5182
KEY PERSONNEL: David Seibert; Education Coordinator
AFFILIATION: Cook County Government
FACILITY TYPE: Research; Educational; Hospital; Clinic; Support group; HIV counseling and testing
STAFF: Paid professional 21; Paid nonprofessional 1; Volunteers 50
YEAR FOUNDED: 1983
FUNDING: Federal government; State government; Local government
OUTREACH: Speakers bureau
NETWORKS: AIDS Foundation of Chicago; Chicago Area AIDS Task Force; Chicago Comprehensive AIDS Prevention Education Program
RESEARCH: Surveillance of AIDS/ARC cases at Cook County Hospital, seroprevalence studies, knowledge and behavioral changes due to education and antibody testing, analysis of seropositives tested by the service
ADDITIONAL INFO: Provides inpatient and outpatient treatment of PWAs, PWARCs, HIV seropositives, and persons at risk of HIV infection. Provides AIDS education, HIV antibody counseling and testing, and support to those affected by HIV and their families, significant others, and friends
AVAILABLE LITERATURE: *AIDS Info: Facts You Should Know*, a brochure of general AIDS information; *Informacion Sobre el SIDA Verdades que ud. Debe Saber*, a Spanish-language flyer of general AIDS information; *AIDS and Drug Use: If You Shoot Drugs, Here's What You Should Know*, an informational brochure for IV drug users; *SIDA y el Uso de Drogas*, a Spanish-language brochure about drugs and IV drug use; *The HIV Antibody Test*, a flyer of information about the test; *El Examen de Anticuerpo HIV*, a Spanish-language flyer describing the test
LANGUAGES: Spanish

274. DuPage County Health Dept
111 N County Farm Rd
Wheaton, IL 60187
(312) 682-7400 x7310
KEY PERSONNEL: Bonnie Jane Adelman; AIDS/Family Planning/STD Coordinator
FACILITY TYPE: Educational; Clinic; HIV counseling and testing
STAFF: Paid professional 6
FUNDING: Federal government; State government; Local government; Private
OUTREACH: Educational programs for community groups, businesses, schools, and health care workers, speakers bureau, outreach to Hispanic community and other minority groups
ADDITIONAL INFO: Provides anonymous, free, confidential counseling and testing
LANGUAGES: Spanish, American Sign Language

275. Englewood Community Health Organization (ECHO)
945 W 69th St
Chicago, IL 60621
(312) 962-5600
KEY PERSONNEL: Anthony Cole; Program Manager, Alcohol/Substance Abuse Services
FACILITY TYPE: Educational; Clinic; Substance abuse treatment
STAFF: Paid professional 90; Paid nonprofessional 20; Volunteers 5
FUNDING: State government; Private; Fees for services or products
OUTREACH: General substance abuse prevention information and basic AIDS education and risk reduction information
NETWORKS: Westside Association and Substance Abuse Network (WASAN) of Chicago
RESEARCH: AIDS and Blacks
ADDITIONAL INFO: ECHO is a residential program for the chronically, mentally ill and substance abusers

276. Franklin-Williamson Bi-County Health Dept
Williamson County Airport
Marion, IL 62959
(618) 993-8111, 439-0951
KEY PERSONNEL: Pam Streuter; Health Educator
AFFILIATION: Southern Illinois AIDS Task Force
FACILITY TYPE: Educational; Clinic; Task force; HIV counseling and testing
YEAR FOUNDED: 1961
FUNDING: Federal government; State government; Local government

OUTREACH: Presentations to schools, school staff, health care workers, church groups, civic groups, general audiences; counseling and education to high risk groups
SEMINARS: Mar 16, 1988—"Workshop for School Teachers;" Mar 3, 1988—"Workshop for County School Administrators;" Jan 1, 1988—"Workshop for Schoolteachers/Principals"
ADDITIONAL INFO: This agency is an HIV counseling and testing site. Provides education at all levels to all groups
LANGUAGES: American Sign Language

277. Gay Community AIDS Project (GCAP)
PO Box 713
Champaign, IL 61820
(217) 337-2928; Hotline: (217) 351-AIDS
KEY PERSONNEL: Bob Browne; Grant Project Administrator
AFFILIATION: Champaign-Urbana Public Health Dept
FACILITY TYPE: Educational; Support group; Fund-raising; Task force
STAFF: Paid nonprofessional
YEAR FOUNDED: 1985
FUNDING: Federal government; State government; Private; Fund-raisers
OUTREACH: Buddy program, speakers bureau, wellness workshops, home callers
NETWORKS: National AIDS Network (NAN); AIDS Action Council; Gay Men's Health Crisis; San Francisco AIDS Foundation (SFAF)
ADDITIONAL INFO: GCAP's objective is to ascertain and express gay community concerns regarding AIDS issues, to educate both gay and non-gay persons about AIDS, to provide support services for persons with AIDS and others adversely affected by AIDS, and to work with other groups and agencies which are dealing with AIDS issues
AVAILABLE LITERATURE: *GCAPsule*, newsletter; 16 fact sheets/brochures are available
LANGUAGES: Spanish, German

278. Hemophilia Foundation of Illinois
332 S Michigan Ave, Ste 812
Chicago, IL 60604
(312) 427-1495
KEY PERSONNEL: Kenneth Schad; Acting Executive Director
FACILITY TYPE: Educational; Hospital; Clinic; Support group; Fund-raising
YEAR FOUNDED: 1949
FUNDING: Federal government; Private; Fund-raisers
OUTREACH: Legal counseling, medical advisory counseling, social workers, educational workshops
NETWORKS: National Hemophilia Foundation
SEMINARS: Nov 15, 1988—"Annual Symposia"
AVAILABLE LITERATURE: *Factor*, a quarterly newsletter; *Hemophilia*, an informational brochure about the foundation

279. Horizons Community Services, Inc
FORMER NAME: Gay and Lesbian Horizons
3225 N Sheffield
Chicago, IL 60657
(312) 472-6469; Gay and Lesbian Helpline: (312) 929-HELP; Toll-free Hotline: (800) AID-AIDS (IL only); Anti-Violence Hotline: (312) 871-CARE
KEY PERSONNEL: Bruce Koff; Executive Director
FACILITY TYPE: HIV counseling and testing; Social service agency
STAFF: Paid professional 8; Paid nonprofessional 7; Volunteers 250
YEAR FOUNDED: 1973
FUNDING: Federal government; State government; Local government; Private; Fund-raisers; Fees for services or products
OUTREACH: Gay and lesbian speakers bureau, youth outreach, AIDS/HIV counseling services, professional training and education
SEMINARS: "Lesbian Wellness Conference;" "Gay and Lesbian Identity Conference"
RESEARCH: Youth and AIDS/HIV
ADDITIONAL INFO: Purpose is to serve all of the gay and lesbian communities in the metropolitan Chicago area
LANGUAGES: Spanish

280. Illinois Alcoholism and Drug Dependence Association (IADDA), AIDS Project
859 W Wellington
Chicago, IL 60657
(312) 525-2798
KEY PERSONNEL: Bella H Selan; Director AIDS Project

FACILITY TYPE: Educational; Clinic
STAFF: Paid professional 2; Paid nonprofessional 2
YEAR FOUNDED: 1986
FUNDING: State government; Private
OUTREACH: Trains substance abuse professionals about AIDS, educates recovering substance abusers in treatment to become community AIDS ambassadors
NETWORKS: Chicago Area AIDS Task Force; Chicago AIDS Foundation; National AIDS Network (NAN); Medical Task Force; National Institute on Drug Abuse
SEMINARS: Numerous ongoing training sessions
RESEARCH: Attempting to trace recovering addicts who have graduated from AHAPA to see whether they relapse sooner or later than a matched control group without an AIDS mission
ADDITIONAL INFO: Addicts Helping Addicts Prevent AIDS (AHAPA) is conducted in 6 residential treatment programs of the Gateway Foundation and the Human Resource Development Institute. HIV Information Exchange and Support Group (HIVIES) was implemented by this agency and 6 of its provider members. These support groups are for persons with a substance abuse history
AVAILABLE LITERATURE: *SIDA Alerta: No Comparta Agujas si no Quiere SIDA*, a brochure of brief AIDS information; *Stop Sharing...*, a card for IV drug users; *If You Want Anonymous, Confidential Testing for HIV, the Virus that Can Cause AIDS...*, a card for anyone wanting HIV testing; *Then...Your Baby May be at Risk for AIDS*, a card for pregnant mothers; *Go Into Drug Treatment Now! Avoid AIDS*, a card urging drug treatment; *Are You at Risk for AIDS Infection?*, a card of questions; (all cards also available in Spanish) *Symptoms of AIDS and ARC*, a card with pictorial symptoms (also available in Spanish); *Social Security Card*, a card of safe sex tips; *AIDS Kills, Avoid Contamination*, a card showing how to clean needles; *Confused?*, a poster for anonymous testing and counseling; *The AIDS Pyramid: Where Do You Fit In?*, a poster of the stages of AIDS infection; *HIVIES is: Human Immunodeficiency Virus Information Exchange Support Group*, a poster showing where the group is located in Chicago; *This Pamphlet Will Not Give You AIDS*, a pamphlet describing AIDS and how you can and cannot become infected; *...Someone Who May Get AIDS From Using Drugs...*, a booklet for anyone who knows someone who is a drug user
LANGUAGES: Spanish

281. Kupona
4611 S Ellis Ave
Chicago, IL 60653
(312) 536-3000
KEY PERSONNEL: Tim Offutt
FACILITY TYPE: Educational; Support group; Client services/case management; Day care

282. Lake County Substance Abuse Program
2400 Belvidere
Waukegan, IL 60085
(312) 360-6770
KEY PERSONNEL: Nicholas R. Mayor; Program Director
FACILITY TYPE: HIV counseling and testing; Substance abuse treatment

283. Lee County Health Dept
144 N Court
Dixon, IL 61021
(815) 284-3371
KEY PERSONNEL: Peggy Meyer; Public Health Nurse
AFFILIATION: Lee County Government
FACILITY TYPE: Clinic; Health department
STAFF: Paid professional 6; Paid nonprofessional 9
YEAR FOUNDED: 1947
FUNDING: State government; Local government; Fees for services or products
OUTREACH: AIDS education

284. Midwest Hispanic AIDS Coalition (MHAC)/Coalicion Hispana Sobre el SIDA del Medioeste
1608 N Milwaukee Ave, Ste 912
Chicago, IL 60680
(312) 252-6888, 996-0034
KEY PERSONNEL: Aida L Giachello; Regional Coordinator
AFFILIATION: Hispanic Health Alliance
FACILITY TYPE: Research; Educational; Support group; Task force

STAFF: Paid professional 2; Paid nonprofessional 2
YEAR FOUNDED: 1988
FUNDING: Federal government; Dues
OUTREACH: Training and technical assistance to midwest organizations, health education workshops, regional group discussions, developing provider data bank, promoting collaboration among groups
RESEARCH: HIV infection and AIDS prevention and education
ADDITIONAL INFO: The Midwest Hispanic AIDS Coalition (MHAC) is a non-profit membership organization of Hispanic and non-Hispanic providers and consumers. The coalition addresses prevention and education issues in the areas of HIV infection and AIDS among Hispanics in Illinois, Michigan, Indiana, Wisconsin, Minnesota, Missouri and Ohio
AVAILABLE LITERATURE: *MHAC News*, a newsletter; *MHAC—Midwest Hispanic AIDS Coalition*, a brochure describing the agency
LANGUAGES: Spanish

285. Peoria City County Health Dept (PCCHD)
2116 N Sheridan Rd
Peoria, IL 61604
(309) 685-6181 x208
KEY PERSONNEL: Shellie Wilkes; STD Program Coordinator
AFFILIATION: Peoria City County Government
FACILITY TYPE: Educational; Clinic; HIV counseling and testing; Health department
STAFF: Paid professional 70; Paid nonprofessional 40; Volunteers 5
YEAR FOUNDED: 1942
FUNDING: State government; Local government; Fees for services or products
OUTREACH: Speakers bureau, distribution of AIDS information to the public, AIDS presentations to organizations and businesses, condom distribution
NETWORKS: Central Illinois Area AIDS Task Force
SEMINARS: Feb 3-4, 1988—"AIDS Education Training Workshop;" Apr 29, 1988—"6th Annual Conference on Advances in Sexually Transmitted Diseases and Reproductive Health"

286. The Reimer Foundation
606 W Barry, Ste 300
Chicago, IL 60657
(312) 935-SAFE
KEY PERSONNEL: Del Barrett; Chairman
FACILITY TYPE: Research; Educational; Fund-raising; Condom distribution
STAFF: Paid nonprofessional 6; Volunteers 87
YEAR FOUNDED: 1987
FUNDING: Federal government; State government; Local government; Private; Fund-raisers; Fees for services or products
ADDITIONAL INFO: The primary goal of this agency is to help in AIDS prevention through safer sex and the distribution of free condoms
AVAILABLE LITERATURE: Posters, pamphlets, cards, video spots, advertisements, and condom displays

287. St Mary's Alcohol/Drug Addiction Treatment Center
1800 E Lakeshore Dr
Decatur, IL 62521
(217) 429-2963
KEY PERSONNEL: Barbara H Hanson; Adminstrator
FACILITY TYPE: HIV counseling and testing; Substance abuse treatment

288. Social Security AIDS Regional Office V
300 S Wacker Dr
Chicago, IL 60606
(312) 353-7065
KEY PERSONNEL: Karen F Brach, Regional Public Affairs Director
FACILITY TYPE: Educational; Client services/case management; Financial assistance
ADDITIONAL INFO: A financial resource for persons with AIDS
AVAILABLE LITERATURE: Information on disability benefits for people with AIDS; *If You Become Disabled*, a 31-page booklet about Social Security benefits available to those who become disabled; *A Guide to Supplemental Security Income*

289. Southern Illinois AIDS Task Force
FORMER NAME: Jackson County AIDS Task Force
PO Box 307
Murphysboro, IL 62901

(618) 684-3143
KEY PERSONNEL: Sheila Patterson; AIDS Educator
AFFILIATION: Jackson County Health Dept
FACILITY TYPE: Task force
STAFF: Paid professional 1; Volunteers 17
YEAR FOUNDED: 1985
FUNDING: Federal government; State government
OUTREACH: A speaker's bureau of educational presentations on AIDS to schools, health care providers, and civic groups in a 3-county area
RESEARCH: AIDS education in schools, AIDS curriculum
ADDITIONAL INFO: Task force members are invited to present papers and talks at area conferences, workshops, and seminars as well as health fairs. They have produced educational modules on AIDS and psychosocial issues, AIDS and the first aiders, AIDS and Illinois legislation and have coordinated support groups for PWAs

290. Substance Abuse and Alcoholism Treatment Center, Inc
701-09 W Roosevelt Rd
Chicago, IL 60607
(312) 829-3002
KEY PERSONNEL: David Johnson; Director
FACILITY TYPE: HIV counseling and testing; Substance abuse treatment

291. Tazewell County Health Dept
RR 1, Box 15
Tremont, IL 61568-0015
(309) 925-5511, 477-2223
KEY PERSONNEL: Sarah Buller Fenton; Communicable Disease Coordinator
AFFILIATION: Tazewell County Government
FACILITY TYPE: HIV counseling and testing; Health department
STAFF: Paid professional 25; Paid nonprofessional 26
YEAR FOUNDED: 1971
FUNDING: State government; Local government; Fees for services or products; Donations
OUTREACH: HIV antibody counseling and testing, referral services, educational services to schools, general public, and special interest groups
NETWORKS: Central Illinois AIDS Task Force
LANGUAGES: German, American Sign Language

292. Test Positive Aware Network, Inc (TPA Network, Inc)
1340 W Irving Park, Ste 259
Chicago, IL 60613
(312) 728-1943; Hotline: (312) 728-1943
KEY PERSONNEL: Christopher S Clason; Executive Director
FACILITY TYPE: Educational; Support group
STAFF: Paid nonprofessional 1; Volunteers 50
YEAR FOUNDED: 1987
FUNDING: Local government; Private; Fund-raisers; Fees for services or products
OUTREACH: Fellowship meetings held every Tuesday and Friday evenings with guest speakers or group discussion on HIV issues
NETWORKS: Chicago Area AIDS Task Force; AIDS Foundation of Chicago; Illinois Media Task Force on AIDS
SEMINARS: Nov 1987—"Chicago AIDS Symposium," Executive Planning Committee; Mar 1989—"Self-Help and Life Threatening Conditions Symposium," Executive Planning Committee
ADDITIONAL INFO: TPA Network is a non-therapeutic support fellowship and information network for people impacted by HIV. The network has over 500 members from across the mid-west
AVAILABLE LITERATURE: *Looking for Positive Support?: Test Positive Aware Network*, a brochure describing the network; *TPA News*, a monthly newsletter; *Fact Sheet #1: Alternative Treatments*, an 11-page brochure describing the various alternative treatments; *Fact Sheet #2: Confidentiality*, a pamphlet discussing whom to tell when you are HIV positive; *Fact Sheet #3: Summary of Meeting Topics*, a calendar; *Fact Sheet #4: Directory of HIV Agencies*, a directory for the greater Chicago metropolitan area; *Fact Sheet #5: Public Aid and Social Security*, a guide for getting through the red tape with directories of Illinois Department of Public Aid Offices and Social Security offices in the Chicago area; *Fact Sheet #6: Physicians and Therapists Listing*, a referral list of physicians, dentists, and therapists; *Fact Sheet #7: TPA News Digest*, a collection of news stories from past *TPA News*
LANGUAGES: Spanish

293. University of Illinois at Chicago, AIDS Outreach Intervention Project
2121 W Taylor St, Rm 555
Chicago, IL 60612
(312) 996-5523
KEY PERSONNEL: Wayne Wiebel; Principal Investigator
AFFILIATION: University of Illinois at Chicago School of Public Health
FACILITY TYPE: Research
STAFF: Paid professional 14; Paid nonprofessional 12
YEAR FOUNDED: 1986
FUNDING: Federal government
OUTREACH: Outreach to active IV drug users and sex partners
NETWORKS: Illinois Alcoholism and Drug Dependence Association; Treatment Alternatives to Street Crime; Illinois Medical Referral; Cook County Hospital; Center for Addictive Problems
SEMINARS: Participates in worldwide conferences presenting results of the study
RESEARCH: Epidemiology of drug abuse and of infectious diseases; qualitative epidemiology; applied urban sociology and anthropology
AVAILABLE LITERATURE: *AIDS Prevention Outreach to IVDU's in Four U.S. Cities*, an informational brochure about a poster presentation for the IV International Conference on AIDS in Stockholm; *Needle Sharing Among Intravenous Drug Abusers: National and International Perspectives, NIDA Research Monograph 80*, pages 137-50, authored by W. Wayne Wiebel, entitled "Combining ethnographic and epidemiologic methods in targeted AIDS interventions: The Chicago Model;" *Patterns and Trends in Substance Abuse, Chicago, Illinois, June 1988*, a booklet describing the trends in Chicago
LANGUAGES: Spanish

INDIANA

294. AIDS Task Force, Inc
1208 E State Blvd
Fort Wayne, IN 46805
(219) 484-2711
KEY PERSONNEL: Jack Ryan; Executive Director
FACILITY TYPE: Educational; Support group; Hospice; Fund-raising; Task force
STAFF: Paid professional 2; Paid nonprofessional 1; Volunteers 400
YEAR FOUNDED: 1985
FUNDING: State government; Private; Fund-raisers
OUTREACH: Speakers bureau, interagency and corporate training
NETWORKS: Indiana Community Action Groups; National AIDS Network (NAN)
SEMINARS: Oct 1987—"AIDS Awareness Week;" Oct 1988—"Medical Society Seminar;" Dec 1988—"Community Seminar"
RESEARCH: Street people, hustlers, prostitutes, deaf students
ADDITIONAL INFO: Provides a library of 60 different video titles for education and various supporting books and brochures
AVAILABLE LITERATURE: *Monthly News Sheet*; 3 brochures available for distribution
LANGUAGES: Spanish, German, French

295. Bartholomew County Health Dept, Counseling and Testing Site
2400 17th St
Columbus, IN 47201
(812) 379-1555
KEY PERSONNEL: Heidi Heim, RN
AFFILIATION: Bartholomew County Government
FACILITY TYPE: Clinic; Task force; HIV counseling and testing; Health department
STAFF: Paid professional 2
YEAR FOUNDED: 1985
FUNDING: Local government
OUTREACH: Educate schools, businesses, and civic groups
NETWORKS: Indiana Community Action Group on AIDS

296. Damien Center
FORMER NAME: Bagladies, Inc
1350 N Pennsylvania
Indianapolis, IN 46202
(317) 632-0123
KEY PERSONNEL: I Michael Shuff; Executive Director
FACILITY TYPE: Research; Educational; Support group; Hospice; Task force; Client services/case management
STAFF: Paid professional 3; Volunteers 150
YEAR FOUNDED: 1987

FUNDING: Federal government; State government; Private; Fund-raisers

OUTREACH: Speakers bureau, interactive theater, consultation to developing AIDS groups in Indiana, liaison with prison system

NETWORKS: National AIDS Network (NAN)

RESEARCH: Volunteers utilization and demographics, issues affecting public policy

ADDITIONAL INFO: Formed in 1987 by the consolidation of AIDS service and education programs previously offered by the gay community, religious community, and health and human service providers. Provides AIDS education, counseling, and support

AVAILABLE LITERATURE: Publishes a newsletter and computer-generated information sheets

LANGUAGES: Spanish, American Sign Language

297. Evansville AIDS Task Force
111 N Spring St
Evansville, IN 47711
(812) 476-5437
KEY PERSONNEL: Larry Rowland

298. Evansville-Vanderburgh County Dept of Public Health
Civic Center Complex, Rm 127
Evansville, IN 47708
(812) 426-5692
KEY PERSONNEL: Jane Hoopes; County Health Officer
AFFILIATION: Evansville-Vanderburgh County Government
FACILITY TYPE: Clinic; HIV counseling and testing; Health department
FUNDING: Federal government; State government; Local government
OUTREACH: STD education, diagnosis and treatment, HIV testing and counseling, HIV referral
ADDITIONAL INFO: Provides tuberculosis clinic, public health nurses, communicable disease clinics, and environmental health programs

299. Gary Health Dept, Counseling and Testing Site
1145 W 5th Ave
Gary, IN 46402
(219) 885-5475
KEY PERSONNEL: Karen Richard; Public Health Advisor
AFFILIATION: Indiana State Government
FACILITY TYPE: Clinic; HIV counseling and testing
STAFF: Paid professional 8
YEAR FOUNDED: 1985
FUNDING: State government
OUTREACH: Presentations to the community on AIDS testing
ADDITIONAL INFO: This clinic provides free and anonymous counseling and testing for the HIV antibody test

300. Indiana State Board of Health AIDS Activity Office
1330 W Michigan St
Indianapolis, IN 46206
(317) 633-0851
KEY PERSONNEL: Dr Judith Johnson; Director, Division of Acquired Diseases
FACILITY TYPE: Health department

301. Justice, Inc
PO Box 2387
Indianapolis, IN 46278
(317) 634-9212
KEY PERSONNEL: Kent Robinson; Legislative Coordinator
FACILITY TYPE: Educational; Legal
STAFF: Paid nonprofessional 1; Volunteers 16
YEAR FOUNDED: 1981
FUNDING: Fund-raisers; Dues
OUTREACH: Distribute AIDS brochures, representation on local and statewide task forces and committees
SEMINARS: Sep 1988—"Together We Can...Strengthening Self and Community"
ADDITIONAL INFO: Lobbies state legislature on AIDS legislation and gay and lesbian rights
AVAILABLE LITERATURE: Quarterly newsletter; *What is AIDS?*, a brochure of AIDS facts; *What is the HIV Test?*, a brochure of information about the HIV test; *What is Safer Sex?*, a brochure about safer sex

302. Madison/Delaware County AIDS Task Force
PO Box 2111
Muncie, IN 47307
(317) 646-9206
KEY PERSONNEL: Donna Dodson; Co-Chairperson
AFFILIATION: Madison/Delaware County Government
FACILITY TYPE: Task force
STAFF: Volunteers 3
FUNDING: Private; Fund-raisers
OUTREACH: Speakers bureau, support groups, buddy system, financial support system
AVAILABLE LITERATURE: *Madison/Delaware County AIDS Task Force, Inc*, a brochure describing the services of the task force; *Play Safer*, a button; *Safer Sex Card*, a pocket card

303. Marion County AIDS Coalition
FORMER NAME: Indiana AIDS Task Force
1350 N Pennsylvania St, Damien Center
Indianapolis, IN 46202
(317) 929-3466
KEY PERSONNEL: Carolyn Sanders, Director
AFFILIATION: Association for Practitioners in Infection Control (APIC)
FACILITY TYPE: Educational; Support group; Task force
FUNDING: Donations
OUTREACH: Provides educational programs, buddy support, counseling, and errand assistance
ADDITIONAL INFO: Founded in 1983 as an educational community service
AVAILABLE LITERATURE: Distributes publications from other agencies

304. Project AIDS Lafayette, Inc (PAL)
FORMER NAME: Dignity/Lafayette AIDS Task Force
PO Box 5375, 810 North St
Lafayette, IN 47903
(317) 742-2305; Hotline: (317) 742-2305
KEY PERSONNEL: John M Roach; Director
FACILITY TYPE: Educational; Support group; Task force
STAFF: Paid professional 1; Volunteers 18
YEAR FOUNDED: 1985
FUNDING: Private; Fund-raisers; Donations
ADDITIONAL INFO: Founded by Dignity/Lafayette, Inc. Offers support, referral, information, educational programs, buddy support, and positive support to individuals and groups regardless of race, color, creed, handicap, sex, or sexual orientation
AVAILABLE LITERATURE: *Services Provided by Project AIDS Lafayette, Inc.*, a flyer describing the services of PAL; *Project AIDS Lafayette A Caring Community Newsletter*, a newsletter

305. Tecumseh Area Planned Parenthood Association, Inc (TAPPA), AIDS Counseling and Testing Program
PO Box 1159, 1016 E Main St
Lafayette, IN 47902
(317) 742-7281
KEY PERSONNEL: Betty Memmer; Counselor
FACILITY TYPE: Educational; Clinic; HIV counseling and testing
STAFF: Paid professional 1.5; Volunteers 2
YEAR FOUNDED: 1987
FUNDING: State government; Private; Fund-raisers; Fees for services or products
OUTREACH: Education and training programs covering all aspects of AIDS and AIDS prevention
NETWORKS: Community AIDS Resource Association (CARA)
ADDITIONAL INFO: Provides free, anonymous HIV counseling and testing to all persons who request the test
AVAILABLE LITERATURE: *The Adventures of the Amazing Mr. Condom*, a comic strip in the Purdue *Exponent*; *AIDS: Don't Play the Game*, a 30-second TV health message; *AIDS: Don't Play the Game*, a brochure with facts about AIDS; *AIDS: Don't Play the Game*, a card for the agency; *Mr. Condom*, a condom (2-pack)

306. Terre Haute AIDS Task Force
201 Cherry St
Terre Haute, IN 47807
(812) 238-8431
KEY PERSONNEL: P Ekstrom; Public Health Communicable Disease Coordinator
FACILITY TYPE: Task force
YEAR FOUNDED: 1986
FUNDING: Private
OUTREACH: Educational presentations

IOWA

307. AIDS Coalition of Northeast Iowa
2530 University Ave
Waterloo, IA 50701
(319) 234-6831
KEY PERSONNEL: Angie Turner; Administrator
FACILITY TYPE: Educational; Support group
STAFF: Volunteers 60
YEAR FOUNDED: 1986
FUNDING: State government
OUTREACH: Present programs to students, community groups and worksites
SEMINARS: Apr 21, 1988—"AIDS: A Look to the Future"
ADDITIONAL INFO: Provides support for PWAs and their families. The coalition has compiled an in-house AIDS resource manual which lists the various services available to PWAs
AVAILABLE LITERATURE: Publishes a quarterly newsletter

308. AIDS Education Committee, Gay Coalition of Des Moines
PO Box 851
Des Moines, IA 50304
(515) 279-2110
KEY PERSONNEL: Allen Vander Linden

309. AIDS Support Group of Quad Cities
Box 4095
Davenport, IA 52808
(319) 322-1563

310. Central Iowa AIDS Project (CIAP)
2116 Grand Ave
Des Moines, IA 50312
(515) 244-6700
KEY PERSONNEL: Nancy Mosman; Chairperson
FACILITY TYPE: Educational
STAFF: Volunteers 110
YEAR FOUNDED: 1985
FUNDING: Federal government; State government; Donations
OUTREACH: Speakers Bureau
NETWORKS: Oct 12-14, 1988—"Central Iowa AIDS Project Conference on HIV and AIDS"
ADDITIONAL INFO: CIAP serves as a networking agency to identify needs and develop direct services to meet those needs. Urges member organizations to take on the responsibility for providing those services once they are developed

311. Hospice of Central Iowa (HCI)
3609 Douglas Ave
Des Moines, IA 50310
(515) 274-3400
KEY PERSONNEL: Kate Colburn; Executive Director
FACILITY TYPE: Educational; Hospice
STAFF: Paid professional 2; Volunteers 264
YEAR FOUNDED: 1978
FUNDING: Federal government; State government; Private; Fund-raisers; Fees for services or products; Grants
OUTREACH: Trains healthcare professionals for working with PWAs, trains people on death, dying and grief
NETWORKS: Central Iowa AIDS Project
SEMINARS: Oct 7, 1987—"Managing Services to People with AIDS;" Mar 31, 1988—"A Day with Hospice"
RESEARCH: Grief issues of survivors of PWAs
AVAILABLE LITERATURE: *Focus on Hospice, Heartline*

312. ICON PWA Fund
711 Navajo St
Council Bluffs, IA 51501
(712) 366-1791
KEY PERSONNEL: Don Randolph

313. Iowa Center for AIDS/ARC Resources and Education (ICARE)
PO Box 2989
Iowa City, IA 52244
(319) 338-2135
KEY PERSONNEL: Gayle Warner; Treasurer
AFFILIATION: United Way Agency
FACILITY TYPE: Educational; Support group; Fund-raising
STAFF: Volunteers 42
YEAR FOUNDED: 1987
FUNDING: Private; Fund-raisers; United Way; DIFFA; Broadway Cares
OUTREACH: Speakers bureau, legislative advisory, brochures and printed materials from other organizations
NETWORKS: National AIDS Network (NAN); National Association of Persons with AIDS (NAPA)
ADDITIONAL INFO: Provides support groups. ICARE is an all-volunteer organization with phone counseling, a buddy system, information on alternative treatment, and financial assistance

314. Iowa City Crisis Intervention Center
FORMER NAME: Johnson County AIDS Coalition
321 E 1st St
Iowa City, IA 52240
(319) 351-0140; Hotline: (319) 351-0140; Toll-free: (800) 798-2289 (IA only)
KEY PERSONNEL: Ken Kauppi; Acting Director
FACILITY TYPE: Educational; Support group
YEAR FOUNDED: 1970
FUNDING: Private
OUTREACH: Suicide prevention workshops, crisis intervention counseling skills workshops
NETWORKS: Johnson County AIDS Coalition
AVAILABLE LITERATURE: Maintains in-house training manuals

315. Iowa City Free Medical Clinic
120 N Dubuque St
Iowa City, IA 52245
(319) 337-4459
KEY PERSONNEL: Ann Rhomberg; HIV Testing Coordinator
FACILITY TYPE: Educational; Clinic; HIV counseling and testing
STAFF: Paid professional 4; Volunteers 200
YEAR FOUNDED: 1971
FUNDING: Federal government; Local government; Private; Fund-raisers; Fees for services or products
ADDITIONAL INFO: Provides free basic medical care for low-income persons and HIV antibody counseling and testing. The clinic is an alternate test site for the state of Iowa and provides anonymous testing
LANGUAGES: Spanish

316. Johnson County AIDS Project
1105 Gilbert Ct
Iowa City, IA 52240
(319) 356-6040
KEY PERSONNEL: Kot Flora; AIDS Program Coordinator
AFFILIATION: Johnson County Health Dept
FACILITY TYPE: Educational; Health department
STAFF: Paid professional 2
YEAR FOUNDED: 1968
FUNDING: Local government
OUTREACH: Educational programs targeted to specific groups

317. Quad Cities AIDS Coalition (QCAC)
605 Main St, Rm 224
Davenport, IA 52803
(319) 326-8618; Hotline: (319) 324-8638
KEY PERSONNEL: Danette Simons; Chairperson
FACILITY TYPE: Educational; Support group; Task force
STAFF: Volunteers 50
YEAR FOUNDED: 1986
FUNDING: State government; Donations
ADDITIONAL INFO: The Quad Cities AIDS Coalition consists of an education committee, a support committee, a publicity committee, and a board of directors. The committees were formed to better organize the QCAC's Health Education and Risk Reduction Program

AVAILABLE LITERATURE: *Quad Cities AIDS Coalition*, an informational brochure; *The Quad Cities AIDS Coalition Phone Line*, a flyer with telephone numbers; *Quad Cities AIDS Support Group*, an informational flyer with telephone numbers

KANSAS

318. Dodge City Family Planning Clinic, Inc
PO Box 1152, 307 Military
Dodge City, KS 67801
(316) 225-1933
KEY PERSONNEL: Twila M Helfrich, RN
AFFILIATION: Kansas Dept of Health and Environment
FACILITY TYPE: Clinic; HIV counseling and testing
STAFF: Paid professional 1; Paid nonprofessional 1
FUNDING: Federal government; Fees for services or products; Donations
OUTREACH: One-to-one counseling, speakers bureau
ADDITIONAL INFO: Provides counseling and testing for HIV antibodies. Gives forums in the surrounding towns
LANGUAGES: Spanish

319. Kansas AIDS Network, Inc (KAN)
PO Box 2728, 1115 W 10th, Ste 8
Topeka, KS 66601
(913) 357-7499; Toll-free: (800) 365-0219
KEY PERSONNEL: Phil D Jones; Executive Director
FACILITY TYPE: Research; Educational
STAFF: Paid professional 1
YEAR FOUNDED: 1985
FUNDING: State government; Local government; Private
OUTREACH: Speakers bureau, educational support
NETWORKS: National AIDS Network (NAN)
SEMINARS: Apr 1987, May 1988, May 1989—"Kansas Regional AIDS Conference"
RESEARCH: Knowledge, attitudes, beliefs, and behaviors for targeted groups, physican survey
ADDITIONAL INFO: This agency is a resource referral network for persons with HIV infections, across the state of Kansas including physicians, dentists, legal assistance, hospice, home health, hospitals, counseling, and education. KAN's purpose is to educate the citizens of Kansas. Distributes free condoms
AVAILABLE LITERATURE: *Network News*, a newsletter; *Safer-Sex Guidelines*, a safer sex card for the wallet; *Facts About AIDS*, an informational brochure; *KAN Brief*, a weekly statistical update
LANGUAGES: American Sign Language

320. Office of Health and Environmental Education, Kansas Dept of Health and Environment
Landon State Office Bldg
Topeka, KS 66620
(913) 296-1216
KEY PERSONNEL: Virginia Lockhart; Director
FACILITY TYPE: Educational
STAFF: Paid professional 4; Paid nonprofessional 6
FUNDING: Federal government; State government
OUTREACH: Consultation and workshops available to schools, community groups, correctional institutions, health care providers, day care centers, nursing homes, and worksites
NETWORKS: Kansas AIDS Network
ADDITIONAL INFO: Operates a 3000-item film and video lending library and a 3500-title literature distribution center. A catalog is available, but services are restricted to Kansas residents and agencies
LANGUAGES: Spanish, Southeast Asian

321. Topeka AIDS Project, Inc (TAP)
PO Box 118
Topeka, KS 66601
(913) 232-3100
KEY PERSONNEL: Lauren Corbett; Clinical Director
FACILITY TYPE: Educational; Support group; Hospice
STAFF: Paid professional 1; Paid nonprofessional 1
YEAR FOUNDED: 1985
FUNDING: State government; Local government; Private
OUTREACH: Speakers bureau, coordination of seminars and conferences
NETWORKS: National AIDS Network (NAN)

SEMINARS: Apr 1988—"Clergy and AIDS;" May 1988—"Regional VA Conference on AIDS;" Jun, 1988—"Kansas Association of Homes for the Aging Workshop/Seminar"
ADDITIONAL INFO: Offers clinical and educational programs. The clinical services are provided to PWAs, PWARCs, HIV positive individuals, and significant loved ones. The educational services are provided to corporations, professionals in health care, and community groups
AVAILABLE LITERATURE: *TAP Update*, a newsletter
LANGUAGES: Spanish, American Sign Language

322. Wichita AIDS Task Force (WATF)
PO Box 2652
Wichita, KS 67201
(316) 265-7994
KEY PERSONNEL: Linda Santiago, Director; Bret-Alan Hubbard
FACILITY TYPE: Support group; Task force
FUNDING: Donations; Grants
OUTREACH: Speakers bureau
NETWORKS: National AIDS Network; National AIDS Housing Caucus; AIDS Action Council
SEMINARS: Jul 24, 1987—"AIDS: A Woman's Issue"
ADDITIONAL INFO: Founded in 1986 to provide services to PWAs, PWARCs, and their significant others

KENTUCKY

323. AIDS Crisis Taskforce/Lexington
PO Box 11442
Lexington, KY 40575
(606) 281-5151
KEY PERSONNEL: Edwin Hackney

324. The Community Health Trust of Kentucky
PO Box 363
Louisville, KY 40201
(502) 634-1789; Gay/Lesbian Hotline: (502) 637-4342
KEY PERSONNEL: Roy Holladay; President
FACILITY TYPE: Educational; Support group; Hospice; Fund-raising
STAFF: Volunteers 50
YEAR FOUNDED: 1984
FUNDING: Private; Fund-raisers
OUTREACH: Safer sex seminars, speakers bureau
NETWORKS: AIDS Education Coalition of Jefferson County
ADDITIONAL INFO: The Community Health Trust maintains the Glade House (a hospice), provides psychological counseling, support groups for HIV positive individuals, social services for getting SSI/Medicaid, and an AIDS buddy system
AVAILABLE LITERATURE: *The Community Health Trust*, a brochure describing the agency
LANGUAGES: Spanish

325. Lexington Fayette County Health Dept (LFCHD)
650 Newtown Pike
Lexington, KY 40508
(606) 252-2371; Hotline: (606) 255-6152; Toll-free: (800) 654-AIDS (KY only)
KEY PERSONNEL: Sanford Joseph; AIDS Manager
AFFILIATION: Lexington Fayette Urban County Government
FACILITY TYPE: Educational; Clinic; Task force; HIV counseling and testing; Health department
STAFF: Paid professional 7
YEAR FOUNDED: 1985
FUNDING: State government; Local government
OUTREACH: Speakers bureau, resource literature for professional, para-professional, and gay groups
NETWORKS: Planned Parenthood; Home Health; University of Kentucky
SEMINARS: Provides various conferences for local health department staff, medical professional seminar through the AIDS Crisis Task Force (ACT Lexington)
RESEARCH: Social marketing of educational objectives
ADDITIONAL INFO: The AIDS program in Lexington, the first to institute anonymous testing in Kentucky, serves as a resource to the northeast Kentucky area

AVAILABLE LITERATURE: *HIV Antibody Counseling Guidelines for Health Care Personnel*, a brochure with guidelines on how to counsel those taking the HIV antibody test; *Antibody Testing*, a brochure that provides the most current information available about AIDS and HIV antibody testing
LANGUAGES: Spanish

326. Lexington Gay Services Organizations
PO Box 11471
Lexington, KY 40511
(606) 231-0335
FACILITY TYPE: Educational
ADDITIONAL INFO: Source of additional AIDS information

327. Northern Kentucky AIDS Task Force
401 Park Ave
Newport, KY 41071
(606) 491-6611
KEY PERSONNEL: Julane Simpson; AIDS Corrdinator
AFFILIATION: Northern Kentucky District Health Dept
FACILITY TYPE: Task force; HIV counseling and testing
YEAR FOUNDED: 1986
FUNDING: Federal government; State government
OUTREACH: AIDS education to community

328. Charles I Schwartz Chemical Dependency Treatment Center
420 S Broadway
Lexington, KY 40508
(606) 255-4268
KEY PERSONNEL: Jeanne Keen; Coordinator
FACILITY TYPE: HIV counseling and testing; Substance abuse treatment

LOUISIANA

329. Baton Rouge MCC/AIDS Project
Box 64996
Baton Rouge, LA 70896
Task Force: 929-8830; Hotline: (800) 342-AIDS
KEY PERSONNEL: Shar Wilkins

330. Central Louisiana AIDS Support Services (CLASS)
PO Box 12251, 1771 Elliott St, Ste B
Alexandria, LA 71315
(318) 443-5216; Hotline: (318) 443-5216
KEY PERSONNEL: Ron Saunders; Director
AFFILIATION: Louisiana AIDS Prevention and Surveillance Project
FACILITY TYPE: Educational; Support group; Task force
STAFF: Paid professional 1; Paid nonprofessional 1; Volunteers 18
YEAR FOUNDED: 1987
FUNDING: State government; Private; Fund-raisers
OUTREACH: Counseling for PWAs and loved ones, educational programs, buddy volunteers, referrals, and hotline
AVAILABLE LITERATURE: Distributes materials from other agencies
LANGUAGES: Spanish

331. Community Relief for People with AIDS
1940 Dauphine St
New Orleans, LA 70116
(504) 948-4568; 943-1460
KEY PERSONNEL: Al McNairn, Director
FACILITY TYPE: Support group
FUNDING: Donations
ADDITIONAL INFO: Established in 1985 to provide funds to PWAs for rent, food, medication, and utilities on an interim basis until their Social Security and Medicare starts

332. Desire Narcotic Rehab Center (DNRC) Inc Drug Free
3307 Desire Pkwy
New Orleans, LA 70126
(504) 945-8885
KEY PERSONNEL: Betty H Wilkerson; Program Coordinator
FACILITY TYPE: HIV counseling and testing; Substance abuse treatment

333. Foundation for Health Education
1219 Barracks St
New Orleans, LA 70116
(504) 928-2270
KEY PERSONNEL: Jim West
FACILITY TYPE: Educational
ADDITIONAL INFO: Source of additional AIDS information

334. Greater Louisiana Alliance for Dignity (GLAD)
PO Box 4523
Shreveport, LA 71104
(318) 222-4523; Hotline: (318) 222-4523
KEY PERSONNEL: Mical De Brow; President
FACILITY TYPE: Educational; Support group; Fund-raising
STAFF: Volunteers 20
YEAR FOUNDED: 1983
FUNDING: Fund-raisers; Donations
OUTREACH: Hotline, support groups for PWAs and families, educational programs

335. Immunological Support Program
5000 Hennessy Blvd
Baton Rouge, LA 70809
(504) 765-8917
KEY PERSONNEL: Libby Leinweber; Coordinator
AFFILIATION: Our Lady of the Lake Hospital
FACILITY TYPE: Educational; Hospital; Support group; Task force; HIV counseling and testing
STAFF: Paid professional 5
FUNDING: Fees for services or products
OUTREACH: Community awareness, pre- and post-test counseling, case management, St Anthony's Home for the homeless ill, family and significant other counseling, HIV testing, PWA counseling
AVAILABLE LITERATURE: *HIV AIDS ARC*, a brochure of general information about services provided to PWAs and PWARCs; *St. Anthon's Home*, a brochure describing the home; *The Baton Rouge AIDS Taskforce*, a flyer describing the task force; *Human Immunodeficiency Virus (HIV) Baton Rouge Community Resources*, a one-page directory; *St. Anthon's Home Philosophy*, a one-page flyer about the purpose of the home; *Common Sense About AIDS*, an AIDS awareness and prevention guide

336. Minority People AIDS Concerns/New Orleans
902 Felicity
New Orleans, LA 70130
(504) 529-2661
KEY PERSONNEL: Leonard Greene

337. New Orleans Health Dept, Delgado (STD) Clinic
320 S Claiborne Ave, 2nd Fl
New Orleans, LA 70112
(504) 525-0086; Information: (504) 525-1251; Main line: (504) 525-8594
KEY PERSONNEL: Gail A Thornton; Program Director
AFFILIATION: New Orleans City Government
FACILITY TYPE: Educational; Clinic; HIV counseling and testing
STAFF: Paid professional 19; Paid nonprofessional 6
YEAR FOUNDED: 1940
FUNDING: Federal government; State government; Local government
OUTREACH: AIDS education and risk reduction programs, diagnosis and treatment of all sexually transmitted diseases
ADDITIONAL INFO: Delgado Clinic serves as the primary care facility for the diagnosis and treatment of all STDs in New Orleans. Provides counseling and testing for the HIV virus
LANGUAGES: Spanish

338. NO/AIDS Task Force
PO Box 2616
New Orleans, LA 70176-2616
(504) 891-3732; Hotline: (504) 522-AIDS; Toll-free: (800) 99-AIDS-9 (LA only)
KEY PERSONNEL: Gretchen W Bosworth; Acting Executive Director
FACILITY TYPE: Educational; Task force
STAFF: Paid professional 7; Volunteers 500
YEAR FOUNDED: 1983
FUNDING: Federal government; Private; Fund-raisers
AVAILABLE LITERATURE: *NO/AIDS Task Force*, an informational card about the task force; *Newslive*, newsletter; educational brochures

339. Project Lazarus

PO Box 3616
New Orleans, LA 70177-3616
(504) 949-3609
KEY PERSONNEL: Katy Quigley; Project Administrator
FACILITY TYPE: Hospice; Residential facility (adults)
STAFF: Paid professional 3; Paid nonprofessional 8.5; Volunteers 49
YEAR FOUNDED: 1985
FUNDING: Private; Fund-raisers; Fees for services or products
OUTREACH: Community education
NETWORKS: Metropolitan AIDS Advisory Committee; New Orleans AIDS Task Force; New Orleans AIDS Project; Louisiana Joint Legislative AIDS Committee
ADDITIONAL INFO: Project Lazarus is a residential program for persons with AIDS or ARC who are rendered homeless because they can no longer live independently or whose family and friends can no longer house and assist them. The project's purpose is to provide a comfortable home-like atmosphere through which continuity of care is facilitated
AVAILABLE LITERATURE: *Someone I Love Has AIDS*, button; *Project Lazarus Statement of Purpose*, a flyer describing the agency; a program and policy manual and newsletter are in the planning stages
LANGUAGES: American Sign Language, Spanish

340. Terrebonne Parish Health Unit

PO Box 309, 600 Polk St
Houma, LA 70361
(504) 857-3601
KEY PERSONNEL: Linda Pellegrin; Nurse Supervisor
FACILITY TYPE: Clinic; Health department
STAFF: Paid professional 10; Paid nonprofessional 12
FUNDING: Federal government; State government; Local government; Fees for services or products

341. Tulane-LSU AIDS Clinical Trials Unit (ACTU)

FORMER NAME: Tulane-LSU AIDS Treatment Evaluation Unit (ATEU)
1430 Tulane Ave, Infectious Disease Setion
New Orleans, LA 70112
(504) 584-3605
KEY PERSONNEL: Jennifer L Istre; Project Coordinator
AFFILIATION: National Institutes of Health/National Institute of Allergy and Infectious Disease (NIH/NIAID)
FACILITY TYPE: Research; Educational; Hospital; Clinic
STAFF: Paid professional 32; Paid nonprofessional 11
YEAR FOUNDED: 1987
FUNDING: Federal government
OUTREACH: Focus is to provide access to alternative investigational treatments under the auspices of the NIH/NIAID AIDS clinical trials group, outreach and educational efforts are aimed at increasing patients and health care providers knowledge of clinical trials and HIV infection
NETWORKS: Delta Regional AIDS Education Training Center; Pediatric AIDS Program at Children's Hospital
SEMINARS: 1987—"AIDS Update," continuing education symposium aimed at Louisiana physicians and other health care providers; 1988—"WorldAIDS Day;" 1989—"Physicians Update Sympsium"
RESEARCH: Primary infection, opportunistic infection, pharmacokinetics of new drugs, biological res ponse modifiers
ADDITIONAL INFO: The Tulane-LSU ACTU was founded in January 1987 by the NIH and is one of 45 sites in a research network which comprises the AIDS Clinical Trials Group. More than 200 patients have been enrolled in investigational drug clinical trials within the first two years of funding, more than 5000 nationwide. The unit sponsors trials for a wide range of drugs and stages of infection. Interested parties are urged to call the ACTU office at (504) 584-3605 for an accurate list of available protocols.
AVAILABLE LITERATURE: *Update: A Quarterly Newsletter of the Tulane-LSU AIDS Clinical Trials Unit*
LANGUAGES: French, Spanish

MAINE

342. AIDS Action of Central Maine

2 Bates St, c/o Blais
Lewiston, ME 04240
FACILITY TYPE: Educational
ADDITIONAL INFO: Source of additional information on AIDS

343. The AIDS Project, Inc (TAP)

FORMER NAME: Gay Health Action Committee
22 Monument Square, 5th Fl
Portland, ME 04101
(207) 774-6877; Hotline: (800) 851-AIDS
KEY PERSONNEL: Robert Mitchell; Executive Director
FACILITY TYPE: Educational; Clinic; Support group; Fund-raising; Task force; HIV counseling and testing
STAFF: Paid professional 5; Volunteers 20
YEAR FOUNDED: 1983
FUNDING: Federal government; State government; Local government; Private; Fund-raisers; Fees for services or products
OUTREACH: Speakers bureau, eductional materials
ADDITIONAL INFO: Founded in 1983 as an educational agency, support group, and an HIV counseling and testing facility. Provides financial support services, counseling, and professional case managers
AVAILABLE LITERATURE: *The AIDS Project Newsletter; TAP Client Newsletter*
LANGUAGES: French

344. The Clinic

200 Main St
Lewiston, ME 04240
(207) 795-4357
AFFILIATION: Androscoggin Home Health Services
FACILITY TYPE: Educational; Clinic; HIV counseling and testing
STAFF: Paid professional 5; Paid nonprofessional 2
YEAR FOUNDED: 1978
FUNDING: Federal government; State government; Private; Fund-raisers; Fees for services or products
OUTREACH: Education to the medical community, high schools, various groups, and high risk individuals, street/clinic, disease intervention specialists available
ADDITIONAL INFO: STD screening clinic providing anonymous HIV counseling and testing. Maintains an information line and a GC screening program

345. Maine Dept of Human Services, Office on AIDS

State House Station 11
Augusta, ME 04333
(207) 289-3747; Toll-Free: (800) 851-2437 ME only
KEY PERSONNEL: Patrick Cote; Program Director
AFFILIATION: Maine State Government
FACILITY TYPE: Educational; HIV counseling and testing
YEAR FOUNDED: 1986
FUNDING: Federal government; State government
OUTREACH: Technical assistance for education programs, policy development, and other areas
NETWORKS: Maine Consortium for Health Professionals in Education; Maine AIDS Allinace
AVAILABLE LITERATURE: *AIDS: If Your HIV Antibody Test Results are Positive*, a brochure of what to do; *Condom Information*, a brochure of information about condoms and how to use them; *AIDS: Information About HIV Antibody Testing*, a brochure that describes the test; *AIDS: Am I at Risk?*, a brochure that is a self-assessment guide; *There's No AIDS Problem in Maine. Right?*, a newspaper pamphlet with AIDS facts and resource information; *Questions and Answers About Acquired Immune Deficiency Syndrome (AIDS)*, a 1987 booklet of questions and answers about AIDS; *AIDS Resource Listing of Materials*, a listing and description of various pamphlets, brochures, and booklets that are available from this agency and others throughout the United States

346. Maine Health Foundation, Inc

PO Box 7329
Portland, ME 04112
KEY PERSONNEL: Don Myer; President
FACILITY TYPE: Educational; Support group; Fund-raising
STAFF: Volunteers 15
YEAR FOUNDED: 1983
FUNDING: Federal government; State government; Private; Fund-raisers
ADDITIONAL INFO: This agency provides direct financial support to PWAs and PWARCs and locates other service organizations that provide additional support.

347. Maine Lesbian/Gay Political Alliance
PO Box 108
Yarmouth, ME 04096
FACILITY TYPE: Educational
ADDITIONAL INFO: Source of additional information on AIDS

MARYLAND

348. AIDS Project of the Cancer Center/Baltimore
22 S Green St
Baltimore, MD 21201
FACILITY TYPE: Research
ADDITIONAL INFO: Source of additional AIDS information

349. American College Health Association (ACHA), Task Force on AIDS
15879 Crabbs Branch Way
Rockville, MD 20855
(301) 963-1100; Chairperson: (804) 924-2670
KEY PERSONNEL: Stephen D Blom; Executive Director
FACILITY TYPE: Research; Educational; Task force
STAFF: Paid professional 14; Paid nonprofessional 6; Volunteers 27
YEAR FOUNDED: 1985
FUNDING: Federal government; Private; Fund-raisers; Fees for services or products
OUTREACH: AIDS education on college campuses, regional workshops, national conferences, education for primary and secondary school teachers, nationwide HIV seroprevalence study on college campuses
NETWORKS: National AIDS Network (NAN); American Council on Education (ACE); National Leadership Coalition on AIDS (NLCA); National Health Council
SEMINARS: Oct 10-11, 1988—"AIDS Prevention in Higher Education," Kansas City; Nov 3-4, 1988—"AIDS Prevention in Higher Education," Orlando; Nov 17-18, 1988—"AIDS Prevention in Higher Education," Austin
RESEARCH: Seroprevalence of HIV, knowledge/attitudes/beliefs of college/university students
ADDITIONAL INFO: Membership is open to health care professionals in higher education institutions
AVAILABLE LITERATURE: *AIDS: What Everyone Should Know*, a brochure of AIDS information; *The HIV Antibody Test*, a brochure describing the test; *Making Sex Safer*, a brochure discussing safer sex; *Safer Sex*, a brochure of safer sex information; *What Are Sexually Transmitted Diseases?*, a brochure describing various STDs; *ACHA Educational Materials Catalog and Order Form*; *AIDS on the College Campus: ACHA Special Report*, a 65-page booklet discussing AIDS and the college student (a revision is in process); *Sexual Decision Making*, a brochure on safer sex; *Women and AIDS*, a brochure for women
LANGUAGES: Spanish

350. Baltimore City Health Dept, Preventive Medicine and Epidemiology Bureau of Sexually Transmitted Diseases
FORMER NAME: Baltimore City Health Dept, Bureau of Disease Control
303 E Fayette St, 5th Fl
Baltimore, MD 21202
(301) 396-4448
KEY PERSONNEL: Sylvia Scher; Training Center Coordinator
FACILITY TYPE: Educational; Clinic
STAFF: Paid professional 100
FUNDING: Federal government; State government; Local government; Grants
OUTREACH: Educational training programs for health professionals
SEMINARS: The Baltimore City STD Prevention/Training Center provides the following courses: Nov 1-4, 1988—"Lab Methods," 24 hours; Nov 7-11, 14-15, 1988—"Intensive Training," 56 hours; Dec 15-16, 1988—"STD Update," 16 hours; Jan 26-27, 1989—"AIDS Update: Diagnosis, Treatment, Management, and Future Trends," 16 hours; Feb 6-9, 1989—"Worksite AIDS Prevention and Awareness Training," 32 hours; Feb 22-24, 1989 "Lab Methods," 24 hours; Mar 6-10, 1989—"Intensive Training," 40 hours; Mar 6-17, 1989—"Comprehensive Training," 80 hours; Mar 30-31, 1989—"Integration of HIV Services in Existing Programs," 16 hours; Apr 5-6, 1989—"AIDS Education for Dental Professionals," 16 hours; Apr 12-14, 1989—"DIS Update," 24 hours; May 4-5, 1989—"AIDS: Related Counseling Strategies and Education," 16 hours; May 18-19, 1989—"STD Update," 16 hours; Jun 14-16, 1989—"Lab Methods," 24 hours; Jul 19-21, 1989—"DIS Update," 24

hours; Sep 11-14, 1989—"First Responders AIDS Awareness and Prevention Training," 32 hours; Sep 18-22, 1989—"Intensive Training," 40 hours; Sep 25-26, 1989—"Intensive Extended Training Core Option," 16 hours; Oct 18-20, 1989—"Lab Methods," 24 hours
RESEARCH: Medication and behavioral impact, STDs
AVAILABLE LITERATURE: *Protect Yourself and Your Partner: AIDS and the AIDS Antibody Test*, a brochure describing the test; *Protect Yourself and Your Partner: Have Safe Sex*, a brochure of safer sex pointers; *The AIDS Antibody Test: What Your Results Mean*, a brochure describing the HIV test

351. Baltimore County Health Dept
401 Bosley Ave, New Courts Bldg, 3rd Fl
Towson, MD 21204
(301) 494-2711; Hotline: (301) 494-AIDS
KEY PERSONNEL: Randy Berger; AIDS Medical Consultant
AFFILIATION: Baltimore County Government
FACILITY TYPE: HIV counseling and testing; Health department
STAFF: Paid professional 10
FUNDING: Federal government; State government; Local government
OUTREACH: Sponsors slide show presentations for community groups
ADDITIONAL INFO: Offers free, anonymous, no appointment needed HIV counseling and testing at 4 sites throughout Baltimore County. Provides case management for people with HIV infection
AVAILABLE LITERATURE: Safer sex/prevention posters; informational video about HIV for detention centers

352. Charles County Health Dept
PO Box 640, Garrett Ave
LaPlata, MD 20646
(301) 934-9577, 932-0557
KEY PERSONNEL: C Devadason; Health Officer
AFFILIATION: Maryland Dept of Health and Mental Hygiene
FACILITY TYPE: Educational; Clinic; HIV counseling and testing
FUNDING: Federal government; State government; Local government; Fees for services or products
OUTREACH: Speakers bureau with videos and printed handouts to schools, community, and civic organizations
SEMINARS: Oct 19, 1988—"Individualized Case Management—A Cost Effective Health Care Program," presented by the Southern Maryland Health Systems Agency in cooperation with local health officers
ADDITIONAL INFO: Provides counseling and testing for HIV (pretest and posttest), HIV risk assessment for clients in STD, family planning, and maternity clinics, drug abuse clinics, and alcohol clinics. Provides up-to-date resource information to PWAs

353. Chase-Brexton Clinic
FORMER NAME: Gay Lesbian Community Center of Baltimore Health Clinic (GLCCB Clinic)
241 W Chase St
Baltimore, MD 21201
(301) 837-2050
AFFILIATION: Gay and Lesbian Community Center of Baltimore
FACILITY TYPE: Clinic; HIV counseling and testing
STAFF: Paid professional 3; Paid nonprofessional 5; Volunteers 100
YEAR FOUNDED: 1979
FUNDING: State government; Local government; Fund-raisers; Donations
OUTREACH: Patient education, community outreach and education
NETWORKS: National Association of Community Health Centers, Inc
ADDITIONAL INFO: Founded as an STD clinic in 1979 and is now an HIV counseling and testing site. Provides seropositive reactor clinics, counseling, women's health clinic

354. Cherry Hill Drug Abuse Rehab
2490 Giles Rd
Baltimore, MD 21225
(301) 396-1646, 396-1647, 396-1648
FACILITY TYPE: HIV counseling and testing; Substance abuse treatment

355. Dorchester County Health Dept, AIDS Health Service Coordination
Route 1, Box 50, Woods Rd
Cambridge, MD 21613
(301) 228-3223
KEY PERSONNEL: Beverly Chapple; AIDS Health Service Coordinator

FACILITY TYPE: Educational; Clinic; Support group; Hospice; HIV counseling and testing; Health department; Substance abuse treatment; Health promotion

STAFF: Paid professional 61; Paid nonprofessional 31; Volunteers 2

FUNDING: Federal government; State government; Local government

OUTREACH: Speakers available to community organizations, schools, and other groups

ADDITIONAL INFO: The AIDS Health Services Coordination includes case management, community education, and any health services already available through the health department such as immunization, family planning, STD, home health, hospice, and mental health and addictions counseling

356. EarthTide, Inc
2901 Druid Park Dr, Ste 104
Baltimore, MD 21215
(301) 225-9635
KEY PERSONNEL: Tony Allen; Co-Director
FACILITY TYPE: Educational; Support group; Residential facility (adults)
STAFF: Paid nonprofessional 7
YEAR FOUNDED: 1987
FUNDING: State government; Local government
OUTREACH: Services provided to schools, churches, agencies, community organizations, neighborhood associations and drug treatment programs; conducts the Black Inter-Community Educational Project (BICEP) and Lady ASSP (AIDS Socials and Safer Sex Parties)
RESEARCH: Teens, drug abusers, and prostitutes
ADDITIONAL INFO: A community-based, nonprofit minority AIDS organization with the philosophy of "Each One, Teach One." Earthtide's goal is to initiate a proactive consciousness around the issue of AIDS throughout minority communities. EarthTide's Supportive Living Housing Program (SLHP) provides room, board and personal care services to, primarily, recovering homeless drug addicts with AIDS—male and female, gay and straight. Other activities include MAPP (Making a Positive Path) Anonymous, a support group for Narcotics Anonymous; Minority Outreach Program; BICEP (Black Inter-Community Education Project), a multifaceted approach to promoting behavioral change and attitudes among women; and Lady ASSP (AIDS Socials and Safer Sex Parties), at-home social activity where women discuss sexuality and relationships in the context of AIDS prevention
AVAILABLE LITERATURE: *Here Lies You If You Don't Protect Yourself!*, a brochure for IV drug users; *One Good Reason Why Women of Color Should Use Condoms, Talk About Safer Sex, and Give Condoms to Other Women*, a safer sex brochure for women; *Teen Talk on AIDS*, a brochure of AIDS information and safer sex tips for teens; *Each One, Teach One*, a brochure describing the agency

357. Health Education Resource Organization (HERO)
101 W Read St, Ste 812
Baltimore, MD 21201
(301) 685-1180; Hotline: (301) 333-AIDS, 945-AIDS; Toll-free: (800) 638-6252 (MD only); TDD (800) 553-3140
KEY PERSONNEL: Roberta Klishis; Director of Client Services
FACILITY TYPE: Educational; Support group; Fund-raising
STAFF: Paid professional 20; Paid nonprofessional 14; Volunteers 300
YEAR FOUNDED: 1983
FUNDING: Federal government; State government; Local government; Private; Fund-raisers
OUTREACH: Provides outreach in high risk areas, education to all drug and alcohol treatment programs, provides educational programs to all professionals in health care upon request
SEMINARS: "AIDS in the Work Place," with United Way; "The State and AIDS," with Johns Hopkins University
RESEARCH: Working with NIDA to follow seroconversion in IV drug abusers
ADDITIONAL INFO: HERO, is a non-profit community group formed in 1983 to provide accurate information and assistance to people concerned about or affected by AIDS and human immunodeficiency virus (HIV) infection
AVAILABLE LITERATURE: *AIDS Doesn't Give a Damn, So We Have to*, an informational brochure about HERO; *AIDS Risk: A Reference Guide*, a safer sex card; *Drug Users: Do Not Share Needles*, a brochure describing how to sterilize needles; *Questions and Answers About the HIV Antibody Test*, a brochure describing the test; *Safe Sex for Men and Women Concerned About AIDS*, a safer sex brochure; *You Don't Have to Be White or Gay to Get AIDS*, a brochure explaining who can get AIDS; *Andrea and Lisa*, a comic book explaining how one contracts AIDS; *AIDS Precautions for the*

First Responder, a general information brochure; *HERO News*, a monthly newsletter; *A Healthy Gift From HERO*, an envelope with a condom, lubricant, safer sex information and instructions on how to use the condom; *Stop Transmission Fluid Leaks*, a poster and matchbook cover with a condom; *You Won't Believe What We Like to Wear in Bed*, two posters, one of two young White men and the other of two young Black men urging the use of condoms; *AIDS Can Blow Your High*, a poster urging the use of clean needles; *Smart Sportswear for the Active Man* and *Life Preserver*, two posters urging the use of condoms

LANGUAGES: Spanish, American Sign Language

358. Howard County Health Dept
3450 Courthouse Drive
Ellicott City, MD 21043
(301) 992-2333
KEY PERSONNEL: Robin Vidrick; Community Health Nurse
AFFILIATION: Howard County Government
FACILITY TYPE: Educational; Clinic
STAFF: Paid professional 10; Paid nonprofessional 2
YEAR FOUNDED: 1932
FUNDING: State government; Local government
OUTREACH: Brochures distributed to numerous community locations, public speaking to community groups, newspaper and cable TV information, outreach to youth through the schools and teen health clinic, outreach to drug and alcohol clients and chronically mentally ill clients
NETWORKS: Red Cross Visiting Nurse Association
SEMINARS: May-Jun 1988—"Training in AIDS for all County Supervisors," day-long training sessions; Sep 5, 1988—"Labor of Love," AIDS benefit concert fundraiser for PWAs sponsored by the Howard County AIDS Alliance; Aug-Sep 1988—"Workshops for Howard County School Teachers," day-long workshops on curriculum implementation; Apr 16, 1988—"The Impact of AIDS on the People of Howard County"
AVAILABLE LITERATURE: Monthly newsletter; distributes materials from other agencies

359. Johns Hopkins Hospital First AIDS Service
600 N Wolfe St, Blalock 1111
Baltimore, MD 21205
(301) 955-3150
KEY PERSONNEL: Richard Chaisson; Director, AIDS Service
AFFILIATION: Johns Hopkins University School of Medicine
FACILITY TYPE: Research; Educational; Hospital; Clinic; Support group; HIV counseling and testing
STAFF: Paid professional 25; Volunteers 15
YEAR FOUNDED: 1985
FUNDING: Federal government; State government; Fees for services or products
OUTREACH: Psychiatric support groups for HIV positive patients and family members
NETWORKS: Maryland State Health Dept; Baltimore City Health Dept; Health Education Resource Organization (HERO)
SEMINARS: Sep 27, 1988—"Economic Impact of AIDS;" Oct 1988—"AIDS in the Workplace;" 1989—"Workshop for Private Practitioners Caring for HIV Infected Individuals"
RESEARCH: Clinical, hematology, immunology, pharmacology, epidemiology, behavioral
ADDITIONAL INFO: Provides full inpatient and outpatient services, utilizing specialties available within the Johns Hopkins Medical Institutions such as neurology, psychiatry, dermatology, social work, etc. The agency is an aerosolized pentamidine clinic and provides screening and referral services
AVAILABLE LITERATURE: American Sign Language, interpreters in various languages available

360. Maryland Dept of Health and Mental Hygiene, AIDS Administration
FORMER NAME: AIDS Administration
201 W Preston St, Rm 308
Baltimore, MD 21201
(301) 225-5019; Hotline: (301) 945-AIDS; Toll-free: (800) 638-6252
KEY PERSONNEL: John P Krick; Chief, Center for AIDS Education
AFFILIATION: Maryland State Government
FACILITY TYPE: Research; Educational; Clinic; Support group; Task force; HIV counseling and testing
STAFF: Paid professional 50
YEAR FOUNDED: 1987
FUNDING: Federal government; State government

OUTREACH: AIDS educational workshops, referral services, program management, literature development
NETWORKS: American College Health Association
SEMINARS: "Intercampus Network Conference and Minority Outreach Conference"
RESEARCH: Knowledge, attitudes, and beliefs surveys
ADDITIONAL INFO: Provides counseling and testing sites, education and outreach, telephone information and referral, epidemiology and patients services, and assists with the Maryland AIDS Drug Assistance Program (MADAP)
AVAILABLE LITERATURE: *Say Yes to Condoms*, a brochure kit; distributes various other publications
LANGUAGES: Spanish

361. Mayor's AIDS Study Group/Baltimore
111 N Calvert
Baltimore, MD 21201
FACILITY TYPE: Research; Educational
ADDITIONAL INFO: Source of additional AIDS information

362. Montgomery County HERO
100 Maryland Ave, 1st Fl
Rockville, MD 20850
(301) 762-3385
KEY PERSONNEL: David Brumbach, Director

363. National AIDS Information Clearinghouse (NAIC)
PO Box 6003
Rockville, MD 20850
Reference: (301) 762-5111; Publications order, dial toll-free: (800) 458-5231
KEY PERSONNEL: Ruthann Bates, Director
AFFILIATION: Centers for Disease Control
FACILITY TYPE: Educational
YEAR FOUNDED: 1987
FUNDING: Federal government
OUTREACH: Provides technical assistance to organizations delivering AIDS and HIV services. On request, tours are conducted of the NAIC facility
NETWORKS: Administered by the CDC's National AIDS Information and Education Program (NAIEP)
ADDITIONAL INFO: NAIC can help to identify organizations such as clinics, hospitals, extended-care facilities, public health departments, commercial enterprises, and religious groups whose work is related to AIDS. Locates hard-to-find educational materials through use of its 2 online databases
AVAILABLE LITERATURE: *NAIC: Your Key Resource*, a clearinghouse for AIDS information brochure; *User's Guide*, describes NAIC and the services it provides; *NAIC Conference Calendar*, listing of upcoming exhibits and conferences; *AIDS Resources Database*; *AIDS Unpublished Educational Materials Database*
LANGUAGES: Spanish, French, Creole, American Sign Language

364. National Institute of Allergy and Infectious Diseases (NIAID)
9000 Rockville Pike
Bethesda, MD 20892
(301) 496-5717
KEY PERSONNEL: Patricia Randall; Chief
FACILITY TYPE: Research
STAFF: Paid professional 700
YEAR FOUNDED: 1948
FUNDING: Federal government
OUTREACH: Professional outreach/technology transfer
AVAILABLE LITERATURE: *Update*, informational pamphlets including "Soluble CD4 Linked to Toxin: Potential New AIDS Treatment," "Transgenic Mice Develop AIDS-Like Disease;" *Backgrounder*, fact sheets covering "New AIDS Virus Gene Discovered," "NIAID AIDS Clinical Trials Program," "NIAID Extramural AIDS Program," "National Cooperative Drug Discovery Groups—AIDS," "National Cooperative Vaccine Development Groups," "NIAID Vaccine Evaluation Units," "Multicenter AIDS Cohort Study (MACS)," "Programs for Excellence in Basic Research on AIDS (PEBRA)," "Genetic Sequence Database and Analysis Unit," "NIAID AIDS Reagent Repository," "NIAID International Efforts in AIDS Research," "NIAID Intramural AIDS Research," "NIAID Intramural AIDS Vaccine Study," "AIDS Outreach and Technology Transfer Program"

365. National Institute of Drug Abuse (NIDA)
5600 Fishers Lane
Rockville, MD 20857
(301) 443-6245; Hotline: (800) 662-HELP
KEY PERSONNEL: Susan B Lachter; Director, Office of Research Communications
AFFILIATION: Alcohol, Drug Abuse, and Mental Health Administration
FACILITY TYPE: Research; Educational
STAFF: Paid professional 178
YEAR FOUNDED: 1974
FUNDING: Federal government
OUTREACH: Training for drug abuse treatment personnel, outreach services to intravenous drug abusers to teach them about AIDS and encourage them to seek treatment for their addiction
RESEARCH: Drug abuse and AIDS, the effects of drugs on the immune system, drug abuse prevention and treatment research
ADDITIONAL INFO: NIDA provides drug-related AIDS information to the general public. Drug users, as well as their significant others can call to get treatment referrals, general information, and names of support groups. NIDA's role is to reduce the spread of the disease in intravenous drug abusers, their sexual partners, and their offspring
AVAILABLE LITERATURE: *NIDA Notes*, a quarterly newsletter; *Research Monograph Series*; *Statistical Series*; various pamphlets
LANGUAGES: Spanish

366. Prince George's County Health Dept, Office on AIDS
3003 Hospital Dr
Cheverly, MD 20785
(301) 386-0348
KEY PERSONNEL: Fran Preneta; AIDS Education Coordinator
AFFILIATION: Prince George County Government
FACILITY TYPE: Educational; Clinic; Support group; Task force; HIV counseling and testing; Client services/case management
STAFF: Paid professional 23; Volunteers 15
YEAR FOUNDED: 1987
FUNDING: Federal government; State government; Local government
OUTREACH: Community AIDS education programs through the speakers bureau, consultations and outreach to community agencies and groups in developing AIDS educational programs, policies, and procedures, staff training
NETWORKS: AIDS Education Coalition; Prince George's County Interdepartmental AIDS Committee
SEMINARS: 1988—"Teens and AIDS," "AIDS in the College Community," "Pediatric AIDS," "AIDS and Drug Abusers," "Understanding and Overcoming Barriers to AIDS Education"
RESEARCH: Knowledge, attitudes, and practices studies, behavior change research
ADDITIONAL INFO: Provides information and education, community outreach, patient services, HIV antibody testing, buddy program, support groups, and partner notification program
AVAILABLE LITERATURE: *You Hold the Key to AIDS Prevention*, a condom card; *You Can Not Get AIDS By...*, a bookmark; *Your Local Office on AIDS*, a brochure about the facility; *AIDS Speakers Bureau*, a pamphlet providing information about the speakers bureau; *AIDS Whys*, a flyer that answers questions about AIDS and gives important information; *AIDS Fact Sheet*; *Patient Orientation Handbook*; *Could I Be Infected With the AIDS Virus?*, a brochure in planning; *Don't Fan Fear...Get the Facts*, a handheld fan; a videotape on AIDS in the minority is in the making
LANGUAGES: American Sign Language

367. Queen Anne's County Health Dept
206 N Commerce St
Centreville, MD 21617
(301) 758-0720
KEY PERSONNEL: Mary Ann Thompson; Communicable Disease Nurse
AFFILIATION: Maryland State Dept of Health and Mental Hygiene
FACILITY TYPE: Educational; Health department
STAFF: Paid professional 3
FUNDING: State government; Local government
OUTREACH: Educational programs, assistance to public schools for AIDS education for staff and students

368. Talbot County Health Dept, AIDS Program
PO Box 480
Easton, MD 21601
(301) 822-2292

KEY PERSONNEL: Robin Ford; Community Health Nurse
FACILITY TYPE: Educational; HIV counseling and testing; Health department
STAFF: Paid professional 1
FUNDING: State government; Local government
OUTREACH: Educational services and programs to any interested group
ADDITIONAL INFO: The main purpose of this program is to offer confidential counseling and testing for HIV antibody

369. University of Maryland Drug Treatment Center Drug-Free Program
721 W Redwood St
Baltimore, MD 21201
(301) 837-3313
KEY PERSONNEL: Nancy B. Levinbook; Program Coordinator
FACILITY TYPE: HIV counseling and testing; Substance abuse treatment

370. University of Maryland Medical School, Infectious Disease Clinic, AIDS Patient Care Program
PO Box 243 UMH, 22 S Greene St
Baltimore, MD 21201
(301) 328-4300
KEY PERSONNEL: Priscilla A Furth, Director, AIDS Patient Care Program
AFFILIATION: University of Maryland Medical School
FACILITY TYPE: Educational; Clinic
STAFF: Paid professional 2; Volunteers 10
YEAR FOUNDED: 1987
FUNDING: State government; Fees for services or products
RESEARCH: Treatment of cryptococal meningitus, APP, influence of psychosocial factors in diagnosis, correlation of serum and salivary antibodies in AIDS
AVAILABLE LITERATURE: *AIDS: A Working Definition*, a 20-minute video providing a definition of AIDS, a description of the population at risk, and overview of the current and projected incidence; *AIDS: Preventing Infection*, a 20-minute video presenting practical measures on how to avoid exposure to HIV and the necessary steps which must be taken to prevent infection; *Nursing and AIDS: Professional and Personal Concerns*, a 20-minute video examining the medical and psychosocial concerns of nurses and nursing assistants working with AIDS patients; *AIDS: Emotional Needs of the Patient and Family*, a 20-minute video exploring psychosocial problems associated with the AIDS patient and the patient's family; *Pediatric AIDS*, a 20-minute video giving an overview of the crisis posed by the alarming increase in the number of children with HIV infection and AIDS

371. West End Drug Abuse Program
2401 W Baltimore St
Baltimore, MD 21223
(301) 945-7706
KEY PERSONNEL: Aldolphus Albertie; Director
FACILITY TYPE: HIV counseling and testing; Substance abuse treatment

372. Wicomico County Health Dept
300 W Carroll St
Salisbury, MD 21801
(301) 749-1244
KEY PERSONNEL: Karen Satterlee; AIDS Coordinator
FACILITY TYPE: Educational; Clinic; Client services/case management; HIV counseling and testing
FUNDING: State government
OUTREACH: Education on transmission, prevention, etc of AIDS, pre- and post-counseling; distributes pamphlets, audiovisuals, and other educational materials; speakers bureau; education to staff of community groups
LANGUAGES: Spanish, Korean, Laotian

MASSACHUSETTS

373. AIDS Action Committee (AAC)
131 Clarendon St
Boston, MA 02116
(617) 437-6200
KEY PERSONNEL: Larry Kessler; Executive Director

FACILITY TYPE: Educational; Support group; Fund-raising; Task force; Public Policy Program; Advocacy; Resource Planning
STAFF: Paid professional 71; Volunteers 1,800
YEAR FOUNDED: 1982
FUNDING: Federal government; State government; Local government; Private; Fund-raisers; Fees for services or products
OUTREACH: Speakers bureau, AIDS education in the workplace, IV drug users education, gay and lesbian outreach, women outreach, Black, Hispanic, and Haitian community outreach
NETWORKS: National AIDS Network (NAN); AIDS Action Council; AIDS Consortium; National AIDS Round table
ADDITIONAL INFO: "AIDS Action is a non-profit corporation committed to combating the epidemic of AIDS and to addressing the needs of those affected, through service, education, advocacy, and outreach." In addition "AIDS Action seeks to serve with a compassionate and caring presence, people of all cultures affected by AIDS and HIV-related disorders, as well as those at risk fo infection."
AVAILABLE LITERATURE: *Monthly Update*, newsletter; Volunteer newsletter; PWA newsletter; *Treatment Issues Newsletter*, *Public Policy Newsletter*, numerous pamphlets, journal articles, buttons, posters, and videos
LANGUAGES: American Sign Language, Spanish, French, Creole, Portuguese, German

374. American Red Cross, Northeast Region
60 Kendrick St
Needham, MA 02194
(617) 449-0773
FACILITY TYPE: Research; Educational
ADDITIONAL INFO: Provides information concerning criteria for blood donor eligibility

375. Clinical AIDS Program/Boston City Hospital
818 Harrison Ave
Boston, MA 02118
(617) 424-5160; Hotline: (617) 424-5916
AFFILIATION: Boston City Hospital
FACILITY TYPE: Research; Educational; Hospital; Clinic; Support group
YEAR FOUNDED: 1986
FUNDING: Federal government; State government; Local government; Fees for services or products
OUTREACH: Care providers for speaking
NETWORKS: Boston AIDS Consoritum
SEMINARS: Monthly—"AIDS Clinical Conferences"
RESEARCH: Clinical drug trials, virology, behavioral sciences, addiction
ADDITIONAL INFO: This agency is a primary care provider for AIDS/ARC patients with liaisons for addiction services, chronic care, home care, and AIDS Action Committee care coordinated with the Pediatric AIDS Program as needed
AVAILABLE LITERATURE: *AIDS Newsletter*, a monthly newsletter
LANGUAGES: French, Spanish

376. Comprehensive Pediatric AIDS Program (CPAP)
Boston City Hospital, Dowling 5 South, 818 Harrison Ave
Boston, MA 02118
(617) 424-5903
KEY PERSONNEL: Deanna Forist; Director
FACILITY TYPE: Hospital; Residential facility (children)
STAFF: Paid professional 12; Volunteers 20
YEAR FOUNDED: 1986
FUNDING: State government; Private; Fund-raisers
OUTREACH: Speakers bureau providing speakers for day care centers, schools, and public health groups
RESEARCH: Alternative drug trials
ADDITIONAL INFO: CPAP "is a residential program which provides a wide range of services for children with HIV-infection and their families. The philosophy of the program is to provide a home-like environment that reflects the individual medical and psychosocial needs of each child and their family."
AVAILABLE LITERATURE: *Comprehensive Pediatric AIDS Program*, a brochure describing the facility; *Children's AIDS Program Information Packet*, a packet containing an introduction, press release, definition of pediatric AIDS, program brochures, and articles

377. Council of Churches of Greater Springfield
152 Sumner Ave
Springfield, MA 01106
(413) 733-2149
KEY PERSONNEL: Rev Ann Geer; Executive Director
FACILITY TYPE: Support group; Task force
STAFF: Paid professional 3; Paid nonprofessional 4; Volunteers 100
YEAR FOUNDED: 1938
FUNDING: Private; Church contributions
OUTREACH: Provides programs on human sexuality and AIDS and pastoral care
NETWORKS: Pastoral Care Committee; Dignilife; Massachusetts Council of Churches
SEMINARS: Oct, 1988— "AIDS Prayer Vigil;" Apr, Sep, 1988— "Human Sexuality"
ADDITIONAL INFO: Hosts a monthly Western Area Church Executive Meeting which provides updates and shares resources with the denominational leaders. Maintains an active legislative lobbying component and works closely with the Massachusetts Council of Churches in Boston.
AVAILABLE LITERATURE: *Pastoral Committee for AIDS of Western Massachusetts*, brochure describing the organization; *Dignilife*, brochure describing the mission of Dignilife; newsletter
LANGUAGES: American Sign Language

378. Dimock Substance Abuse Treatment Services
55 Dimock St
Roxbury, MA 02119
(617) 442-2121
KEY PERSONNEL: Jonathan Robinson; Program Director
FACILITY TYPE: HIV counseling and testing; Substance abuse treatment

379. Fenway Community Health Center (FCHC)
FORMER NAME: AIDS Action Project
16 Haviland St
Boston, MA 02115
(617) 267-0900
KEY PERSONNEL: Martha W Moon; Family Nurse Practitioner
FACILITY TYPE: Research; Educational; Clinic; Support group; Fundraising; HIV counseling and testing
STAFF: Paid professional 50; Paid nonprofessional 20; Volunteers 20
YEAR FOUNDED: 1971
FUNDING: Federal government; State government; Local government; Private; Fund-raisers; Fees for services or products
OUTREACH: Speakers bureau, networking, education
NETWORKS: Boston AIDS Consortium; Mayor's Committee on AIDS; Governor's Task Force on AIDS; Massachusetts Nurses Association Committee on AIDS; Massachusetts League of Community Health Centers
SEMINARS: Apr 9, 1988—"2nd Women and AIDS Conference;" Oct 1989—"3rd Women and AIDS Conference"
RESEARCH: Behavioral-epidemiologic studies of HIV infection in homosexually active males
ADDITIONAL INFO: Provides primary care and treatment for HIV infection
AVAILABLE LITERATURE: *Fenway Research*, a quarterly newsletter; *Women Are Getting AIDS Too*, a brochure for women; *Remember Our Names*, a poster

380. Haitian Committee on AIDS in Massachusetts
177 Harvard St
Dorchester, MA 02124
(617) 436-2848
FACILITY TYPE: Educational; Support group
ADDITIONAL INFO: Provides information, referrals, support, and emergency assistance to Haitian persons with AIDS and their families

381. La Ahanza Hispana, Inc
409 Dudley St
Roxbury, MA 02119
(617) 427-7175
KEY PERSONNEL: Luis Prado; Executive Director
AFFILIATION: United Way Massachusetts Bay
FACILITY TYPE: Educational; Clinic; Support group; Task force
STAFF: Paid professional 20; Paid nonprofessional 50; Volunteers 3
YEAR FOUNDED: 1969
FUNDING: State government; Local government; Private; Fund-raisers; Fees for services or products

OUTREACH: Substance abuse counseling, advocacy, prevention, education for youth and adults
NETWORKS: Boston Consortium at Harvard University School of Public Health; Latino Health Network; HOPE; Project Star; Governor's Task Force on AIDS
RESEARCH: Hispanic population, health, morbidity, mortality, services
LANGUAGES: Spanish

382. Lifeline Institute, Inc
664 Main St
Amherst, MA 01002
(413) 253-2822
KEY PERSONNEL: Tetty E Gorfine, Director
FACILITY TYPE: Educational
FUNDING: Donations; Grants; Dues
OUTREACH: Speakers bureau, workshops, conferences
NETWORKS: Western Massachusetts AIDS Consortium
SEMINARS: Oct 19-20, 1985 and Oct 18-19, 1986—"Celebrating Our Unity and Diversity;" Feb 3, 1985—"Myths and Realities of AIDS"
ADDITIONAL INFO: Founded in 1984 as an educational agency

383. Massachusetts AIDS Task Force
150 Tremont St
Boston, MA 02111
(617) 727-2700
FACILITY TYPE: Educational
ADDITIONAL INFO: Established by Governor Dukakis and Human Services Secretary Manual Carballo in the summer of 1983 to review and assess the state's monitoring, educational, and treatment efforts relating to AIDS

384. Massachusetts Center for Disease Control, Division of Communicable Disease Control
305 South St
Boston, MA 02130
(617) 522-3700; Hotline: (617) 727-9080; Collect: (617) 522-4090
KEY PERSONNEL: Laureen Kunches; AIDS Program Manager
AFFILIATION: Massachusetts Dept of Public Health
FACILITY TYPE: Research; Educational; Clinic; Support group; HIV counseling and testing
STAFF: Paid professional 62
FUNDING: Federal government; State government
OUTREACH: Educational services, resource development, referral services
ADDITIONAL INFO: Provides individual counseling and HIV antibody testing through the free and anonymous alternative testing site program. Conducts AIDS case surveillance and epidemiology
AVAILABLE LITERATURE: *AIDS Newsletter*
LANGUAGES: Spanish

385. Massachusetts Dept of Public Health, Health Resource Office
150 Tremont St, 9th Fl
Boston, MA 02111
(617) 734-4246; AIDS Hotline: 424-5916; (800) 235-2331 (in Massachusetts only); AIDS Action Line: 536-7733
KEY PERSONNEL: Nancy Weiland, Director; Steve Wroblewski, State AIDS Coordinator
FACILITY TYPE: Educational
FUNDING: State government
LIBRARY: Contains a variety of journals, reprints, pamphlets, and reports covering all aspects of AIDS. Open to in-house use
OUTREACH: Education to the general public, speakers, surveys, and reports
ADDITIONAL INFO: Founded in 1985 as a means of providing as much information as possible to the general public on all aspects of AIDS
AVAILABLE LITERATURE: *The AIDS Epidemic: A Survey of Massachusetts Activity*, a 2-page chronology; *AIDS: Updated Information for Physicians and Health Care Providers*, a 14-page booklet with information on AIDS (April, 1985); *AIDS: Updated Information for Dentists and Dental Auxiliaries*, a 16-page booklet with information about AIDS for dentists (June, 1986); *Public Health Fact Sheet*, a 2-page pamphlet giving current facts about AIDS; *Governor's Task Force on AIDS Policies and Recommendations*, a 50-page booklet covering all of the state's policies on AIDS as it pertains to schools and health care facilities (January, 1987); *Report on AIDS and the Needle-Using Drug Abuser*, a 36-page report on AIDS and drug abusers; *AIDS Educational Activities*, a 2-page report on AIDS education in Massachusetts; *AIDS Research Contracts*, a 4-page

report on contracts awarded with amounts for 1985, 1986, and 1987; *Dukakis Announces Grants to Expand Home Health Services to AIDS Victims*, a 3-page news release describing a $240,000 grant for AIDS home health services; *Memorandum on HIV Testing*, a 5-page memo covering the October 13, 1986 Massachusetts law designed to assure confidentiality of the AIDS antibody test results

386. Mayor's Liaison to Lesbian and Gay Community/Boston
Boston City Hall
Boston, MA 02201
(617) 725-3485
AFFILIATION: Mayor's Task Force on AIDS
FACILITY TYPE: Educational; Public interest group

387. Meridian House
408 Meridian St
East Boston, MA 02128
(617) 569-7310
KEY PERSONNEL: Susan A Elberger; Executive Director
FACILITY TYPE: HIV counseling and testing; Substance abuse treatment

388. Newton Health Dept
492 Waltham St
West Newton, MA 02165-1999
(617) 552-7058
KEY PERSONNEL: J David Naparstek; Commissioner of Health
AFFILIATION: Newton City Government
FACILITY TYPE: Educational; Health department
STAFF: Paid professional 29; Paid nonprofessional 11
YEAR FOUNDED: 1688
FUNDING: Local government; Fees for services or products
OUTREACH: Home visits, speakers bureau, educational seminars
NETWORKS: Massachusetts Dept of Public Health
SEMINARS: Jun 19, 1987—"AIDS Affects Us All;" Dec 8, 1987—"School AIDS Education Curriculum;" Jan 12, 1988—"AIDS—What Our Children Need to Know;" Jun 14, 1988—"AIDS in the Workplace;" Jun 24, 1988—"An Outreach to Youth"
AVAILABLE LITERATURE: *Policy Statements for School and Day Care Attendance*, a brochure; *A Community Responds: A Model Program for Middlesex County Communities*, an informational brochure
LANGUAGES: Translators available for most languages

389. NUVA Inc Outpatient Alcohol and Drug Counseling
3 Emerson Ave
Gloucester, MA 01930
(508) 283-0000
KEY PERSONNEL: James P Means; Clinical Director
FACILITY TYPE: HIV counseling and testing; Substance abuse treatment

MICHIGAN

390. Calhoun County AIDS Education Steering Committee
190 E Michigan Ave
Battle Creek, MI 49017
(616) 966-1210
KEY PERSONNEL: Bruce Parsons; Administrator
AFFILIATION: Calhoun County Health Dept
FACILITY TYPE: Educational; Health department
STAFF: Volunteers 18
YEAR FOUNDED: 1987
FUNDING: Donations
OUTREACH: Educational programs provided to the community as requested

391. Children's Immune Disorder (CID)
614 W McNichols
Detroit, MI 48046
(313) 469-0412
KEY PERSONNEL: Martha Poquette

392. Gay and Lesbian Community Information Center/Detroit
940 W McNichols
Detroit, MI 48203
(313) 345-2722
KEY PERSONNEL: Bill Ashley, Co-Director; John Cook, Co-Director

FACILITY TYPE: Educational
FUNDING: Maintained and supported by Chosen Books (gay, lesbian, and feminist bookstore)
OUTREACH: Informational referral
ADDITIONAL INFO: Founded in 1984 as an informational referral agency for the Detroit area. Have on hand personal contacts for emergencies, hotlines, hospitals, doctors, tests, therapists, educational materials, and speakers

393. Genesee County Health Dept
310 W Oakley St
Flint, MI 48503-3996
(313) 257-3585
KEY PERSONNEL: Robert Pestronk; Health Officer
FACILITY TYPE: Educational; Clinic; HIV counseling and testing; Health department
STAFF: Paid professional 140
FUNDING: Federal government; State government; Local government; Private; Fees for services or products; Donations
OUTREACH: Speakers bureau, education offered in clinic, substance abuse and community settings
NETWORKS: Genesee County AIDS Task Force
SEMINARS: Nov 13, 1987—"Genesee County Health Dept Staff AIDS Update;" Nov 19, 1987—"Update for Police, Corrections, Court and EMT Personnel;" "May 23, 26, 27, 1988—"Genesee County Employee AIDS Update;" Sep 23, 30, 1988—"Flint City Employees AIDS Update"
RESEARCH: Legal issues
ADDITIONAL INFO: This facility has been an AIDS counseling and testing site since June 1985. Provides counseling, testing, education, referrals, networking with other agencies involved in AIDS continuum of care. Provides off-site clinics in substance abuse, gay, care, low-socioeconomic/minority areas
AVAILABLE LITERATURE: *AIDS Alert Newsletter*, *AIDS Clinical Digest*, a bimonthly newsletter; pamphlets dealing with general and youth AIDS education, substance abuse, women, gay populations and safe sex, AIDS information cards, assorted books describing the AIDS epidemic
LANGUAGES: American Sign Language

394. Grand Rapids AIDS Task Force (GRATF)
PO Box 6603
Grand Rapids, MI 49516-6603
(616) 459-9177; Hotline (616) 459-9177
KEY PERSONNEL: James Gardner; Chairman of the Board
FACILITY TYPE: Educational; Support group; Hospice; Fund-raising; Task force
STAFF: Paid nonprofessional 1; Volunteers 100
YEAR FOUNDED: 1985
FUNDING: Private; Fund-raisers; Donations
OUTREACH: Information and referral, financial assistance, non-emergency transportation, hospital-home visitation, buddy program, psychosocial programs, spiritual counseling, educational programs
ADDITIONAL INFO: Formed with the primary goal of caring for the mental, physical, material and spiritual needs of persons with AIDS, as well as their families, and to educate the general public about AIDS in the West Michigan, Kent County area
AVAILABLE LITERATURE: *Information Booklet on Services Offered by the Grand Rapids AIDS Task Force*
LANGUAGES: Spanish

395. Health Education Association, Detroit (HEAD)
PO Box 670055
Royal Oak, MI 48067
(313) 883-6049
KEY PERSONNEL: Chet Simpson; President
FACILITY TYPE: Support group
STAFF: Volunteers 10
YEAR FOUNDED: 1985
FUNDING: Donations
ADDITIONAL INFO: HEAD is a not-for-profit Michigan corporation "organized to provide temporary financial assistance to persons with the acquired immune deficiency syndrome." It "has concentrated its efforts on direct financial assistance to persons with AIDS in meeting their day-to-day needs of housing and utilities, clothing and transportation, prescription and other medical expenses, home care services, etc."

396. Hemophilia Foundation of Michigan (HFM)
411 Huron View Blvd, Ste 101
Ann Arbor, MI 48103
(313) 761-2535; Toll-free: (800) 482-3041 (MI only)
KEY PERSONNEL: Trish Kennedy; Health Educator
AFFILIATION: National Hemophilia Foundation
FACILITY TYPE: Research; Educational; Clinic; Support group; Fund-raising
STAFF: Paid professional 6.5; Paid nonprofessional 2; Volunteers 21
FUNDING: Federal government; State government; Private; Fund-raisers; Fees for services or products; United Way of MI
OUTREACH: Supports 8 diagnostic clinics in Michigan, sponsors support groups, counsels patients/families on the management of hemophilia and AIDS, sponsors 3-week summer camp for children with hereditary bleeding disorders, conducts annual meetings and educational symposia
NETWORKS: Michigan Dept of Public Health; Governors AIDS Expert Committee; Wellness Networks
SEMINARS: Jun 11, 1988—"You're Invited" (annual business meeting), Ann Arbor; Spring 1989—"Annual Business Meeting," Ann Arbor
RESEARCH: Provides funds for research through treatment centers and university research institutes as provided by the United Way of Michigan and approved by local Medical Advisory Committee and the Hemophilia Foundation of Michigan Board of Directors
ADDITIONAL INFO: The Hemophilia Foundation of Michigan exists to promote opportunities for improving the quality of life for those affected by hereditary bleeding disorders
AVAILABLE LITERATURE: *Agency Fact Sheet*; *Hemophilia Update*, a periodic newsletter to educate and update families and professionals; *The Artery*, a quarterly newsletter of information provided by the Hemophilia Foundation; *1987 Annual Report: Hemophilia Foundation of Michigan a United Way Agency*; *Clotting Agents are Lifesavers*, a general brochure about hemophilia; *Comprehensive Care for Hemophilia and von Willebrand's Disease*, a general brochure; *A Little Quiz*, a quiz about hemophilia; *A Story About a Special Summer Camp for Kids with Hemophilia*, a brochure describing the summer camp for kids with hemophilia

397. Jackson County Health Dept
410 Erie St
Jackson, MI 49203
(517) 788-4477, 788-4375
KEY PERSONNEL: Suzanne Carl; Nursing Supervisor
AFFILIATION: Michigan Dept of Public Health
FACILITY TYPE: Educational; Clinic; HIV counseling and testing; Health department
STAFF: Paid professional 3
YEAR FOUNDED: 1986
FUNDING: State government
OUTREACH: Speakers bureau
NETWORKS: Wellness Network; Friends—Persons with AIDS Alliance; United Community Services of Metro Detroit; AIDS Related Communication Coalition

398. Kalamazoo County AIDS Prevention Program
418 W Kalamazoo Ave
Kalamazoo, MI 49007
(616) 383-8850; Hotline: (616) 383-8881
KEY PERSONNEL: Julie Linn; Coordinator
AFFILIATION: Kalamazoo County Human Services Dept
FACILITY TYPE: Educational; HIV counseling and testing; Health department
STAFF: Paid professional 5
YEAR FOUNDED: 1986
FUNDING: State government; Local government
OUTREACH: Presentations, professional consultations, material distribution, counseling and testing (anonymous and confidential)
NETWORKS: Kalamazoo AIDS Coordinating Consortium
AVAILABLE LITERATURE: *Facts About AIDS*, a brochure

399. Michigan Organization for Human Rights (MOHR)
19641 W Seven Mile Rd
Detroit, MI 48219-2721
(313) 537-6647
KEY PERSONNEL: Jeffery L Swanson; Acting Executive Director
FACILITY TYPE: Advocacy; Lobbying
STAFF: Paid professional 5
YEAR FOUNDED: 1977
FUNDING: State government; Local government; Private; Fund-raisers

OUTREACH: Operates the Detroit area lesbian and gay community center; produce and distribute *Lambda Report*, a cable TV program
AVAILABLE LITERATURE: *MOHR News and Information*, newsletter

400. Special Office on AIDS Prevention (SOAP), Center for Health Promotion, Michigan Dept of Public Health
3423 N Logan
Lansing, MI 48909
(517) 335-8371; Hotline: (800) 872-AIDS
KEY PERSONNEL: Randall S Pope; Chief
FACILITY TYPE: Educational
STAFF: Paid professional 16
YEAR FOUNDED: 1986
FUNDING: Federal government; State government
OUTREACH: Counseling training, universal precaution training
NETWORKS: Michigan State Medicare Society Task Force; AIDS Related Communication Coalition; Greater Detroit Area Health Council Task Force
AVAILABLE LITERATURE: *AIDS Prevention and Control Activities*, a 1988 informational pamphlet; *AIDS and Everyone*, a 1987 health update pamphlet of general information; *AIDS in the Workplace*, a 1987 health update pamphlet with information on AIDS in the workplace; *AIDS Update*, a newsletter; *AIDS in Michigan: A Report to the Governor and the Legislature, February 1987*; *Perinatal AIDS in Michigan: A Report of the Maternal and Infant Task Force on AIDS, June 1988*

401. Venereal Disease Action Coalition (VDAC)/United Community Services of Metropolitan Detroit
1212 Griswold
Detroit, MI 48226-1899
(313) 226-9496
KEY PERSONNEL: Judy Lipshutz; Coordinator
AFFILIATION: AIDS Related Communication Coalition (ARCC)
FACILITY TYPE: Educational
STAFF: Paid professional 2; Paid nonprofessional 1
YEAR FOUNDED: 1982
FUNDING: Federal government; State government
OUTREACH: Speakers bureau, updates for professionals, teens, general population, social and civic groups with a special focus on minorities and populations at risk
NETWORKS: AIDS Related Communication Coalition (ARCC); Client-Centered Community-Based AIDS Care Management
RESEARCH: Women at risk, preteens/parents AIDS education, adolescents, male attitudes and beliefs surrounding AIDS prevention and intervention
ADDITIONAL INFO: Provides technical assistance and consultation on AIDS education, services and policies to VDAC members and others upon request. Provides training for peer counselors with Ann Arbor Planned Parenthood. Participated and directed the American Social Health Association previewing of "Sex, Drugs, and AIDS" for 1000 Detroit area high school students
AVAILABLE LITERATURE: Bimonthly newsletter; *AIDS Resource Directory*, a directory for the state of Michigan

402. Vida Latina
4124 W Vernor
Detroit, MI 48209
(313) 843-2437
KEY PERSONNEL: Felix Carpio; Acting Coordinator
FACILITY TYPE: Educational; Support group; HIV counseling and testing
STAFF: Paid professional 2; Paid nonprofessional 2; Volunteers 1
YEAR FOUNDED: 1988
FUNDING: Federal government
AVAILABLE LITERATURE: *AIDS...Can Attack Anyone/SIDA es AIDS Y...Puede Atacar a Cualquiera*, a series of bilingual (English and Spanish) leaflets in a folded envelope packet, marked confidential, covering "Where do you go for information and services?," "Latinos and AIDS," "Children and AIDS," "Signs of Danger," "What is the difference between being positive and having ARC or AIDS?," "How to know if a person is infected?," "If you know someone who might be infected with the AIDS virus or who already has AIDS, then...," "How to protect your family," "Who can get infected with the AIDS virus," "Where can the virus be found?," "What causes AIDS?," "What is AIDS?," "Don't let fear hold you back!," "Protect your partner," "Let's talk about condoms," "What a woman can do so she won't become infected," "Ways a woman can become infected," "What a homosexual can do to avoid getting infected," "How a male homosexual can get

infected," "What a man should do to avoid becoming infected," "Ways a man can become infected," "How to protect yourself and others if you inject (shoot) intravenous drugs," "How a person who injects (shoots) drugs becomes infected"

403. Washtenaw County Public Health Division, AIDS Counseling and Testing Clinic
555 Towner Blvd
Ypsilanti, MI 48198
(313) 485-2181
KEY PERSONNEL: Vicki Nighswander; AIDS Clinic Coordinator
AFFILIATION: Washtenaw County Public Health Division
FACILITY TYPE: Educational; Clinic; HIV counseling and testing
STAFF: Paid professional 4
FUNDING: State government; Local government
OUTREACH: Referrals for positive testers, weekly presentations at the Washtenaw County Jail, school health outreach, education to high risk individuals, prostitutes, substance abusers
NETWORKS: Washtenaw AIDS Education Network (WAEN); Wellness Networks, Inc., Huron Valley
SEMINARS: Aug 1988—"Safer Sex for Gay Men;" Oct 1988—"Family Night Out"
RESEARCH: Mental health of HIV positive persons
ADDITIONAL INFO: Provides anonymous, confidential, and free pre- and post-counseling and testing for HIV antibody. Provides education to everyone in the community, especially to high risk groups
AVAILABLE LITERATURE: *AIDS Counseling and Testing Clinic*, a brochure describing the facility and services

404. Wayne County Health Dept
Wayne Westland Complex
Westland, MI 48185
(313) 467-3300
KEY PERSONNEL: Diane Casey, RN
AFFILIATION: Wayne County Government
FACILITY TYPE: Educational; Clinic; Health department
STAFF: Paid professional 6
FUNDING: Federal government; State government; Local government
OUTREACH: Community education
ADDITIONAL INFO: Provides numerous inservice training sessions and conferences for the community and state
AVAILABLE LITERATURE: Distributes materials from other agencies

405. Wellness House of Michigan
PO Box 03827
Detroit, MI 48203
(313) 865-AIDS
KEY PERSONNEL: Will R Whitmer, Executive Director
FACILITY TYPE: Support group
ADDITIONAL INFO: Founded in 1985 to provide a residence for PWAs who have been displaced by family, friends, or landlords and who are no longer able financially to support themselves
AVAILABLE LITERATURE: *Cradle With Care*, a 2-fold brochure describing the services of the Children's Immune Disorder; *Poppers, Your Health and AIDS: Can You Afford the Risk?*, a 3-fold brochure discussing poppers and AIDS; *When a Friend Has AIDS*, a 2-fold brochure of what to do and say; *Play Safe*, a 2-fold sexually explicit brochure on safe sex; *Should I Have the Test?*, a 2-fold brochure of questions and answers about the HTLV III blood test; *Helping with AIDS*, a 2-fold brochure resource list; *Guidelines for Persons Who Have Developed Antibody to HTLV-III*, a 2-fold brochure that answers some questions about testing positive; *AIDS: It's Everybody's Business*, a 2-fold brochure of information about AIDS; *Update: Information on AIDS*, a 2-fold brochure of general AIDS information; *Healthy Sex is Fun Sex*, a 2-fold brochure on safe sex

406. Wellness Networks, Inc/Flint
PO Box 438
Flint, MI 48501
(313) 232-2417; Hotline: (313) 232-0888
KEY PERSONNEL: Robert Bader; Volunteer Coordinator
AFFILIATION: Wellness Networks, Inc.
FACILITY TYPE: Educational; Support group; Fund-raising
STAFF: Paid professional 1; Paid nonprofessional 1; Volunteers 76
YEAR FOUNDED: 1986

FUNDING: Private; Fund-raisers
ADDITIONAL INFO: Provides educational inservices, AIDS information and referral on the telephone and through several groups. Works with 5 local hospitals, Genesee County Health Dept, Saginaw County Health Dept, several area churches, Genesee County Commission on Substance Abuse, Genesee County Mental Health, and several hospices

407. Wellness Networks, Inc/Huron Valley (WNI-HV)
PO Box 3242
Ann Arbor, MI 48106
(313) 572-WELL
KEY PERSONNEL: Scott Plakun; President
FACILITY TYPE: Educational; Support group
STAFF: Volunteers 150
YEAR FOUNDED: 1985
FUNDING: State government; Private; Fund-raisers
OUTREACH: Speakers bureau, booth at local events

408. Wellness Networks, Inc (WNI)
PO Box 1046
Royal Oak, MI 48068
(313) 547-3783; Hotline: (313) 547-9040; Toll-free: (800) 872-AIDS (MI only)
KEY PERSONNEL: Scott Walton; Executive Director
AFFILIATION: National AIDS Network (NAN)
FACILITY TYPE: Educational; Support group; Fund-raising; Referral
STAFF: Paid professional 4; Volunteers 300
YEAR FOUNDED: 1984
FUNDING: State government; Private; Fund-raisers
OUTREACH: Hospital visitation, speakers bureau, sup port services, practical support, buddy program
NETWORKS: Wellness Networks/Flint; Wellness Net works/Huron Valley (Ann Arbor); Wellness Net works/Grand Traverse Area (Traverse City); Wellness Networks/K.A.R.E.S. (Kalamazoo)
AVAILABLE LITERATURE: *Wellness Newsletter*, bimonthly newsletter
LANGUAGES: Spanish

MINNESOTA

409. The Aliveness Project Center For Living
730 E 38th St
Minneapolis, MN 55407
(612) 822-7946; Hotline: (612) 822-3016; TTY
KEY PERSONNEL: Steven Katz; Administrator
AFFILIATION: National Association of People with AIDS (NAPWA)
FACILITY TYPE: Educational; Support group; Task force; Coalition
STAFF: Volunteers 400
YEAR FOUNDED: 1986
FUNDING: Private; Fund-raisers
OUTREACH: Education to hospitals, schools, Red Cross, com munity groups, people at risk, people of color, women, and children
NETWORKS: National AIDS Network (NAN); National Association of People With AIDS (NAPWA)
RESEARCH: Alternative and holistic medicine
AVAILABLE LITERATURE: Newsletter and buttons
LANGUAGES: American Sign Language

410. Hennepin County Medical Center (HCMC)
701 Park Ave S
Minneapolis, MN 55415
(612) 347-2693
KEY PERSONNEL: Margaret Simpson; Infectious Disease Director
AFFILIATION: Hennepin County Government
FACILITY TYPE: Research; Educational; Hospital; Clinic
YEAR FOUNDED: 1887
FUNDING: Federal government; State government; Local government

411. Metropolitan Visiting Nurses Association (MVNA)
250 S 4th St
Minneapolis, MN 55415
(612) 348-2700
KEY PERSONNEL: Carol Dinndorf; Supervisor
AFFILIATION: Minneapolis Health Dept
FACILITY TYPE: Hospice; Home care
STAFF: Paid professional 50
YEAR FOUNDED: 1902

FUNDING: Federal government; State government; Local government; Fees for services or products; United Way

NETWORKS: Minnesota AIDS Project; Hennepin County Medical Center AIDS Clinic

ADDITIONAL INFO: Provides home care for PWAs including IV therapy regardless of ability to pay. Includes nurses, HHA/Homemakers companion, and personal care attendants

412. Olmsted County Health Dept
1650 4th St SE
Rochester, MN 55904
(507) 285-8370; Hotline: (507) 285-8508
KEY PERSONNEL: Arvid J Houglum; Director of Public Health
AFFILIATION: Minnesota Dept of Health
FACILITY TYPE: HIV counseling and testing; Health department
STAFF: Paid professional 50; Paid nonprofessional 20
YEAR FOUNDED: 1912
FUNDING: Federal government; State government; Local government; Fees for services or products
OUTREACH: AIDS educational programs, AIDS Task Force
SEMINARS: Performs HIV testing within the department's sexually transmitted disease clinics by appointment. Organized an AIDS Task Force to educate the public on AIDS
AVAILABLE LITERATURE: Several publications in the process of being produced
LANGUAGES: Cambodian, Vietnamese

413. Red Door Clinic
527 Park Ave
Minneapolis, MN 55415
(612) 347-3300; Hotline: (612) 347-AIDS
KEY PERSONNEL: Margaret Hagen; Nursing Supervisor
AFFILIATION: Hennepin County Community Health Dept
FACILITY TYPE: Clinic
STAFF: Paid professional 12; Paid nonprofessional 4
YEAR FOUNDED: 1972
FUNDING: Local government
OUTREACH: Community education services
AVAILABLE LITERATURE: Distribute various pamphlets and posters

414. Saint Paul Division of Public Health
555 Cedar St, Rm 111
Saint Paul, MN 55101
(612) 292-7735
KEY PERSONNEL: Mary Sonnen; Program Director
FACILITY TYPE: Research; Educational; Clinic; Support group; HIV counseling and testing
STAFF: Paid professional 3; Paid nonprofessional 1.5
YEAR FOUNDED: 1985
FUNDING: State government; Local government; Donations
OUTREACH: Paid and volunteer speakers bureau to Ramsey County
RESEARCH: Seroprevalence
ADDITIONAL INFO: Maintains an HIV counseling and testing program. Operates within a sexually transmitted disease clinic that has been operating since 1972
LANGUAGES: Southeast Asian dialects, American Sign Language

415. Saint Paul Urban Indian Health Board
1021 Marion St
Saint Paul, MN 55117
(612) 487-3315
KEY PERSONNEL: William L Burnes; Executive Director
FACILITY TYPE: Clinic
STAFF: Paid professional 10
YEAR FOUNDED: 1978
FUNDING: Federal government; State government; Local government; Private; Fund-raisers; Fees for services or products
OUTREACH: Health education, family dynamics, chemical dependency information
ADDITIONAL INFO: Services that are provided include a medical clinic, behavioral health care, chemical dependency services, pre-natal clinic, community education, health professional training, family planning, and traditional care

AVAILABLE LITERATURE: *Family Planning*, a brochure on family planning; *Horizon: An American Indian Chemical Dependency Program*, a brochure describing the program; *Prenatal Care*, a brochure describing the service that is provided in cooperation with Health Start; *Family/Child Enrichment Program*, a brochure describing the program; *St. Paul Urban Indian Health Board*, an informational brochure; a monthly newsletter is also published
LANGUAGES: Native American dialects

416. Social Security Administration/Minneapolis
1811 Chicago Ave
Minneapolis, MN 55404
(612) 349-3787
KEY PERSONNEL: Josh E Melssen, District Manager
FACILITY TYPE: Educational
ADDITIONAL INFO: A source of general information and financial aid
AVAILABLE LITERATURE: *If You Become Disabled*, a 31-page booklet presenting information on applying for disability from the SSA; *Your Social Security*, a 35-page booklet outling what Social Security means; *SSI for Aged, Disabled, and Blind People*, a 15-page booklet with general information on Social Security
LANGUAGES: Spanish

MISSISSIPPI

417. Jackson Metropolitan Community Church
6069 Old Canton Rd, Ste 166
Jackson, MS 39211
(601) 956-8211
KEY PERSONNEL: Sam Edelman-Richard; Pastor
AFFILIATION: Universal Fellowship of Metropolitan Community Churches
FACILITY TYPE: Educational; Support group; Religious
STAFF: Paid professional 1; Volunteers varies
YEAR FOUNDED: 1983
FUNDING: Private; Fund-raisers
OUTREACH: Weekly Bible studies, seminars, workshops, special programs
SEMINARS: Summer 1987—"Homosexuality and the Bible," a 12-week series; Spring 1988—"Women, Men, and the Bible;" Sep 1987, Jun 1988—"AIDS Vigil of Prayer"
ADDITIONAL INFO: Provides counseling, networking, referrals for services, support groups as needed, and social activities which are drug and alcohol free. Works with gay and lesbian people and their parents and families
AVAILABLE LITERATURE: Publishes a newsletter
LANGUAGES: Spanish, American Sign Language

418. Mississippi Gay/Lesbian Alliance (MGLA)
FORMER NAME: Mississippi Gay Alliance
PO Box 8342
Jackson, MS 39284-8342
Hotline: (601) 353-7611; Toll-free: (800) 537-0851 (MS only)
KEY PERSONNEL: Eddie Sandifer; Executive Director
FACILITY TYPE: Educational; Support group; Fund-raising; Task force
STAFF: Paid nonprofessional 1; Volunteers 304
YEAR FOUNDED: 1973
FUNDING: State government; Fund-raisers
AVAILABLE LITERATURE: *This Month in Mississippi*, a monthly magazine
LANGUAGES: Spanish, American Sign Language

419. Mississippi State Dept of Health, AIDS/HIV Prevention Program
PO Box 1700
Jackson, MS 39209
(601) 960-7723; Hotline: (800) 826-2961
KEY PERSONNEL: Lydia D. Patterson; Director
AFFILIATION: Mississippi State Dept of Health
FACILITY TYPE: Health department
STAFF: Paid professional 5
FUNDING: Federal government; State government
OUTREACH: Speakers bureau, counseling and testing sites, coundeling and testing training to health care workers
NETWORKS: Statewide AIDS Task Force

SEMINARS: Apr, 1988, 1989—"Minority AIDS Conference"
AVAILABLE LITERATURE: *Teens and AIDS*, a brochure of basic information about AIDS for teens, parents, and school personnel; *HIV (AIDS Virus) Infection*, a brochure about AIDS; *What You Should Know About AIDS*, the CDC pamphlet of facts about the disease, how to protect yourself and your family and what to tell others

MISSOURI

420. AIDS Project/Springfield
309 N Jefferson, 254 Landmark Bldg
Springfield, MO 65806
(417) 864-5594
KEY PERSONNEL: Kenny Cowan; Office Coordinator
FACILITY TYPE: Research; Educational; Support group; Fund-raising
STAFF: Paid nonprofessional 1; Volunteers 40
YEAR FOUNDED: 1985
FUNDING: State government; Private; Fund-raisers
OUTREACH: Public education, telephone referral, in-house education
NETWORKS: Greene County Health Dept; American National Red Cross
ADDITIONAL INFO: This facility provides a wide range of services including support groups, spiritual counseling, bereavement counseling, limited financial support, buddy system, food, transportation assistance, assistance with Medicaid/Medicare applications, assistance with disability, and health and nutritional education.
AVAILABLE LITERATURE: *Surgeon General's Report on Acquired Immune Deficiency Syndrome; AIDS Project/Springfield*, a brochure about the facility; *Sex and You: It's Your Choice...It's Your Life*, a brochure of safer sex guidelines; *When a Friend has AIDS*, a brochure of what to say and what to do; *What You Should Know About AIDS*, a CDC booklet of facts; *AIDS: A Guide for Survival*, a 91-page book published by the Harris County Medical Society and Houston Academy of Medicine; *You Can Do Something About AIDS*, a 126-page book published by the Stop AIDS Project and distributed free by Sasha Alyson; *Beyond Fear*, a video; *A Letter From Brian*, a video; *Can AIDS be Stopped*, a video; *Killer in the Village*, a video; *Sex, Drugs and AIDS*, a video; *AIDS Hits Home—AIDS in Search of a Miracle*, a video; *Dr. Rosenfeld Interviews Dr. Fauci about AIDS*, a video; *AIDS: Changing the Rules*, a video

421. Columbia/Boone County Health Dept
PO Box N, 600 E Broadway
Columbia, MO 65205
(314) 874-7355
KEY PERSONNEL: Linda Hancik; Chief, Bureau of Personal Health Services
AFFILIATION: Columbia/Boone County Government
FACILITY TYPE: Clinic; HIV counseling and testing; Health department
STAFF: Paid professional 31
FUNDING: Federal government; State government; Local government; Donations

422. Four-State Community AIDS Project (CAP)
PO Box 3476
Joplin, MO 64803-3476
(417) 625-2486; Hotline: (417) 625-2486
KEY PERSONNEL: Deanne Ashley; Director
FACILITY TYPE: Educational; Support group
STAFF: Volunteers 20
YEAR FOUNDED: 1987
FUNDING: Private; Fund-raisers
OUTREACH: Provides the latest information about AIDS, HIV, HIV antibody testing, and available testing facilities, distributes information from other organizations and agencies
NETWORKS: United States Conference of Mayors
SEMINARS: Jul 1987—"Volunteer Training Program," Joplin; Jan 21, 1988—"AIDS in the Workplace," Joplin; Sep 1988—"Volunteer Training Program," Joplin; Oct 1988—"Of Interest to Parents," Joplin, co-sponsored with the Joplin Health Dept and Planned Parenthood
ADDITIONAL INFO: CAP is a non-profit organization established to educate community groups and individuals about AIDS, to provide direct services to people with AIDS or related conditions, and to give support to friends and family of people with AIDS in the greater Joplin area

AVAILABLE LITERATURE: *Update*, a periodically published newsletter; *Community AIDS Project*, a brochure describing CAP

423. Gay Services Network, Inc
PO Box 32592
Kansas City, MO 64111
Hotline: (816) 931-4470
KEY PERSONNEL: Geoff Segebarth; President
FACILITY TYPE: Educational
STAFF: Volunteers 32
YEAR FOUNDED: 1974
FUNDING: Private; Fund-raisers
OUTREACH: Periodic educational programs for the gay community, AIDS/safer sex programs, distribute condoms
NETWORKS: National Gay and Lesbian Task Force (NGLTF)
SEMINARS: 1987—"Safer Sex,", Kansas City (held 6 times during the year; Apr 1988—"Broken Walls, Broken Silence," Kansas City (a program of songs)
ADDITIONAL INFO: Operates the GAY TALK telephone hotline. Provides AIDS and safer sex information through outreach programs at bars, businesses, etc. Uses trained volunteers to staff tables that give one-on-one information as well as free condoms

424. Good Samaritan Project
3940 Walnut St
Kansas City, MO 64111
(816) 561-8784; Hotline: (816) 561-8780; Teens Toll-free: (800) 234-TEEN
KEY PERSONNEL: Virginia Allen; Executive Director
FACILITY TYPE: Educational; Support group
STAFF: Paid professional 5.5; Volunteers 587
YEAR FOUNDED: 1985
FUNDING: Private; Fund-raisers; Grants
OUTREACH: Speakers bureau, library and resource center, Teens' Teaching AIDS Prevention (Teens TAP)
NETWORKS: National AIDS Network (NAN); Greater Kansas City Hospice Coalition; Regional Home Health Care Association
SEMINARS: 1988—"KC AIDS Symposium;" 1988—"Bixby Institute Conference on AIDS;" 1989—"Regional AIDS and Adolescents Conference"
ADDITIONAL INFO: Good Samaritan Project is a community-based AIDS service organization that offers information and education resources and provides direct services and support to people with AIDS, people with AIDS-Related Complex, those with a positive antibody test, and their families, friends, and loved ones in the Greater Kansas City area and surrounding communities
AVAILABLE LITERATURE: *Safer Sex, Your Responsibility, Your Choice*, a safer sex brochure; *Good Samaritan Project: A Community Response to the Care and Support of Persons Affected by AIDS*, an informational brochure about the agency; *Warning: This Brochure May Save Your Life*, an educational brochure for teens with a button; *When a Friend Has AIDS*, a brochure of what to say and what to do; *AIDS: Good News*, a brochure of facts of how you do not catch AIDS; *AIDS and Drugs*, a brochure for the IV drug user; *Disease Does Not Discriminate*, a brochure for minorities; a newsletter
LANGUAGES: Spanish, American Sign Language

425. Heart of America Human Services
PO Box 2696
Kansas City, MO 64142
FACILITY TYPE: Support group
ADDITIONAL INFO: Source of additional AIDS information

426. Kansas City Free Health Clinic
FORMER NAME: Westport Free Health Clinic
5119 E 24th St
Kansas City, MO 64127
(816) 231-4481; Hotline: (816) 231-8895
KEY PERSONNEL: David Arnold; President
FACILITY TYPE: Educational; Clinic; Support group; HIV counseling and testing
STAFF: Paid professional 3; Volunteers 250
FUNDING: State government; Private; Fund-raisers
OUTREACH: Media awareness, safe sex seminars, outreach to male prostitutes, escorts, transvestite prostitutes, and homeless, street education outreach program for IV drug abusers and prostitutes, HIV counseling and testing, nursing clinic, legal assistance and social services

ADDITIONAL INFO: Kansas City Free Health Clinic is a not-for-profit corporation that provides services and education to people with AIDS and AIDS-related illnesses, and to people who have been exposed to the virus

AVAILABLE LITERATURE: *A.I.D.S. Related Services*, an informational brochure; *Mediform*, a fact sheet that disseminates alternative treatment information; *Client Referral Sheet, HIV Positive*, an informational sheet; *Kansas City Free Health Clinic Newsletter*

427. Mid-Missouri AIDS Project (MMAP)

PO Box 1371, 811 E Cherry St, Ste 320
Columbia, MO 65205
(316) 875-2437
KEY PERSONNEL: John Hawkins; Director
FACILITY TYPE: Educational; Support group; Hospice; Fund-raising
STAFF: Paid professional 1; Volunteers 20
YEAR FOUNDED: 1986
FUNDING: State government; Local government; Private; Fund-raisers; Fees for services or products
OUTREACH: Speakers bureau, hotline
ADDITIONAL INFO: Provides support groups for PWAs and significant others, buddy program, hotline, and a speakers bureau. Involved in the AIDS Awareness Day on the University of Missouri, Columbia campus
LANGUAGES: American Sign Language

428. Saint Joseph/Buchanan County Community Health Clinic

FORMER NAME: Public Health Clinic of Saint Joseph
904 S 10th St
Saint Joseph, MO 64503
(816) 271-4725; Hotline: (816) 271-7913
KEY PERSONNEL: Penney Moore, RN
FACILITY TYPE: Clinic; HIV counseling and testing
FUNDING: State government; Local government
OUTREACH: Public speaking
NETWORKS: Good Samaritan Support Group; Community Task Force on AIDS
SEMINARS: Nov 1988—"Round Table Meeting for Exchange of Information on Services Available"
ADDITIONAL INFO: Provides pretest counseling, testing, post-test counseling, referral provided by appointment at no charge. Offers the same services through the prenatal clinic
AVAILABLE LITERATURE: *AIDS*, a bookmark with brief AIDS facts and important telephone numbers for Northwest Missouri; *Women and AIDS*, a 1988 Missouri Dept of Health brochure; *What You Should Know About AIDS*, a CDC pamphlet about AIDS; *AIDS and Children: Information for Parents of School-Age Children*, a 1986 American National Red Cross pamphlet for parents; *AIDS and the Safety of the Nation's Blood Supply*, a 1987 American National Red Cross pamphlet; *Caring for the AIDS Patient at Home*, a 1986 American National Red Cross pamphlet; *AIDS: The Facts*, a 1986 American National Red Cross pamphlet with brief facts; *AIDS and Your Job—Are There Risks?*, a 1986 American National Red Cross pamphlet on AIDS in the workplace; *If Your Test for Antibody to the AIDS Virus is Positive*, a 1986 American National Red Cross pamphlet for those who test positive; *AIDS, Sex, and You*, a 1986 American National Red Cross pamphlet of how to protect yourself from AIDS; *Gay and Bisexual Men and AIDS*, a 1986 American National Red Cross pamphlet for gays and bisexuals

429. Saint Louis Effort for AIDS (EFA)

4050 Lindell Blvd
Saint Louis, MO 63108
(314) 531-2847; Hotline: (314) 531-7400
KEY PERSONNEL: Mark Kalk; Director of Education
FACILITY TYPE: Educational; Clinic; Support group; Fund-raising
STAFF: Paid professional 1; Volunteers 300
YEAR FOUNDED: 1985
FUNDING: Private; Fund-raisers; Fees for services or products
OUTREACH: Speakers bureau, clergy training seminars, hotline, library facility, publications, volunteer training seminars, sponsorship of social events for volunteers
NETWORKS: AIDS Action Council; National AIDS Network (NAN); Missouri AIDS Caucus; Lambda Legal Defense and Education Fund
ADDITIONAL INFO: Provides support services for PWAs and PWARCs and their significant others, including legal aid, financial aid, support groups, buddies, hotlines, grants, and educational materials

AVAILABLE LITERATURE: *Frontline*, a monthly newsletter; pamphlets and posters; *AIDS: Learn, Protect and Enjoy*, an audiovisual presentation
LANGUAGES: American Sign Language

430. Saline County Nursing Service

76 W Arrow
Marshall, MO 65340
(816) 886-3434
KEY PERSONNEL: Billie F Vardiman; Administrator
AFFILIATION: Saline County Government
FACILITY TYPE: Educational 3; Hospital 3; Clinic; HIV counseling and testing; Health department
STAFF: Paid professional 2
YEAR FOUNDED: 1952
FUNDING: Federal government; State government; Local government; Donations
OUTREACH: Available for local public health programs, education on all subjects including AIDS
NETWORKS: Inter-Agency Council
SEMINARS: Jun 1988—"AIDS Seminar," held with local hospital for county education
ADDITIONAL INFO: Provides counseling and testing for HIV

MONTANA

431. Billings AIDS Support Network

PO Box 1748
Billings, MT 59103
(406) 245-2029; Hotline: (406) 252-1212 (24 hrs)
KEY PERSONNEL: Mary Hernandez, President
AFFILIATION: National AIDS Network (NAN); Montana AIDS Coalition; Out in Montana; Billings AIDS Task Force; Helena AIDS Support Network
FACILITY TYPE: Educational; Support group; Fund-raising; HIV counseling and testing
STAFF: Volunteers 7
YEAR FOUNDED: 1986
FUNDING: State government; Private; Fund-raisers
OUTREACH: Speakers bureau; fund-raisers at local gay bar
NETWORKS: National AIDS Netwok (NAN)
SEMINARS: Nov 1987—ROGAM Inservice; Mar 1988—Hospice Inservice; Mar 1988—Montana AIDS Conference for Gays/Safe Sex Workshop; Oct 1988—Volunteer Training; Feb 1989—"AIM for the Heart," a public forum; Mar 1989—Volunteer Workshop
ADDITIONAL INFO: Services offered include a 24-hour hotline; one-on-one counseling; support group for people with AIDS, ARC, or HIV-positive test result; support group for family and friends dealing with AIDS; speakers bureau and inservices on AIDS and prevention; annual training for current and new volunteers; information and referrals; information on HIV testing at Deering Clinic
AVAILABLE LITERATURE: *AIDS is Preventable*, brochure offering tips for prevention; *AIDS: What Everyone Needs To Know*, brochure outlining facts about AIDS
LANGUAGES: Spanish

432. Yellowstone City-County Health Dept, Deering Community Health Center

123 S 27th St
Billings, MT 59101
(406) 256-6821; BASN: (406) 252-1212
FACILITY TYPE: Educational; Clinic; Support group; Task force; HIV counseling and testing
STAFF: Paid professional 2; Volunteers 10
YEAR FOUNDED: 1987
FUNDING: Federal government; State government; Local government
OUTREACH: Support groups for HIV positive, family and friends
NETWORKS: Billings AIDS Task Force (BATF); Billings AIDS Support Network (BASN)
SEMINARS: Oct 29, 1988—"Train the Volunteers"
ADDITIONAL INFO: Provides HIV testing
LANGUAGES: Spanish

NEBRASKA

433. American Red Cross AIDS Education Coalition of Nebraska (ARCAEC)
3838 Dewey Ave
Omaha, NE 68105
(402) 341-2723 x120
KEY PERSONNEL: Bob Power; Coordinator of AIDS Education
AFFILIATION: American National Red Cross
FACILITY TYPE: Educational
STAFF: Volunteers 35-45
YEAR FOUNDED: 1985
FUNDING: Private
OUTREACH: Serves as an educational network for various businesses, organizations, and projects throughout Nebraska
NETWORKS: VA Medical Center; Lutheran Metro Ministries; American Red Cross—Lancaster County; United Methodist Ministries; Nebraska Civil Liberties Union; Pottawattamie County Red Cross; Douglas County Health Dept; AIDS Interfaith Network; Clarkson Hospital; Imperial Court of Nebraska; Nebraska Conference United Church of Christ; Bergan Mercy Hospital; Omaha Archdiocese; Lancaster County Health Dept; University of Nebraska—Lincoln Adult Education; Metro Omaha Medical Society; Metropolitan Community Church; Family Home Care; KETV Channel 7; Nebraska AIDS Project (NAP); Consultation Services; Nebraska League for Nurses; Creighton University Health Dept; National Council of Jewish Women; Nebraska State Health Dept; KMTV Channel 3; University of Nebraska Medical Center AIDS Education/Training; Galen and Nellie Inc; Viral Syndrome Clinic of the University of Nebraska Medical Center; Midland Lutheran College; Hyland Plasma Center; Parents and Friends of Lesbians and Gays (PFLAG)
SEMINARS: Sep 1989—"Conference for Business Leaders"
ADDITIONAL INFO: Established to bring all state groups together and move on the AIDS problem. ARCAEC's aim is to keep everyone informed and holds regular meetings in gay bars
AVAILABLE LITERATURE: *Nebraska AIDS Update*, a quarterly newsletter

434. Douglas County Health Dept, Epidemiology Section/AIDS Activity
1819 Farnam St, Rm 401
Omaha, NE 68183
(402) 444-7214
KEY PERSONNEL: Carol Allensworth; Epidemiology Section Supervisor
AFFILIATION: Douglas County Government
FACILITY TYPE: Health department
STAFF: Paid professional 3.5; Paid nonprofessional .5; Volunteers .2
YEAR FOUNDED: 1854
FUNDING: Federal government; State government; Local government
OUTREACH: HIV counseling and testing program, making general information available, speakers bureau, consultation service, surveillance
NETWORKS: Nebraska AIDS Project; American Red Cross; AIDS Education Coalition of Nebraska
SEMINARS: Mar 1988—"Attacking AIDS: An Approach for Omaha—Minority Conference," Omaha; Oct-Nov 1987—"AIDS Awareness Campaign," Omaha (including Town Hall meeting); Jan, Feb, Apr, Jun 1988—"HIV Counseling and Sex Partner Referral Workshops," Omaha
AVAILABLE LITERATURE: *AIDS Facts About Blacks*, AIDS facts as they pertain to Blacks; *AIDS Facts About Hispanics*, AIDS facts as they pertain to Hispanics; *AIDS Prevention*, a flyer of safer sex tips; *Who's At High Risk*, a flyer of statistics pertaining to high risk groups; *Dispelling Myths*, a flyer of facts about AIDS; *Nation's Blood Supply*, a flyer of facts about the blood supply and AIDS; *AIDS: Not Just a White Disease*, a flyer giving statistics by race

435. Grand Island/Hall County Dept of Health
105 E 1st
Grand Island, NE 68801
(308) 381-5175
KEY PERSONNEL: Mary Henn; Health Educator and AIDS Coordinator
AFFILIATION: Nebraska Dept of Health
FACILITY TYPE: Educational; Clinic; HIV counseling and testing
STAFF: Paid professional 3
YEAR FOUNDED: 1985
FUNDING: Federal government; State government; Local government

OUTREACH: AIDS education to 5th-8th graders in Hall County public schools, AIDS education to Kearney, NE, public school staff, information of blood and body fluid precautions and AIDS education for nursing homes, detox centers, and school nurses
SEMINARS: "Education for Rural Nebraska"
ADDITIONAL INFO: Provides free confidential counseling and testing

436. Nebraska AIDS Education and Training Center
4048 Swanson Center, Univ of Nebraska Medical Center
Omaha, NE 68105
(402) 559-6681
KEY PERSONNEL: Lanyce Keel; Coordinator
AFFILIATION: University of Nebraska Medical Center
FACILITY TYPE: Educational
STAFF: Paid professional 2
YEAR FOUNDED: 1988
FUNDING: Federal government
OUTREACH: Education and training to professionals
NETWORKS: Mountain Plains Regional AIDS Education and Training Center
SEMINARS: 1988—"AIDS '88 Regional Conference," co-sponsored with the National Hospice Organizations; 1989—"Train the Trainer Workshop for Health Care Professionals"
RESEARCH: AZT and EL721 clinical trials
ADDITIONAL INFO: Established to provide education and training about AIDS to doctors, dentists, dental personnel, physician assistants, nurses, public health workers, social workers and emergency medical technicians in Nebraska
AVAILABLE LITERATURE: *The Nebraska AIDS Experience—A Shared Journey*, a videotape

437. Nebraska AIDS Project
PO Box 3512
Omaha, NE 68103
(402) 342-4233, 6-11pm
KEY PERSONNEL: Raymond Hoffman

NEVADA

438. Aid for AIDS of Nevada
2116 Paradis Rd
Las Vegas, NV 89104
(702) 369-6162; Hotline: (702) 369-5637
KEY PERSONNEL: Sandra Long; Executive Director
FACILITY TYPE: Educational; Support group; Fund-raising; Client services/case management
STAFF: Paid professional 3; Paid nonprofessional 1; Volunteers 130
YEAR FOUNDED: 1984
FUNDING: State government; Local government; Private; Fund-raisers

439. Nevada AIDS Foundation
FORMER NAME: Northern Nevada AIDS Foundation; Northern Nevada AIDS Task Force
PO Box 478
Reno, NV 89504
(702) 329-2437; Hotline: (702) 329-2437
KEY PERSONNEL: Linda Broughton; Executive Director
FACILITY TYPE: Educational; Support group; Fund-raising
STAFF: Paid professional 1; Volunteers 15
YEAR FOUNDED: 1985
FUNDING: Federal government; Private; Fund-raisers
OUTREACH: Speakers bureau, distributes publications
AVAILABLE LITERATURE: Publishes a newsletter; *AIDS*, a brochure of AIDS information; *The Residence Program*, a brochure about the residence program

440. Nevada Hispanic Services, Inc
FORMER NAME: Centro de Informacion Latino Americano
PO Box 11735, 190 E Liberty St
Reno, NV 89510
(702) 786-6003
KEY PERSONNEL: Al Bravo; Substance Abuse Counselor
FACILITY TYPE: Educational
STAFF: Paid professional 2; Paid nonprofessional 4; Volunteers 2
YEAR FOUNDED: 1985
FUNDING: State government; Local government; Private; Fund-raisers; Fees for services or products

OUTREACH: Provides material, information and or referrals to Hispanic individuals in order to prevent drug/alcohol addiction and use

RESEARCH: AIDS Education to Hispanics

ADDITIONAL INFO: Provides service to Non-English speaking Hispanics in the areas of interpretation, translation, voter registration, information, referral, English classes, advocacy and job placement

AVAILABLE LITERATURE: Newsletter being planned for 1989

LANGUAGES: Spanish

441. State of Nevada Health Division
505 E King St, Rm 200
Carson City, NV 89710
(702) 885-4800; Hotline: (800) 842-AIDS
KEY PERSONNEL: Sandra Ziegler; AIDS Coordinator
FACILITY TYPE: Educational; Health department
FUNDING: Federal government; State government
AVAILABLE LITERATURE: *Nevada State Health Division: AIDS Program*, an 8-page resource booklet

442. WestCare Family Services Division
401 S Highland Dr
Las Vegas, NV 89106
(702) 385-2090
KEY PERSONNEL: Willie Smith; Clinical Services Director
FACILITY TYPE: HIV counseling and testing; Substance abuse treatment

NEW HAMPSHIRE

443. Citizen Alliance Gay/Lesbian Rights, AIDS Education
PO Box 756
Concord, NH 03229
(603) 228-2355
KEY PERSONNEL: Celeste Gosselin

444. Feminist Health Center of Portsmouth STD Clinic
FORMER NAME: New Hampshire Feminist Health Center
232 Court St
Portsmouth, NH 03801
(603) 436-7588
KEY PERSONNEL: Mara Lamstein, Coordinator
FACILITY TYPE: Educational; Clinic
FUNDING: State government
OUTREACH: Speakers bureau
ADDITIONAL INFO: Founded in 1980 as an STD clinic for men and women

445. HIV Counseling and Testing Service, Feminist Health Center—Portsmouth
FORMER NAME: New Hampshire Feminist Health Center
PO Box 456, 559 Portsmouth Ave
Greenland, NH 03840
(603) 436-7588
KEY PERSONNEL: Mary Halleck; Coordinator STDs, HIV services
FACILITY TYPE: Clinic; HIV counseling and testing
STAFF: Paid professional 10; Paid nonprofessional 17
YEAR FOUNDED: 1984
FUNDING: State government; Private; Fund-raisers; Fees for services or products

446. The Latin American Center
521 Maple St
Manchester, NH 03104
(603) 669-5661; Hotline: (603) 647-6960
KEY PERSONNEL: Jeff Goodrich; AIDS Program Coordinator
AFFILIATION: Greater Manchester Association of Social Service Agencies
FACILITY TYPE: Educational
STAFF: Paid professional 5; Volunteers 1
YEAR FOUNDED: 1972
FUNDING: Federal government; Private; Fund-raisers; Fees for services or products
OUTREACH: AIDS presentations to Hispanic community by trained Hispanic presenters, reference library on AIDS in Spanish, Spanish-language AIDS information hotline

NETWORKS: Manchester Dept of Health; Elliot Hospital; Bureau of Disease Control, Concord, NH

SEMINARS: Jan, 1989—"Dance with AIDS Information;" Mar, 1989—"Hispanic AIDS Poster Contest"

LANGUAGES: Spanish

447. New Hampshire AIDS Foundation (NHAF)
789 Maple St
Manchester, NH 03104
(603) 595-0218
KEY PERSONNEL: Dan Dunham; Secretary
FACILITY TYPE: Educational; Support group; Fund-raising
STAFF: Volunteers 200
YEAR FOUNDED: 1987
FUNDING: State government; Private; Fund-raisers; Fees for services or products
OUTREACH: AIDS education lectures to high schools, colleges, public and private groups and clubs
NETWORKS: American National Red Cross; National Association of Social Workers (NASW); AIDS Response; AIDS Action Committee (AAC); National AIDS Network (NAN)
SEMINARS: 1987-1988—"Buddy Training Seminars"
ADDITIONAL INFO: Provides buddies, support groups, pharmacy, and living expenses for 35 clients at various levels of need

448. New Hampshire Buddy System
PO Box 1570
Concord, NH 03301
KEY PERSONNEL: Lawrence Fontaine

449. New Hampshire Division of Public Health Services, Bureau of Disease Control, AIDS Program
6 Hazen Dr, Health and Human Services Bldg
Concord, NH 03301
(603) 271-4477; AIDS Hotline: (800) 872-8909; Toll-free: (800) 852-3345 ext 4477
KEY PERSONNEL: Joyce Cournoyer; AIDS Program Chief
AFFILIATION: New Hampshire State Government
FACILITY TYPE: Educational; Health department
STAFF: Paid professional 2
FUNDING: Federal government; State government
OUTREACH: Education, antibody counseling and testing, information clearinghouse, technical assistance
SEMINARS: "HIV Counseling and Partner Referral Course"
AVAILABLE LITERATURE: *Women and AIDS*, a brochure for women; *What is the Test?*, a brochure describing the test and what it tells you; *AIDS: A Resource Guide for New Hampshire*, a 47-page guide

450. Strafford County Prenatal and Family Planning Program (The Clinic)
PO Box 791, 50 Chestnut St
Dover, NH 03820
(603) 749-2346
KEY PERSONNEL: Tess Hall; Health Education Coordinator
FACILITY TYPE: Educational; Clinic
STAFF: Paid professional 32
YEAR FOUNDED: 1969
FUNDING: Federal government; State government; Local government; Private; Fees for services or products
OUTREACH: Health and sexuality education
SEMINARS: Apr 2, 9, 23, 1987—"Teaching Family Life/Health Education to Adolescents;" May 1987—"AIDS: Our Community Responds;" Mar 31, 1988—"AIDS Education: Professional Education and Training Workshop;" Nov 4, 1987—"The School's Role in AIDS Education;" Oct 23, 31, Nov 4, 1987, Nov 2, 1988—"Film Festival"
ADDITIONAL INFO: A complete medical, educational, and referral agency providing services for reproductive and sexual health regardless of race, creed, age, gender, color, national origin, handicap or sexual orientation
AVAILABLE LITERATURE: *The Clinic*, a brochure describing the clinic; *Mutual Caring/Mutual Sharing*, a sexuality education curriculum for adolescents

NEW JERSEY

451. AIDS Education Project, New Jersey Lesbian and Gay Coalition
PO Box 1431
New Brunswick, NJ 08903
(210) 992-5666; Helpline: 596-0767
KEY PERSONNEL: Norman Clevely, Coordinator
FACILITY TYPE: Educational
ADDITIONAL INFO: Source of additional AIDS information

452. AIDS Resource Foundation for Children, Saint Clare's Home for Children
182 Roseville Ave
Newark, NJ 07107
(201) 483-4250
KEY PERSONNEL: Terry Zealand; Executive Director
AFFILIATION: Saint Clare's Home for Children
FACILITY TYPE: Educational; Support group; Hospice; Fund-raising
STAFF: Paid professional 25; Paid nonprofessional 3; Volunteers 27
YEAR FOUNDED: 1985
FUNDING: State government; Local government; Private; Fund-raisers
OUTREACH: Provides education to community groups, at-risk groups, schools, and professionals
NETWORKS: Pediatric AIDS Committee of Newark and Jersey City
AVAILABLE LITERATURE: *AIDS Resource Foundation for Children Newsletter*
LANGUAGES: Spanish, Japanese

453. American Red Cross of Northern New Jersey
PO Box 838, 106 Washington St
East Orange, NJ 07019
(201) 676-0800
KEY PERSONNEL: Kay Ham; Director of Health and Safety Services
AFFILIATION: American National Red Cross
FACILITY TYPE: Educational; Task force
STAFF: Paid professional 1; Paid nonprofessional 2
YEAR FOUNDED: 1881
FUNDING: Fund-raisers; Fees for services or products
OUTREACH: Presentations to corporations on AIDS in the workplace, AIDS education for youth using student workbooks, teacher materials, videos, and other visuals
NETWORKS: American Red Cross Chapters in Trenton, New Brunswick, Warren County, Bergen County, Essex County, and Hudson County
SEMINARS: Jun 29, 1988—"AIDS and the Workplace—Strategies for New Jersey Businesses"
ADDITIONAL INFO: Provides massive campaigns of educational information for all aspects of the community. The intended purpose is to eliminate the fear of AIDS and make sure the facts are presented, especially in the safety of the blood supply of the nation
AVAILABLE LITERATURE: *AIDS: The Facts*, a 1987 brochure of facts about AIDS; *AIDS and Your Job—Are There Risks?*, a 1988 brochure on AIDS in the workplace; *If Your Test for Antibody to the AIDS Virus is Positive*, a 1986 brochure on what testing positive means; *What Every Parent Should Know About AIDS*, 1987 general information for parents; *AIDS and the Safety of the Nation's Blood Supply*, a 1987 brochure describing the safety of the nation's blood supply; *AIDS and Children: Information for Parents of School-Age Children*, a 1986 brochure of general information for parents; *AIDS and Children: Information for Teachers and School Officials*, a 1986 brochure for teachers on AIDS in the schools; *Gay and Bisexual Men and AIDS*, a 1986 general information brochure; *Facts About AIDS and Drug Abuse*, a 1986 general information brochure about AIDS and how it relates to drug use; *Caring for the AIDS Patient at Home*, a 1986 brochure with advice on how to care for the AIDS patient; *See Beyond Fear: You Can't Get AIDS by Shaking Hands or By Hugging, In Restaurants or in Restrooms*, a 1986 bright red and black poster; *Don't Listen to Rumors About AIDS, Get the Facts*, a poster with picture of Patti LaBelle urging individuals to get the facts

454. Atlantic City Health Dept
35 S Martin Luther King Blvd
Atlantic City, NJ 08401
(609) 347-6457; Hotline: (609) 347-6456
KEY PERSONNEL: James L Budd; Health Officer
AFFILIATION: Atlantic City Government
FACILITY TYPE: HIV counseling and testing; Health department
STAFF: Paid professional 7

FUNDING: Federal government; State government; Local government
OUTREACH: AIDS education, HIV counseling and testing
ADDITIONAL INFO: Provides HIV counseling and testing in a 5-county area of southern New Jersey

455. Caribbean Haitian Council, Inc (CAHACO)
410 Central Ave
East Orange, NJ 07018
(201) 678-5059
KEY PERSONNEL: Ernst Olibrice, Director
FACILITY TYPE: Educational; Support group
FUNDING: State government
LIBRARY: Contains governmental publications on AIDS and is open to the public
OUTREACH: Counseling, referrals to medical centers
NETWORKS: New Jersey AIDS Advisory Council
ADDITIONAL INFO: Founded in 1980 as a gay and lesbian community center
LANGUAGES: French, Creole

456. CURA (Community United for the Rehabilitation of the Addicted)
61 Lincoln Park
Newark, NJ 07104
(201) 622-3570
FACILITY TYPE: Educational; Substance abuse treatment
ADDITIONAL INFO: Source of AIDS information

457. East Orange Health Dept, HIV Counseling and Testing Site
143 New St
East Orange, NJ 07017
(201) 266-5498; Hotline: (201) 266-5454
KEY PERSONNEL: Arlene Gudis; Coordinator
AFFILIATION: East Orange City Government
FACILITY TYPE: Educational; Clinic; Support group; HIV counseling and testing
STAFF: Paid professional 7; Paid nonprofessional 1
YEAR FOUNDED: 1988
FUNDING: Federal government; State government; Local government
OUTREACH: Counseling and testing in regional drug treatment centers, sexually transmitted disease clinics, family planning clinics, and on site
ADDITIONAL INFO: The program is one of 10 sites for counseling and testing and reports to the New Jersey State Health Dept. Provides AIDS education on-site and off-site upon request
AVAILABLE LITERATURE: Distributes materials from the New Jersey State Dept of Health
LANGUAGES: Spanish

458. Hispanic Association of Ocean County, Inc
203 2nd St
Lakewood, NJ 08701
(201) 367-0619
KEY PERSONNEL: Ruth Centeno; AIDS Coordinator
FACILITY TYPE: Educational; Social service agency
STAFF: Paid professional 2
FUNDING: State government; Local government; Private; Fund-raisers
OUTREACH: Workshops provided to general public through local cable program
NETWORKS: Hispanic AIDS Sub-Committee of New Jersey; Latino AIDS Caucus
ADDITIONAL INFO: Focuses its work on Hispanics. Sponsors workshops for incarcerated Hispanics in New Jersey on a regular basis as well as providing education to the general public
AVAILABLE LITERATURE: Currently producing a video on AIDS aimed towards Caribbean Hispanics
LANGUAGES: Spanish

459. Hyacinth Foundation AIDS Project
FORMER NAME: Hyacinth Foundation/New Jersey AIDS Project
211 Livingston Ave
New Brunswick, NJ 08901
(201) 246-0204; Toll-free: (800) 433-0254
KEY PERSONNEL: Karl Manger; Director of Services
FACILITY TYPE: Educational; Support group; Client services/case management
STAFF: Paid professional 9; Paid nonprofessional 2; Volunteers 400
YEAR FOUNDED: 1985
FUNDING: State government; Private; Fund-raisers

OUTREACH: AIDS hotline, speakers bureau, publications, media contacts

NETWORKS: National AIDS Network (NAN); New Jersey Lesbian and Gay Coalition

SEMINARS: Jan 29, 1988—"AIDS: A Professional Approach," Jersey City; 2-day volunteer training sessions throughout the year in various cities

RESEARCH: Blue Project: studying risk factors of gay men in married relationships and bisexual men

ADDITIONAL INFO: The Hyacinth Foundation AIDS Project is committed to the belief that there can be quality of life after an AIDS or ARC diagnosis. It has built a network of services for all individuals affected by the AIDS crisis including people with AIDS or ARC, those who test positive for HIV, family members and friends, and the worried well

AVAILABLE LITERATURE: *Hyacinth Foundation*, a calling card; *How to Use a Condom (Rubber) for Safer Sex*, a folded card of instructions; *AIDS Project*, a brochure describing the service; *Speakers Bureau*, a brochure outlining the service; *Men and AIDS*, a general information brochure about AIDS for men; *When a Friend Has AIDS*, a brochure of suggestions on what to say and what to do; *Women at Risk*, a brochure of general information for women; *The Hyacinth Foundation AIDS Project*, a flyer with brief information and telephone numbers; *Hyacinth Foundation AIDS Project Newsletter*, a quarterly newsletter

LANGUAGES: Spanish

460. Jersey City Mayor's AIDS Task Force

586 Newark Ave
Jersey City, NJ 07306
(201) 547-5168

KEY PERSONNEL: Robert Vogt; Assistant Health Officer

AFFILIATION: Jersey City Mayor's Office

FACILITY TYPE: Educational; Task force

STAFF: Volunteers varies

YEAR FOUNDED: 1987

FUNDING: Local government

OUTREACH: Speakers bureau

SEMINARS: Jul 6, 1988—"Annual Celebration in Existence"

AVAILABLE LITERATURE: *AIDS Directories for Citizens of Jersey City and Hudson County*, a brochure describing the services

LANGUAGES: Spanish

461. La Casa de Don Pedro, Inc

21-23 Broadway
Newark, NJ 07104
(201) 483-2703

KEY PERSONNEL: Hector Miranda; Alcoholism Coordinator

FACILITY TYPE: Educational; Clinic; Support group; Client services/case management; Substance abuse treatment

YEAR FOUNDED: 1984

FUNDING: Local government; Fees for services or products

NETWORKS: Saint Michael Hospital—C.U.R.A., Inc.; National Council on Alcoholism

RESEARCH: AIDS pharmacy, resources, rights

ADDITIONAL INFO: This facility is an "alternative" out-patient pharmacy facility for alcoholics and drug users. It distributes information on AIDS prevention to schools and private organizations.

AVAILABLE LITERATURE: Distributes literature from other organizations

LANGUAGES: Spanish

462. LaHara Steele Productions

705 Downing Ct
Willingboro, NJ 08046
(609) 871-3318

KEY PERSONNEL: Joseph R. Steele; Executive Producer

FACILITY TYPE: Research; Educational; Fund-raising; Substance abuse treatment

STAFF: Paid professional 2; Paid nonprofessional 2; Volunteers 2

YEAR FOUNDED: 1986

FUNDING: Private; Fund-raisers; Fees for services or products

OUTREACH: Music appreciation workshop with live solo duet and group performers

NETWORKS: Politico Congress of Black Women

SEMINARS: Feb 25, 1989—"Workshop," a workshop on music therapy with music and a musical show

RESEARCH: Music therapy

ADDITIONAL INFO: LaHara Steele is a dynamic force in the educational battle to inform young people of the dangers of drug use and abuse. It combines music with positive messages. The rap song, *The Faces of Heroin*, is being used by treatment centers and educational programs throughout America, such as Rutgers University, Hampton Hospital and Discovery House.

AVAILABLE LITERATURE: *The Faces of Heroin*, a rap song; *The Faces of Heroin*, a poster with the words of the rap song and illustrations; *AIDS Education Song*

LANGUAGES: Spanish

463. L.I.F.T., Inc, AIDS Education/Prevention Program for Minorities

225 N Warren St
Trenton, NJ 08618
(609) 392-8688

KEY PERSONNEL: Joseph R Steele; Program Coordinator

FACILITY TYPE: Research; Educational; Fund-raising; Task force

YEAR FOUNDED: 1987

FUNDING: Federal government; State government; Local government; Private; Fund-raisers

OUTREACH: AIDS workshops and training, literature distribution, surveys

SEMINARS: Workshops for Trenton Public School System; Monthly "Share Day" program for staff in-service and daycare parents in-service

RESEARCH: Drug abuse program; Halfway House

464. New Brunswick Counseling Center

84 New St
New Brunswick, NJ 08901
(201) 246-4025

KEY PERSONNEL: Ronald Trautz; Clinical Supporter

FACILITY TYPE: HIV counseling and testing; Substance abuse treatment

465. New Jersey Buddies

61 Church St
Teaneck, NJ 07666
Hotline: (201) 837-8125

KEY PERSONNEL: Frank Smith; AIDS Coordinator

FACILITY TYPE: Educational; Support group

STAFF: Paid professional 1; Paid nonprofessional 1; Volunteers 260

YEAR FOUNDED: 1985

FUNDING: State government; Fund-raisers; Donations

OUTREACH: Educational buddy training, speakers bureau, community outreach

ADDITIONAL INFO: "New Jersey Buddies, a non-profit community based support organization, founded in 1985, is dedicated to offering PWAs, and the community, support and education."

AVAILABLE LITERATURE: *The Reality of Hope*, a brochure describing the agency; *A Resource Guide for Living With AIDS*, a 1989 booklet for PWAs; *New Jersey Buddies Companion*, a quarterly newsletter

LANGUAGES: Spanish

466. South Jersey AIDS Alliance (SJAA)

1616 Pacific Ave, Ste 201
Atlantic City, NJ 08401
(609) 347-8799; Toll-free: (800) 432-AIDS

KEY PERSONNEL: Michelle Brunetti; Coordinator

FACILITY TYPE: Educational; Support group; Fund-raising; Task force; Client services/case management

STAFF: Paid professional 3; Volunteers 42

YEAR FOUNDED: 1985

FUNDING: Federal government; State government; Local government; Private; Fund-raisers

OUTREACH: Minority outreach education to Black and Hispanic communities, speakers bureau

SEMINARS: Jan, Aug 1987, Jan 1988—"Volunteer Training"

AVAILABLE LITERATURE: *Because We Care*, a brochure describing the agency

LANGUAGES: Spanish

467. VA Medical Center

Tremont Ave and S Center St
East Orange, NJ 07019
(201) 676-1000 ext 1271

KEY PERSONNEL: Robert J. Powers; Chief

FACILITY TYPE: HIV counseling and testing; Substance abuse treatment

NEW MEXICO

468. AIDS/ARC Home Care Program, Adult/In-Home Based Services Bureau, Social Services Div, Human Services Dept, State of New Mexico
PO Box 2348, P.E.R.A. Bldg, Rm 321
Santa Fe, NM 87504-2348
(505) 827-4483
KEY PERSONNEL: James D Waltner; Physician Administrator
AFFILIATION: State of New Mexico
FACILITY TYPE: Home care
STAFF: Paid professional 1
YEAR FOUNDED: 1987
FUNDING: Federal government; State government
OUTREACH: Case management, private duty nursing, homemaker/personal care, adult day program
RESEARCH: Health care delivery systems for HIV-related illnesses
ADDITIONAL INFO: A/AHCP, a 2176 Medicaid Waiver program for HIV-related diseases, was approved by the HCFA
AVAILABLE LITERATURE: *Fact Sheet*
LANGUAGES: Spanish, Native American dialects

469. AIDS Impact Drop-in Support Group/Albuquerque
722 Silver St
Albuquerque, NM 87102
FACILITY TYPE: Support group
ADDITIONAL INFO: Source of additional AIDS information

470. AIDS Prevention Program
1190 St Francis Dr
Santa Fe, NM 87503
(505) 827-0086; Hotline: (800) 454-AIDS
KEY PERSONNEL: Jane Wilson; Health Program Manager
AFFILIATION: New Mexico State Health and Environment Dept
FACILITY TYPE: Educational; HIV counseling and testing; Health department
STAFF: Paid professional 13; Paid nonprofessional 5
YEAR FOUNDED: 1986
FUNDING: Federal government; State government
OUTREACH: Train the counselor, train the trainer
NETWORKS: New Mexico AIDS Task Force; New Mexico AIDS Consortium
ADDITIONAL INFO: Provides a variety of programs including surveillance, seroprevalence, public education, counseling and testing, health education and risk reduction and minority outreach
AVAILABLE LITERATURE: *Get the Facts About AIDS and How It Can Be Prevented*, a brochure of basic AIDS facts; *How to Lower Your Risks of AIDS*, a brochure of AIDS prevention information; *How to Avoid AIDS if You "Get Around a Lot"*, a brochure of AIDS information and safer sex tips; *AIDS and the Navajo: Facts About the Disease*, a brochure for Navajos with AIDS facts; *Si de Verdad los Quiere Protejalos*, a Spanish-language comic book about AIDS; *People Like Us*, a video; *Gentes como nosotros*, a Spanish-language video
LANGUAGES: Spanish

471. New Mexico AIDS Services, Inc (NMAS)
209A McKenzie St
Santa Fe, NM 87108
(505) 984-0911; 266-0911
KEY PERSONNEL: Don Schmidt, Executive Director; Ron McDaniels, President
FACILITY TYPE: Educational; Support group
FUNDING: Federal government; State government; Local government; Donations
LIBRARY: Contains various materials and handouts on all aspects of AIDS and AIDS services and is open to the general public
OUTREACH: Provides risk reduction education including "Health Awareness Parties" and "Bonding With Health," provides education to teams by assisting them in specific AIDS cases, and educational in-service training pertaining to AIDS
NETWORKS: National AIDS Network

ADDITIONAL INFO: Founded in 1985 as an educational and emotional support agency. Programs include emotional support and counseling, case management and home care, gay men's health, and referral
AVAILABLE LITERATURE: *AIDS: Shooting Up and Your Health*, a 1-fold brochure on IV drug use and AIDS, hepatitis-B, and endocarditis; *AIDS: What Everyone Should Know*, a 3-fold brochure with general information about AIDS; *AIDS: What Every Student Should Know*, a 2-fold brochure with AIDS information for students including safe sex guidelines; *AIDS Guidelines for Risk Reduction*, a 3-fold brochure with detailed guidelines on safe sex; *AIDS Fact Sheet*, a 1-page list of AIDS facts; *New Mexico AIDS Services Newsletter*, a monthly newsletter with information about the organization and reports of upcoming conferences
LANGUAGES: Spanish

472. New Mexico Public Health Div, District IV Health Office
200 E Chisum
Roswell, NM 88201
(505) 624-6050
KEY PERSONNEL: Paula Miller; Health Educator
AFFILIATION: New Mexico State Public Health Div
FACILITY TYPE: Educational; Clinic
STAFF: Paid professional 10
YEAR FOUNDED: 1920
FUNDING: Federal government; State government
OUTREACH: Public and school health education workshops and seminars
SEMINARS: On-going education at all district schools
LANGUAGES: Spanish

NEW YORK

473. AIDS Center of Queens County, Inc (ACQC)
113-20 Jamaica Ave
Richmond Hill, NY 11418
(718) 847-1966; Hotline: (718) 847-1966
KEY PERSONNEL: Gary Maffei; Executive Director
FACILITY TYPE: Educational; Support group; Fund-raising; Task force
STAFF: Paid professional 7; Paid nonprofessional 3; Volunteers 200
YEAR FOUNDED: 1986
FUNDING: State government; Local government; Private; Fund-raisers
OUTREACH: Distributes educational literature, condoms, and bleech kits, speakers bureau, distributes information at health fairs
NETWORKS: AIDS Service Delivery Consortium—NYC; Gay Men's Health Crisis (GMHC) Budget Working Committee; New York AIDS Coalition; Human Resource Agency's Executives Concerned About AIDS
SEMINARS: Oct 1987, 1988—"Service Providers Symposium;" Jun 1988—"Memorial Service"
ADDITIONAL INFO: ACQC serves Queens County residents. The agency is an independent, community based, non-profit organization primarily funded by the New York State Dept of Health, AIDS Institute, and private donations
AVAILABLE LITERATURE: *ACQC Journal: The Newsletter of the AIDS Center of Queens County*, a quarterly newsletter; distributes various brochures, fact sheets and posters
LANGUAGES: Spanish, American Sign Language

474. AIDS Comprehensive Family Care Center
FORMER NAME: Children and Youth AIDS Hotline
1300 Morris Park Ave, Rm F-401
Bronx, NY 10461
(212) 430-4227, 430-3652; Hotline: (212) 430-3333
KEY PERSONNEL: Toni Cabat; Project Coordinator
AFFILIATION: Albert Einstein College of Medicine
FACILITY TYPE: Research; Educational; Hospital; Clinic; Support group
STAFF: Paid professional 25; Volunteers 40
YEAR FOUNDED: 1981
FUNDING: Federal government; State government; Local government; Fees for services or products
OUTREACH: Speakers bureau, consultation, referral services, education
RESEARCH: HIV and children, HIV and women/pregnancy, prenatal transmission, treatment of HIV in children
AVAILABLE LITERATURE: *Children Can Get AIDS Too: Questions and Answers*, a brochure of AIDS facts; *Recommended Precautions for Caregivers of Children with AIDS*, a brochure of recommendations; *Children Have AIDS Too*, poster
LANGUAGES: Spanish, French, Hebrew, German

475. AIDS Council of Northeastern New York, Inc (ACNENY)
307 Hamilton St
Albany, NY 12210
(518) 434-4686; Hotline: (518) 445-2439
KEY PERSONNEL: Mary C Freeman; Executive Director
AFFILIATION: New York State Dept of Health, AIDS Institute
FACILITY TYPE: Educational; Support group; Fund-raising; Client services/case management
STAFF: Paid professional 15; Volunteers 150
YEAR FOUNDED: 1981
FUNDING: State government; Private; Fund-raisers
OUTREACH: Educational outreach services are provided within in a 17-county area from Columbia to Franklin and Clinton in the north country
AVAILABLE LITERATURE: *Updates*, quarterly newletter; *Support and Services for People Who Test Positive for the HIV Antibody*, a brochure of recommendations, resources, and referrals; *AIDS Management: Through Community Services*, a brochure describing the agency

476. AIDS Education and Resources Center, School of Allied Health Professions
FORMER NAME: Training Program in AIDS for Health Professionals
SUNY at Stony Brook, Health Sciences Center, Level 2-075
Stony Brook, NY 11794-8206
KEY PERSONNEL: Rose A Walton; Project Director
AFFILIATION: SUNY at Stony Brook School of Allied Health Professions
FACILITY TYPE: Educational
STAFF: Paid professional 7; Paid nonprofessional 3
YEAR FOUNDED: 1986
FUNDING: Federal government; State government; Private
OUTREACH: Health professionals education and resources, health professions student education, community education
RESEARCH: Affective education strategies for health care workers
AVAILABLE LITERATURE: *The Bridge*, a quarterly newsletter giving information on AIDS research, education, care, and services

477. AIDS Education and Service Coordination Project
111 Westfall Rd
Rochester, NY 14692
(716) 274-6114
KEY PERSONNEL: Susan Cowell; AIDS Coordinator
AFFILIATION: Monroe County Government
FACILITY TYPE: Educational; Fund-raising
STAFF: Paid professional 3; Paid nonprofessional 1
YEAR FOUNDED: 1988
FUNDING: State government
OUTREACH: Training of county staff, administers 3 community grants for minority AIDS education, administers support for the Rochester Area Task Force on AIDS (RATFA)
NETWORKS: Rochester Area Task Force on AIDS (RATFA)
RESEARCH: Evaluation of teaching methods and risk reduction efforts
ADDITIONAL INFO: The RATFA Strategic Planning Committee developed a 5-year plan for the region. The recommendations include increasing the involvement of local government
AVAILABLE LITERATURE: *AIDS in the Rochester/Finger Lakes Region—1988*, a report to the community on AIDS; *AIDS Action Plan: Five Year Agenda for Rochester and the Finger Lakes Region, Executive Summary*, a 1987 plan of action in summary; *AIDS Action Plan: Five Year Agenda for Rochester and the Finger Lakes Region*, the full report; distributes materials published by the New York AIDS Institute

478. AIDS Epidemiology Program/Albany
Empire State Plaza, Corning Tower, Rm 668
Albany, NY 12237
(518) 474-6730
KEY PERSONNEL: Benedict I Truman, Director
AFFILIATION: New York State Dept of Health
FACILITY TYPE: Educational; Clinic
FUNDING: Federal government; State government
LIBRARY: Provides public information on AIDS
RESEARCH: Conducts epidemiologic research on AIDS
ADDITIONAL INFO: Founded in 1983 as a collection agency for the AIDS registry, field data, and AIDS epidemiology studies
AVAILABLE LITERATURE: *AIDS Surveillance Monthly Update*

479. AIDS Institute
Corning Tower Bldg, Rm 359 Empire State Plaza
Albany, NY 12237
(518) 473-7238; Hotline, New York State: (800) 541-AIDS; Hotline, New York City: (718) 485-8111; HIV Counseling Hotline: (800) 872-2777; ADAP Hotline: (800) 542-2437
KEY PERSONNEL: James Bulger; Executive Deputy Director
AFFILIATION: New York State Dept of Health
FACILITY TYPE: Research; Educational; HIV counseling and testing
STAFF: Paid professional 200
YEAR FOUNDED: 1983
FUNDING: Federal government; State government; Private
OUTREACH: Anonymous HIV counseling and testing, community service programs, community-based organizations, AIDS drug assistance program, education and training
NETWORKS: New York City AIDS Service Delivery Consortium
SEMINARS: Provides general workshops—"HIV Counseling and Testing and Training," "AIDS Overview," "Women and Pediatric AIDS," "Long-Term Care"
RESEARCH: Men's Project, a federally funded cohort study of gay and bisexual men in a low incidence area for AIDS
ADDITIONAL INFO: Founded in 1983 to coordinate New York State's AIDS prevention and service efforts. The AIDS Drug Assistance Program was initiated in 1987 to provide AZT and other FDA-approved drugs to persons with AIDS
AVAILABLE LITERATURE: *Having a Baby?: Have a Test for AIDS Virus First*, an informational brochure; *Va a Tener un Bebe?: Sometase Primero a una Prueba para Detectar el Virus del SIDA*, an informational brochure on having a baby in Spanish; *AIDS Does Not Discriminate*, informational brochure; *What Parents Need to Tell Children About AIDS*, a booklet of facts; *Lo que los Padres Deben decir asus Hijos Sobre el SIDA*, a booklet in Spanish about AIDS; *Do You Have Questions About AIDS?*, a brochure about the institute; *Quiere usted Preguntar Algo Sobre el SIDA?*, a Spanish-language brochure about the institute; *Women and AIDS*, an informational brochure for women; *Las Mujeres y el SIDA*, a Spanish-language informational brochure for women; *AIDS Service Programs*, an informational card with telephone numbers; *Llame para Informarse Mejor*, a Spanish-language informational card with telephone numbers; *HIV Counseling and Testing Program*, an informational card about the HIV antibody test; *Programas de Servicio a la Comunidad*, a Spanish-language informational card about the HIV antibody test; *100 Questions and Answers: AIDS*, a booklet of questions and answers; *100 Preguntas y Respuestas: SIDA*, a Spanish-language booklet of questions and answers on AIDS; *AIDS and HIV Counseling and Testing*, a brochure about the HIV antibody test; *Servicios de Analisis y Orientacion Sobre el SIDA y el VIH*, a Spanish-language brochure about the HIV antibody test; *Don't Die of Embarrassment*, a series of posters each with the message given by a prominent person—Cher, Richard Belzer, Whoopi Goldberg, Esai Morales
LANGUAGES: Spanish

480. AIDS Prevention Research Center
622 W 113th St
New York, NY 10025
(212) 854-3035, 854-4078
KEY PERSONNEL: Adam Gordon; CSW Staff Associate
AFFILIATION: Columbia University School of Social Work
FACILITY TYPE: Research; Educational
STAFF: Paid professional 6
YEAR FOUNDED: 1754
FUNDING: Federal government
NETWORKS: American Health Foundation; Cornell University Medical College; Beth Israel Medical Center
ADDITIONAL INFO: The center is dedicated to the development and testing of interventions to prevent the spread of AIDS and HIV infection among minority group members through the reduction of intraveneous drug use and unsafe sexual behavior
AVAILABLE LITERATURE: Published in various journals

481. AIDS Resource Center, Inc
24 W 30th St
New York, NY 10001
(212) 481-1270
KEY PERSONNEL: Douglas H Dornan; Executive Director
FACILITY TYPE: Support group; Hospice; Fund-raising; Task force; Residential facility (adults)
STAFF: Paid professional 25; Paid nonprofessional 30; Volunteers 150
YEAR FOUNDED: 1983

FUNDING: Federal government; State government; Local government; Private; Fund-raisers

OUTREACH: Speakers bureau, workshops on housing, developmental and technical assistance for other groups interested in housing

NETWORKS: New York City AIDS Service Delivery Consortium; National AIDS Network (NAN)

SEMINARS: Apr 27, 1988—"Supportive Housing for Homeless People with AIDS: The Need—The Options—The Opportunity," a technical assistance workshop

ADDITIONAL INFO: The AIDS Resource Center has helped to develop permanent, affordable housing for homeless people with AIDS. Operates the Bailey House, opened in 1986, and offers a Scattered Site Apartment Program.

AVAILABLE LITERATURE: *AIDS...A Compassionate Pastoral Response*, an informational brochure; *AIDS Resource Center*, a card outlining what the agency provides; *AIDS Resource Center, Inc* , a brochure giving details about the agency; *Supportive Housing for People with AIDS*, an informational flyer; *News from the AIDS Resource Center*, a newsletter

LANGUAGES: Spanish

482. AIDS Rochester, Inc (ARI)

20 University Ave
Rochester, NY 14605
(716) 232-3580; Hotline: (716) 232-4430
KEY PERSONNEL: Jackie Nudd; Executive Director
FACILITY TYPE: Educational; Support group; Fund-raising; Task force
STAFF: Paid professional 10; Paid nonprofessional 3; Volunteers 205
YEAR FOUNDED: 1983
FUNDING: State government; Private; Fund-raisers
OUTREACH: Educational in service programs for any agency or group, outreach with the community and outlying counties
NETWORKS: Baden Street; Planned Parenthood; RATFA; Action for a Better Community; Puerto Rican Youth Development
SEMINARS: May 19-20, 1987—"AIDS," a community health care conference
ADDITIONAL INFO: The goals of this agency are education, service, media representation, and professional referrals. Offers advocacy, buddies, clothing and food cupboards, crisis intervention, educational programs, grants, hotline, interpreters, newsletter, referrals, support groups, and transportation
AVAILABLE LITERATURE: *AIDS Rochester, Inc.*, an informational brochure; annual report, quarterly newsletter, volunteer newsletter, and client newsletter
LANGUAGES: Spanish, American Sign Language

483. AIDS Task Force of Central New York

627 W Genesee St
Syracuse, NY 13204
(315) 475-2430; Hotline: 475-AIDS
KEY PERSONNEL: Bradley R Cohen, Executive Director; Lucinda Cawley, Education Coordinator; Ray Durr, Support Services Coordinator; Terry Martin, Office Manager
FACILITY TYPE: Educational; Support group; Task force
FUNDING: State government; Donations; Grants
LIBRARY: Contains materials on AIDS, psychology, death and dying, substance abuse, and homosexuality and is open to interested persons
OUTREACH: Speakers bureau, counseling
NETWORKS: National AIDS Network; New York State AIDS Network
SEMINARS: Produces several seminars and symposia throughout the year
ADDITIONAL INFO: Founded in 1983 to provide accurate and up-to-date information about AIDS to people at high risk, health and human service professionals, and the general public and to insure that support services for people affected by AIDS are available and accessible
AVAILABLE LITERATURE: *Needles, Drugs and AIDS*, a 2-fold brochure on AIDS and drugs; *Children with AIDS: Guidelines for Parents and Caregivers*, a 10-page pamphlet with general information on AIDS as it pertains to children; *Guidelines for Safer and Healthier Sex*, a 3-fold brochure on safe sex; *When a Friend Has AIDS*, a 2-fold brochure on recommendations of what to do; *Resource List*, a 4-page pamphlet of books and videos about AIDS. The task force also provides a folder of materials from other agencies including *Safe Sex; Women Need to Know About AIDS; AIDS: Get the Facts; Ask the Experts About AIDS and the Blood Supply* (American Red Cross); *AIDS: Information for Gay Men*; reprints of articles are included in the folder

484. AIDS Task Force of National Council of Churches

475 Riverside Dr, Rm 572
New York, NY 10015
(212) 870-2421
FACILITY TYPE: Support group
ADDITIONAL INFO: A support group for AIDS patients and friends

485. AIDS-Related Community Services (ARCS)

FORMER NAME: Mid-Hudson Valley AIDS Task Force
214 Central Ave, Lower Level
White Plains, NY 10606
(914) 993-0606; AIDSline: (914) 993-0607
KEY PERSONNEL: John Egan; Executive Director
FACILITY TYPE: Educational; Support group; Client services/case management
STAFF: Paid professional 26; Volunteers 165
YEAR FOUNDED: 1983
FUNDING: State government; Local government; Private; Fund-raisers
OUTREACH: Speakers bureau, workshops, conferences, media events, educational presentations to communities, agencies, etc, AIDSline
NETWORKS: New York City AIDS Service Delivery Consortium
ADDITIONAL INFO: Founded to provide education, support groups, counseling, buddies, AIDSline and other support services in the counties of Westchester, Rockland, Putnam, Dutchess, Sullivan, Orange, and Ulster
AVAILABLE LITERATURE: *Here to Help*, a poster with telephone numbers; *Here to Help*, a brochure describing the services of the agency; *ARCS News*, a newsletter
LANGUAGES: Spanish, French

486. American Management Association (AMA)

135 W 50th St
New York, NY 10020
(212) 586-8100
KEY PERSONNEL: Don Bohl; Group Editor
FACILITY TYPE: Educational; Professional
AVAILABLE LITERATURE: *AIDS: The New Workplace Issues*

487. American Run for the End of AIDS (AREA)

2350 Broadway
New York, NY 10024
FACILITY TYPE: Educational
ADDITIONAL INFO: Source of additional AIDS information

488. Association for Drug Abuse Prevention and Treatment, Inc (ADAPT)

85 Bergen St
Brooklyn, NY 11201
(718) 834-9585
KEY PERSONNEL: Celeste Derr; Education Director
FACILITY TYPE: Educational; Support group; Substance abuse treatment
STAFF: Paid professional 15; Volunteers 200
YEAR FOUNDED: 1980
FUNDING: Local government; Private; Fund-raisers
OUTREACH: Outreach and education to IV drug users, alternatives to incarceration program, support groups for PWAs, PWARCs, HIV positive individuals, their care partners, women, Hispanics, the bereaved, and those at risk of getting AIDS, IV league buddies, referrals, public information, training around the issues of AIDS and IV drug use and treatment for staff of hospitals, drug treatment facilities, and AIDS organizations
ADDITIONAL INFO: ADAPT's goals are to provide education and outreach services to the intravenous drug user (IVDU) community about AIDS, the AIDS/IV link, and risk-reduction methods; provide public education about AIDS and the AIDS/IV link; identify special needs of current and ex-IVDUs and advocate for services and funds to meet those needs; and to assist in the coordination of state and local resources for AIDS prevention and treatment, especially for IVDUs.
AVAILABLE LITERATURE: *ADAPT*, a flyer describing the organization; *Safety Kit*, a safer sex information with a condom; *AIDS: Sindrome de Immunidad Deficiente Adquirida (SIDA)*, an informational brochure of AIDS facts; *AIDS: The Mainline Message from ADAPT*, a brochure of basic AIDS facts; *Esta Cansado de Usar Drogas? Venga a ADAPT*, a flyer advertising ADAPT; *Tired of Using Drugs; Reach Out to ADAPT*, a flyer advertising ADAPT; *AIDS es Mortal*, a flyer aimed at drug users; *AIDS is Deadly*, a flyer for drug users
LANGUAGES: Spanish

489. Beekman Downtown Hospital
170 William St
New York, NY 10038
FACILITY TYPE: Clinic; Hospital
ADDITIONAL INFO: Source of AIDS information

490. Bellevue Hospital Methadone Maintenance Tretment Program
27th St and 1st Ave C and D Bldg Ground Fl
New York, NY 10016
(212) 561-3201
KEY PERSONNEL: Joseph Annesi; Administrator
FACILITY TYPE: HIV counseling and testing; Substance abuse treatment

491. Betances Health Unit, Inc
281 E Broadway
New York, NY 10002
(212) 227-8401
KEY PERSONNEL: Andrea Cowan; Development Assistant
FACILITY TYPE: Educational; Clinic; Fund-raising
STAFF: Paid professional 16; Paid nonprofessional 19; Volunteers 2
YEAR FOUNDED: 1970
FUNDING: State government; Private; Fees for services or products
OUTREACH: Emergency Nutrition Enrichment Project (ENEP), Shelter Health Assessment, Prevention and Education (SHAPE) Project
NETWORKS: Henry Street Settlement; American Red Cross; Educational Alliance; Grand Street Settlement
SEMINARS: Provides six nutrition education seminars per month and six health education seminars at shelters served by SHAPE per month
ADDITIONAL INFO: This is a non-profit community based family medical practice providing primary health care services including prenatal care, podiatry, gynecology, homeopathic medicine, plus alternative therapies such as acupuncture and massage. The social work staff assists with HIV positive individuals and PWAs and their families.
LANGUAGES: Spanish, French, Chinese, Russian, Arabic

492. Beth Israel Medical Center
1st Ave and 16th St
New York, NY 10003
(212) 420-4184
KEY PERSONNEL: Errol A Chin-Loy; AIDS Coordinator
AFFILIATION: Mount Sinai Hospital
FACILITY TYPE: Hospital; HIV counseling and testing
YEAR FOUNDED: 1890
FUNDING: Local government; Private; Fees for services or products
OUTREACH: Outreach through drug programs by the AIDS coordinator for substance abuse, Karpas health information service of education to the general public, AIDS coordinator education to the local agencies
NETWORKS: New York City Management AIDS Advisory Council; Gay Men's Health Crisis; New York Hospital Association; Premier Hospitals Alliance; UJA-Federation of Jewish Philanthropies
SEMINARS: Oct 19, 1988—"AIDS Education Forum;" Sep 16, 1987—"AIDS: A Community Update"
RESEARCH: AIDS treatment evaluation
ADDITIONAL INFO: Beth Israel is a designated AIDS center under the New York State Dept of Health
AVAILABLE LITERATURE: *Are You Hooked on IV Drugs?*, an informational brochure; *Te Estas Inyectando?*, an informational brochure in Spanish
LANGUAGES: Language bank

493. Beth Simchat Torah
31 Bethune St
New York, NY 10014
(212) 869-3486 day; 924-8899 night
FACILITY TYPE: Support group
ADDITIONAL INFO: Provides spiritual support, fellowship, and assistance to gay and Jewish people with AIDS at home and in the hospital

494. Bronx Municipal Hospital Center
Pelham Pkwy and Eastchester Rd
Bronx, NY 10461
(212) 430-5455
FACILITY TYPE: Clinic
ADDITIONAL INFO: A clinic with ambulatory and emergency room services

495. Brooklyn AIDS Task Force
22 Chapel St
Brooklyn, NY 11201
(718) 596-4781; Hotline: (718) 852-8042
FACILITY TYPE: Educational; Support group; Fund-raising
STAFF: Paid professional 7; Volunteers 30
YEAR FOUNDED: 1986
FUNDING: State government; Local government
OUTREACH: Training programs, forums, speakers bureau, case management, crisis intervention
NETWORKS: Greenpoint/Williamsberg Resource Committee; Brooklyn Teen Pregnancy Network
SEMINARS: Jul 9, 1987—"AIDS: A Community Planning Symposium," Brooklyn; Oct 24, 1987—"AIDS: It Will Take All of Us, A Community Responds," Brooklyn; Nov 19, 1988—"Empowerment: A Prescription for Women's Health," Brooklyn
AVAILABLE LITERATURE: *Brooklyn AIDS Task Force Community Service Program*, an informational brochure about the service; *Anyone Can Get AIDS*, answers to a child's questions about AIDS; *Needle Sharing Equals AIDS Sharing*, a bumper sticker; *If You Share Needles You Share AIDS*, a bumper sticker; *The Sun Will Come Out Tomorrow If You Use a Condom Today*, a bumper sticker; *A Condom Is Another Way of Saying I Care*, a bumper sticker; *AIDS Warrior on the Go*, a bumper sticker; *Do You Know Where Your Condom Is?*, a bumper sticker; *What Is It?*, a child's coloring book about AIDS; *Que es Eso?*, a child's coloring book about AIDS in Spanish; *Qu'est—ce Que c'Est?*, a child's coloring book about AIDS in French; *Win a Free Trip to Life/Practice Safer Sex*, a pen; *Prevention/A Chance for a Brighter Life*, a cigarette lighter; *Top Secret*, a condom case; *AIDS?*, a refrigerator magnet with telephone number; *Caring is Learning the Facts About AIDS*, a refrigerator magnet with telephone numbers
LANGUAGES: French, Spanish, Creole

496. Brownsville Clinic
564 Hopkinson Ave
Brooklyn, NY 11212
(718) 385-4000
KEY PERSONNEL: Bruce Stewart; Director
FACILITY TYPE: HIV counseling and testing; Substance abuse treatment

497. Bushwick Clinic
1149-55 Myrtle Ave
Brooklyn, NY 11206
(718) 574-1400
KEY PERSONNEL: Fele Reyes; Director
FACILITY TYPE: HIV counseling and testing; Substance abuse treatment

498. Cabrini Medical Center
227 E 19th St
New York, NY 10003
(212) 995-6000
AFFILIATION: Stuyvesant Polyclinic
FACILITY TYPE: Hospital
YEAR FOUNDED: 1892
FUNDING: Federal government; State government; Private; Fund-raisers
OUTREACH: Health information center, distributes AIDS brochures, lectures and Workshops
ADDITIONAL INFO: Cabrini Medical Center offers general medical, surgical acute care services and emergency services. Cabrini is affiliated with Stuyvesant Polyclinic, which offers assessments and comprehensive primary and specialty care for patients with AIDS and ARC. Cabrini's Infectious Disease Dept conducts research. The Cabrini Hospice accepts terminally ill individuals who have a prognosis of six months or less.
AVAILABLE LITERATURE: Maintains a language bank

499. Chinatown Health Clinic
89 Baxter St
New York, NY 10013
FACILITY TYPE: Clinic
ADDITIONAL INFO: Source of AIDS information

500. Community Health Project (CHP)
208 W 13th St
New York, NY 10011
(212) 675-3559
KEY PERSONNEL: Rona Affoumado; Executive Director
AFFILIATION: National Association of Community Health Centers
FACILITY TYPE: Educational; Clinic; Support group
STAFF: Paid professional 16; Volunteers 150
YEAR FOUNDED: 1983
FUNDING: Local government; Private; Fund-raisers; Fees for services or products
OUTREACH: Educational seminars, training, technical assistance, consultation
NETWORKS: Robert Wood Johnson AIDS Services Consortium of New York; AIDS Budget Working Group; New York City AIDS Task Force; New York State AIDS Task Force; New York City Health and Hospitals Corp
RESEARCH: Early intervention and treatment of HIV asymptomatic seropositive patients, behavior modification, and stress reduction techniques
ADDITIONAL INFO: CHP is a community-based primary care clinic for HIV/AIDS associated medical and psychosocial problems. As of June 30, 1988, the project had more than 1600 registered patients
AVAILABLE LITERATURE: *Check-Up*, a quarterly newsletter
LANGUAGES: American Sign Language, Spanish

501. Comprehensive Alcoholism Treatment Center
937 Fulton St
Brooklyn, NY 11238
(718) 789-1212
KEY PERSONNEL: Robert Sage; Vice President
FACILITY TYPE: HIV counseling and testing; Substance abuse treatment

502. Albert Einstein College of Medicine
Bronx Psychiatric Center 1500 Waters Pl
Bronx, NY 10461
(212) 409-9450
KEY PERSONNEL: John Langrod; Director
FACILITY TYPE: HIV counseling and testing; Substance abuse treatment

503. Fund for Human Dignity
FORMER NAME: NGTF/Fund For Human Dignity
666 Broadway, Ste 410
New York, NY 10012
(212) 529-1600; Hotline: (800) 221-7044
KEY PERSONNEL: Sherrie Cohen; Executive Director
FACILITY TYPE: Educational; Advocacy
STAFF: Paid professional 5; Paid nonprofessional 6; Volunteers 70
YEAR FOUNDED: 1974
FUNDING: Private; Fund-raisers
OUTREACH: National gay and lesbian crisisline that answers questions about AIDS and lesbian and gay issues; maintains a clearinghouse of gay and lesbian educational materials
SEMINARS: Jul 24, 1988—"The First National Lesbian and Gay Education Conference: Initiatives Toward a National Education Agenda for Our Culturally Diverse Community"
RESEARCH: Gay and lesbian education, anti-homophobia education, gay positive curricula
AVAILABLE LITERATURE: *The National AIDS Resource Directory*, a nationwide directory of AIDS service organizations, testing sites, etc.; distributes and produces other publications

504. Gay and Lesbian Community Center/Buffalo
647 W Delavan Ave
Buffalo, NY 14222
(716) 886-1274
FACILITY TYPE: Educational
ADDITIONAL INFO: Source of additional AIDS information

505. Gay Men's Counseling Service/Sayville
201 Foster Ave
Sayville, NY 11782
FACILITY TYPE: Support group
ADDITIONAL INFO: Source of additional AIDS information

506. Gay Men's Health Crisis, Inc (GMHC)
PO Box 274, 132 W 24th St
New York, NY 10011
(212) 807-6655; Hotline: 807-7035
KEY PERSONNEL: Richard Donne, Executive Director
FACILITY TYPE: Educational
FUNDING: Federal government; State government; Local government; Donations; Grants
LIBRARY: Contains publications about AIDS and safe sex. Open to interested persons
OUTREACH: Speakers bureau, conduct AIDS prevention and safe sex workshops
SEMINARS: Participate in many symposia and seminars
RESEARCH: Studying the changes in sexual behavior from high-risk to low-risk
ADDITIONAL INFO: Founded in 1982 as an educational and support agency for persons with AIDS and ARC including crisis intervention counseling, group therapy, buddy program, and legal, financial, and health care advocacy
AVAILABLE LITERATURE: *Health Letter*, a bimonthly newsletter with information about AIDS and safe sex; *Medical Answers About AIDS*, a 42-page booklet prepared by Lawrence Mass with complete questions and answers about all aspects of AIDS and safe sex; *Women Need to Know About AIDS*, information for women about AIDS; *An Ounce of Prevention is Worth a Pound of Cure*, safe sex guidelines. Other publications available from GMHC include: *AIDS Hotline; AIDS Problem List/Nursing Care Plan; Condom* poster; *Early Symptoms of AIDS and ARC; GMHC Annual Report; GMHC Recreation Therapy Services; GMHC Services; Healthy Sex is Great Sex* poster; *Infection Precautions for PWAs; Infections Frequently Associated with AIDS; Information for Gay Men; Information for the General Public; Information for NYS Correctional Facilities; Kaposi's Sarcoma; Legal Aspects of AIDS; Overview of Psycho-Social Issues; Pin Card* (safe sex guidelines with safety pin); *Safer Sex Comix; Safer Sex Guidelines* (written in "street" language); *Strategies for the Worried Well; The Volunteer; Treatment of Opportunistic Infections; What Everyone Should Know About AIDS; What is GHMC; What You Should Know About Insurance*; and *When a Friend Has AIDS*
LANGUAGES: Spanish, Chinese

507. God's Love We Deliver, Inc (GLWD)
PO Box 1776, Old Chelsea Station
New York, NY 10011
(212) 874-1193; Hotline: (212) 874-1424
KEY PERSONNEL: Ganga Stone; President
FACILITY TYPE: Client services/case management; Food supply
STAFF: Paid professional 15; Volunteers 120
YEAR FOUNDED: 1986
FUNDING: State government; Private; Fund-raisers
NETWORKS: AIDS Budget Working Committee; National AIDS Network (NAN)
ADDITIONAL INFO: Provides hot meals for homebound PWAs
AVAILABLE LITERATURE: Publishes a newsletter and pamphlets
LANGUAGES: American Sign Language, Spanish

508. Haitian Coalition on AIDS (HCA)
50 Court St, Ste 605
Brooklyn, NY 11201
(718) 855-0972
KEY PERSONNEL: Marie M Saint Cyr, Director
FACILITY TYPE: Support group
FUNDING: Grants
OUTREACH: Workshops on AIDS prevention, education for family members and loved ones of PWAs
NETWORKS: AIDS Institute of New York
ADDITIONAL INFO: Founded in 1983 to serve the Haitian community of New York by providing AIDS information
AVAILABLE LITERATURE: Flyers about AIDS for the Haitian community
LANGUAGES: Creole

509. Haitian Women's Program, American Friends Services Committee
15 Rutherford Place
New York, NY 10003
(212) 598-0965
KEY PERSONNEL: Patricia Benoit; Co-Director
FACILITY TYPE: Educational
STAFF: Paid professional 2.5; Volunteers 5
YEAR FOUNDED: 1982
FUNDING: State government; Private; Fund-raisers
OUTREACH: Workshops in community center, churches, and hospitals
AVAILABLE LITERATURE: Provides booklets, pamphlets, and video tapes in Creole and English
LANGUAGES: Creole, French

510. Health Education AIDS Liaison, Inc (HEAL)
PO Box 1103, Old Chelsea Station
New York, NY 10113
(212) 674-4673; Hotline: (212) 674-HOPE
KEY PERSONNEL: Frank Russo; Executive Director
FACILITY TYPE: Research; Educational; Support group
STAFF: Paid professional 1; Volunteers 15
YEAR FOUNDED: 1982
FUNDING: Private; Donations
OUTREACH: Support group, healing kitchen, At Peace with HIV program, explorations in immunity
RESEARCH: Tracking and studying the affects of hypnotherapy on HIV positive persons and studying the effects of a combined fully integrated program on individuals with AIDS, ARC, and HIV
ADDITIONAL INFO: HEAL is a support group which educates and informs people about AIDS and AIDS concerns on alternative and holistic therapies AIDS
AVAILABLE LITERATURE: *HEAL*, a newsletter; various flyers about the organization and articles in newspapers
LANGUAGES: Spanish

511. HEALTH WATCH Information and Promotion Service
3020 Glenwood Rd
Brooklyn, NY 11210
(718) 434-5411
KEY PERSONNEL: Norma J Goodwin; President
FACILITY TYPE: Educational
STAFF: Paid professional 5; Paid nonprofessional 2; Volunteers varies
YEAR FOUNDED: 1984
FUNDING: Federal government; State government; Private; Fees for services or products
OUTREACH: Educational information related to AIDS, cancer, hypertension, heart disease, diabetes, obesity and teenage pregnancy
SEMINARS: Oct 1988—"Diabetes in the Black Population: The Current State of Knowledge;" Mar 1989—"Imperatives for Action;" Oct 1989—"Achieving Heart Health in the Black Population"
RESEARCH: Black and other ethnic minority health improvement, especially regarding AIDS, cancer, hypertension, heart disease, diabetes, obesity, and teenage pregnancy
ADDITIONAL INFO: Formed in 1984 with initial research and development support from the National Cancer Institute, and additional support from the New York State Science and Technology Foundation
AVAILABLE LITERATURE: *HEALTH WATCH News*, a regular newsletter; *If You're Black You Should Be Reading This*, a cancer awareness brochure; *The Real Deal About AIDS*, an informative brochure for teenagers; *Your Teenagers Don't Have to Get AIDS*, a brochure for parents

512. Hispanic AIDS Forum
853 Broadway, Ste 2007
New York, NY 10003
(212) 870-1902; 870-1864
FACILITY TYPE: Support group
ADDITIONAL INFO: Source of additional information on AIDS for Hispanics

513. Human Sexuality Program, Dept of Health Education
239 Green St, 6th Fl
New York, NY 10003
(212) 998-5793
KEY PERSONNEL: Ronald Moglia; Director
AFFILIATION: New York University, School of Education, Health, Nursing and Arts Professions

FACILITY TYPE: Educational
STAFF: Paid professional 6
FUNDING: Private; Fees for services or products
OUTREACH: Consultant to the public educational institutions
NETWORKS: Sex Information and Education Council of the U.S. (SIECUS)
RESEARCH: AIDS education integrated in health/family life education in public schools
ADDITIONAL INFO: Grants advanced degrees in human sexuality, health education, and public health

514. Institute for Human Identity (IHI)
118 W 72nd St, 1st Fl
New York, NY 10023
(212) 799-9432
KEY PERSONNEL: Patti Geier, Clinical Coordinator; Henry Weinhoff, Administrator
FACILITY TYPE: Support group
FUNDING: Fees for services or products; Donations
LIBRARY: Contains books dealing with therapy and lesbian/gay-related issues, gay and lesbian newspapers, magazines, and journals. For staff and clients to use in-house
OUTREACH: Speaking engagements, training sessions for gay counselors, workshops on various issues
SEMINARS: Apr 4, 1987—"Toward an Affirmative Identity": A conference on psychotherapy for lesbians and gays
ADDITIONAL INFO: Founded in 1973 as a therapy and counseling center for the lesbian, gay, and bisexual community offering individual, couple, and group therapy on a sliding fee scale

515. Interfaith Medical Center
555 Prospect Pl
Brooklyn, NY 11238
(718) 935-7277
KEY PERSONNEL: Nancy Seddio; Chief
FACILITY TYPE: Educational; Hospital; Clinic; Support group
YEAR FOUNDED: 1986
FUNDING: Federal government; State government; Local government
ADDITIONAL INFO: Treats both medical and mental health aspects of PWAs, PWARCs, significant others, and those individuals from the high-risk groups who worry that they may contract AIDS
AVAILABLE LITERATURE: Speakers bureau

516. Jefferson County Committee on AIDS Information (JCCAI)
1020 State St
Watertown, NY 13601
(315) 782-4410; Hotline: (315) 782-9514
KEY PERSONNEL: Jerry S Moore; Chairman
AFFILIATION: American Red Cross, Jefferson County Chapter
FACILITY TYPE: Educational; Support group
STAFF: Volunteers 22
YEAR FOUNDED: 1986
FUNDING: Private
OUTREACH: Speakers bureau, resource bibliography, AIDS community discussion forum project
NETWORKS: AIDS Task Force of Central New York

517. Kaleidoscope
13206 W 125th St
New York, NY 10027
(212) 678-1277
KEY PERSONNEL: Sandra Tatum; Director
FACILITY TYPE: HIV counseling and testing; Substance abuse treatment

518. Lincoln Hospital Acupuncture Clinic
349 E 140th St
Bronx, NY 10454
(212) 993-3100
KEY PERSONNEL: Ana Oliveira; Clinic Supervisor
AFFILIATION: Lincoln Hospital
FACILITY TYPE: Clinic
STAFF: Paid professional 21
YEAR FOUNDED: 1972
FUNDING: Fees for services or products
OUTREACH: Speakers on substance abuse and AIDS

ADDITIONAL INFO: Provides acupuncture treatment for substance abuse and AIDS, ARC, and HIV positive. Also provides herbal treatments and conducts Chi Cong classes for immune deficient patients
AVAILABLE LITERATURE: Published articles on acupuncture
LANGUAGES: Spanish, Portuguese

519. Long Island Association for AIDS Care, Inc (LIAAC)
FORMER NAME: Long Island AIDS Project
PO Box 2859
Huntington Station, NY 11746
(516) 385-2451; Hotline: (516) 385-AIDS
KEY PERSONNEL: Gail Barouh; Executive Director
FACILITY TYPE: Educational; Support group; Client services/case management
STAFF: Paid professional 13; Paid nonprofessional 3; Volunteers 300
YEAR FOUNDED: 1984
FUNDING: State government; Local government; Private; Fund-raisers; Grants
OUTREACH: Educational programs to people at risk, caregivers, health care workers, corporations, churches, educational institutions, religious groups, public and private health and service agencies, and community groups
NETWORKS: Nassau County AIDS Care Consortium
ADDITIONAL INFO: Provides a hotline, buddy program, support groups, crisis intervention, case management, legal clinic, activities program, hospital visitation, and general client advocacy
AVAILABLE LITERATURE: *Long Island Association for AIDS Care*, an informational brochure; safer sex card, posters, newsletter
LANGUAGES: Spanish

520. Lower Eastside Service Center, Inc, AIDS Prevention Program
46 E Broadway
New York, NY 10002
(212) 431-4160 ext 230
KEY PERSONNEL: Christopher Dustow; AIDS Coordinator
FACILITY TYPE: Research; Substance abuse treatment
STAFF: Paid professional 1; Volunteers 1
YEAR FOUNDED: 1987
FUNDING: State government; Private; Fees for services or products
OUTREACH: Commercials on TV, lectures on AIDS to other service organizations, lectures on AIDS to community groups
NETWORKS: New York City AIDS Forum; Lower East Side AIDS Task Force; Lower East Side Mental Health Consortium
SEMINARS: Dec 1988-Apr 1989—"Workshop series on AIDS for Professionals"
ADDITIONAL INFO: The AIDS Prevention Program serves the clients who are registered within the Lower Eastside Service Center, which is a multi-modality drug treatment agency serving mostly former IV drug users. The program addresses all concerns regarding HIV infection to full-blown AIDS. Services are for clients and significant others. Provides therapy
AVAILABLE LITERATURE: *AIDS: Information for Drug Users and Concerned Others*, a brochure of guidelines for drug users; *AIDS (SIDA): Informacion para Usadores de Drogas y Personas Interesadas*, a Spanish-language brochure of guidelines for drug users (also available in Chinese)
LANGUAGES: Spanish, Chinese

521. Memorial Sloan-Kettering Cancer Center
1275 York Ave
New York, NY 10021
(212) 794-7177
KEY PERSONNEL: Elizabeth Anderson, Director
FACILITY TYPE: Clinic
ADDITIONAL INFO: An infectious disease clinic for individuals diagnosed with AIDS/ARC opportunistic infections; diagnostic assessment clinic for symptomatic individuals

522. Metropolitan AIDS Project (MAP)
1901 First Ave
New York, NY 10029
(212) 360-5554
KEY PERSONNEL: Susan Katz, Director
FACILITY TYPE: Clinic; Support group
ADDITIONAL INFO: An interdisciplinary team using a bio-psychosocial approach in caring for PWAs, their families, and care partners

523. Minority Task Force on AIDS
475 Riverside Dr, Rm 456
New York, NY 10115
(212) 749-1214
AFFILIATION: New York City Council of Churches
FACILITY TYPE: Support group
ADDITIONAL INFO: Source of additional information on AIDS

524. Momentum AIDS Outreach Program
619 Lexington Ave
New York, NY 10022
(212) 935-2200
KEY PERSONNEL: Peter Avitabile; Executive Director
AFFILIATION: Saint Peters Church
FACILITY TYPE: Educational; HIV counseling and testing
STAFF: Paid professional 12; Volunteers 250
YEAR FOUNDED: 1985
FUNDING: State government; Local government; Private; Fund-raisers
OUTREACH: AIDS education seminars, safer sex and risk reduction workshops, volunteer training and orientation, outreach to religious communities
NETWORKS: Mayor's Voluntary Action Committee AIDS Task Force; New York Committee on AIDS Funding
ADDITIONAL INFO: Provides an average of 350 meals per week to PWAs and their families, individual and family counseling, financial entitlement advocacy, free take-home groceries, and clothing at 6 sites in New York City
AVAILABLE LITERATURE: *Love for People Living with AIDS: Momentum AIDS Outreach Program*, a brochure describing the services of the agency; *Momentum AIDS Outreach Program*, a brochure of information about the program
LANGUAGES: Spanish

525. Montefiore MMTP Unit 2
2005 Jerome Ave
Bronx, NY 10453
(212) 583-0600
KEY PERSONNEL: Iris Newman; Administrative Coordinator
FACILITY TYPE: HIV counseling and testing; Substance abuse treatment

526. Nassau County Medical Center, AIDS Program
2201 Hempstead Tpke
East Meadow, NY 11554
(516) 542-2506
KEY PERSONNEL: Bruce Agins; AIDS Program Director
AFFILIATION: Nassau County Government
FACILITY TYPE: Hospital
FUNDING: Local government
AVAILABLE LITERATURE: *NCMC Services to Persons with AIDS*, a brochure describing the services that are available; *News*, a newsletter

527. National League for Nursing, Inc (NLN)
10 Columbus Cir
New York, NY 10019
(212) 582-1022; (800) 847-8480
FACILITY TYPE: Research; Educational
STAFF: Paid professional 50; Paid nonprofessional 50
FUNDING: Fees for services or products; Dues
AVAILABLE LITERATURE: *AIDS Guidelines for Schools of Nursing*, an informational brochure; *Nursing and Health Care*, a monthly journal. Publishes over 40 other titles per year covering all aspects of nursing

528. New Jewish Agenda (NJA)
64 Fulton St, Ste 1100
New York, NY 10038
(212) 227-5885
KEY PERSONNEL: David Coyne, Executive Director
FACILITY TYPE: Educational
FUNDING: Donations; Grants
ADDITIONAL INFO: Founded in 1980 as an educational group for the Jewish community, with AIDS work a small and new group. Major focus has been on Middle East peace, Central America, feminism, economic and social justice, and disarmament
AVAILABLE LITERATURE: Produces a national newsletter

529. New York City Commission on Human Rights and Discrimination Unit
52 Duane St, 7th Fl
New York, NY 10007
(212) 566-1826; 566-5446; 566-7638
KEY PERSONNEL: Keith O'Connor, Director; Mitchell Karp, Attorney; Katy Taylor, Deputy Director
FACILITY TYPE: Educational; Legal
FUNDING: State government
OUTREACH: Education specialist provides training on discrimination issues; produces written materials and videos
NETWORKS: Interagency Task Force on AIDS for NYC
SEMINARS: Various seminars concerning AIDS
ADDITIONAL INFO: Founded in 1983 as a human rights agency to defend the rights of PWAs
AVAILABLE LITERATURE: *AIDS and People of Color: The Discriminatory Impact*, a 21-page report of the commission on AIDS and discrimination; *NYC Commission on Human Rights Report on Discrimination Against People with AIDS, November 1983—April 1986*, a 47-page report reviewing the individual cases of discrimination that resulted from AIDS. Also publishes pamphlets on discrimination in the workplace, produces videos on discrimination and distributes a poster, *AIDS Discrimination is Illegal*
LANGUAGES: Spanish, Creole

530. New York City Dept of Health, AIDS Education Unit
125 Worth St, Box 46
New York, NY 10013
(212) 566-8290; 566-8292
KEY PERSONNEL: Ravinia Hayes-Cozier, Director
FACILITY TYPE: Educational
OUTREACH: Programs to educate IV drug users and their significant others about AIDS. *AIDS: A Resource Guide for New York City*, Includes general information on AIDS patient services, counseling, advocacy and emotional support, home care, financial assistance, legal services, human rights and complaint resolution, hospital patient representatives, hospital social work contact list, outpatient mental health services, and AIDS support groups
SEMINARS: AIDS Forum; Clinical Investigator's Meeting
ADDITIONAL INFO: Founded in 1985 as an educational unit of the New York City Dept of Health, giving information about AIDS to everyone
AVAILABLE LITERATURE: *AIDS: Facts About Acquired Immunodeficiency Syndrome*, a 4-page brochure with general information about AIDS; *AIDS and Shooting Drugs*, a 1-page brochure about AIDS and drug shooting; *AIDS: What Everyone Should Know*, a 2-fold brochure in English and Spanish presenting facts about AIDS including how it is spread, who is at risk, protection, and risk of transmitting AIDS during pregnancy; *Kids and AIDS*, a 1-page brochure about children with AIDS; *AIDS: the Antibody Test*, a 1-page brochure about the AIDS blood test; *AIDS and Straight People*, a 1-page brochure on AIDS and straight people; *Women Can Get AIDS Too*, a 1-page brochure on women and AIDS; *AIDS in Your Neighborhood*, a single-page pamphlet with general information on AIDS; *Women and AIDS*, a 2-fold brochure in English and Spanish; *Children and AIDS*, a 2-fold brochure in English and Spanish; *Shooting Up and AIDS*, a 2-page pamphlet discussing IV drug users and AIDS; *AIDS Surveillance Update*, a 7-page booklet of AIDS statistics for New York; *AIDS Education*, a 2-page brochure outlining New York City's AIDS education programs; *AIDS: A Resource Guide for New York City*, a 39-page booklet of resources in New York City of interest to PWAs; *AIDS: A Special Report on Acquired Immunodeficiency Syndrome*, a 39-page booklet for New York City schools; *AIDS and Drugs*, a 2-page brochure on drugs and AIDS
LANGUAGES: Spanish

531. New York City Dept of Health, Division of AIDS Program Services
125 Worth St, Box A/1
New York, NY 10013
(212) 566-7103; Hotline: (718) 485-8111
KEY PERSONNEL: Peggy Clarke; Assistant Commissioner
AFFILIATION: New York City Dept of Health
FACILITY TYPE: Research; Educational; Task force; HIV counseling and testing; Client services/case management
STAFF: Paid professional 350
YEAR FOUNDED: 1987
FUNDING: Federal government; State government; Local government; Private

OUTREACH: Outreach to IV drug users, communities with high IV drug use, Black and Hispanic communities, Haitian communities, gay and bisexual men, gay and bisexual men of color, and lesbian and gay adolescents
NETWORKS: New York City Interagency Task Force on AIDS
SEMINARS: Conducts numerous training workshops throughout the year including "Municipal Conference on AIDS" and "Religious Conference on AIDS"
RESEARCH: HIV seroprevalence, behavior change, effect of prevention and education programs on knowledge, attitude and behavior of persons reached
AVAILABLE LITERATURE: *AIDS: A Resource Guide for New York City*, a 44-page directory; *AIDS Education*, an informational brochure in English and Spanish; *Needle Talk*, a video program on AIDS and IV drug users; *CHI: City Health Information*, a newsletter; *Bill and Brenda/Carlos y Carla*, bilingual comic book on IV drug use and AIDS; *People Helping People*, an informational brochure; *AIDS: the Antibody Test*, a bilingual brochure on the HIV antibody test; *AIDS and Drugs*, a brochure for IV drug users; *El SIDA (AIDS) y Las Drogas*, brochure for IV drug users; *AIDS—What Everyone Should Know*, a bilingual informational brochure; *Women and AIDS*, a bilingual brochure for women; *Shooting Up and AIDS*, a bilingual brochure for IV drug users; *AIDS in Your Neighborhood*, a bilingual general information brochure; *AIDS in NYC—You Can Get Help*, a bilingual brochure of places to get help; *AIDS—The Straight Facts*, a bilingual brochure of AIDS facts; *Condoms, Safer Sex, and AIDS*, a bilingual safer sex brochure; *Get the Facts...Not AIDS*, a brochure for teens about AIDS; *Eating Right and AIDS*, a bilingual brochure about good eating habits; *AIDS Does Not Discriminate*, a flyer; *AIDS Hotline Wallet Card*; *AIDS, Sex and Drugs: Don't Pass It On*, a poster; *Don't Let AIDS Deal You a Losing Hand*, a poster; *He Can Only Strike You If You Let Him*, a poster; *Las Mujeres Tambien Pueden Contraer El AIDS*, a poster; *Women Can Get AIDS Too*, a poster; *AIDS Gets Around*, a poster available in English, Spanish, Creole, or Chinese; *Don't Leave Home Without Your Rubbers*, a poster; *Don't Die of Embarrassment*, a poster; *No Se Muera de la Pena*, a poster; *Bang. Your're Dead*, a poster; *Talk About AIDS Before It Hits Home*, a poster; *Hable del AIDS Antes que Toque a su Puerta*, a poster; *You Can't Live on Hope*, a poster; *No Se Puede Vivir de Esperanzas*, a poster; *Charlie Brought Home a Case of AIDS*, a poster;
LANGUAGES: Spanish, Creole, Chinese, American Sign Language

532. New York State Dept of Health, AIDS Prevention Program
677 S Salina St
Syracuse, NY 13202
(315) 428-4728
KEY PERSONNEL: Howard Lavigne; AIDS Education Training Specialist
AFFILIATION: New York State Dept of Health, AIDS Institute
FACILITY TYPE: Educational
STAFF: Paid professional 1
YEAR FOUNDED: 1986
FUNDING: Federal government
OUTREACH: Presents educational programs to organizations, schools, businesses, prisons, and civic groups
AVAILABLE LITERATURE: *AIDS and HIV Counseling and Testing*, 1987 brochure on the HIV test; *How to Use a Condom (Rubber)*, explicit pocket guide to using a condom; *What Parents Need to Tell Children About AIDS*, a 1987 brochure of AIDS facts for parents; *Safe Sex*, illustrated brochure of safer sex practices; *Coping With AIDS: Psychological and Social Considerations in Helping People with HTLV-III Infection*, a 1987 16-page booklet about AIDS; *What You Should Know About AIDS*, a brochure of AIDS facts; *100 Questions and Answers: AIDS*, a 1988 booklet of questions and answers; *Women and AIDS*, a brochure of AIDS facts for women; *HIV Counseling and Testing Program*, a card of testing facts with telephone numbers; *AIDS Service Programs: Call for Facts, Call for Help*, a card with telephone numbers; *AIDS: Information for N.Y.S. Correctional Services Department Employees*, a pamphlet for employees of correctional institutions; *AIDS: Protect Yourself and Those You Care About*, a safer sex brochure; *If You're Pregnant...Your Baby Might be Born with AIDS/Cree Estar Embarazada?...su Bebe Puede Nacer con SIDA (AIDS)*, a card of AIDS information for those who are pregnant; *Having a Baby?: Have a Test for AIDS Virus First*, a brochure for those comtemplating children; *AIDS Does Not Discriminate*, a brochure of 10 facts about AIDS; *Programa de Analisis y Orientaction Sobre el VIH*, a Spanish-language brochure about the HIV test; *AIDS: Informacion para los Empleodos del Departamento de Servicios Correccionales*

del Estadode Nueva York, a Spanish-language brochure for employees of correctional institutions; *Don't Die of Embarrassment*, a safer sex poster; *HIV Antibody Testing (Prueba del Anticuerpo VIH)*, a card with testing center telephone numbers

533. New York State Dept of Health, HIV Counseling and Testing Program
677 S Salina St
Syracuse, NY 13202
(315) 428-4728; Hotline: (315) 428-4736
KEY PERSONNEL: Janet Osborn; Regional Coordinator
AFFILIATION: New York State Dept of Health, AIDS Institute
FACILITY TYPE: Educational; HIV counseling and testing
STAFF: Paid professional 5
YEAR FOUNDED: 1985
FUNDING: State government
OUTREACH: Speakers bureau, education, counseling, testing
AVAILABLE LITERATURE: Distributes various pamphlets and posters from the state and other agencies; *AIDS and HIV Counseling and Testing*, a brochure about the HIV test

534. North East Neighborhood Association (NENA)
279 E 3rd St
New York, NY 10009
(212) 477-8500
FACILITY TYPE: Clinic

535. North Shore University Hospital Drug Treatment and Education Center
400 Community Dr
Manhasset, NY 11030
(516) 562-3010
KEY PERSONNEL: John Imhof; Director
FACILITY TYPE: HIV counseling and testing; Substance abuse treatment

536. Northern Lights Alternatives, Inc
78 W 85th St, Ste 5E
New York, NY 10024
(212) 877-4846, 337-8747
KEY PERSONNEL: Victor Phillips; National Director
FACILITY TYPE: Educational; Hospital; Support group; Fund-raising
STAFF: Paid professional 3; Volunteers 20
YEAR FOUNDED: 1986
FUNDING: Private; Fund-raisers
OUTREACH: Disseminates information, conducts AIDS Mastery seminar, children with AIDS care program
NETWORKS: Mayor's Task Force on AIDS; New York Consortium of AIDS Organizations
ADDITIONAL INFO: The purpose of Northern Lights Alternatives is to create programs which will help to educate, inform, and inspire people with AIDS (PWAs) and the general community—by providing facts and responding to needs as they arise during the AIDS crisis.
AVAILABLE LITERATURE: *Northern Lights Alternatives*, a brochure describing the services of the group; various one-page flyers announcing services and events

537. Office of Gay and Lesbian Health Concerns (OGLHC)
125 Worth St, Box 67
New York, NY 10013
(212) 566-4995; Hotline: (212) 691-9377
KEY PERSONNEL: Ron Vachon; Director
AFFILIATION: New York City Dept of Health
FACILITY TYPE: Educational; HIV counseling and testing; Substance abuse treatment
STAFF: Paid professional 7
YEAR FOUNDED: 1983
FUNDING: Local government
OUTREACH: Outreach and education to lesbians and gay men who do not normally use community services, AIDS education and prevention outreach program targeting gay and bisexual men of color
NETWORKS: National Lesbian/Gay Health Foundation; National AIDS Network (NAN); National Coalition of Gay STD Services; AIDS Action Council
SEMINARS: Apr 29, 1988, Apr 28, 1989—"10 percent of Those We Serve," focusing on special treatment needs of lesbians and gay men affected by alcoholism and other addictions; May 20-22, 1988—"First National Conference on Homophobia"

RESEARCH: Lesbian and gay alcoholism and other addictions to be published as "The Treatment of Alcoholism in Lesbians and Gay Men: A Survey of Mainstream Agencies"
ADDITIONAL INFO: Founded as a health service agency concerned with access to and quality of health and human services for lesbian and gay New Yorkers, including services for AIDS, alcoholism, STDs, gynecological/reproductive health, parenting, and youth health needs
AVAILABLE LITERATURE: *Lavender Health*, a newsletter; *For Men Who Have Sex With Men*, a safer sex wallet card; *Do You Want to GLOE?*, a card presenting information about Gay and Lesbian Outreach and Education; *Gay and Lesbian Health Concerns*, an informational brochure
LANGUAGES: American Sign Language

538. People with AIDS Coalition, Inc (PWA Coalition)
31 W 26th St
New York, NY 10010
(212) 532-0290; Hotline: (212) 532-0568
KEY PERSONNEL: Christopher L Babick; Deputy Director
AFFILIATION: National Association of People With AIDS (NAPWA)
FACILITY TYPE: Educational; Support group
STAFF: Paid professional 8; Volunteers 95
YEAR FOUNDED: 1985
FUNDING: State government; Local government; Private; Fund-raisers
OUTREACH: Support groups for women, PWARCs, mothers, Spanish speaking PWAs/PWARCs; meal program, hotline, public forums, singles teas
NETWORKS: New York State AIDS Network; AIDS Action Council; National AIDS Network (NAN); New York City AIDS Service Delivery Consortium; AIDS Institute; New York City AIDS Budget Working Committee
ADDITIONAL INFO: The PWA Coalition philosophy is self-empowerment. Encourages PWAs/PWARCs to take an active role in the treatment they choose. Provides up-to-date information on all alternative treatments. All services and literature are free to PWAs/PWARCs
AVAILABLE LITERATURE: *Newsline*, a monthly magazine with articles about living with AIDS including a resource directory; *Surviving and Thriving with AIDS: Hints for the Newly Diagnosed*, a collection of articles in book form about living with AIDS and helpful tips for the newly diagnosed. Spanish-language edition of this book is also available

539. PWA Health Group
31 W 26th St
New York, NY 10010
(212) 532-0280
KEY PERSONNEL: Tom Wilcox; Office Manager
FACILITY TYPE: Client services/case management
STAFF: Paid professional 2; Paid nonprofessional 4; Volunteers 5
YEAR FOUNDED: 1987
FUNDING: Donations
ADDITIONAL INFO: Provides alternative products to people with AIDS
LANGUAGES: Portuguese

540. Regional AIDS Education Training Center
BOCES, Health Education Center
Yorktown Heights, NY 10598
(914) 245-2700
KEY PERSONNEL: Kenneth L Packer; Regional AIDS Education Coordinator
AFFILIATION: New York State Education Dept
FACILITY TYPE: Educational
STAFF: Paid professional 2; Paid nonprofessional 1
YEAR FOUNDED: 1988
FUNDING: State government
OUTREACH: Teacher training about AIDS information, helping districts meet the AIDS education mandate, assistance to districts in forming Health (AIDS) Advisory Councils, AIDS information training for Health Advisory Councils, technical assistance to district health and AIDS education curriculum writing committees and health coordinators, updating educators on new information, media, materials, and teaching techniques for AIDS education, parent (PTA) information services about AIDS
NETWORKS: Westchester Consortium for AIDS Education
SEMINARS: Jan 17, 1989—"Conference on Teaching AIDS to Black and Hispanic in School Youth;" Apr 12, 1989—"Conference on Counseling Techniques with Student PWAs or Students with PWAs in Their Family"

ADDITIONAL INFO: This program is part of the activities of a regional health education center. It also provides help to districts on substance abuse prevention, and curriculum development in other areas of health education.
AVAILABLE LITERATURE: *Pulse Beats*, monthly newsletter on education for health

541. Roosevelt Hospital and AIDS Clinic
428 W 59th St
New York, NY 10019
FACILITY TYPE: Hospital; Clinic
ADDITIONAL INFO: Source of additional AIDS information

542. Southern Tier AIDS Program, Inc (STAP)
65 Broad St
Johnson City, NY 13790
(607) 798-1706; Hotline: (607) 723-6520
KEY PERSONNEL: Mary F Dean; Executive Director
FACILITY TYPE: Educational; Support group
STAFF: Paid professional 3; Paid nonprofessional 1; Volunteers 65
YEAR FOUNDED: 1984
FUNDING: State government; Donations
OUTREACH: AIDS education for health professionals, social service providers, business, industry, schools, and general public
ADDITIONAL INFO: Founded as an educational agency with community service its primary goal
AVAILABLE LITERATURE: Publishes a newsletter
LANGUAGES: Spanish

543. Stamp Out AIDS, Inc
240 W 44th St
New York, NY 10036
(212) 354-8899
KEY PERSONNEL: John Glines; Project Director
FACILITY TYPE: Fund-raising
STAFF: Volunteers varies
YEAR FOUNDED: 1986
FUNDING: Private
NETWORKS: National AIDS Network (NAN)
ADDITIONAL INFO: Raises money through the sale of stamps and buttons. Distributes money through grants to AIDS service organizations for direct services to PWAs and PWARCs
AVAILABLE LITERATURE: *Stamp Out AIDS*, stamps and buttons

544. Starting Point
132-6 W 125th St
New York, NY 10027
(121) 678-1212
KEY PERSONNEL: Lucy Miro-Quesada; Director
FACILITY TYPE: HIV counseling and testing; Substance abuse treatment

545. Stuyvesant Polyclinic Adult Medical Clinic
137 2nd Ave
New York, NY 10003
FACILITY TYPE: Clinic
ADDITIONAL INFO: Source of AIDS information

546. Third Horizon
2195 3rd Ave
New York, NY 10035
(212) 678-1223
KEY PERSONNEL: Doris Hammonds; Director
FACILITY TYPE: HIV counseling and testing; Substance abuse treatment

547. Village Nursing Home AIDS Day Treatment Program (AIDS DTP)
133 W 20th St
New York, NY 10011
(212) 633-1616
KEY PERSONNEL: Leah Mason-Beck; Director
AFFILIATION: Village Nursing Home
FACILITY TYPE: Client services/case management; Day care
STAFF: Paid professional 10; Volunteers 30
YEAR FOUNDED: 1988
FUNDING: Local government; Private; Fund-raisers
OUTREACH: Pamphlets and community board meetings

NETWORKS: National AIDS Network (NAN); New York AIDS Coalition; Coalition on AIDS Funding
ADDITIONAL INFO: Provides a missing link between hospital and home. Designed to sustain and enhance self-help and independent living skills in men and women experiencing physical, psychiatric or neurological disability associated with AIDS
AVAILABLE LITERATURE: *When Home is Not Enough*, a brochure describing the daycare facility; *Village Nursing Home AIDS Program: Adult Day Care*, a flyer giving some history about the program
LANGUAGES: Spanish

548. West Side AIDS Project
593 Columbus Ave
New York, NY 10024
(212) 877-6020
KEY PERSONNEL: Judy Wenning; Director
AFFILIATION: Goddard-Riverside Community Center
FACILITY TYPE: Educational; Support group; HIV counseling and testing; Client services/case management
STAFF: Paid professional 2; Volunteers 6
YEAR FOUNDED: 1986
FUNDING: Local government; Private
OUTREACH: Educational presentations for community residents and agencies
NETWORKS: National AIDS Network (NAN); Upper Manhattan Task Force on AIDS
AVAILABLE LITERATURE: *Friends: When You Need a Friend or Want to be One.../Amigos: Un Amigo en las Buenas y en las Malas...*, a bilingual brochure describing the agency
LANGUAGES: Spanish

549. Westchester County Dept of Health
112 E Post Rd
White Plains, NY 10601
(914) 285-5100; Hotline: (914) 285-6015; Espanol: (914) 285-5210
KEY PERSONNEL: Anita S Curran; Commissioner of Health
AFFILIATION: New York State Health Dept
FACILITY TYPE: Health department
STAFF: Paid professional 464
YEAR FOUNDED: 1930
FUNDING: Federal government; State government
OUTREACH: Training services for employees and staff of E.M.S., parole, social service, home care, prisons, probation, group homes, school teachers, students, PTAs, board members, and other staffs of other community agencies
NETWORKS: New York State Health Dept
SEMINARS: May 12, 1988—"The Care of AIDS Patients Outside the Hospital," sponsored by Bethel Springvale Inn, Inc., Bethel Methodist Home, Subcommittee on Education for Long Term Care, Commission's Task Force on AIDS Westchester County Dept of Health, Hudson Valley Health Systems Agency, Lower Hudson Valley Region, New York State Public Health Association
RESEARCH: AIDS education for targeted high risk groups—continuity of care via commission's task force on AIDS
AVAILABLE LITERATURE: *The AIDS Virus: What You Should Know/El Virus del SIDA: Lo Que Usted Debe Saber*, a dual-language brochure with AIDS information; *AIDS Awareness*, a newspaper insert for the Gannett Westchester Rockland newspapers containing a variety of information on AIDS, a glossary, and a directory of resources
LANGUAGES: Spanish, French, Chinese, Italian, Filipino, German

550. Western New York AIDS Program (WNYAP)
FORMER NAME: Buffalo AIDS Task Force, Inc
220 Delaware Ave, Ste 512
Buffalo, NY 14202
(716) 847-2441; Hotline: (716) 847-2437
KEY PERSONNEL: Ronald Silverio; Executive Director
FACILITY TYPE: Educational; Support group; Fund-raising; Task force; Client services/case management
STAFF: Paid professional 12; Volunteers 125
YEAR FOUNDED: 1983
FUNDING: State government; Private; Fund-raisers
OUTREACH: Speakers bureau, training of trainers pro gram, risk-reduction workshops
NETWORKS: AIDS Service Organizations Consortium of Western New York; AIDS Educators Network of Western New York

AVAILABLE LITERATURE: *Western New York AIDS Program Newsletter*, a monthly newsletter
LANGUAGES: Spanish, Arabic, American Sign Language

NORTH CAROLINA

551. AIDS Control Program
PO Box 2091
Raleigh, NC 27602
(919) 733-7301
KEY PERSONNEL: David Volly; Supervisor
FACILITY TYPE: Educational; Task force; HIV counseling and testing
STAFF: Paid professional 18
YEAR FOUNDED: 1986
FUNDING: Federal government; State government
OUTREACH: Surveillance, HIV counseling and testing, partner notification, health education, risk reduction

552. The AIDS Services Project (TASP)
FORMER NAME: The AIDS Support Network of LGHP
PO Box 3203
Durham, NC 27705-1203
(919) 688-5777
KEY PERSONNEL: Jill Duvall; Project Coordinator of LGHP/TASP
AFFILIATION: Lesbian and Gay Health Project (LGHP)
FACILITY TYPE: Educational; Support group
STAFF: Paid professional 3; Volunteers 50
YEAR FOUNDED: 1987
FUNDING: State government; Private; Fund-raisers; Grants
OUTREACH: Buddy program, support groups, social service advocacy, crisis intervention, access to legal counseling, emergency assistance fund, health care provider referrals, speakers bureau
NETWORKS: North Carolina AIDS Service Organization Coalition (NCASOC)
ADDITIONAL INFO: Provides education, information, health care provider referrals, support for gay and lesbian community concerning generic health issues
AVAILABLE LITERATURE: *LGHP Newsletter*, distributes pamphlets and audiovisuals from other agencies

553. AIDS Task Force of Winston-Salem
PO Box 2982
Winston-Salem, NC 27102
(919) 723-5031

554. Duke University AIDS Clinical Trials Unit
PO Box 3238 Duke Univ Medical Center
Durham, NC 27710
(919) 684-5260
KEY PERSONNEL: John Bartlett; Clinical Research Director
AFFILIATION: Duke University Medical Center
FACILITY TYPE: Research; Educational; Hospital; Clinic
STAFF: Paid professional 10
YEAR FOUNDED: 1987
FUNDING: Federal government; Private; Fees for services or products
RESEARCH: Antiviral and immunomodulatory agents

555. ERASE
PO Box 1296
Greenville, NC 27835
(919) 756-8453

556. GROW AIDS Resource Project
PO Box 4535
Wilmington, NC 28406
(919) 675-9222
KEY PERSONNEL: Leo J Teachout; Executive Director
FACILITY TYPE: Educational; Support group; Fund-raising
STAFF: Paid nonprofessional 1; Volunteers 40
YEAR FOUNDED: 1983
FUNDING: Private; Fund-raisers
OUTREACH: Speakers bureau, safer sex workshops, information and referral file, gay and lesbian switchboard, discrimination documentation project, social and community activities
NETWORKS: North Carolina AIDS Services Coalition; Southeastern North Carolina AIDS Task Force; National AIDS Network (NAN)

ADDITIONAL INFO: Organized to promote crisis intervention, counseling programs, and support for people with sexual orientation concerns, to develop affirmative programs to enhance human dignity, and to defind human and civil rights
AVAILABLE LITERATURE: *Backgrounds*, a newsletter; *Play Safe, Stay Healthy, Use Condoms*, a safer sex card; *GROW*, an informational card; *AIDS: What You Do About It May Save Your Life*, a brochure of AIDS facts and preventive measures; *AIDS Resource Project/AIDS Risk Reduction Guidelines*
LANGUAGES: Spanish

557. Lesbian and Gay Health Project (LGHP)
PO Box 3203
Durham, NC 27705-1203
(919) 683-2182
KEY PERSONNEL: Karen Winstead; AIDS Educator Organizer
FACILITY TYPE: Educational; Support group
STAFF: Paid professional 1.5; Volunteers 50
YEAR FOUNDED: 1982
FUNDING: Private; Fund-raisers
ADDITIONAL INFO: LGHP provides health care referrals, education and an AIDS support network
AVAILABLE LITERATURE: *Lesbian and Gay Health Project*, a brochure describing the project; *Lesbian and Gay Health Project: Guidelines for AIDS Risk Reduction*, a brochure of AIDS facts and safer sex guidelines; *North Carolina Lesbian and Gay Health Project*, a newsletter

558. Metrolina AIDS Project (MAP)
PO Box 32662
Charlotte, NC 28232
(704) 333-2437; Hotline: (704) 333-2437
KEY PERSONNEL: David Prybylo; AIDS Educator
FACILITY TYPE: Educational; Support group; Fund-raising
STAFF: Paid professional 3; Paid nonprofessional 1; Volunteers 200
YEAR FOUNDED: 1985
FUNDING: State government; Local government; Private; Fund-raisers
OUTREACH: PWA support group, HIV positive/ARC support group, family-friends-partners support group, buddy support program, bereavement group, Dennis fund for emergency financial assistance, social services, hotline, risk reduction workshops, speakers bureau
ADDITIONAL INFO: The mission of MAP is to provide care for those affected by AIDS in the community.
AVAILABLE LITERATURE: *MAP*, a newsletter; *Metrolina AIDS Project*, a flyer outlining the services of MAP; *History of Metrolina AIDS Project*

559. NC AIDS Control Program
PO Box 2091
Raleigh, NC 27602-2091
(919) 733-7301
KEY PERSONNEL: David Jolly; Supervisor
AFFILIATION: North Carolina State Government
FACILITY TYPE: Educational
STAFF: Paid professional 25
YEAR FOUNDED: 1986
FUNDING: Federal government; State government
OUTREACH: State and regional workshops for health care workers and community-based organizations, community-based risk reduction projects for gay men and IV drug users, minority education project
AVAILABLE LITERATURE: *AIDS in the Black Community: The Facts*, a brochure with AIDS facts as they pertain to the Blacks; *AIDS: Information for North Carolina Legislators*, a brochure of AIDS facts targeted for legislators; *How to Use a Condom (Rubber)*, a small pocket size brochure with explicit instructions on how to use a condom; *What Women Should Know About AIDS*, a 1988 brochure for women; *What Everyone Should Know About AIDS*, a 1987 brochure of general AIDS information; *Information for Persons with a Positive HIV Antibody Test Result*, a 1987 brochure for those who test positive

560. Stanly County Task Force
945 N 5th St
Albemarle, NC 28001
(704) 982-9171
KEY PERSONNEL: Deborah Bennett; Health Educator
AFFILIATION: Stanly County Health Dept
FACILITY TYPE: Task force
YEAR FOUNDED: 1987

OUTREACH: Provides speakers to local businesses, schools and community groups, distributes pamphlets and brochures

ADDITIONAL INFO: The task force is composed of representatives from the Stanly County Health Dept, Dept of Social Services, school personnel, mental health, ministers, doctors, dentists, hospital personnel, policemen, firemen, emergency personnel, hospices, and the local media

561. The Sycamore Center
101 W Sycamore St, No 410
Greensboro, NC 27401
(919) 275-9341
KEY PERSONNEL: Timothy Daughtry; Executive Director
FACILITY TYPE: HIV counseling and testing; Substance abuse treatment

562. Triad Health Project (THP)
PO Box 5716
Greensboro, NC 27435
(919) 275-1654
KEY PERSONNEL: David E Clough; Executive Director
FACILITY TYPE: Support group; Fund-raising; Task force
STAFF: Paid nonprofessional 1; Volunteers 100
YEAR FOUNDED: 1986
FUNDING: Private; Fund-raisers
OUTREACH: Educational outreach, information distribution, support groups, advocacy, buddy program, liasion, referral
ADDITIONAL INFO: THP is a community-based, nonprofit, volunteer organization with the primary goal of providing support services to PWAs and to individuals whose lives have been touched by AIDS

563. VA Cooperative Studies No. 298: Treatment of AIDS and AIDS-Related Complex
508 Fulton St
Durham, NC 27705
(919) 286-6950
KEY PERSONNEL: Patricia M Spivey; Study Coordinator
AFFILIATION: Veterans Administration
FACILITY TYPE: Research; Hospital; Clinic
FUNDING: Federal government
RESEARCH: Response of patients with ARC to AZT or placebo
ADDITIONAL INFO: An AZT trial program with treatment centers located at VA Medical Centers in New York, Miami, Houston, Los Angeles, San Francisco, DC, and at the Walter Reed Army Medical Center in DC

564. Western North Carolina AIDS Project (WNCAP)
PO Box 2411, 2 Wall St, Ste 220
Asheville, NC 28802
(704) 252-7489; (704) 252-7489
KEY PERSONNEL: Rocco Patt; Executive Director
FACILITY TYPE: Educational; Support group
STAFF: Paid nonprofessional 1; Volunteers 21
YEAR FOUNDED: 1987
FUNDING: Private; Fund-raisers
OUTREACH: Educational programs, support for PWAs and PWARCs, hotline for crisis intervention, networking
ADDITIONAL INFO: WNCAP is a non-profit organization of volunteers who are collectively seeking positive means for dealing with the AIDS epidemic. Provides counseling and referrals, hotline, informative brochures, AIDS information days, information booth, speakers bureau, safer sex workshops, support groups, peer counselors, buddy support programs, and direct support
AVAILABLE LITERATURE: *Facing Today's Challenge*, an informational brochure about the project; *Goal Statement*, a description of the goals of the project

NORTH DAKOTA

565. AIDS Advisory Council
FORMER NAME: AIDS Task Force
State Health Dept
Bismarck, ND 58501
KEY PERSONNEL: Stephen McDonough; Chairman
AFFILIATION: North Dakota State Health Dept
FACILITY TYPE: Educational
STAFF: Volunteers 25
YEAR FOUNDED: 1985

FUNDING: Federal government
SEMINARS: Sep 20, 1987—"HIV Counseling Training," Fort Yates; Oct 5-6, 1987—"HIV Counseling Training," Bismarck; Oct 3, 1987—"Safer Sex Workshop," Bismarck; Oct 18, 1987—"Buddy System Workshop," Bismarck; Oct 8, 1987—"Safer Sex Workshop," Fargo; Aug 11, 1988—"Be a Buddy Workshop," Fargo; Jul 8, 1988—"Be a Buddy Workshop," Williston; May 16, 1988—"Train the Trainer Workshop," Fargo; May 18, 1988—"Train the Trainer Workshop," Bismarck
AVAILABLE LITERATURE: *AIDS and North Dakota: A Plan for Action*, a 1987 131-page booklet describing how the State of North Dakota is planning for AIDS education, testing, etc.

566. North Dakota State Health Dept and Consolidated Laboratories
State Capitol
Bismarck, ND 58505
(701) 224-2378; Hotline: (800) 472-2180
KEY PERSONNEL: Eileen M Dockter; AIDS Program Coordinator
AFFILIATION: North Dakota State Dept of Health and Consolidated Laboratories
FACILITY TYPE: Educational; Task force
STAFF: Paid professional 6
FUNDING: Federal government
AVAILABLE LITERATURE: *Safer Sex*, a pocket card listing what is and is not safe sex; *Women and AIDS*, a brochure for women; *AIDS Facts*, a brochure of AIDS facts; *Now I'm Positive*, a brochure with answers for people who test positive for the AIDS virus; *AIDS and North Dakota: A Plan for Action*, a 131-page long range plan for the State of North Dakota; *Living Positive: AIDS Support Group*, a video for those who have tested positive

OHIO

567. AIDS Volunteers of Cincinnati (AVOC)
PO Box 19009
Cincinnati, OH 45219
(513) 421-AIDS
KEY PERSONNEL: Linda Seiter; Executive Director
FACILITY TYPE: Educational; Support group
STAFF: Paid professional 1; Paid nonprofessional 1
YEAR FOUNDED: 1983
FUNDING: Private
NETWORKS: National AIDS Network (NAN)
SEMINARS: 1989—"Attidudinal Healing Workshop"
ADDITIONAL INFO: AVOC was formed in 1983 in response to the AIDS epidemic in Cincinnati. The first executive director was hired in January, 1989.
AVAILABLE LITERATURE: *AVOC Newsletter*, a bi-monthly news letter

568. American Red Cross, Columbus Area Chapter
995 E Broad St
Columbus, OH 43205
(614) 253-7981
KEY PERSONNEL: Carolyn Hanks; AIDS Education Coordinator
AFFILIATION: American Red Cross
FACILITY TYPE: Educational; HIV counseling and testing
STAFF: Paid professional 8; Paid nonprofessional 3; Volunteers 5
YEAR FOUNDED: 1951
FUNDING: Private
OUTREACH: Support groups for HIV positive individuals, PWAs, PWARCs, family, friends, and acquaintances, educational services for community groups, schools, and worksites
NETWORKS: AIDS Provider Coalition
SEMINARS: Apr 20, Oct 6, 1988, Apr, Oct 1989—"Community Facilitator Training Day; Apr 21-22, 1988—"Workplace Facilitator Training and Trainer Training," Columbus; Jul 22-23, 1988—"Minority Facilitator Training," Columbus; Jun 11-16, 1989—"All Ohio Red Cross Training Institute," Columbus
ADDITIONAL INFO: Provides HIV antibody testing for individuals other than blood donors
AVAILABLE LITERATURE: Provides American Red Cross brochures, posters, buttons, and stickers

569. Athens AIDS Task Force
18 N College St
Athens, OH 45701
(614) 592-4397
KEY PERSONNEL: Eva Fotis; Project Coordinator

FACILITY TYPE: Educational; Support group; Fund-raising; Task force
STAFF: Paid professional 1; Paid nonprofessional 1
YEAR FOUNDED: 1984
FUNDING: State government; Private
OUTREACH: Support groups for PWAs and PWARCs, friends forum, HIV positive and wellness group, limited financial assistance for emergency needs
NETWORKS: National AIDS Network (NAN); Ohio AIDS Coalition
SEMINARS: May 17-23, 1988—"AIDS Awareness Week;" "The Church's Response to AIDS," a workshop held periodically consisting of a panel discussion led by PWAs, friends and families

570. Auglaize County AIDS Task Force
Corner of Wood and Lima St
Wapakoneta, OH 45895
(419) 738-3410
KEY PERSONNEL: Janet Bassitt; Public Health Educator
AFFILIATION: Auglaize County Health Dept
FACILITY TYPE: Task force
STAFF: Volunteers 30
YEAR FOUNDED: 1987
FUNDING: Fund-raisers
OUTREACH: Speakers bureau

571. Canton City AIDS Task Force
218 Cleveland Ave SW, City Hall, 3rd Fl
Canton, OH 44702
(216) 489-3231
KEY PERSONNEL: Robert Pattison, Health Commissioner
AFFILIATION: Canton City Health Dept
FACILITY TYPE: Educational; Clinic; Support group; Task force
ADDITIONAL INFO: Provides education, testing, counseling, referrals, buddies, and housing

572. Canton City Health Dept
218 Cleveland Ave SW
Canton, OH 44702
(216) 489-3322, 489-3231
KEY PERSONNEL: Jenilyn Reo; Nursing Director
AFFILIATION: Canton City Government
FACILITY TYPE: HIV counseling and testing; Health department
STAFF: Paid professional 46
YEAR FOUNDED: 1840
FUNDING: Federal government; State government; Local government
OUTREACH: Speakers bureau, counseling and testing for HIV antibody
AVAILABLE LITERATURE: *Counseling and Testing Site for HIV (AIDS) Antibodies*, an informational brochure; distributes materials from other agencies

573. Case Western Reserve University
2074 Abington Rd
Cleveland, OH 44106
(216) 844-3227
KEY PERSONNEL: Michael M Lederman, Director
AFFILIATION: Univ Hospitals of Cleveland
FACILITY TYPE: Educational; Hospital; Clinic
OUTREACH: Telephone answering service by staff physicians
ADDITIONAL INFO: An educational resource agency

574. Cincinnati Health Dept, AIDS Program
3101 Burnet Ave
Cincinnati, OH 45229
(513) 352-3138; Hotline: (513) 352-3138
KEY PERSONNEL: Michael Ritchey; Director
AFFILIATION: Cincinnati City Government
FACILITY TYPE: Educational; Clinic; Support group
STAFF: Paid professional 7
YEAR FOUNDED: 1982
FUNDING: Federal government; State government; Local government; Fees for services or products

575. Cleveland AIDS Foundation
11900 Edgewater Dr, Ste 907
Lakewood, OH 44107
FACILITY TYPE: Educational
ADDITIONAL INFO: Source of additional AIDS information

576. Cleveland Area AIDS Task Force
2074 Abington Rd
Cleveland, OH 44106
(216) 844-1000
KEY PERSONNEL: E S Bowerfind, Coordinator
AFFILIATION: Univ Hospital of Cleveland
FACILITY TYPE: Educational; Task force
ADDITIONAL INFO: Provides counseling, referrals, buddies, and housing

577. Cleveland City, Dept of Health and Human Resources
1925 Saint Clair Ave
Cleveland, OH 44114
(216) 664-2324; Toll-free: (800) 332-AIDS
KEY PERSONNEL: Nancy McCormick; AIDS Coordinator
AFFILIATION: Cleveland City Government
FACILITY TYPE: Educational; Clinic; Support group; HIV counseling and testing
STAFF: Paid professional 2
FUNDING: State government; Local government
OUTREACH: Educational programs, support groups for PWAs, PWARCs, HIV positive individuals, worried well
NETWORKS: AIDS Commission of Greater Cleveland; Ohio Dept of Health Counseling and Testing Sites
LANGUAGES: Spanish

578. Cleveland/Cuyahoga County AIDS Task Force
2074 Abington Rd
Cleveland, OH 44106
(216) 664-2324
KEY PERSONNEL: Kevin Blanchett, Coordinator
FACILITY TYPE: Educational; Task force
ADDITIONAL INFO: Provides counseling, referrals, buddies, and housing

579. Columbus AIDS Task Force
1500 W 3rd Ave, Ste 329
Columbus, OH 43212
(614) 488-2437; Toll-free: (800) 332-AIDS (OH only)
KEY PERSONNEL: Gloria J T Smith; Executive Director
FACILITY TYPE: Educational; Support group; Task force
STAFF: Paid professional 4; Paid nonprofessional 2; Volunteers 380
YEAR FOUNDED: 1984
FUNDING: State government; Local government; Private; Fund-raisers
OUTREACH: Client case management, free legal services for PWAs and PWARCs, weekly support groups for PWAs, PWARCs, HIV positive individuals, and significant others, speakers bureau, safer sex workshops, hotline
NETWORKS: National AIDS Network (NAN)
SEMINARS: Seminars and conferences throughout the year; safer sex workshops
ADDITIONAL INFO: Focuses on the AIDS health crisis and all persons affected by it
AVAILABLE LITERATURE: *Women and AIDS*, an informational brochure for women; *Facts the Public Should Know About AIDS*, an informational brochure of general AIDS facts; *Support Group for Persons testing HIV/HTLV-3 Positive*, a brochure for those who test positive; *Needles, AIDS, and You*, a brochure for the IV drug user; *Buddy Support Program*, an informational pamphlet; *Keep Columbus Beautiful*, a condom poster; *This Four-Letter Word Will Scare You to Death*, an AIDS poster; *You Will See...at the Bar Tonight Because They Play Safe*, a safer sex poster; *People Who Play Safe...Are Still Here*, a safer sex poster; *Some Diseases Are Getting Away with Murder*, an AIDS poster; monthly newsletter

580. Columbus Health Dept
181 S Washington Blvd
Columbus, OH 43215
(614) 222-7772; Hotline: (614) 464-2437
KEY PERSONNEL: Joni Scolieri; Test Site Coordinator
AFFILIATION: Columbus City Government
FACILITY TYPE: Clinic; Support group; HIV counseling and testing
STAFF: Paid professional 12; Paid nonprofessional 3; Volunteers 10
YEAR FOUNDED: 1985
FUNDING: Federal government; State government; Local government
OUTREACH: Speakers bureau, health fairs, prostitute outreach
RESEARCH: Behavioral change

ADDITIONAL INFO: This agency provides anonymous, confidential counseling and testing for HIV infection, data collection and analysis, and support groups for HIV positive individuals.

AVAILABLE LITERATURE: *AIDS in the Workplace*, an informational brochure; *HIV Infection—Antibody Testing*, a brochure about the test

581. Combined Health District/Dayton
451 W 3rd St
Dayton, OH 45402
FACILITY TYPE: Educational
ADDITIONAL INFO: Source of additional AIDS information

582. Community Drug Board
FORMER NAME: Summit County Community Drug Board
725 E Market
Akron, OH 44305
(216) 434-4141; Hotline: (216) 535-5181
KEY PERSONNEL: Jackie Figler; Coordinator of Volunteer Services
AFFILIATION: Summit County Mental Health Board
FACILITY TYPE: Clinic; Support group
STAFF: Paid professional 60; Paid nonprofessional 7; Volunteers 150
YEAR FOUNDED: 1973
FUNDING: Federal government; State government; Local government; Private; Fund-raisers; Fees for services or products
OUTREACH: Women's outreach, speakers bureau, AIDS education
NETWORKS: Multi County AIDS Network; AIDS Holistic Services
SEMINARS: Feb 12, 1988—"AIDS Update," with Multi-County AIDS Network; Jun, Sep 1988—"Buddy Training," with Multi-County AIDS Network
RESEARCH: Substance abusers and AIDS
ADDITIONAL INFO: Provides a support group for the significant others of PWAs. Maintains an AIDS hotline
AVAILABLE LITERATURE: *Multi-County AIDS Network*, a brochure describing the network; *Invitation to Wholeness*, a brochure describing an AIDS Holistic services program
LANGUAGES: Spanish, American Sign Language

583. Cordelia Martin Health Center, Neighborhood Health Association, Inc
905 Nebraska Ave
Toledo, OH 43607
(419) 255-7883
KEY PERSONNEL: Delores Busby; Outreach Worker
AFFILIATION: Cordelia Martin Health Center
FACILITY TYPE: Clinic
STAFF: Paid professional 20; Paid nonprofessional 22
YEAR FOUNDED: 1969
FUNDING: State government; Local government; Fees for services or products
OUTREACH: Health care for the homeless
ADDITIONAL INFO: Provides comprehensive primary health and dental care services for adults and children. Sliding fees charged for services based upon the federal poverty guidelines. Center accepts all forms of insurance, including medicaid, general relief, and medicare
AVAILABLE LITERATURE: Provides fact sheets on AIDS

584. Dayton Area AIDS Task Force (DAATF)
PO Box 3214
Dayton, OH 45401
(513) 223-2437
KEY PERSONNEL: Peggy Minnich; President
FACILITY TYPE: Task force
STAFF: Volunteers 50
YEAR FOUNDED: 1984
FUNDING: Fund-raisers; Fees for services or products
OUTREACH: Speaker's Bureau, buddy support program, emergency and social service needs

585. Dayton Free Clinic and Counseling Center
1133 Salem Ave
Dayton, OH 45406
(513) 278-9481
KEY PERSONNEL: Victor McCarley, Director
FACILITY TYPE: Clinic
FUNDING: Donations; Grants
LIBRARY: Contains materials pertaining to AIDS for staff use

NETWORKS: Teen Pregnancy/Parenting Coalition; Freedom of Choice Network; Black AIDS Task Force; United Way of Greater Dayton
ADDITIONAL INFO: Founded in 1970 as a clinic and counseling center providing counseling, pregnancy testing, medical clinic services, and education

586. Erie County General Health District AIDS Task Force
PO Box 375, 420 Superior St
Sandusky, OH 44870
(419) 626-5623
KEY PERSONNEL: Donald Ledwell; Health Commissioner
AFFILIATION: Erie County General Health Dept
FACILITY TYPE: Educational; Task force; HIV counseling and testing
STAFF: Paid professional 2; Volunteers 39
YEAR FOUNDED: 1986
FUNDING: Local government; Donations
OUTREACH: Speakers bureau, consultation, information and referral, resource library, posters, pamphlets, case management of PWAs and PWARCs
SEMINARS: 73 programs given in 1987 and 43 given in the first half of 1988
RESEARCH: Safety of blood supply, case studies of sexual partners of persons at risk or PWAs and PWARCs, effectiveness of state mandated testing programs, treatment research, behavioral change studies—what educational/marketing methods are effective, case studies of life expectancies under new and experimental treatment programs
AVAILABLE LITERATURE: *AIDS*, a flyer of brief AIDS information; *Don't Open Yourself to AIDS*, a poster

587. Greater Cincinnati AIDS Task Force
Mail Location 560, 231 Bethesda Ave
Cincinnati, OH 45267-0563
(513) 872-4701
KEY PERSONNEL: Evelyn V Hess, Chairman; Mary Nordlund, Coordinator
AFFILIATION: Univ of Cincinnati Medical Center
FACILITY TYPE: Educational; Clinic; Task force
FUNDING: State government; Grants
LIBRARY: Information from various agencies concerning AIDS available to professionals, health professionals, patients, families, and the public
OUTREACH: Community talks, lectures, counseling services
NETWORKS: AIDS Volunteers of Cincinnati (AVOC)
RESEARCH: Research on virology, immunology, and reproductive immunology
ADDITIONAL INFO: Founded in 1982 as an educational task force for the greater Cincinnati area

588. Health Issues Taskforce of Cleveland
2250 Euclid Ave
Cleveland, OH 44115
(216) 621-0766
KEY PERSONNEL: Gary K Reynolds; Executive Director
FACILITY TYPE: Educational; Support group
STAFF: Paid professional 3; Volunteers 250
YEAR FOUNDED: 1983
FUNDING: Donations; Grants
OUTREACH: Speakers bureau, buddy program, crisis intervention counseling, direct financial assistance, housing, resources directory and referrals, individual and group support counseling, educational materials, safer sex programs for gays, bisexual men, Blacks, Hispanics
NETWORKS: Ohio AIDS Coalition; National AIDS Network (NAN); AIDS Action Council
ADDITIONAL INFO: The task force is a community-based AIDS service organization serving greater Cleveland. Coordinates its work with other community organizations and government agencies to provide a unified city response to the HIV epidemic
AVAILABLE LITERATURE: *AIDS: Facts not Fiction*, a general information brochure about AIDS; *AIDS Knows No Color*, a general brochure for Blacks and Hispanics; *When a Friend Has AIDS*, a brochure of suggestions on what to say and what to do; *Never Share Your Works*, a brochure for IV drug users; *Play Safely/Safer Sex*, a safer sex wallet card; *Health Issues Taskforce Newsletter*, a bimonthly newsletter; Spanish-language versions of some brochures are available

589. HIV Education and Counseling Center
FORMER NAME: HTLV-III Test Site
3101 Burnet Ave
Cincinnati, OH 45229
(513) 352-3138
KEY PERSONNEL: Michael Ritchey, Health Activities Coordinator; Ronn Rucker, Health Education Counselor; Deb Tripp, Counselor Coordinator; I Schwarberg, Health Education Counselor
AFFILIATION: A Clement Health Center, Cincinnati Health Dept
FACILITY TYPE: Educational; Clinic
FUNDING: Grants
LIBRARY: Contains reprints of brochures and educational materials printed by AIDS Volunteers of Cincinnati, and videotapes. Open to all interested persons
OUTREACH: Speakers bureau
NETWORKS: AIDS Volunteers of Cincinnati
SEMINARS: Feb 18-19, May 19-20, Nov 17-18, 1987—"AIDS Update": A 2-day seminar for interdisciplined health providers
ADDITIONAL INFO: Founded in 1985 as an educational and testing agency for AIDS. Currently in the process of developing and training local support groups as well as in-house home care training programs for visiting nurses

590. Joshua House
FORMER NAME: Joshua Foundation
PO Box 13192
Columbus, OH 43213
(614) 235-1070
KEY PERSONNEL: Michael Graham; Director
FACILITY TYPE: Residential facility (adults)
STAFF: Paid professional 4; Volunteers 35
YEAR FOUNDED: 1987
FUNDING: Local government; Private; Fund-raisers; Grants
OUTREACH: Meeting room, food pantry, and laundry facility are available to all PWAs and PWARCs in Columbus and Franklin County
NETWORKS: National AIDS Network (NAN); National Assocation of People With AIDS (NAPWA)
RESEARCH: Sexual identity/sexual expression issues of persons suffering from severe health alterations due to HIV
ADDITIONAL INFO: The mission of Joshua House is to provide residence for individuals diagnosed with HIV, including, but not limited to, AIDS/ARC, by a licensed physician, with emphasis on the psychosocial, physical, and spiritual well-being of each resident

591. Kent State University AIDS Task Force
College of Education
Kent, OH 44242
(216) 672-7977
KEY PERSONNEL: Jacob Gayle, PhD

592. Lake County AIDS Task Force
105 Main St, Administration Bldg
Painesville, OH 44077
(216) 357-2554; Hotline: (216) 354-AIDS
KEY PERSONNEL: Rae Grady; AIDS Program Coordinator
AFFILIATION: Lake County General Health District
FACILITY TYPE: Educational; Support group; Task force
STAFF: Paid professional 1; Volunteers 38
YEAR FOUNDED: 1986
FUNDING: State government; Local government; Private
OUTREACH: Training for emergency personnel, policy, firefighters, health care workers, and educators, consultation in policy development
NETWORKS: American National Red Cross; Catholic Service Bureau
SEMINARS: Presented over 100 training sessions
RESEARCH: Counseling for HIV positive individuals
AVAILABLE LITERATURE: Distributes pamphlets, brochures, and posters from other agencies

593. Lesbian-Gay Community Service Center of Greater Cleveland
FORMER NAME: Gay Education and Awareness Resource
PO Box 6177
Cleveland, OH 44101
(216) 522-1999; Hotline: (216) 781-6736
KEY PERSONNEL: Audrey Wertheim; Director of Services
FACILITY TYPE: Support group; Fund-raising
STAFF: Paid professional 1; Paid nonprofessional 4; Volunteers 80
YEAR FOUNDED: 1974

FUNDING: State government; Local government; Private; Fund-raisers; Fees for services or products
OUTREACH: Drop in center for PWAs, PWARCs, and HIV positive men and women, forums and workshops to explore holistic resources and options, experimental treatments and trials, alternative therapies, and legal positions
SEMINARS: May 19, 1988—"AIDS in the Gay Community;" Aug 9, 1988—"Report from The International Lesbian-Gay Health Conference"
ADDITIONAL INFO: This center was originally formed as a research and education foundation and is now "a multi-service agency providing programs, meeting space, awareness and advocacy for all Clevelanders."
AVAILABLE LITERATURE: *Lesbian-Gay Community Service Center of Greater Cleveland*, a brochure describing the center with appliction form; *The Living Room*, a brochure describing a new AIDS program for PWAs, PRWARCs, and HIV positive men and women

594. Mahoning County Area AIDS Task Force
FORMER NAME: Youngstown AIDS Task Force
PO Box 1143, City Hall, 7th Fl
Youngstown, OH 44501
(216) 742-8766
KEY PERSONNEL: Neil H Altman; President, AIDS Task Force
AFFILIATION: Youngstown Health Dept
FACILITY TYPE: Educational; Clinic; Support group; Fund-raising; Task force; HIV counseling and testing
STAFF: Volunteers 100
YEAR FOUNDED: 1987
FUNDING: Federal government; State government; Private; Fund-raisers; Dues
OUTREACH: Speakers bureau, HIV antibody counseling and testing, educational programs, minority outreach, support groups
NETWORKS: Multi County AIDS Network; National AIDS Network (NAN)
SEMINARS: 1987, 1988—"Speakers Bureau Training Seminars"
AVAILABLE LITERATURE: *Resource Directory*
LANGUAGES: Spanish, American Sign Language

595. Medical College of Ohio
C S No 10008
Toledo, OH 43699
(419) 381-3741
KEY PERSONNEL: Ann Donabedian, Contact
FACILITY TYPE: Educational; Clinic; Support group
ADDITIONAL INFO: Provides education, testing, and counseling for AIDS

596. Montgomery County (Ohio) Health Dept
PO Box 972
Dayton, OH 45422
(513) 225-6462
KEY PERSONNEL: Rosemary Grant, Contact
FACILITY TYPE: Educational; Clinic; Support group
ADDITIONAL INFO: Provides education, testing, and counseling on AIDS

597. Northeast Ohio Task Force on AIDS (NEOTFA)
FORMER NAME: Akron City AIDS Task Force; Akron Area Task Force on AIDS
PO Box 44309-2138, 251 E Mill St
Akron, OH 44309-2138
(216) 762-AIDS
KEY PERSONNEL: Donald J Manson; President
AFFILIATION: Akron Health Dept
FACILITY TYPE: Educational; Support group; Fund-raising; Task force; HIV counseling and testing
STAFF: Paid nonprofessional 1; Volunteers 20
YEAR FOUNDED: 1985
FUNDING: State government; Local government; Private; Fund-raisers
OUTREACH: Community education, school education, employee seminars, outreach to gay bars, bath house owners, bartenders, university groups, support groups for PWAs, PWARCs, HIV positive individuals, friends and family
NETWORKS: National AIDS Network (NAN); AIDS Action Council; American Foundation for AIDS Research (AmFAR); Health Issues Task Force

SEMINARS: Provide in-service seminars to businesses; "AIDS and You," for law enforcement personnel, firefighters, paramedics, clergy, health care professionals, mental health professionals; meetings with Akron and Canton area gay bar and bath owners and managers

ADDITIONAL INFO: Provides services to Summit, Stark, Portage, Medina, and Wayne Counties. Its purpose is to provide education, prevent transmission, help those who are infected with the AIDS virus, and to deal with the increasing consequences of AIDS in our communities

AVAILABLE LITERATURE: *NEOTFA News*, a newsletter; *NEOTFA*, an informational brochure about the task force; *Information for People of Color*, an informational brochure of AIDS facts for Asians, Blacks, Latinos, and Native Americans

598. Ohio AIDS Coalition (OAC)
PO Box 10034
Columbus, OH 43201
(614) 445-8277
KEY PERSONNEL: Howard Fradkin; Chair
FACILITY TYPE: Task force
STAFF: Volunteers 4
YEAR FOUNDED: 1984
FUNDING: State government; Private; Fund-raisers; Fees for services or products
SEMINARS: Ohio AIDS Coalition Healing Weekends for PWAs and PWARCs, 2 in 1988, 3 projected in 1989; sponsor statewide AIDS walk and memorial service
ADDITIONAL INFO: OAC is a coalition of AIDS task forces and service organizations across the state. The goals are to provide networking, support, consultation, and statewide programming to individual groups and to the state government.

599. Ohio Dept of Health, AIDS Unit
246 N High St, 8th Fl
Columbus, OH 43266-0588
(614) 466-5480; Hotline: (800) 332-AIDS (OH only)
KEY PERSONNEL: Robert Campbell; Supervisor
FACILITY TYPE: Research; Educational; Clinic; HIV counseling and testing; Health department
STAFF: Paid professional 16; Volunteers 4
YEAR FOUNDED: 1986
FUNDING: Federal government; State government
OUTREACH: Health education and speaker referrals, consultants to the gay, minority, and IV drug use communities
NETWORKS: National AIDS Network (NAN); Ohio AIDS Coalition (OAC)
SEMINARS: Mar 1988—"AIDS in Ohio's Black and Hispanic Communities;" May 14-22, 1988—AIDS Awareness Week;" May 17, 1988—"Ohio, Working Together to Prevent AIDS;" Nov 1988—"Infection Control Practitioner Conference;" Nov 4, 1988—"Conference of Local AIDS Task Forces;" Oct 1988—"2nd Minority Conference"
RESEARCH: Knowledge, attitudes, and behaviors of general public, health care providers and persons at risk, participating in CDC 30-city serosurvey in Cleveland
ADDITIONAL INFO: Helps sponsor "Healing Weekends" for PWAs, PWARCs, and others twice per year where physical, emotional, and relational healing are addressed
AVAILABLE LITERATURE: *AIDS In the Black Community*, a brochure for Blacks; *Children and AIDS*, a brochure for parents; *Ohio Working Together to Prevent AIDS*, stamps with the Hotline telephone number; *Progress*, a newsmagazine; *Ohio Dept of Health Recommendations for Clinical Management of Individuals with HTLV-3 Infection*; *Safer Sex, Condoms and AIDS*, a safer sex brochure with condom information; *AIDS Facts for Life*, a wallet card of safer sex tips; *Ohio Dept of Health Policy Regarding Mandatory (Involuntary) AIDS Antibody Testing*, a pamphlet discussing the policy; *A Guide for Living with the AIDS Virus*, a pamphlet about the AIDS virus and living with being HIV positive; *Acquired Immune Deficiency Syndrome (AIDS) Data for Ohio and the United States*, a fact sheet with statistics; *Some Facts About AIDS*, an informational brochure; *Ohio AIDS Education Package*, a curriculum package; *AIDS Information Manual*, a multi-page notebook of information about all aspects of AIDS

600. Ohio Dept of Health, Bureau of Preventive Medicine, Communicable Disease Division, AIDS Activities Unit
PO Box 118
Columbus, OH 43266-01118

(614) 466-5480; Hotline: (800) 332-AIDS
KEY PERSONNEL: Rachelle Randolph; Health Planning Coordinator
AFFILIATION: Ohio State Health Dept
FACILITY TYPE: Health department
STAFF: Paid professional 25
YEAR FOUNDED: 1887
FUNDING: Federal government; State government
OUTREACH: Statewide conferences, counselor training programs, AIDS advisory committee, Hispanic program, minority program, speakers bureau, hotline, KAB surveys, adolscent program, counseling and teting sites, surveillance
NETWORKS: National AIDS Network (NAN); National Minority AIDS Council; Ohio Public Health Association
SEMINARS: Has an active conference program throug hout the year
AVAILABLE LITERATURE: *AIDS Kills: Avoid Contamination*, a card with information on how to clean needles; *SIDA es Mortal: Evite Contaminacion*, a Spanish-language card on how to clean needles; *AIDS Facts for Life*, a card of facts about AIDS; *AIDS Among Minorities*, a card with minority statistics and AIDS; *Women and AIDS*, a brochure of facts about AIDS and women; *Children and AIDS: What Should Parents Know?*, a brochure of brief AIDS information; *AIDS in the Black Community*, AIDS information for Blacks; *Some facts about AIDS*, a brochure of AIDS information; *A Guide for Living with the AIDS Virus*, a booklet for those who have the virus; *Ohio Health Promotion Network: AIDS*, a booklet listing and describing various resources from other facilities in the United States; *Ohio AIDS Education Package*, a booklet with information for health educators, school teachers, school administrators, medical personnel, and other concerned individuals explaining in lay terms the infection process, the consequences of infection, and infection risks with the primary purpose being to alleviate unwarranted fear of AIDS infection; *You Can Get AIDS: AIDS Does Not Discriminate*, a poster; *You Can Get AIDS: Bad Habits Die Hard*, a poster for drug users; *You Can Get AIDS: Be Safe, Be Informed, Don't Kill Our Future*

601. Social Health Association, Dayton
184 Salem Ave
Dayton, OH 45406
(513) 220-6622
KEY PERSONNEL: Cheryl Morrisey; Health Promotion Specialist
FACILITY TYPE: Educational; Support group
STAFF: Paid professional 4; Paid nonprofessional 1; Volunteers 2
YEAR FOUNDED: 1948
FUNDING: Private; Donations
OUTREACH: Teen pregnancy/STD/AIDS prevention programs in the schools, support groups for the family and friends of PWAs, distributes information
NETWORKS: Dayton Area AIDS Task Force

602. Southern Ohio AIDS Task Force
PO Box 1287
Portsmouth, OH 45662
(614) 353-3339
KEY PERSONNEL: Vince Engel, Coordinator
FACILITY TYPE: Educational; Task force
ADDITIONAL INFO: Provides counseling, referrals, buddies, and housing

603. Special Immunology Unit (SIU)
2074 Abington Rd
Cleveland, OH 44106
(216) 844-7890
KEY PERSONNEL: Robert Plona; Advanced Clinical Nurse
AFFILIATION: University Hospitals of Cleveland
FACILITY TYPE: Research; Educational; Hospital; Clinic
YEAR FOUNDED: 1988
FUNDING: Fees for services or products
NETWORKS: Health Issues Taskforce

604. Toledo Area AIDS Task Force, Inc
151 N Michigan St, Ste 322
Toledo, OH 43624
(419) 242-4777; Information Line: (419) 242-AIDS
KEY PERSONNEL: Gert Heitz; Program Director
FACILITY TYPE: Educational; Support group; Task force
STAFF: Paid professional 2.5; Volunteers 30
YEAR FOUNDED: 1986
FUNDING: Private; Fund-raisers; Fees for services or products

OUTREACH: Street outreach to IV drug users, prostitutes, gay men in gay bars, general population
ADDITIONAL INFO: This agency has a Board of Trustees that is representative of the community: clergy, health educators, social workers, public health nurse, gays/lesbians, people of color, etc. Provides educational sessions at the request of colleges, schools, churches, and others
LANGUAGES: Spanish

605. Toledo City Health Dept
635 N Erie St
Toledo, OH 43624
(419) 245-1785
KEY PERSONNEL: Chuck Gains
FACILITY TYPE: Educational; Clinic; Support group
ADDITIONAL INFO: Provides education, testing, and counseling for AIDS

OKLAHOMA

606. AIDS Support Program, Inc (ASP)
FORMER NAME: Oklahoma AIDS Foundation
PO Box 57531
Oklahoma City, OK 73157-2057
(405) 840-2437
KEY PERSONNEL: Cynthia Scott; Director
FACILITY TYPE: Educational; Support group; Fund-raising; HIV counseling and testing
STAFF: Paid professional 1; Paid nonprofessional 1; Volunteers 40
YEAR FOUNDED: 1986
FUNDING: State government; Private; Fund-raisers
OUTREACH: Speakers bureau, support groups for PWAs, PWARCs, HIV positive individuals, and their friends and families
NETWORKS: National AIDS Network (NAN)
ADDITIONAL INFO: Provides a group home, general support groups, HIV positive group, PWA group, buddy system, speakers bureau, and is an anonymous testing site
AVAILABLE LITERATURE: Newsletter for support groups

607. Garfield County Health Dept
2501 Mercer Dr
Enid, OK 73701
(405) 233-0650
KEY PERSONNEL: Kirk Mosley; Medical Director
AFFILIATION: Garfield County Government
FACILITY TYPE: Clinic; Task force; HIV counseling and testing; Health department
STAFF: Paid professional 14; Paid nonprofessional 8; Volunteers 35
FUNDING: State government; Local government; Fees for services or products
OUTREACH: Speakers bureau, literature distribution for the task force, educational presentations, seminars
SEMINARS: 1987—"Seminar on AIDS for Church Staffs;" 1987—"Workshop for Counselors, Teachers Providing AIDS Education"
ADDITIONAL INFO: This agency is an STD clinic and provides HIV counseling and testing
AVAILABLE LITERATURE: *AIDS: A New Disease, Facts That Everyone Should Know*, a brochure of AIDS facts

608. Oasis Community Center, AIDS Hotline
2135 NW 39th St
Oklahoma City, OK 73112
FACILITY TYPE: Support group
ADDITIONAL INFO: Source of additional AIDS information

609. Oklahoma State Health Dept, AIDS Division
PO Box 53551
Oklahoma City, OK 73152
Hotline: (800) 522-9054; Toll-free: (800) 522-9054
KEY PERSONNEL: Ron Toth; Director of AIDS Division
AFFILIATION: Oklahoma State Health Dept
FACILITY TYPE: Educational
STAFF: Paid professional 13
FUNDING: Federal government; State government
OUTREACH: Community AIDS education programs, speakers bureau training, HIV counseling training, HIV/AIDS epidemiology services

AVAILABLE LITERATURE: *100 Common Questions and Answers About AIDS*, a brochure of general AIDS information
LANGUAGES: Spanish

610. Tulsa AIDS Task Force
1711 S Jackson, Unit FF
Tulsa, OK 74107
(918) 743-4093
KEY PERSONNEL: Kevin Gabel

OREGON

611. Carper House, Inc
1085 W 6th Ave
Eugene, OR 97402
(503) 342-7716
KEY PERSONNEL: Richard Carper; Founder
FACILITY TYPE: Support group; Hospice; HIV counseling and testing
STAFF: Paid professional 7; Paid nonprofessional 4
YEAR FOUNDED: 1988
FUNDING: Private; Fund-raisers; Fees for services or products
OUTREACH: Presentations to the community on hospices and what it is like living the experience
SEMINARS: Sep 1988—"Sweden, International Tour"
ADDITIONAL INFO: The resident remains the main decision maker over his/her own treatment and life. Provides nutritional meals, counseling, therapeutic programs, and monitoring medications

612. Cascade AIDS Project, Inc (CAP)
408 SW 2nd St, Ste 412
Portland, OR 97204
(503) 223-5907; Hotline: (503) 223-AIDS; Toll-free: (800) 777-2437 (OR only)
KEY PERSONNEL: Patrick Miner; Administrative Assistant
FACILITY TYPE: Educational; Support group; Fund-raising; Client services/case management
STAFF: Paid professional 12; Volunteers 550
YEAR FOUNDED: 1986
FUNDING: Federal government; State government; Local government; Private; Fund-raisers
OUTREACH: Emotional support through the PAL project (personal active listener), support groups for PWAs, PWARCs, HIV positive individuals, concerned lovers, family members and friends, conseling, home health care, community health nurse, transportation, public assistance, financial aid, food and household supplies, information and referral, speakers bureau, safer sex workshops, literature distribution
NETWORKS: Oregon AIDS Task Force; Coalition for AIDS Education; National AIDS Network (NAN)
ADDITIONAL INFO: The Cascade AIDS Project is a community-based, non-profit organization founded to serve the direct needs of those living with AIDS as well as the educational needs of the community
AVAILABLE LITERATURE: *Impact*, agency newsletter; *PWA Connection*, newsletter for PWAs; *Captions*, a volunteer newsletter; *You Can Make a Difference*, a brochure about the agency; *Great Northwest Sex*, a safer sex brochure; *Using a Condom*, instructions on how to use a condom; *Myths and Facts About AIDS*, a brochure of AIDS facts and myths; *Just the Facts*, a flyer for those who have tested positive; *Safer Sex Guidelines*, tips for safer sex including a condom; *We Can Live Together*, an AIDS poster

613. Douglas County Health and Social Services Health Center
621 W Madrone St
Roseburg, OR 97470
(503) 440-3500
KEY PERSONNEL: Linda Whiat; Health Educator
AFFILIATION: Douglas County Government
FACILITY TYPE: Educational; Clinic; Health department
STAFF: Paid professional 134; Volunteers 500
FUNDING: Federal government; State government; Local government; Fees for services or products
OUTREACH: AIDS education on a county-wide basis to schools, businesses, county governmental departments, state and federal facilities, and community groups

SEMINARS: 1988—"AIDS and Substance Abuse"
ADDITIONAL INFO: This facility is an alternative test site for HIV antibody testing. Provides mental health support services and limited primary medical care for PWAs

614. Gay and Lesbian Alliance (GALA)
PO Box 813
Roseburg, OR 97470-0166
(503) 672-4126; Hotline: (503) 672-4126; Community Center: (503) 679-9144
KEY PERSONNEL: Jim Hopper; Administrative Assistant
FACILITY TYPE: Research; Educational; Support group; Fund-raising; Task force
STAFF: Volunteers 15
YEAR FOUNDED: 1981
FUNDING: Private; Fund-raisers; Grants
OUTREACH: Youth group, HIV support group, gayline, community center
NETWORKS: MCC Roseburg; Douglas County AIDS/ARC Council; Ruby House
RESEARCH: Violence against gays and lesbians, gay and lesbian history, gay and lesbian outreach
ADDITIONAL INFO: GALA is an all-volunteer organization focused on developing community gay and lesbian education. The community center is a source of additional AIDS information
AVAILABLE LITERATURE: *Gay Ol' Times*, a newsletter

615. Good Samaritan Hospital AIDS Task Force
NW 23rd St
Portland, OR 97120
(503) 229-7711
FACILITY TYPE: Hospital; Task force
ADDITIONAL INFO: Source of additional AIDS information

616. Mid-Oregon AIDS/Health/Education and Support Services, Inc (MASS)
1115 Madison St NE, No 510
Salem, OR 97303
Hotline: (503) 363-4963
KEY PERSONNEL: Patricia Jackson; Secretary
FACILITY TYPE: Educational; Support group; Hospice
STAFF: Volunteers 25
YEAR FOUNDED: 1985
FUNDING: Local government; Private; Fund-raisers
OUTREACH: Educational meetings that are open to the public
ADDITIONAL INFO: Serves the counties of Marion, Park, Benton, Linn, and Yamhill. MASS is primarily an educational group that takes part in many AIDS awareness programs including a booth at the state fair
AVAILABLE LITERATURE: Distribute brochures from other agencies, meeting notices and buttons
LANGUAGES: Spanish

617. Multnomah County Health Division AIDS Program
426 SW Stark
Portland, OR 97204
(503) 248-3406; Hotline: (503) 248-3816
KEY PERSONNEL: Jeanne Gould; Program Manager
AFFILIATION: Multnomah County Health Division
FACILITY TYPE: Research; Educational; Clinic
STAFF: Paid professional 5
YEAR FOUNDED: 1986
FUNDING: State government; Local government; Fees for services or products
OUTREACH: General community education, outreach and education to schools, out of school youth, health care providers, minorities, gay and bisexual men
NETWORKS: Oregon Hispanic AIDS Program; Oregon Minority AIDS Coalition; Cascade AIDS Project
RESEARCH: Effective interaction strategies for IV drug users, cost containment through nursing case management
LANGUAGES: Works with all languages through a contract with the language bank

618. Oregon AIDS Task Force, Research and Education Group
PO Box 40104
Portland, OR 97240-0104
(503) 229-7126
KEY PERSONNEL: James H Sampson; Executive Director

FACILITY TYPE: Research; Educational; Fund-raising; Task force
STAFF: Paid professional 5; Volunteers 7
YEAR FOUNDED: 1988
FUNDING: Private; Fund-raisers; Fees for services or products
OUTREACH: Community seminars, presentations to business and industry, and health care related groups
NETWORKS: Physicians Association for AIDS Care
SEMINARS: "AIDS Update 1988"
RESEARCH: Clinical research projects related to HIV disease
ADDITIONAL INFO: Provides an alternative setting for clinical research projects
AVAILABLE LITERATURE: *For Clinical Studies of HIV Disease*, a brochure describing the Oregon AIDS Task Force

619. Phoenix Rising
FORMER NAME: Town Council Foundation
333 SW 5th, Ste 404
Portland, OR 97204
(503) 223-8299
KEY PERSONNEL: Helen Lottridge; Executive Director
FACILITY TYPE: Educational; Support group; HIV counseling and testing
STAFF: Paid professional 22; Paid nonprofessional 1; Volunteers 10
YEAR FOUNDED: 1979
FUNDING: Private; Fund-raisers; Fees for services or products
OUTREACH: Speakers bureau, confronting homophobia, counseling services, information and referral, gay youth services
AVAILABLE LITERATURE: Publishes a quarterly newsletter
LANGUAGES: American Sign Language

620. Ruby House
PO Box 182
Dillard, OR 97432
(503) 679-9913
KEY PERSONNEL: Billy Russo; House Manager
FACILITY TYPE: Hospice
STAFF: Volunteers 10
YEAR FOUNDED: 1988
FUNDING: State government; Private; Fund-raisers; Fees for services or products
OUTREACH: Daycare for PWAs
NETWORKS: Douglas County AIDS/ARC Council; Gay and Lesbian Alliance
ADDITIONAL INFO: This hospice consists of a 13-room house, 6 bedrooms, 2 baths, for total care

621. Shanti in Oregon, Inc
752 Jefferson
Eugene, OR 97402
(503) 342-5088
KEY PERSONNEL: Scott Meisner; Executive Director
FACILITY TYPE: Support group
STAFF: Paid professional 1; Paid nonprofessional 2; Volunteers 60
YEAR FOUNDED: 1986
FUNDING: Local government; Private; Fund-raisers
OUTREACH: Education on the psychosocial issues of AIDS, emotional and practical support
NETWORKS: Willamette AIDS Council of Eugene, OR
SEMINARS: Apr, Sep 1988—"Emotional Support Volunteer Training;" Jun 1988—"Practical Support Training;" Jan, May, Oct 1989—"Emotional Support Training"
ADDITIONAL INFO: Shanti in Oregon is a volunteer-based community agency providing emotional and practical support services to persons with HIV or AIDS, and to their families, friends and loved ones. Trains volunteers in other communities throughout Oregon in setting up and operating support service programs. Provides drug outreach education and services, and performs financial, legal and other advocacy for clients
AVAILABLE LITERATURE: *Shanti in Oregon, Inc.*, a brochure describing the agency
LANGUAGES: Spanish, French

622. University of Oregon Health Sciences Center, Division of Infectious Diseases
3181 SW Sam Jackson Park Rd
Portland, OR 97201
(503) 279-7735; Hotline for Professionals: (800) 562-AIDS
KEY PERSONNEL: James D Simons; HIV/AIDS Program Manager
AFFILIATION: Oregon State Division of Higher Education

FACILITY TYPE: Research; Educational; Hospital; Clinic; Support group; Task force
YEAR FOUNDED: 1988
FUNDING: Federal government; State government; Local government; Private; Fees for services or products
OUTREACH: Statewide professional education through NIH/PHS grant, schools of medicine, nursing, and dentistry
NETWORKS: National AIDS Network (NAN); International Society for AIDS Education
RESEARCH: Clinical trials, treatment pilot programs
ADDITIONAL INFO: Serves Washington, Alaska, Montana, Idaho, and Oregon and is funded by a 3-year grant. Serves to evaluate, develop and implement HIV/AIDS education and training for health care professionals
LANGUAGES: Full range of interpreters available

623. Western Health Clinics
3777 SE Milwaukie Blvd
Portland, OR 97202
(503) 234-1777
KEY PERSONNEL: Calvin Hightower; Regional Director
FACILITY TYPE: HIV counseling and testing; Substance abuse treatment

624. Willamette AIDS Council (WAC)
329 W 13th Ave, Ste D
Eugene, OR 97401
(503) 345-7089; Business: (503) 683-5936
KEY PERSONNEL: Sally Sheklow; General Manager
FACILITY TYPE: Educational
STAFF: Paid professional 2; Volunteers 20
YEAR FOUNDED: 1985
FUNDING: State government; Private; Fund-raisers
OUTREACH: Telephone helpline, speakers bureau, safer sex workshops, resource library, condom and poster distribution, information tables at Saturday markets and special events and fairs
NETWORKS: Community AIDS Consortium; Oregon Women's AIDS Network; National AIDS Network (NAN)
SEMINARS: Spring 1988—"Challenges and Changes: Women's Role in the AIDS Epidemic"
RESEARCH: Risk reduction among gay/bisexual men (survey conducted in 1987)
AVAILABLE LITERATURE: *The Care and Feeding of Dental Dams*, a flyer with descriptive information for women on the use of the dental dam; *Love Safely*, a balloon; *Love Safely*, a button; *Love Safely*, a packaged condom with instructions on how to use it and information on safer sex; *No Sex Without Latex*, a packaged condom with instructions on how to use it
LANGUAGES: Spanish, American Sign Language

PENNSYLVANIA

625. Action AIDS, Inc
PO Box 1625
Philadelphia, PA 19105
(215) 732-2155
KEY PERSONNEL: Anna Forbes; Director of Community Relations, Action AIDS
FACILITY TYPE: Educational; Support group; Client services/case management
STAFF: Paid professional 20; Volunteers 400
YEAR FOUNDED: 1986
FUNDING: Federal government; Local government; Private; Fund-raisers
OUTREACH: Minority outreach, educational committees, safer sex seminars for men and women, speakers bureau
NETWORKS: Philadelphia AIDS Advocacy Coalition; Philadelphia AIDS Consortium; National AIDS Network (NAN)
ADDITIONAL INFO: Volunteer-based organization providing a wide variety of services including a buddy system, public advocacy, education, and support groups and counseling for PWAs, PWARCs, HIV positive individuals, parents and relatives of PWAs, lovers, spouses, family and friends of PWAs, women affected by AIDS, and recovering substance abusers
AVAILABLE LITERATURE: *Action AIDS*, an informational brochure; *Accion contra SIDA*, an informational brochure in Spanish; *Action AIDS Insider*, a newsletter; *Action AIDS Newsletter*
LANGUAGES: Spanish

626. AIDS Activities Coordinating Office (AACO)
FORMER NAME: AIDS Control Program
City Hall Annex, 13th Fl
Philadelphia, PA 19107
(215) 686-5070; Hotline: (215) 875-6560
KEY PERSONNEL: David Fair; Executive Assistant
AFFILIATION: Philadelphia Dept of Public Health
FACILITY TYPE: Educational; Clinic; Health department
STAFF: Paid professional 50; Paid nonprofessional 10
YEAR FOUNDED: 1987
FUNDING: Federal government; State government; Local government
OUTREACH: Speakers bureau, case management, residential services, mental health services, home health care, transportation, educational out reach
NETWORKS: National AIDS Network (NAN)
SEMINARS: Hold many conferences, workshops, and meetings
ADDITIONAL INFO: This is a coordinating agency that brings all other groups together for a common purpose of education and support. It has an Agency Services Division, Medical Affairs, Policy and Planning Division, Surveillance Unit, AIDS Prevention Services Division, and Administration Unit. The following agencies hold Dept of Health/AACO contracts to provide AIDS-related services: Action AIDS, Inc, centralized case mangement services for people with HIV infection; AIDS Library of Philadelphia, a volunteer-based resource center; BEBASHI, Blacks Educating Blacks About Sexual Health Issues; Choice AIDS Hotline; Congreso de Latinos, Inc, HIV testing and counseling; Episcopal Community Services; Family Planning Council of Southeastern Pennsylvania; Gaudenzia, Inc, residential services; Marian Homes, Inc., residential services; Philadelphia Community Health Alternatives; Philadelphia Health Management Corporation AIDS Prevention Project; Philadelphia Home Care; We the People with AIDS/ARC, advocacy and mutual support organization.
AVAILABLE LITERATURE: *The AACO Report*, newsletter; *Questions and Answers About AIDS*, a 1987 booklet of questions and answers; *Directory of AIDS-Related Resources in the Philadelphia Area*, a one page directory; *AIDS is a Fatal Disease*, brochure; *Nobody Can Give You AIDS*, an informational brochure; *11 Questions Frequently Asked by Physicians*; *What You Must Know About AIDS*, a *Readers Digest* reprint; *AIDS? Me?*, a brochure for the clinic; *Shooting Drugs and AIDS*, brochure for drug users; *Safer Sex*, an informational brochure; *AIDS: The Facts*, an informational brochure; *When a Friend Has AIDS*, a brochure of what to say and what to do; *Caring for the AIDS Patient at Home*, a Red Cross brochure; *AIDS and Your Job*, a Red Cross brochure; *If Your Test for Antibody to the AIDS Virus is Positive*, a Red Cross brochure; *AIDS and Children: for Teachers*, a Red Cross brochure for teachers; *How to Use a Condom*, a sheet of instructions; *How to Use a Condom (Rubber)*, a wallet card; *Facts About AIDS: How to Protect Yourself and Your Family*, a one sheet flyer; *Understanding AIDS*, tear-off sheets; *Understanding AIDS*, the Surgeon General's mailing; *Entendiendo El SIDA (AIDS)*, the Surgeon General's mailing in Spanish; *What You Should Know About AIDS*, informational brochure; *AIDS Comic Books*; *Many Teens are Saying No*, a brochure on abstinence in regards to sex; *About AIDS and Shooting Drugs*; *What Young People Should Know About AIDS*; *AIDS: Think About It/Pienselo*, an English and Spanish brochure; *Talking with Your Teenager About AIDS*; *Talking with Your Child About AIDS*; *AIDS: Risk, Prevention, Understanding*, an informational brochure; *How You Won't Get AIDS*, an CDC brochure; *What About AIDS Testing*, a CDC brochure; the following posters are available: *A Man Who Shoots Up Can Be Very Giving...He Can Give You and Your Baby AIDS*; *Most Babies with AIDS Are Born to Mothers or Fathers Who Have Shot Drugs*; *Guess Who Else Can Get AIDS if You Shoot Drugs*; *When You Share Needles You Could Be Shooting up AIDS*; *Protect Your Loved Ones...Protect Yourself, Use a Condom*, in English or Spanish; *Look Who Can Get AIDS...Protect Yourself, Use a Condom*, in English or Spanish; *This is How You Can Get AIDS*, a cartoon in English or Spanish; *Anyone Can Get AIDS...Protect Yourself, Use a Condom*, in English or Spanish; *You Won't Get AIDS...*, a series of four posters from CDC; *A Matter of Life*, a videotape

627. AIDS Council of Erie County, Inc
4718 Lake Pleasant Rd
Erie, PA 16504
(814) 825-0881; (800) 445-6262
KEY PERSONNEL: Jackie Tammaro

628. AIDS Intervention Project/Altoona
PO Box 352
Altoona, PA 16603
(814) 946-5411; (800) 445-6262
KEY PERSONNEL: Bonnie Ashcroft

629. AIDS Task Force of the Lehigh Valley
723 Chew St, Allentown Health Bureau
Allentown, PA 18102
(215) 437-7742
KEY PERSONNEL: Anne Taylor; Coordinator
AFFILIATION: Allentown Health Bureau
FACILITY TYPE: Task force
STAFF: Paid professional 1; Volunteers 65
YEAR FOUNDED: 1985
FUNDING: Federal government; State government; Private
OUTREACH: Speakers bureau, help in creation of an AIDS policy for schools, prisons, and worksites
SEMINARS: May 28, 1988— "Hispanic Leadership Conference on AIDS;" Sep 1988—"The Technical Issues of AIDS"
ADDITIONAL INFO: The AIDS Task Force of the Lehigh Valley is a coalition of community agencies founded in 1985. The current membership of 75 individuals represents the participation of 50 organizations. The Task Force is divided into 4 working committees, a speakers bureau, and an executive committee
AVAILABLE LITERATURE: *AIDS: The Virus, The Disease, The Social Dilemma*, an instructor's guide
LANGUAGES: Spanish

630. Allegheny County Health Dept
3333 Forbes Ave
Pittsburgh, PA 15213
(412) 578-8026
KEY PERSONNEL: N Mark Richards, Director
FACILITY TYPE: Educational; Clinic
ADDITIONAL INFO: Monitors reported cases of AIDS, provides public speakers to professional and lay groups, and provides HIV antibody testing and counseling

631. American Red Cross, Erie
4961 Pittsburgh Ave
Erie, PA 16509
(814) 833-0942
AFFILIATION: American National Red Cross
FACILITY TYPE: Educational
STAFF: Paid professional 10; Paid nonprofessional 3; Volunteers 500
YEAR FOUNDED: 1881
FUNDING: Private; Fund-raisers; Fees for services or products
NETWORKS: AIDS Council of Erie County, Inc
AVAILABLE LITERATURE: Provides publications from the national headquarters of the American National Red Cross

632. ANAWIM: AIDS Pastoral Care
PO Box 362
Pittsburgh, PA 15230
(412) 782-4023
KEY PERSONNEL: Charlene Fregeolle, Co-coordinator; Mariana Blanco, Co-coordinator
AFFILIATION: Dignity, Pittsburgh
FACILITY TYPE: Support group; HIV counseling and testing Religious
STAFF: Volunteers 6
YEAR FOUNDED: 1984
FUNDING: Private; Fund-raisers; Donations
NETWORKS: Pittsburgh Interagency Council on AIDS (PICA)
ADDITIONAL INFO: Provides pastoral care in hospital and at home, social services, supportive counseling with PWAs, families, and friends, and memorial services

633. BEBASHI (Blacks Educating Blacks About Sexual Health Issue)
1528 Walnut St, Ste 1414
Philadelphia, PA 19102
(215) 546-4140
KEY PERSONNEL: Rashidah Lorraine Hassan; Executive Director
FACILITY TYPE: Educational; Support group; HIV counseling and testing
STAFF: Paid professional 10; Paid nonprofessional 7; Volunteers 100
YEAR FOUNDED: 1985
FUNDING: Federal government; State government; Local government; Private; Fund-raisers; Fees for services or products
OUTREACH: Outreach AIDS education to children, women, drug users, gay and bisexual men of color, low income housing
NETWORKS: National AIDS Network (NAN); Minority AIDS Council; National Black Caucus on AIDS; Philadelphia Consortium on AIDS
RESEARCH: Knowledge, attitudes and behavior studies among specific population groups
ADDITIONAL INFO: Provides HIV counseling to individuals affected by the epidemic
AVAILABLE LITERATURE: *AIDS in the Black Community*, a brochure for Blacks; *State of Black Phila—1987*, a brochure of statistics; distributes brochures from other organizations
LANGUAGES: Spanish, Arabic

634. Berks AIDS Health Crisis (BAHC)
PO Box 8626
Reading, PA 19603
(215) 375-2242
KEY PERSONNEL: Katharyn Waldman-Anderson; Administrator
FACILITY TYPE: Educational; Support group; Fund-raising; Task force
STAFF: Paid professional 2; Volunteers 10
YEAR FOUNDED: 1985
FUNDING: State government; Private; Fund-raisers
OUTREACH: Speakers bureau
ADDITIONAL INFO: Provides support for PWAs and significant others
LANGUAGES: Spanish

635. Congreso de Latinos Unidos, Inc
704 W Girard Ave
Philadelphia, PA 19123
(215) 625-0550; Hotline: (800) 228-4201
KEY PERSONNEL: Carmen Paris; Program Director
FACILITY TYPE: Educational; Social service agency
STAFF: Paid professional 20; Paid nonprofessional 42
YEAR FOUNDED: 1977
FUNDING: Federal government; State government; Local government
OUTREACH: Outreach and education through Programa Esfuerzo
ADDITIONAL INFO: Provides an array of services to the Philadelphia Puerto Rican/Latino community. The Programa Esfuerzo provides AIDS education and outreach to the Hispanic community
AVAILABLE LITERATURE: *Congreso de Latinos Unidos, Inc*, a brochure describing the agency; *Boletin del Congreso*, a newsletter; *How to Use a Condom (Rubber)*, a small folded pocket card; *AIDS/SIDA: Informese*, an American Red Cross brochure of AIDS facts; *Caring for the AIDS Patient at Home*, an American Red Cross patient care brochure; *Safer Sex: Avoiding AIDS Virus Transmission*, a brochure of general guidelines for safer sex; *AIDS: The Facts*, a brochure of general AIDS facts; *Datos Sobre el SIDA*, a brochure of detailed AIDS information; *La Vida de la Mujer Latina y su Bebe Estanen Peligro AIDS*, a general brochure for the Hispanic community; *Preguntas y Respuestas: el SIDA (AIDS)*, a brochure of general AIDS information; *What You Should Know About AIDS*, a booklet of facts about the disease; *Programa Esfuerzo*, a flyer describing an AIDS education prevention program (in English and Spanish); *Entendiendo el SIDA (AIDS)*, The CDC booklet of AIDS information in Spanish
LANGUAGES: Spanish

636. Counseling Associates
152 Cambridge Rd
King of Prussia, PA 19406
(215) 272-0800
KEY PERSONNEL: Vincent F Miraglia; Director
FACILITY TYPE: HIV counseling and testing; Substance abuse treatment

637. Hemophilia Center of Western Pennsylvania (HEWP)
812 5th Ave
Pittsburgh, PA 15219
(412) 622-7200
KEY PERSONNEL: Margaret V Ragni; Director
AFFILIATION: National Hemophilia Foundation
FACILITY TYPE: Research; Educational; Clinic; Support group
STAFF: Paid professional 7
YEAR FOUNDED: 1972
FUNDING: Federal government; State government
OUTREACH: Education on AIDS prevention and risk reduction

SEMINARS: May 13, 1987—"Region III Federal Hemophilia Meeting;" Jun 17, 1988—"Region III Coordinating Workshop for AIDS Protocol"

RESEARCH: AIDS and the hemophiliac person, hematologic problems

ADDITIONAL INFO: Provides state-funded comprehensive hemophilia care programs and offers expertise in management of hemalogic, orthopedic, genetic, AIDS, and hepatitis-related problems.

AVAILABLE LITERATURE: *Hemophilia Newsnotes*, a quarterly newsletter

638. Home Nursing Agency, AIDS Intravention Project of Central Pennsylvania
PO Box 352, 201 Chestnut Ave
Altoona, PA 16603
(814) 946-5411; Hotline: (800) 445-6262
KEY PERSONNEL: Nancy L Truscott; Psychiatric Nurse Clinician
AFFILIATION: Home Nursing Agency (HNA)
FACILITY TYPE: Educational; Support group; Hospice; Fund-raising; Task force
STAFF: Volunteers 50
YEAR FOUNDED: 1986
FUNDING: Fund-raisers
OUTREACH: Speakers bureau, outreach to schools, churches, civic groups, occupational groups, senior citizens, radio stations, television stations
NETWORKS: WJACTV
SEMINARS: Apr 1987—"Confronting AIDS in the Community;" Jan 22-24, 1988—"Volunteer Training Workshop;" Jun 1988—"Safer Sex"
ADDITIONAL INFO: Provides counseling, volunteers for speaking engagements, support for PWAs, PWARCs, HIV positive individuals, and their families, safer sex seminars, and other services to the community
AVAILABLE LITERATURE: Pamphlets in the development stage

639. Northeast AIDS Council of Pennsylvania, Inc (NAC)
PO Box 751
Scranton, PA 18501-0751
(717) 342-6907; Hotline: (717) 342-6907
KEY PERSONNEL: Barry MaKemes; President
FACILITY TYPE: Educational; Support group
STAFF: Volunteers varies
YEAR FOUNDED: 1987
FUNDING: Fund-raisers; Donations
OUTREACH: Speakers bureau, referrals, hotline
ADDITIONAL INFO: Offers buddies, support groups, socialization for PWAs, PWARCs, and HIV positive individuals, and education to the community.

640. PALS
PO Box 783
Erie, PA 16512
(814) 868-9704
KEY PERSONNEL: Father Jeff Hamblin

641. Pennsylvania Dept of Health, Division of Acute Infectious Disease Epidemiology, AIDS Program
PO Box 90, Health and Welfare Bldg
Harrisburg, PA 17108
(717) 787-3350; Hotline: (800) 692-7254
KEY PERSONNEL: George Schelzel; AIDS Program Manager
AFFILIATION: Pennsylvania Dept of Health
FACILITY TYPE: Educational; HIV counseling and testing; Health department
STAFF: Paid professional 12; Paid nonprofessional 5
FUNDING: Federal government; State government
OUTREACH: Funding of minority programs, surveys
ADDITIONAL INFO: Provides education, counseling and testing, and epidemiology
AVAILABLE LITERATURE: *Facts About AIDS*, a brochure for 12th grade reading level; *Questions and Answers About AIDS*, a brochure for 7th grade reading level; *AIDS Update*, a newsletter; posters and wallet-size cards with telephone numbers

642. Persad Center, Inc
121 S Highland Ave, 817 Highland Bldg
Pittsburgh, PA 15206
(412) 441-0857
KEY PERSONNEL: James Huggins; Associate Director

FACILITY TYPE: Educational; Clinic; Support group; Fund-raising
STAFF: Paid professional 8
YEAR FOUNDED: 1972
FUNDING: State government; Private; Fund-raisers; Fees for services or products
OUTREACH: Professional education programs tailored to the needs of agencies and groups, educational programs focusing on helping health and mental health professionals to become sensitive to the special needs of HIV infected people and their significant others
NETWORKS: Pittsburgh Interorganization Council on AIDS
SEMINARS: Presents numerous programs throughout the year
ADDITIONAL INFO: Persad Center is a comprehensive mental health center specializing in services to sexual minorities, including lesbians, gay men, transsexuals, transvestites, and persons experiencing sexual or gender identity confusion. Offers an AIDS services program
AVAILABLE LITERATURE: *Persad Center, Inc*, an informational brochure; *AIDS Related Services at Persad Center, Inc*, a brochure outlining what services are available; a newsletter

643. Philadelphia Community Health Alternatives/The Philadelphia AIDS Task Force (PCHA/PATF)
1216 Walnut St
Philadelphia, PA 19107
(215) 545-8686; Hotline: (215) 732-AIDS
KEY PERSONNEL: Francis J Stoffa, Jr; Executive Director
FACILITY TYPE: Educational; Clinic; Support group; Fund-raising; Task force; HIV counseling and testing
STAFF: Paid professional 13; Volunteers 500
YEAR FOUNDED: 1979
FUNDING: Federal government; Local government; Private; Fund-raisers
OUTREACH: Professional and community education on medical, psychosocial, psychological, political aspects, infection control, safe sex, and legal topics, outreach to Blacks, Hispanics, and Asians, condom distribution
NETWORKS: National AIDS Network (NAN); Pennsylvania AIDS Advocacy Coalition; Philadelphia AIDS Advocacy Coalition
RESEARCH: Research on HIV testing, treatment modalities including medicines and therapies, education, and outreach
ADDITIONAL INFO: This agency was an STD clinic until 1981 when the AIDS Task Force was formed by a group of physicians. Serves as an HIV test site
AVAILABLE LITERATURE: Newsletter; *Questions and Answers*, an informational brochure; *Blacks and AIDS*, a brochure for Blacks; *PCHA Services*, an informational brochure; *Straight Talk, Infection Control Guidelines*, a safer sex brochure; *Women and AIDS*, a brochure for women; *When a Friend Has AIDS*, a brochure giving tips on what to say and what to do; *Volunteering*, a brochure about volunteering with the task force; *Education*, a brochure about AIDS education; *The John Locke Patient Support Fund*, an informational brochure about the fund; *Safe Sex Card*, a wallet-sized card; subway placards
LANGUAGES: Spanish

644. Pitt Men's Study (PMS)
PO Box 7319
Pittsburgh, PA 15213
(412) 624-2008
KEY PERSONNEL: Anthony Silvestre; Director of Community Programs
AFFILIATION: University of Pittsburgh
FACILITY TYPE: Research
STAFF: Paid professional 40; Paid nonprofessional 10
YEAR FOUNDED: 1983
FUNDING: Federal government
OUTREACH: Public education and policy consultation
NETWORKS: Multicenter AIDS Cohort Study (MACS)
RESEARCH: Natural history of HIV—data collected from 2000 bisexual and gay men for epidemiological study, test results, and information and educational services offered to volunteers on an ongoing basis
ADDITIONAL INFO: This is a National Institutes of Health-funded project that involves a consent form, questionnaire, and blood draw with the purpose to measure the prevalence of antibody to HIV among gay and bisexual men in the Pittsburgh area. In addition, over 1000 participants are interviewed and receive a physical exam every six months

AVAILABLE LITERATURE: *A Crisis in Perspective: A Guide to AIDS Research*, an informational brochure; *News and Notes*, a quarterly newsletter

645. Pittsburgh AIDS Task Force (PATF)
141 S Highland Ave, Ste 304
Pittsburgh, PA 15206
(412) 363-6500; Hotline: (412) 363-AIDS; Toll-free: (800) 282-AIDS (PA only)
KEY PERSONNEL: Kerry R Stoner; Executive Director
FACILITY TYPE: Educational; Support group; Fund-raising; Task force
STAFF: Paid professional 4; Paid nonprofessional 2; Volunteers 200
YEAR FOUNDED: 1985
FUNDING: State government; Local government; Private; Fund-raisers
OUTREACH: Speakers bureau, people of color committee, resource library, AIDS prevention for gay and bisexual men, and women
ADDITIONAL INFO: The purpose of this task force is to address the specific health, social and emotional needs of its principal clients, those having AIDS, ARC, or any of the other clinical consequences of HIV infection; to address the associated needs of the families, partners, and friends of the organization's principal clients; to develop programs that will provide assistance to the populations at risk; and to support educational programs for the public at large
AVAILABLE LITERATURE: *Update*, a quarterly newsletter; *Take One*, a brochure; *Women and AIDS*, a brochure for women; *We Welcome Your Participation*, a brochure about the agency; *AIDS and the Law in Pennsylvania*, an informational brochure; *Safe Sex is Coming*, a poster

646. Social Security Administration/Upper Darby
6801 Ludlow St, 1st Fl
Upper Darby, PA 19082
(215) 734-1450
KEY PERSONNEL: Michael L Martin; Branch Manager
FACILITY TYPE: Educational; Social service agency
FUNDING: Federal government

647. South Central AIDS Assistance Network/Harrisburg
PO Box 11573
Harrisburg, PA 17108-1573
(717) 236-4772
KEY PERSONNEL: Rodger Beatty

648. York Area AIDS Coalition (YAAC)
PO Box 509, c/o York City Bureau of Health
York, PA 17405
(717) 849-2297; Hotline: (717) 845-3656
KEY PERSONNEL: Sharon Niesley; Chairperson
AFFILIATION: York City Bureau of Health
FACILITY TYPE: Educational; Task force
STAFF: Volunteers 30
YEAR FOUNDED: 1987
FUNDING: State government; Fees for services or products
OUTREACH: Speakers bureau, community-wide presentations with multiple visual aid resources, county-wide distribution of AIDS education posters
SEMINARS: May 24, 1988—"AIDS: It's York's Problem, Too," a conference attracting 200 professionals from multiple fields
RESEARCH: York City Bureau of Health is conducting a survey of area medical providers to determine availability of HIV testing and counseling, along with awareness levels of related issues
ADDITIONAL INFO: The York Area AIDS Coalition is a task force of individuals representing various groups and organizations, as well as interested citizens throughout the York area, who are concerned about the issues of AIDS and its attendant problems
AVAILABLE LITERATURE: *York Area AIDS Coalition*, a brochure describing YAAC; *AIDS: It's York's Problem Too*, a poster with telephone numbers for additional information
LANGUAGES: Spanish

649. York City Bureau of Health
PO Box 509, 1 Market Way West
York, PA 17405
(717) 849-2252; Hotline: (717) 845-3656
KEY PERSONNEL: David L Hawk; Director
AFFILIATION: York City Government
FACILITY TYPE: HIV counseling and testing; Health department
STAFF: Paid professional 22
YEAR FOUNDED: 1985

FUNDING: Federal government; State government; Local government
OUTREACH: Public education, HIV antibody counseling and testing
NETWORKS: York Area AIDS Coalition; Tri-Community Coordinating Council on AIDS
SEMINARS: May 24, 1988—"AIDS: It's York's Problem Too"
AVAILABLE LITERATURE: *HIV-Antibody Testing in York*, a brochure explaining the test
LANGUAGES: Spanish

650. York Health Corp
132 S George St
York, PA 17401-1465
(717) 845-2209
KEY PERSONNEL: Stuart N Pullen; Executive Director
AFFILIATION: York Area AIDS Coalition
FACILITY TYPE: HIV counseling and testing; Health department
STAFF: Paid professional 18; Paid nonprofessional 10
YEAR FOUNDED: 1970
FUNDING: Federal government; Fees for services or products
OUTREACH: Speakers bureau, outreach to women
ADDITIONAL INFO: Provides free HIV counseling and testing, diagnoses and treatment of HIV related conditions
LANGUAGES: Spanish

RHODE ISLAND

651. Rhode Island Dept of Health, AIDS Program
75 Davis St
Providence, RI 02908
(401) 277-2362
KEY PERSONNEL: Edward Martin, Chief Administrator of AIDS Program
FACILITY TYPE: Research; Educational; Clinic; Task force; HIV counseling and testing
STAFF: Paid professional 11; Paid nonprofessional 3
FUNDING: Federal government; State government
OUTREACH: Education to minority communities, counseling and education during testing for HIV, workplace and public sector education, organizing conferences for various groups
NETWORKS: Rhode Island Project AIDS; Centers for Disease Control; The Urban League; Providence Ambulatory HCF
SEMINARS: Provides regular seminars for police, nurses, and dental personnel; regular counseling certification programs
RESEARCH: Seroprevalence of infants born in Rhode Island
ADDITIONAL INFO: Founded in 1984 to provide education and outreach to high risk groups. Provides counseling, testing and referral to the community, IV drug users, minorities, and women
AVAILABLE LITERATURE: *AIDS Counseling and Testing for HIV Antibody: The Facts*, a brochure describing the test; *Children and AIDS*, a brochure containing facts about AIDS and its affect on children; *Sex and AIDS*, a general brochure of AIDS information and safe sex guidelines

652. Rhode Island Project/AIDS (RIP/AIDS)
22 Hayes St, Rm 124
Providence, RI 02908
(401) 277-6545; Hotline: (401) 277-6502; Spanish Hotline: (800) 442-7432
KEY PERSONNEL: William Lynn McKinney; Interim Executive Director
FACILITY TYPE: Educational; Support group
STAFF: Paid professional 8; Volunteers 350
YEAR FOUNDED: 1985
FUNDING: State government; Private; Fund-raisers; Fees for services or products
OUTREACH: Outreach efforts to bars, civic and political organizations, and various high risk groups, speakers bureau
NETWORKS: National AIDS Network (NAN)
SEMINARS: Jan 12, 1988—"AIDS in the Workplace"
ADDITIONAL INFO: Serves all of Rhode Island and southeastern Massachusetts with over 500 speaking engagements yearly. The center's primary focus is AIDS education
AVAILABLE LITERATURE: Various publications about AIDS in general, safer sex, and testing
LANGUAGES: Spanish

SOUTH CAROLINA

653. AIDS Support Network of Spartanburg (ASNS)
PO Box 4786
Spartanburg, SC 29305-4796
(803) 596-3400
KEY PERSONNEL: Jim Womack; Coordinator
AFFILIATION: Palmetto AIDS Life Support Services (PALSS)
FACILITY TYPE: Educational; Support group
STAFF: Volunteers varies
FUNDING: Private; Fund-raisers
OUTREACH: Provide community educational programs by volunteer health professionals
ADDITIONAL INFO: Provides buddies to HIV infected persons and their families, support groups and education to the community

654. Carolina AIDS Research and Education Project (CARE)
University of South Carolina School of Public Health
Columbia, SC 29208
(803) 777-4845
KEY PERSONNEL: Francisco S Sy; Director
FACILITY TYPE: Research
STAFF: Volunteers 3
YEAR FOUNDED: 1987
FUNDING: Private
OUTREACH: Academic and continuing education courses on AIDS for interdisciplinary professionals and students; develops, implements and evaluates AIDS education programs for specific groups and institutions, distribute current AIDS information through seminars, conferences, film presentations, and publications
SEMINARS: Aug 1, 1987—"First International Conference on AIDS Education;" Aug 2-4, 1988—"Second International Conference on AIDS Education;" Sep 11-14, 1989—"Third International Conference on AIDS Education;" Jul 1988—"First International Interdisciplinary Course on AIDS Education;" Jul 1989—"Second International Interdisciplinary Course on AIDS Education"
RESEARCH: Interdisciplinary research on various aspects of AIDS and AIDS education
ADDITIONAL INFO: CARE's objectives include stimulating and conducting interdisciplinary AIDS research, developing innovative educational strategies for AIDS prevention and control, promoting and providing quality AIDS education programs, and serving as a resource group on current development and information about AIDS
AVAILABLE LITERATURE: *AIDS Doesn't Care Who It Kills...But We CARE*, a brochure describing CARE

655. Palmetto AIDS Life Support Services
PO Box 12124
Columbia, SC 29211
(803) 779-7257; (800) 868-PALS; 577-AIDS
KEY PERSONNEL: Bill Edens

656. Spartanburg County Health Dept
PO Box 4217, 151 E Wood St
Spartanburg, SC 29305-4217
(803) 596-3334
KEY PERSONNEL: Fred Morgan; Epidemiologist
AFFILIATION: Spartanburg County Health Dept of the Dept of Health and Environmental Control of South Carolina
FACILITY TYPE: Health department
STAFF: Paid professional 2
YEAR FOUNDED: 1925
FUNDING: State government
NETWORKS: Spartanburg AIDS Support Network
LANGUAGES: Spanish

657. Wateree Community Actions, Inc (WCAI)
PO Box 1838, 13 S Main St
Sumter, SC 29150
(803) 775-4354
KEY PERSONNEL: Rubye J Johnson; Executive Director
FACILITY TYPE: Educational
YEAR FOUNDED: 1967
FUNDING: Federal government; State government; Private; Fund-raisers
ADDITIONAL INFO: The purpose of Community Actions is to stimulate all available local, state, private and federal sources to aid low-income families and low-income individuals of all ages in obtaining skills, knowledge and motivation, and to secure the opportunities needed for them to become fully self-sufficient
AVAILABLE LITERATURE: *Annual Report: Keys to Self-Sufficiency*

SOUTH DAKOTA

658. Brown County Health Dept
25 Market St
Aberdeen, SD 57401
(605) 622-2373, 622-2435
KEY PERSONNEL: Greg Welch; Communicable Disease Control Regional Supervisor
AFFILIATION: South Dakota Health Dept
FACILITY TYPE: Clinic; Health department
STAFF: Paid professional 3
FUNDING: Federal government; State government
OUTREACH: Secondary and college level training, train the trainer sessions for all elementary and secondary schools in South Dakota
ADDITIONAL INFO: Provides STD services within a 20 county area of northeastern South Dakota including epidemiology and educational efforts

659. Eastern Dakota AIDS Network (EDAN)
PO Box 220
Sioux Falls, SD 57101
Hotline: (605) 332-4599
KEY PERSONNEL: Greg Carey; AIDS Coordinator
FACILITY TYPE: Educational; Support group
STAFF: Volunteers 12
YEAR FOUNDED: 1986
FUNDING: Private; Fund-raisers
OUTREACH: Coordinates communications among service groups in Eastern South Dakota
ADDITIONAL INFO: EDAN is a community-based volunteer organization that provides a communication point for all groups working with AIDS
AVAILABLE LITERATURE: *Together*, a newsletter; *Safer Sex*, a brochure

660. South Dakota Dept of Health, Communicable Disease Program, AIDS Surveillance and Prevention Project
523 E Capitol
Pierre, SD 57501
(605) 773-3364; Hotline: (800) 592-1861 SD only
KEY PERSONNEL: Randy D Louchart; Coordinator of AIDS Project
AFFILIATION: South Dakota Dept of Health
FACILITY TYPE: Educational; Health department
STAFF: Paid professional 22
FUNDING: Federal government; State government
RESEARCH: AIDS transmission, cure and vaccine
AVAILABLE LITERATURE: *Communicable Disease Bulletin*, monthly newsletter; *AIDS/HIV Statistical Update*, a biweekly newsletter

661. South Dakota Dept of Health, Communicable Disease Program, Pierre Area Regional Field Office
523 E Capitol
Pierre, SD 57501
(605) 773-3364; Hotline: (800) 592-1861
KEY PERSONNEL: Chuck Hall; Regional Supervisor
AFFILIATION: South Dakota Dept of Health
FACILITY TYPE: Educational; HIV counseling and testing
STAFF: Paid professional 3
FUNDING: Federal government
OUTREACH: Provides communicable disease education and intervention for South Dakota

TENNESSEE

662. Aid to End AIDS Committee (ATEAC)/Memphis
PO Box 40389
Memphis, TN 38174
(901) 272-7827; Hotline: 726-4299
KEY PERSONNEL: Tom Stewart, President
FACILITY TYPE: Educational; Support group
FUNDING: Donations

OUTREACH: Speakers bureau, counseling for persons with AIDS and their loved ones, safe sex meetings

ADDITIONAL INFO: Founded in 1985 as a service for persons with AIDS, ARC, their families and friends in the Memphis area. Services include a buddy program, emotional support, hospital and home visits, practical support, and referrals

AVAILABLE LITERATURE: *Aid to End AIDS Committee*, a 2-fold brochure describing the committee; *What Every Teenager Should Know About AIDS*, a 3-fold brochure that discusses "What is AIDS?," "How AIDS is not transmitted," "Who gets AIDS?," "Should I avoid a person with AIDS?," "What is being done to find a cure?," "Is there a test?," and "What are the signs of AIDS?." A glossary and test is included; *AIDS Update*, a quarterly newspaper presenting information on AIDS, statistics, and education

663. AIDS Response Knoxville (ARK)
PO Box 3932
Knoxville, TN 37927
(615) 523-AIDS; Hotline: (615) 523-AIDS
KEY PERSONNEL: Lynda Nemon; Executive Director
FACILITY TYPE: Educational; Support group; Fund-raising
STAFF: Paid professional 1; Volunteers 40
YEAR FOUNDED: 1985
FUNDING: Private; Fund-raisers; Grants

664. Carroll County Health Dept
126 W Paris St
Huntingdon, TN 38344
(901) 986-9147
KEY PERSONNEL: Betty Forbess; Nursing Supervisor/AIDS Education Coordinator
AFFILIATION: Tennessee Dept of Health and Environment
FACILITY TYPE: Clinic; Health department
STAFF: Paid professional 5; Paid nonprofessional 5
FUNDING: State government; Local government

665. Chattanooga Council on AIDS Resources, Education, and Support (CARES)
PO Box 8402, 715 E 11th St
Chattanooga, TN 37411
(615) 266-2422; Hotline: (615) 265-2273
KEY PERSONNEL: Kenton Dickerson; Executive Director
FACILITY TYPE: Educational; Support group; Hospice; Fund-raising; HIV counseling and testing
STAFF: Paid professional 1; Volunteers 25
YEAR FOUNDED: 1986
FUNDING: State government; Private; Fund-raisers; Donations
OUTREACH: Presentations to local organizations and schools about AIDS prevention, cooperates with the Hamilton County Health Dept Minority AIDS Program
ADDITIONAL INFO: Provides counseling, support, and educational services to the Southwest Tennessee area. The program is volunteer oriented
AVAILABLE LITERATURE: Monthly newsletter

666. Mid Cumberland Regional Health Office, Tennessee Dept of Health and Environment
Ben Allen Rd
Nashville, TN 37216
(615) 262-6100
KEY PERSONNEL: Jerry Narramore; Director, Communicable Disease Control
AFFILIATION: Tennessee Dept of Health and Environment
FACILITY TYPE: HIV counseling and testing; Health department
STAFF: Paid professional 38
YEAR FOUNDED: 1976
FUNDING: State government
OUTREACH: Provides HIV counseling and testing, partner notification, dental, health and nutritional services, provides education to groups, schools and medical staffs of hospitals and institutions
ADDITIONAL INFO: Provides educational seminars to the region
LANGUAGES: French, Spanish, Farsi

667. Nashville Council on AIDS Resources, Education and Services (Nashville CARES)
PO Box 25107
Nashville, TN 37202
(615) 385-1510, 385-AIDS
KEY PERSONNEL: Sander Potter; Executive Director

FACILITY TYPE: Educational; Support group; Social service agency
STAFF: Paid professional 4; Volunteers 120
YEAR FOUNDED: 1985
FUNDING: State government; Fund-raisers
OUTREACH: Educational presentations, consultation for development of agency policies and employee education, distribution of AIDS literature, telephone education and referrals, community wide conferences, agency inservices, and volunteer training
NETWORKS: National AIDS Network (NAN); AIDS Action Council; Tennessee Council on Social Welfare
AVAILABLE LITERATURE: *Nashville CARES Newsletter*, a monthly newsletter; *Our Caring Message*, a brochure about the agency

668. Tennessee Dept of Health and Environment, AIDS Program
1233 SW Ave
Johnson City, TN 37605-2966
(615) 929-5927
KEY PERSONNEL: Carolyn S Sliger; Regional AIDS Coordinator
AFFILIATION: Tennessee State Government
FACILITY TYPE: Educational; Clinic; Support group; HIV counseling and testing
STAFF: Paid professional 2
YEAR FOUNDED: 1986
FUNDING: Federal government; State government
OUTREACH: Educational programs to include 8 counties for various organizations
SEMINARS: Oct 19, 1988—"Update on AIDS;" Nov 9-10, 1988—"Counseling and Testing Training"
RESEARCH: Diet and nutrition related to HIV positive
ADDITIONAL INFO: Provides free, anonymous counseling and testing

669. Tri-Cities AIDS Project, Inc (TAP)
PO Box 231
Johnson City, TN 37605
(615) 282-2416; Hotline: (615) 282-2416
KEY PERSONNEL: Laura Shelton; Chair
FACILITY TYPE: Educational; Support group; Fund-raising
STAFF: Volunteers 15
YEAR FOUNDED: 1986
FUNDING: Federal government; Private; Fund-raisers
OUTREACH: Educational outreach, condom distribution
NETWORKS: Tennessee AIDS Council
SEMINARS: Oct 1987—"AIDS and Youth"
RESEARCH: Education and usage of services
ADDITIONAL INFO: Provides referrals to appropriate services, including Medicaid, social security, legal, medical, and gay support
LANGUAGES: Spanish, American Sign Language

670. University of Tennessee, Memphis, The Health Science Center
FORMER NAME: UTCHS (University of Tennessee Center for the Health Sciences)
956 Court Ave, Rm F210 Coleman Bldg
Memphis, TN 38163
(901) 528-5942
KEY PERSONNEL: Linda Pifer; Associate Director of Pediatrics and Clinical Laboratory Sciences
AFFILIATION: University of Tennessee, Memphis
FACILITY TYPE: Research; Educational
STAFF: Paid professional 2
YEAR FOUNDED: 1981
FUNDING: Private
RESEARCH: Antibody testing statistical work, research on pneumocystis and toxoplasma gonuii in AIDS
ADDITIONAL INFO: Provides free pneumocystis antigen and antibody titers to all physicians on labs requesting this test on patients sera
AVAILABLE LITERATURE: Published research papers on AIDS education and research papers on AIDS and P Carinii (pneumocystis)

671. Vanderbilt AIDS Project (VAP)
Medical Ctr N, Ste CCC5319
Nashville, TN 37232
(615) 331-8059; Hotline: (615) 322-AIDS
KEY PERSONNEL: Dr Gene A Copello; Director
FACILITY TYPE: Research; Educational; Support group; Fund-raising; HIV counseling and testing Consultation on policy development
STAFF: Paid professional 5; Paid nonprofessional 1; Volunteers 150
YEAR FOUNDED: 1985
FUNDING: Federal government; Private; Fund-raisers; Fees for services or products

NETWORKS: East Central AIDS Education and Training Center; Tennessee AIDS Council; National AIDS Network (NAN)
SEMINARS: Sponsors 15-20 seminars per year
RESEARCH: Behavior change; program evaluation; policy analysis; attitudes/values
AVAILABLE LITERATURE: *The Source*, a news service
LANGUAGES: American Sign Language, Spanish

TEXAS

672. Abilene AIDS Task Force
PO Box 6903
Abilene, TX 79608
(915) 891-2400
KEY PERSONNEL: Gregory Johnson, MD

673. AIDS ARMS Network
PO Box 190945, 2727 Oak Lawn, Ste 222
Dallas, TX 75219
(214) 521-5191
KEY PERSONNEL: Warren W Buckingham III; Project Director
FACILITY TYPE: Client services/case management
STAFF: Paid professional 17; Volunteers 50
YEAR FOUNDED: 1986
FUNDING: Federal government; Private; Fund-raisers
NETWORKS: AIDS Interfaith Network; AIDS Resource Center; Care Line Inc; Care Team Health Service; City of Dallas Health and Human Services; Community Council of Greater Dallas; Dallas County Dept of Human Services/Welfare; Dallas County Health Dept; Dallas County Mental Health/Mental Retardation; Dallas Hospice Care; Darco Drug Services, Inc; Episcopal Church of Saint Thomas the Apostle Greater Dallas Community of Churches; Help is Possible, Inc; Holy Trinity Catholic Church; Home Health Services of Dallas; Ministry to Catholic Homosexuals and Their Families; National Association of PWAs/PWA Coalition; Oak Lawn Counseling Center; Office of Civil Rights; Open Arms, Inc/Bryan's House; Positive AIDS in Recovery; Parkland Memorial Hospital; Professional Care, Inc; Salvation Army; Social Security Administration; Texas Board of Pardons and Parole; Texas Dept of Human Services, Adult Protection Services; Trinity Ministry to the Poor; University of Texas Southwestern Medical Center at Dallas; Veteran's Administration Medical Center; Visiting Nurse Association
ADDITIONAL INFO: Founded to coordinate financial, home care, emotional, and spiritual support for PWAs, PWARCs, or any other HIV-related illnesses
AVAILABLE LITERATURE: *AIDS ARMS Network: The Project, the People, the Process*, a brochure describing the agency
LANGUAGES: Spanish, American Sign Language

674. AIDS Coordinating Committee/Dallas
5740 Prospect, Ste 2004
Dallas, TX 75206
(214) 823-2891
KEY PERSONNEL: Jesse Gonzalez, Coordinator
AFFILIATION: Robert Wood Johnson Foundation AIDS Health Services Program
FACILITY TYPE: Support group
ADDITIONAL INFO: Source of additional AIDS information and services

675. AIDS/Denton, Inc
FORMER NAME: AIDenton, Inc
NT Box 13427
Denton, TX 76203
(817) 382-3813; Hotline: (817) 383-3540
KEY PERSONNEL: Rev Dr Jack P Busby; Campus Minister
AFFILIATION: AIDS Interfaith Network
FACILITY TYPE: Educational; Referral
STAFF: Volunteers 30
YEAR FOUNDED: 1988
FUNDING: Private; Dues
OUTREACH: Speakers bureau, personal interviews, classroom presentations
SEMINARS: 1989—"Workshop for Persons Who Minister to PWAs"
ADDITIONAL INFO: AIDS/Denton began as a coalition of five men who were PWAs, all but one of whom have since died. In April 1988, a retired physician brought together the first group of interested volunteers. Since that time, the group has received legal and

IRS exemption status (non-profit). Currently the group is working with Tarrant County (Fort Worth Health Dept) and Denton Public Health in an effort to coordinate some much-needed testing for Denton County.
AVAILABLE LITERATURE: Distributes educational materials from other organizations
LANGUAGES: Spanish, Polish

676. AIDS Foundation Houston, Inc (AFH)
FORMER NAME: KS/AIDS Foundation
3927 Essex Lane
Houston, TX 77027
(713) 627-6796; Hotline: (713) 524-2437
KEY PERSONNEL: Evelyn Cox; Director of Education
AFFILIATION: National AIDS Network (NAN)
FACILITY TYPE: Educational; Client services/case management
STAFF: Paid professional 23; Paid nonprofessional 5; Volunteers 600
YEAR FOUNDED: 1981
FUNDING: Federal government; State government; Local government; Private; Fund-raisers
OUTREACH: Speakers bureau provides presentations to civic clubs, churches, medical professionals, schools and businesses. Prepares educational programs for businesses
NETWORKS: National AIDS Network (NAN); Texas AIDS Network; AIDS Action Council; Greater Montrose Business Guild; Houston Chapter of Commerce
SEMINARS: Oct 1987—"Living with AIDS in Houston;" Apr 1988—"Women and AIDS;" Oct 1988—"Living with AIDS in Houston"
RESEARCH: The AFH is committed to educating the general public, health care professionals and those at high risk; preventing disease and promoting health; providing vital support services to people with AIDS (PWAs), their families and loved ones. AFH is currently developing a school curriculum and working on an AIDS in the workplace program to encompass all aspects from the building of a philosophy to an educational resources center. Works with substance abusers
AVAILABLE LITERATURE: *AIDS Foundation Houston*; *AIDS: Reducing the Risk*; *When a Friend Has AIDS*, tips on what to say and what to do; *AIDS: What Everyone Needs to Know*, an informational brochure; *HIV Antibody Testing*, a brochure discussing the HIV antibody test; *Stone Soup Food Pantry*, a brochure about the food pantry program; *Protejase Contra AIDSSIDA*, a general informational brochure in Spanish; *AIDS/SIDA y el Sexo Seguro*, a safer sex brochure in Spanish; *Peligra Grave: AIDS/SIDA y las Drogas*, a brochure about drugs and AIDS in Spanish; *AIDS: It's a Black Problem, Too*; *Some Straight Answers About AIDS and IV Drugs*, a brochure for IV drug users; *AIDS and Safer Sex*, a safer sex brochure; *Lifeline*, a newsletter; *AIDS: A Guide for Survival*, a book about AIDS published by the Harris County Medical Society and the Houston Academy of Medicine; *AIDS Legal Hotline*, a brochure about the hotline; *AIDS: The Facts*, an American Red Cross brochure; *Surgeon General's Report on Acquired Immune Deficiency Syndrome*; *Informe del Jefe del Servicio de Salud Publica de los Estados Unidos sobre el Sindrome de Immuno Deficiencia Adquirida (AIDS)*, the Surgeon General's report in Spanish; *What You Should Know About AIDS*, an informational brochure; *A Facts and Resource Guide for the Texas Gulf Coast About AIDS*
LANGUAGES: Spanish

677. AIDS Interfaith Network (AIN)
6525 Inwood Rd
Dallas, TX 75209
(214) 358-4724
KEY PERSONNEL: Charles Carnahan; Director
AFFILIATION: Interfaith
FACILITY TYPE: Educational; Support group; Hospice; Client services/case management; Religious; Home care
STAFF: Paid professional 1; Volunteers 50
YEAR FOUNDED: 1986
FUNDING: Private; Fund-raisers
OUTREACH: Care teams to provide respite care to PWAs and families, counseling, spiritual and sacramental care, referral services
NETWORKS: AIDS ARM Network
SEMINARS: Feb 1988—"Second Hope/Help Conference for Church Professionals," Dallas; Jul 16-17, 1988—"AIDS Awareness Weekend," Dallas
ADDITIONAL INFO: The AIDS Interfaith Network (AIN) is an ecumenical organization designed to meet the spiritual and emotional needs of persons with AIDS, ARC and HIV infections, and their loved ones

AVAILABLE LITERATURE: *Gift*, a newsletter for members; *A.I.D.S.: A Compassionate Pastoral Response to People in Crisis*, a brochure describing the goals of AIN

678. AIDS Legal Hotline/Houston
1236 W Gray
Houston, TX 77019
(713) 528-7702
KEY PERSONNEL: Helen M Gros; Executive Director
AFFILIATION: Clark Read Foundation, Inc
FACILITY TYPE: Legal
YEAR FOUNDED: 1986
FUNDING: Private
OUTREACH: Legal education programs for attorneys who participate in the referral panel
NETWORKS: Houston American Civil Liberties Union (Houston ACLU); Human Rights Foundation; Clark Read Foundation, Inc
AVAILABLE LITERATURE: *Texas AIDS Legal Handbook*

679. AIDS Resource Center
3920 Cedar Springs
Dallas, TX 75219
(214) 521-5124; Hotline: (214) 559-2437
KEY PERSONNEL: John Thomas; Executive Director
AFFILIATION: Robert Wood Johnson Foundation AIDS Health Service Program
FACILITY TYPE: Educational; Fund-raising
STAFF: Paid professional 6
YEAR FOUNDED: 1985
FUNDING: Fund-raisers; Fees for services or products
OUTREACH: Education and information, referrals, speakers bureau, publications, hotline, food pantry, visitation to persons with AIDS, clothing bank, volunteer training, discrimination complaints, legal services, patient advocacy, pet pals, pentamadine mist
AVAILABLE LITERATURE: *AIDS Update*, monthly newsletter; *AIDS Resource Center*, brochure about the center; *The Truth About AIDS: Pass it On*, a multipacket brochure with fact sheets on "All about AIDS," "Transmission," "Facts and Answers," "Reduce Your Risk," and "How You Can Help;" posters and billboards also provided

680. AIDS Services
1702 Horne Rd
Corpus Christi, TX 78416
(512) 851-7298
KEY PERSONNEL: Kathy Thomas, RN
AFFILIATION: Corpus Christi-Nueces County Dept of Public Health
FACILITY TYPE: Educational; Clinic; HIV counseling and testing
STAFF: Paid professional 4; Volunteers 5
YEAR FOUNDED: 1986
FUNDING: State government
OUTREACH: Community education to high risk groups, testing, general community education
ADDITIONAL INFO: Provides community education to high risk groups with a focus on minorities, as well as general community education, testing for HIV, pre- and post-test counseling, and AIDS epidemiology
LANGUAGES: Spanish

681. AIDS Services of Austin (ASA)
FORMER NAME: Austin AIDS Project
PO Box 4874
Austin, TX 78765
(512) 472-2273; Info-line: (512) 472-2437; TDD: (512) 472-8745
KEY PERSONNEL: Janna Zumbrun; Executive Director
FACILITY TYPE: Educational; Support group; Fund-raising; Client services/case management
STAFF: Paid professional 8; Paid nonprofessional 1; Volunteers 300
YEAR FOUNDED: 1985
FUNDING: Federal government; State government; Local government; Private; Fund-raisers
OUTREACH: AIDS education for the general public, risk reduction education for target groups, info-line, AIDS in the workplace education for employers and employees, TDD phone line and AIDS education workshops for the deaf
ADDITIONAL INFO: Provides direct services of case management, health assessment and education, nutrition education, food bank, volunteer assistance, support groups, temporary emergency financial assistance, and in-home nurse aide care

AVAILABLE LITERATURE: *ASA Quarterly*, a newsletter; *ASA Messenger*, a newsletter; *AIDS Services of Austin*, an informational brochure; *AIDS in the Workplace*, a brochure; *AIDS in the Workplace Manual*, a manual for employers
LANGUAGES: American Sign Language

682. Amarillo Bi-City County Health Dept
PO Box 1971, 411 S Austin St
Amarillo, TX 79186
(806) 371-1100
KEY PERSONNEL: Larry Tipping; Epidemiologist
FACILITY TYPE: Research; Educational; Clinic; HIV counseling and testing
STAFF: Paid professional 41
FUNDING: Federal government; State government; Local government; Fees for services or products
OUTREACH: AIDS education programs
NETWORKS: Panhandle AIDS Support Organization (PASO)
RESEARCH: Working with the low dose interferon study
ADDITIONAL INFO: Provides counseling, testing, and case investigation. The interferon study is funded by a local corporation. The program provides educational programs to police and fire departments and corporations, training on pre- and post-test counseling for HIV testing to volunteers for PASO
LANGUAGES: Spanish, Laotian

683. The Austin PWA Coalition
PO Box 50255
Austin, TX 78763
(512) 477-2502
KEY PERSONNEL: Jeffrey Decker; President
AFFILIATION: National Association of People with AIDS (NAPWA)
FACILITY TYPE: Research; Educational; Support group
STAFF: Volunteers 4
YEAR FOUNDED: 1987
FUNDING: Private; Fund-raisers
NETWORKS: AIDS Services of Austin; Austin Lesbian Gay Caucus
RESEARCH: Community research initiative
AVAILABLE LITERATURE: Publishes a newsletter

684. Catholic Diocese of Dallas
3915 Lemmon Ave, Ste 201
Dallas, TX 75219
(214) 522-5961
KEY PERSONNEL: Bob Shortall
AFFILIATION: Robert Wood Johnson Foundation AIDS Health Services Program
FACILITY TYPE: Support group
ADDITIONAL INFO: Source of additional AIDS information and services

685. Catholic Schools of Dallas
PO Box 190507, 3915 Lemmon Ave, Ste 202
Dallas, TX 75219
(214) 528-2360
KEY PERSONNEL: Shaun Underhill; Assistant Superintendent of Schools
AFFILIATION: Catholic Diocese of Dallas
FACILITY TYPE: Educational; Religious
STAFF: Paid professional 700
YEAR FOUNDED: 1890
FUNDING: Private; Fund-raisers
OUTREACH: Curriculum for grades K-12, information sessions for parents, inservice for teachers
SEMINARS: Apr, 1988—"AIDS Symposium for Catholic School Educators;" Fall 1988—"Information Sessions for Parents," held at each local campus
AVAILABLE LITERATURE: *AIDS: A Catholic Educational Approach*

686. The Children's Home
PO Box 600732
Houston, TX 77260
(713) 523-7868
KEY PERSONNEL: Mary P Hennessy; Administrator
FACILITY TYPE: Residential facility (children)
STAFF: Volunteers 5
YEAR FOUNDED: 1986
FUNDING: Private; Fund-raisers

OUTREACH: Work with families of children who have been in foster care

ADDITIONAL INFO: Provides housing, medical, and psychological services for children who are HIV positive or have AIDS/ARC

687. Coastal Bend AIDS Foundation, Inc (CBAF)
PO Box 331416, 616 S Tancahua
Corpus Christi, TX 78404-1416
(512) 883-5815; Hotline: (512) 883-2273
KEY PERSONNEL: Judy J Hales; President
FACILITY TYPE: Educational; Support group; Fund-raising; Client services/case management
STAFF: Paid professional 4; Volunteers 90
YEAR FOUNDED: 1986
FUNDING: State government; Private; Fund-raisers
OUTREACH: Buddy program, speakers bureau, education to local school districts, safer sex workshops, food bank, clothing bank
NETWORKS: National AIDS Network (NAN); Texas AIDS Network; South Texas AIDS Network
ADDITIONAL INFO: The CBAF is a non-profit, non-political, non-denominational service organization that is devoted solely to providing support services to PWAs and PWARCs
AVAILABLE LITERATURE: Quarterly newsletter; Buddy pamphlets; CBAF services and AIDS information pamphlets
LANGUAGES: American Sign Language

688. Community Clinic, Inc/San Antonio
FORMER NAME: San Antonio Free Clinic
210 West Olmos
San Antonio, TX 78212
(512) 821-5522; 821-6407
KEY PERSONNEL: Priscilla King, Director
FACILITY TYPE: Clinic
FUNDING: State government; Donations; Grants
LIBRARY: Provides an information service
ADDITIONAL INFO: Founded in 1970 as an STD clinic

689. Dallas County Health Dept, AIDS Prevention Project
1936 Amelia Ct
Dallas, TX 75235
(214) 920-7916; Hotline: (214) 351-4335
KEY PERSONNEL: Anne Freeman; Program Manager
AFFILIATION: Dallas County Government
FACILITY TYPE: Educational; Support group; HIV counseling and testing
STAFF: Paid professional 17; Paid nonprofessional 3; Volunteers 50
YEAR FOUNDED: 1983
FUNDING: Federal government; Local government; Private
OUTREACH: Outreach to openly gay men, closeted gay and bisexual men, IV drug users, prostitutes, Blacks, Hispanics, adolescents, hearing impaired, and singles, counseling on HIV status and risk reduction, radio and television spots
NETWORKS: Dallas AIDS ARMS Network; Dallas AIDS Coordinating Committee; APHA; National AIDS Network; Society for Epidemiologic Research
SEMINARS: Nov 1987—"AIDS and Youth"
RESEARCH: Behavior change initiators and ways to maintain behavior change
ADDITIONAL INFO: Provides preventive education on AIDS and is an HIV antibody counseling and testing site
AVAILABLE LITERATURE: *Adapt, Enjoy, Survive*, a pocket card on safe sex; *AIDS: The Equal Opportunity Syndrome*, a brochure with general AIDS information and a black and white poster; *Share a Needle and You Can Share AIDS*, a poster with needle sharing crossed out; *AIDS Is Killing Dallas's Drug Users*, a brochure available in English and Spanish on how not to share needles; *Safe Sex*, a safer sex brochure; *Women, Children and AIDS*, a pictorial brochure for hearing and reading impaired; *What You Think You Know About AIDS*, a brochure for adolescents; *Safer Sex*, an explicit brochure that is also available in Spanish; *The Test*, a brochure used for pre-test counseling; *AIDS and the Health Care Worker*, a brochure outlining precautions; *Follow the Steps*, a brochure with recommendations for persons with a HIV positive test; *SIDA y su Familia*, a 20-minute video in Spanish with general AIDS information; *AIDS, A Guide for Survival*, a 91-page paperback book produced by the Dallas County Medical Society and Dallas Academy of Medicine covering a broad range of AIDS topics from transmission to medication to ethics; distributes brochures from other agencies
LANGUAGES: Spanish, American Sign Language

690. DARCO, Drug Services, Inc
FORMER NAME: DARCO Drug Treatment Center
2708 Inwood
Dallas, TX 75235
(214) 956-7181
KEY PERSONNEL: Roy Griffin; Outreach Coordinator
FACILITY TYPE: Research; Educational; Clinic
STAFF: Paid professional 14; Paid nonprofessional 4
YEAR FOUNDED: 1985
FUNDING: Federal government; State government; Local government; Private; Fees for services or products
OUTREACH: AIDS prevention outreach to IV drug users and their sexual partners
NETWORKS: National AIDS Demonstration Research Project of the National Institute on Drug Abuse
RESEARCH: Relative efficacy of various treatment approaches to effect behavioral changes and reduced risk for AIDS
ADDITIONAL INFO: Provides outpatient drug treatment services including methodone-assisted treatment
LANGUAGES: Spanish

691. El Paso City-County Health District, Sexually Transmitted Disease Clinic, Tillman Center
222 S Campbell
El Paso, TX 79901
(915) 541-4511; Hotline: (915) 541-4266
KEY PERSONNEL: Miguel Escobedo; Program Director
FACILITY TYPE: Educational; Clinic; Task force; HIV counseling and testing
STAFF: Paid professional 9
FUNDING: Federal government; State government; Local government; Private; Fees for services or products
OUTREACH: Alternate site for HIV testing, presentations to high schools and middle schools
NETWORKS: El Paso AIDS Task Force
SEMINARS: Aug, 1988—"AIDS and the Hispanic Community"
ADDITIONAL INFO: Conducts HIV counseling and testing
LANGUAGES: Spanish

692. Episcopal Diocese of Dallas
6525 Inwood Rd
Dallas, TX 75209
(214) 352-0410
KEY PERSONNEL: Rev Ted Karpf
AFFILIATION: Robert Wood Johnson Foundation AIDS Health Services Program
FACILITY TYPE: Support group
ADDITIONAL INFO: Source of additional AIDS information and services

693. Fort Worth Counseling Center, AIDS Project
659 S Jennings
Fort Worth, TX 76104
(817) 335-1994
KEY PERSONNEL: Thomas Bruner; Executive Director
FACILITY TYPE: Educational; Support group; HIV counseling and testing
STAFF: Paid professional 3; Paid nonprofessional 2; Volunteers 25
YEAR FOUNDED: 1984
FUNDING: State government; Fund-raisers; Fees for services or products; Donations
OUTREACH: Safer sex workshops, AIDS awareness seminars, public speaking, hospital visitation program
NETWORKS: Fort Worth Public Health Dept; AIDS Coordinating Council; John Peter Smith Hospital
SEMINARS: Provides Safer Sex workshops, AIDS awareness weekends and support group meetings
ADDITIONAL INFO: Provides HIV/AIDS support groups, buddy program, safer sex workshops, information and referral, education and training, HIV antibody testing, practical assistance programs, and hospital visitation teams
AVAILABLE LITERATURE: *Mental Health Services*, a flyer describing the services; *The AIDS Project*, a flyer explaining the services that are available

694. Fort Worth Public Health Dept
1800 University Dr
Fort Worth, TX 76107
(817) 870-7346; Hotline: (817) 870-7346

KEY PERSONNEL: Diane Richey; AIDS Education Specialist
AFFILIATION: Fort Worth City Government
FACILITY TYPE: Clinic
STAFF: Paid professional 7; Paid nonprofessional 3
FUNDING: Federal government; State government; Local government; Fees for services or products
OUTREACH: Inservice workshops related to HIV for health care professionals, target risk groups
NETWORKS: AIDS Coordinating Council of Tarrant County
ADDITIONAL INFO: This agency is a preventive medicine clinic for non-symptomatic HIV positive persons Texas
AVAILABLE LITERATURE: *AIDS Perspectives*, a newsletter of local statistics and announcements
LANGUAGES: Spanish

695. Foundation for Human Understanding
PO Box 190712, 3920 Cedar Springs Rd
Dallas, TX 75219
(214) 528-0144
AFFILIATION: Robert Wood Johnson Foundation AIDS Health Services Program
FACILITY TYPE: Educational; Fund-raising
YEAR FOUNDED: 1983
FUNDING: Private; Fund-raisers

696. Harris County Health Dept
2501 Dunstan
Houston, TX 77005
(713) 526-1841
KEY PERSONNEL: MA DePoe; AIDS Coordinator
AFFILIATION: Harris County Government
FACILITY TYPE: Educational; Clinic; HIV counseling and testing; Health department
STAFF: Paid professional 16
FUNDING: Federal government; Local government; Fees for services or products
OUTREACH: Speakers bureau, patient education, testing/counseling, audiovisual loan program, information/referral
NETWORKS: Houston-Harris County Panel on AIDS; Montrose Clinic; American National Red Cross
ADDITIONAL INFO: Provides educators for the criminal justice system to educate inmates, parolees, and probationers
AVAILABLE LITERATURE: *AIDS Resources for Greater Houston*, an alphabetized directory of agencies that provide AIDS-related services in the Houston area; *Guide to AIDS Educational Materials*, a listing of printed and audiovisual materials
LANGUAGES: Spanish, Vietnamese

697. Hispanic AIDS Committee for Education and Resources (HACER)
1139 W Hildebrand, Ste B
San Antonio, TX 78201
(512) 732-3108
KEY PERSONNEL: Jose C Hernandez; Project Coordinator
FACILITY TYPE: Educational
STAFF: Paid professional 2; Volunteers 15
YEAR FOUNDED: 1987
FUNDING: State government; Private; Donations
OUTREACH: Resource library, materials in Spanish, educational presentations for Hispanics, home visitation and Hispanic focus groups
NETWORKS: Southwest Hispanic AIDS Coalition; San Antonio AIDS Alliance
ADDITIONAL INFO: Provides Spanish-language public service announcements, and pamphlets. The Hispanic HIDS Committee for Education and Resources is a private, non-profit organization established to educate the Hispanic in Texas about the threat of AIDS
AVAILABLE LITERATURE: *H.A.C.E.R.: Hispanic AIDS Committee for Education and Resources*, a brochure describing the agency; *El SIDA/AIDS: Lo Que Toda Mujer Necesita Saber/What a Woman Needs to Know*, a bilingual booklet giving AIDS facts for women; a flyer with the HACER telephone number; *AIDS and Food Handlers*, a bilingual informational flyer; *Hablando Claro, Compadre*, a poster; *Rabbits Have a Certain Reputation: But Rabbits Don't Get AIDS, Humans Do*, a poster; *Los Conejos Tienen Cierta Reputacion: Pero el SIDA/AIDS no Infecta a los Conejos, y a los Humanos, si*, a poster
LANGUAGES: Spanish

698. Houston/Harris County Panel on AIDS
FORMER NAME: Mayor's Task Force on AIDS
PO Box 1562
Houston, TX 77251
(713) 247-1156
KEY PERSONNEL: Tom Portwood; Secretary
AFFILIATION: Houston Mayor's Office
FACILITY TYPE: Task force
STAFF: Paid professional 2
YEAR FOUNDED: 1987
FUNDING: Local government
SEMINARS: Jun 2, 1988—"The Dimensions of AIDS," Houston

699. Houston Health and Human Services Dept, Bureau of Epidemiology—AIDS Surveillance and Seroprevalence Programs
FORMER NAME: AIDS Surveillance Program/Houston
8000 N Stadium Dr
Houston, TX 77054
(713) 794-9320; Hotline: (713) 794-9181
KEY PERSONNEL: Lauri Andress; Public Information Officer
AFFILIATION: Houston City Government
FACILITY TYPE: Educational; Health department
FUNDING: Federal government; State government; Local government; Grants
OUTREACH: Education to patients at the city's 7 health centers as well as to public and private agencies
NETWORKS: US Dept of Health and Human Services; Texas Dept of Health; Centers for Disease Control
SEMINARS: Nov 11, 1987—"AIDS Education for Houston Area Youth;" Apr 8, 1988—"World Health Day Conference," included AIDS education in the Hispanic community; Jun 9, 1988—"Understanding AIDS;" Jun 24, 1988—"AIDS, It's a Black Problem, Too"
ADDITIONAL INFO: A member of the internationally known Texas Medical Center since 1965. The department's major function is to provide Houstonians with basic preventive health services and education, administration of programs for the elderly, human services policy planning and enforcement of environmental regulations
AVAILABLE LITERATURE: *AIDS Information Update*, an informational newsletter; *Epidemiology Notes*, a monthly newsletter; *The Health of Houston: Births, Deaths and Other Selected Measures of Public Health 1982-1986, Citywide Measures*, a statistical report; *The Health of Houston: Births, Deaths and Other Selected Measures of Public Health 1984-1986, Health Service Area Measures*, a statistical report; *AIDS Alert*, an informational brochure in Spanish and English; distributes other materials from other agencies
LANGUAGES: Spanish

700. Humanite Society AIDS Information and Referral Service
520 Heights Blvd, No 1
Houston, TX 77007
(713) 462-4296
KEY PERSONNEL: John Maine; Public Information Director
FACILITY TYPE: HIV counseling and testing; Substance abuse treatment

701. Institute for Immunological Disorders
7407 N Freeway
Houston, TX 77076
(713) 691-3531
FACILITY TYPE: Research; Clinic
ADDITIONAL INFO: Source of additional AIDS information

702. Light of Love Metropolitan Community Church (MCC)—Midland/Odessa
PO Box 11152
Midland, TX 79702
(915) 687-6117; TDD for Deaf: (915) 697-3272
KEY PERSONNEL: LisaDawn McCabe; Paster
AFFILIATION: Universal Fellowship of Metropolitan Community Churches (UFMCC)
FACILITY TYPE: Religious
STAFF: Paid professional .5; Volunteers 5
FUNDING: Private; Dues
OUTREACH: AIDS referral service
ADDITIONAL INFO: Organized HIV testing for 1986 and 1987. A proposal was submitted for 1989

AVAILABLE LITERATURE: *ALERT*, a newsletter of UFMCC; *God, Gays and the Gospel*, UFMCC videotape; *What the Bible Does and Does Not Say About Homosexuality*, a brochure; *AIDS: Is It God's Judgement*, brochure; *AIDS: A Christian Response*
LANGUAGES: Spanish, American Sign Language

703. Midway Complex Alcoholism Program
1601 Vanda St
Lubbock, TX 79403
(806) 766-0310 ext 0252
KEY PERSONNEL: Charlotte Foster; Program Director
FACILITY TYPE: HIV counseling and testing; Substance abuse treatment

704. Montrose Clinic
1200 Richmond
Houston, TX 77006
(713) 528-5531; Hotline: (713) 528-5531
KEY PERSONNEL: Thomas J Audette; Executive Director
FACILITY TYPE: Educational; Clinic; HIV counseling and testing
STAFF: Paid professional 4; Paid nonprofessional 27; Volunteers 146
YEAR FOUNDED: 1981
FUNDING: Federal government; State government; Local government; Private; Fund-raisers; Fees for services or products
OUTREACH: Speakers bureau for medical, civic, social, and educational institution professionals
ADDITIONAL INFO: The Clinic is an alternative HIV antibody testing site for Houston
AVAILABLE LITERATURE: Distributes literature from various agencies
LANGUAGES: Spanish

705. Montrose Counseling Center (MCC)
900 Lovett Blvd, Ste 203
Houston, TX 77006
(713) 529-0037
KEY PERSONNEL: Robert H Hodge; Interim Executive Director
FACILITY TYPE: Clinic; Support group; HIV counseling and testing
STAFF: Paid professional 24; Paid nonprofessional 3; Volunteers 5
YEAR FOUNDED: 1978
FUNDING: State government; Fund-raisers; Fees for services or products
OUTREACH: Speakers bureau, trainers on AIDS and substance abuse
SEMINARS: Every Spring—"Women's Weekend;" Every Fall—"Living With AIDS," Houston
ADDITIONAL INFO: This agency is an alcohol/drug treatment program licensed by the Texas Commission on Alcohol and Drug Abuse
AVAILABLE LITERATURE: Publishes a newsletter
LANGUAGES: American Sign Language

706. Narcotics Withdrawal Centers, Inc
4949 W 34th St, No 111
Houston, TX 77092
(713) 956-7712
KEY PERSONNEL: John Nawrocki; Program Administrator
FACILITY TYPE: HIV counseling and testing; Substance abuse treatment

707. Oak Lawn Counseling Center
5811 Nash St
Dallas, TX 75235
(214) 351-1502; 559-0898
KEY PERSONNEL: Jackie Baker, Coordinator
AFFILIATION: Robert Wood Johnson Foundation AIDS Health Services Program
FACILITY TYPE: Clinic
ADDITIONAL INFO: Source of additional AIDS information and services

708. Omega House
2615 Waugh, Ste 286
Houston, TX 77006
(713) 523-1139
FACILITY TYPE: Hospice
ADDITIONAL INFO: A hospice for AIDS patients

709. Open Arms, Inc
PO Box 191402
Dallas, TX 75219
(214) 559-3946
KEY PERSONNEL: Stefanie Held; Executive Director
AFFILIATION: AIDS ARMS Network
FACILITY TYPE: Support group; Residential facility (children)
STAFF: Paid professional 6; Paid nonprofessional 2; Volunteers 50
YEAR FOUNDED: 1988
FUNDING: State government; Local government; Private; Fund-raisers
NETWORKS: AIDS ARMS Network
ADDITIONAL INFO: Founded as a women's support group. Provides support, telephone counseling, respite child care, and when needed, residential child care
AVAILABLE LITERATURE: *Women Touched by the AIDS Virus*, a brochure for women; *Open Arms, Inc*, a pamphlet about the agency
LANGUAGES: Spanish, American Sign Language

710. Panhandle AIDS Support Organization, Inc (PASO)
4101 W 34th St, Ste C
Amarillo, TX 79109
(806) 358-2853
KEY PERSONNEL: Donna Gerhardt; Executive Director
FACILITY TYPE: Educational; Support group; HIV counseling and testing
STAFF: Paid professional 1; Volunteers 50
YEAR FOUNDED: 1987
FUNDING: Private; Fund-raisers
OUTREACH: Public education, anonymous testing, programs for corporations, small businesses, and schools
SEMINARS: Nov 11-13, 1988—"Buddy Project Program;" Mar 1989—"Public AIDS Forum"
ADDITIONAL INFO: PASO is a support service providing the citizens of Amarillo and the Texas Panhandle with educational information about AIDS and help to those coping with the illness. Serves the 26 counties in the Texas Panhandle and maintains support groups for HIV positive, PWAs and PWARCs and their families, friends, and significant others
AVAILABLE LITERATURE: *PASO*, a brochure describing the agency
LANGUAGES: Spanish, American Sign Language

711. Parkland Memorial Hospital AIDS Clinic
5201 Harry Hines Blvd
Dallas, TX 75235
(214) 590-5632
KEY PERSONNEL: Stephen D Nightingale; Medical Director
FACILITY TYPE: Research; Educational; Hospital; Clinic; Support group
STAFF: Paid professional 10; Paid nonprofessional 3; Volunteers 1
YEAR FOUNDED: 1985
FUNDING: State government; Local government; Fund-raisers; Fees for services or products

712. People with AIDS Coalition Houston, Inc (PWACH, Inc)
FORMER NAME: It's OK/People with AIDS Coalition Houston
800 Rosine, No 204
Houston, TX 77019
(713) 522-5428
KEY PERSONNEL: Bruce W Cook; President
FACILITY TYPE: Educational; Support group
STAFF: Volunteers 30
YEAR FOUNDED: 1976
FUNDING: Private; Fund-raisers
OUTREACH: Speaking on "Impact of AIDS on the Individual," referrals for service and support
NETWORKS: National AIDS Network (NAN); National Association of People with AIDS (NAPWA)
SEMINARS: Nov 1988—"Alternative Therapies"
ADDITIONAL INFO: Provides household goods, clothing, roommate referral and treatment information
AVAILABLE LITERATURE: *People With AIDS Coalition Newsletter*

713. People with AIDS Coalition of Dallas, Inc (PWA Coalition of Dallas, Inc)
PO Box 4338
Dallas, TX 75208-9985
(214) 941-0523
KEY PERSONNEL: Mike Merdian; President
AFFILIATION: National Association of People with AIDS (NAPWA)

FACILITY TYPE: Educational; Support group
STAFF: Paid professional 3
YEAR FOUNDED: 1987
FUNDING: Federal government; State government; Local government; Private; Fund-raisers
OUTREACH: Housing, employment, advocacy, networking, education
SEMINARS: Feb 17-19, 1989—"AIDS and Deafness: A Community's Challenge," Dallas, presented by the Dallas County Deaf AIDS Task Force
ADDITIONAL INFO: "All programs of the coalition seek to motivate a person with AIDS or ARC to retain or gain control of his or her own well-being, and to be active in that pursuit."
AVAILABLE LITERATURE: *PWA Newsline*, bimonthly newsletter; *Purpose and History of the Organization*, a pamphlet describing the facility
LANGUAGES: American Sign Langauge

714. San Antonio AIDS Alliance
FORMER NAME: San Antonio AIDS Task Force
1747 Citadel Plaza, Ste 104
San Antonio, TX 78209
(512) 822-4333
KEY PERSONNEL: Janet Alyn; Acting Director
FACILITY TYPE: Educational
STAFF: Paid professional 1; Volunteers 2
YEAR FOUNDED: 1987
FUNDING: Private; Fund-raisers
OUTREACH: Affiliate members provide information about AIDS in the workplace, professional staff training, school-based AIDS information programs, specific outreach in Hispanic and Black communities, programs for high risk groups such as IV drug users, juvenile offenders, and gays
SEMINARS: Oct, 1987—"AIDS in the Workplace"
AVAILABLE LITERATURE: Publishes a general services brochure and a local directory
LANGUAGES: Spanish

715. San Antonio AIDS Foundation
FORMER NAME: San Antonio Tavern Guild AIDS Foundation
3530 Broadway
San Antonio, TX 78209
(512) 821-6218
KEY PERSONNEL: Papa Bear; President
FACILITY TYPE: Educational; Support group; Hospice; Task force
STAFF: Paid professional 2; Paid nonprofessional 5; Volunteers 9
YEAR FOUNDED: 1986
FUNDING: State government; Private
ADDITIONAL INFO: This agency provides free distribution of videos, weekly mailing of latest AIDS information to doctors, free distribution of AIDS literature, food stamp processing, food bank distribution center, commodities application processing and distribution, social security processing, SSI application and processing, aerosol pentamidine treatments, direct patient assistance, individual counseling, pastoral care, free distribution of condoms, AIDS advocacy action, and soup kitchen.
AVAILABLE LITERATURE: Monthly newsletter
LANGUAGES: Spanish, American Sign Language

716. San Antonio AIDS Medical Foundation
PO Box 2231
San Antonio, TX 78298
(512) 733-1853
FACILITY TYPE: Research; Educational
ADDITIONAL INFO: Source of additional AIDS information

717. Shanti/Houston
PO Box 3045
Houston, TX 77253
FACILITY TYPE: Support group
ADDITIONAL INFO: Source of additional AIDS information

718. Social Security Administration, El Paso
PO Box 9994, 1414 Geronimo
El Paso, TX 79990
(915) 541-7490
FACILITY TYPE: Social service agency
STAFF: Paid professional 44; Volunteers 2
YEAR FOUNDED: 1935
FUNDING: Federal government

OUTREACH: Newspaper, radio, and television ads, pamphlet distribution, mailing projects, speakers bureau
AVAILABLE LITERATURE: Numerous pamphlets and leaflets are available for distribution
LANGUAGES: Spanish, American Sign Language

719. Southwest AIDS Committee, Inc (SWAC)
916 E Yandell
El Paso, TX 79902
(915) 533-5003
KEY PERSONNEL: Terry D Call; Executive Director
FACILITY TYPE: Educational; Support group; Hospice; Fund-raising; Client services/case management
STAFF: Paid professional 4; Paid nonprofessional 1; Volunteers 80
YEAR FOUNDED: 1984
FUNDING: Federal government; State government; Private; Fund-raisers; Fees for services or products
OUTREACH: Speakers Bureau, case management, food bank, referrals, advocacy, legal fund
NETWORKS: Hospice of El Paso; Texas Technical School of Medicine HIV Clinic; Visiting Nurses Association; National AIDS Network (NAN); El Paso AIDS Task Force; AIDS Action Council
SEMINARS: Held seminars on "Women, Children and AIDS," "Children and AIDS," "Gay Men's Health Project"
ADDITIONAL INFO: Provides complete client services, medical equipment loan closet, housing, emergency housing. Developing a multidisciplinary AIDS care facility
AVAILABLE LITERATURE: Newsletters, videos, pamphlets, buttons, and posters
LANGUAGES: Spanish

720. Triangle AIDS Network, Inc
PO Box 12279
Beaumont, TX 77726
(409) 832-8338; Hotline: (409) 724-2437
KEY PERSONNEL: Rosemary Sanderfer; Executive Director
FACILITY TYPE: Educational; Support group; Hospice; Fund-raising
STAFF: Paid professional 2; Volunteers 20
YEAR FOUNDED: 1987
FUNDING: State government; Local government; Private
OUTREACH: Speakers bureau, volunteer training, legal counseling, referrals, professional social service counseling, family and PWA support services
SEMINARS: Nov 1987, 1988—"AIDS Seminar"
ADDITIONAL INFO: Maintains family support groups, PWA support groups, hotline, respite care, buddies, indigent patient care, and a speakers bureau
AVAILABLE LITERATURE: *AIDS and Children*, an American National Red Cross brochure of information for parents of school-age children; *AIDS and Women*, a brochure for women about AIDS; *Questions and Answers About STDs*, a brochure of general information for young adults; *AIDS and the Black Community*, a brochure of general information for Blacks; *AIDS and the IV Drug User*, a brochure for IV drug users telling what to do and what not to do; *Herpes*, a general brochure about herpes; *AIDS and Safer Sex*, a flyer of safer sex guidelines; *What Everyone Should Know about Chlamydia*, an informational brochure; *Viral Hepatitis*, an informational brochure; *Caring for the AIDS Patient at Home*, an American National Red Cross brochure of tips on how to care for PWAs at home; *Peligro Grave: AIDS/SIDA y las Drogas*, a Spanish-language brochure about drugs and AIDS; *What Gay and Bisexual Men Should Know About AIDS*, a booklet of AIDS facts; *What You Should Know About AIDS*, a CDC booklet on AIDS; *AIDS and Your Job: Are there Risks?*, an American National Red Cross brochure about AIDS in the workplace
LANGUAGES: Spanish, American Sign Language

721. West Texas AIDS Foundation (WesTAF)
PO Box 93120
Lubbock, TX 79493
(806) 747-AIDS
KEY PERSONNEL: Frank Bailey; President
FACILITY TYPE: Educational; Support group; Fund-raising; HIV counseling and testing
STAFF: Volunteers 50
YEAR FOUNDED: 1986
FUNDING: Private; Fund-raisers
OUTREACH: Educational programs for civic groups, schools, medical entities, and teachers

NETWORKS: Hospice of Lubbock; Great Plains Home Care, Inc; Great Plains Health Services, Inc
ADDITIONAL INFO: Provides a variety of services including food bank, medical assistance, direct financial assistance, HIV counseling and testing, PWA support group, Shanti Buddy Program, and HIV positive support group
AVAILABLE LITERATURE: *Phoenix*, a quarterly newsletter
LANGUAGES: American Sign Language

UTAH

722. AIDS Coalition of Northern Utah
1961 Washington Blvd
Ogden, UT 84401
KEY PERSONNEL: Gordon B James; Chairperson
FACILITY TYPE: Educational
STAFF: Volunteers 25
YEAR FOUNDED: 1987
FUNDING: Fund-raisers
OUTREACH: Speakers bureau, library
SEMINARS: Oct 1988—"Workshop for Community Leaders"
AVAILABLE LITERATURE: Distribute materials from the American National Red Cross

723. AIDS Project Utah
PO Box 2576, 457 E 300 South, Carriage House
Salt Lake City, UT 84110-2576
(801) 359-2438; Salt Lake City Hotline: (801) 359-2437; Ogden Hotline: (801) 776-8274
KEY PERSONNEL: Richard Starley; Director
FACILITY TYPE: Educational; Support group; Fund-raising; Task force
STAFF: Paid professional 1; Volunteers 75
YEAR FOUNDED: 1985
FUNDING: Private; Fund-raisers
OUTREACH: Community education program, risk reduction workshops, presentations to general public and highly impacted communities, conference displays, literature distribution
NETWORKS: Utah AIDS Consortium; Utah AIDS Alliance; Gay/Lesbian Community Council of Utah
AVAILABLE LITERATURE: Internal newsletter to volunteers and donors
LANGUAGES: Spanish

724. Southwest Utah District Health Dept, Health Clinic
354 East S St, Ste 301
Saint George, UT 84770
(801) 673-4179
KEY PERSONNEL: Margrie K Ence; Nursing Director
FACILITY TYPE: Clinic
STAFF: Paid professional 20; Paid nonprofessional 10; Volunteers 2
YEAR FOUNDED: 1972
FUNDING: State government; Local government; Fees for services or products
ADDITIONAL INFO: Provides counseling and referral.
LANGUAGES: Spanish

VERMONT

725. Vermont CARES
38 Converse Court
Burlington, VT 05401
(802) 863-AIDS
KEY PERSONNEL: Terje Anderson

726. Vermont Dept of Health
PO Box 70, 60 Main St
Burlington, VT 05402
(802) 863-7286; Hotline: (800) 882-AIDS; Toll-free: (800) 642-3323
KEY PERSONNEL: Deborah Kutzko; Program Manager
FACILITY TYPE: Educational; Task force; HIV counseling and testing; Health department
FUNDING: Federal government
OUTREACH: AIDS education provided to schools, churches, police departments, etc..., HIV counseling and testing site, AIDS hotline, AIDS surveillance
NETWORKS: Centers for Disease Control

ADDITIONAL INFO: Provides funding for the Vermont Committee on AIDS Resources and Education Service (VT CARES), Vermont Regional Hemophilia Center, Vermont/New Hampshire Red Cross, Planned Parenthood, and Brattleboro AIDS Project
AVAILABLE LITERATURE: *AIDS Resource Manual*, published by the Vermont AIDS Task Force and the Vermont Dept of Health; *Don't Forget Your Rubbers*, a poster for safer sex; *Vermont Disease Control Bulletin*, a newsletter

VIRGINIA

727. The AIDS Support Group/Charlottesville
PO Box 2322
Charlottesville, VA 22902
(804) 979-7714
KEY PERSONNEL: Jim Heilman

728. American Red Cross, Roanoke Valley Chapter
352 Church Ave SW
Roanoke, VA 24016
(703) 985-3535
KEY PERSONNEL: Steven T Smith; Director, Community Services
AFFILIATION: American National Red Cross
FACILITY TYPE: Educational; Fund-raising
STAFF: Paid professional 4; Volunteers 6
YEAR FOUNDED: 1914
FUNDING: Fund-raisers; Fees for services or products
OUTREACH: AIDS education programs for youth, community, and workplace
NETWORKS: Roanoke AIDS Project; Red Cross Virginia AIDS Coalition
SEMINARS: Mar, Aug 1988—"Red Cross AIDS Facilitator Training"
AVAILABLE LITERATURE: Distributes posters and educational materials from the national headquarters

729. Children's Hospice International (CHI)
1101 King St, Ste 131
Alexandria, VA 22314
(703) 684-0330; Hotline: (800) 2-4-CHILD
KEY PERSONNEL: Patricia Dailey; Executive Assistant
FACILITY TYPE: Research; Educational; Support group; Fund-raising
STAFF: Paid professional 4; Volunteers 3
YEAR FOUNDED: 1983
FUNDING: Private; Fund-raisers; Fees for services or products
OUTREACH: Education-training program
SEMINARS: Sep 15-16, 1988—"Fourth Annual Pediatric Hospice Conference," Philadelphia; Oct 31-Nov 4, 1988—"International Conference on Children and Death," Athens, Greece
AVAILABLE LITERATURE: *Publications of Children's Hospice International*, a flyer describing 72 various publications, audio cassettes, and films covering grief and bereavement, hospice care, programs, support, hospice issues, children and dying, family and trauma issues, pain and symptom management, patient education, AIDS, and other special topics
LANGUAGES: Spanish

730. City of Richmond Community Mental Health Center
501 N 9th St
Richmond, VA 23219
(804) 643-5301; Hotline: (804) 780-8003
KEY PERSONNEL: Jeffrey Hyler; Clincian/Crisis Intervention
AFFILIATION: Richmond Community Services Board
FACILITY TYPE: HIV counseling and testing; Mental health agency
STAFF: Paid professional
YEAR FOUNDED: 1971
FUNDING: Federal government; State government; Local government; Fees for services or products
OUTREACH: AIDS training for staff and clinicians, education, distribution of education materials
SEMINARS: "AIDS: Death and Dying Issues," "AIDS: In the Workplace"
LANGUAGES: American Sign Language, Spanish, Korean, Indian

731. Richmond AIDS Information Network
1721 Hanover Ave
Richmond, VA 23220
(804) 358-6343
FACILITY TYPE: Educational
ADDITIONAL INFO: Source of additional AIDS information

732. Tidewater AIDS Crisis Taskforce (TACT)
814 W 41st St
Norfolk, VA 23508
(804) 423-5859, 877-1300; Hotline: (804) 440-5400
KEY PERSONNEL: Mary Ann Moore
FACILITY TYPE: Educational; Support group; Task force
STAFF: Paid professional 3; Volunteers 218
YEAR FOUNDED: 1983
FUNDING: Federal government; State government; Private; Fund-raisers; Fees for services or products
OUTREACH: Educational programs for the public and targeted groups, support services and referrals for PWAs, PWARCs, and HIV positive individuals
NETWORKS: Regional AIDS Taskforce; Minority AIDS Network; Care Virginia; National AIDS Network (NAN)
RESEARCH: Participating in the Virginia Department of Health Knowledge, Attitude and Behavior Survey conducted by the Virginia Commonwealth University
ADDITIONAL INFO: TACT is a not-for-profit organization devoted to combating the spread of HIV and to helping those persons who are already infected with the virus
AVAILABLE LITERATURE: *Tidewater AIDS Crisis Taskforce*, a brochure describing the agency; *What You Should Know About the Virus*, a brochure of basic facts about AIDS; *Safer Sex*, a brochure of safer sex guidelines

WASHINGTON

733. AIDS Clinic, Harborview Medical Center
325 9th Ave
Seattle, WA 98104
(206) 223-3241
KEY PERSONNEL: Sara Pascoe; Nurse Practitioner
AFFILIATION: University of Washington
FACILITY TYPE: Research; Educational; Hospital; Clinic; HIV counseling and testing; Client services/case management
STAFF: Paid professional 4; Paid nonprofessional 1; Volunteers 15
YEAR FOUNDED: 1984
FUNDING: Federal government; Private; Fees for services or products
OUTREACH: Conferences for medical providers
RESEARCH: Treatment of HIV, oral manifestations of HIV, CNS manifestations of HIV
ADDITIONAL INFO: Works closely with the University of Washington and provides comprehensive medical services
AVAILABLE LITERATURE: *Introduction to Clinic*, a brochure about the clinic; monthly staff meeting minutes
LANGUAGES: Interpreters available

734. AIDS Project/Seattle
610 3rd St
Seattle, WA 98199
FACILITY TYPE: Educational
ADDITIONAL INFO: Source of additional AIDS information

735. AIDS Spiritual Assistance
PO Box 12216
Seattle, WA 98112
(206) 325-2421
KEY PERSONNEL: Ed Perry, Coordinator
FACILITY TYPE: Support group
ADDITIONAL INFO: A network to assist patients, lovers, friends, and families in spiritual matters, especially in relation to AIDS; Monday through Friday, 12pm-5pm

736. American Red Cross, Seattle-King County Chapter
1900 25th Ave S
Seattle, WA 98144
(206) 323-2345
KEY PERSONNEL: Bob Barrie; AIDS Projects Administrator
AFFILIATION: American National Red Cross
FACILITY TYPE: Educational
STAFF: Paid professional 5; Paid nonprofessional 1; Volunteers 26
YEAR FOUNDED: 1881
FUNDING: Federal government; State government; Private; Fees for services or products

OUTREACH: Education for grades 5-12, community, civic, church education, worksite education, health professional education, minority peer education project
NETWORKS: Seattle AIDS Network; AIDS Prevention Project Roundtable; Dept of Health Social Services AIDS Task Force; Governor's AIDS Task Force
SEMINARS: Conduct many forums and workshops throughout the state covering teens and parents, youths, professionals, and nurses
AVAILABLE LITERATURE: *Seattle Area AIDS Resources*, a brochure listing the available resources; *National AIDS Awareness Test*, a video; *AIDS in the Workplace: An Epidemic of Fear*, a video; *A Bad Way to Die*, a video; *Beyond Fear: The Virus, the Individual and the Community*, a video; *Sex, Drugs and AIDS*, a video; *Answers About AIDS*, a video; *AIDS Answers for Young People*, a video; *What is AIDS*, a video for late grade school to early junior high school; *The Subject is AIDS*, a video for teens; *A Letter from Brian*, a video for high school students; *Don't Forget Sherrie*, a video for minority students; *AIDS: Everything You and Your Family Need to Know but Were Afraid to Ask*, a video; *AIDS and Your Job: Are there Risks?*, a brochure; *AIDS: The Facts*, a brochure; *AIDS, Sex, and You*, a brochure; *AIDS and Children*, a brochure for parents of school-age children; *AIDS and Children*, a brochure for teachers and school officials; *Facts about AIDS and Drug Abuse*, a brochure; *If Your Test for Antibody to the AIDS Virus is Positive*, a brochure; *Caring for the AIDS Patient at Home*, a brochure; *Gay and Bisexual Men and AIDS*, a brochure; *Surgeon General's Report on AIDS*, a booklet; *Answers about AIDS*, a brochure; *What Every Parent Should Know About AIDS*, a brochure; *Informate de lo que es el SIDA*, a brochure; *AIDS Resource*, a bookmark with AIDS information telephone numbers; *Beyond Fear*, a packet of information and poster for workplace or group; *LaBelle Poster*, Patti LaBelle endorsing AIDS education; *Can't Get AIDS Poster*, 4 panels indicating that AIDS cannot be spread casually; *AIDS Prevention Program for Youth*, student text; *AIDS Prevention Program for Youth*, a teacher/leader text; *Confronting AIDS*, a public health, health care and research text
LANGUAGES: Uses a language bank with over 70 languages

737. Association of People Living With AIDS (APLWA)
1128 13th Ave, no 105
Seattle, WA 98122
(206) 329-3382
KEY PERSONNEL: Milton Farquhar; Public Relations Director
AFFILIATION: National Association of People with AIDS (NAPWA)
FACILITY TYPE: Educational; Support group; Fund-raising; Client services/case management; Coalition
STAFF: Volunteers 10
YEAR FOUNDED: 1987
FUNDING: Private; Fund-raisers; Donations
OUTREACH: Community outreach, benefit coordination, referral source, hospital visitation, allopathic and naturopathic referrals
NETWORKS: AIDS Action Council; National AIDS Network (NAN); National Minority AIDS Council
SEMINARS: Attend many conferences and make many presentations
AVAILABLE LITERATURE: A study on funeral homes in Seattle-King County; Newsletter; Safer sex push pins
LANGUAGES: Spanish

738. Blood Sisters
PO Box 12152
Seattle, WA 98102
(206) 328-8979
KEY PERSONNEL: Carol Sterling, Coordinator
AFFILIATION: Chicken Soup Brigade
FACILITY TYPE: Support group
ADDITIONAL INFO: Lesbians organizing blood donations for, and on behalf of, gay men with AIDS

739. Catholic Community Services Homecare ("Chore Services")
PO Box 22043, Randolph Carter Center
Seattle, WA 98122
(206) 324-2013
KEY PERSONNEL: Jill L Nave; Service Coordinator and Community Aide Supervisor
FACILITY TYPE: Client services/case management
STAFF: Paid professional 7; Paid nonprofessional 3; Volunteers 5
YEAR FOUNDED: 1984
FUNDING: State government
OUTREACH: Provides training to those interested in providing homecare services through the program

NETWORKS: Northwest AIDS Foundation
ADDITIONAL INFO: Provides free non-medical homecare services to PWAs and PWARCs who meet the state's financial eligibility criterion of low income

740. Chicken Soup Brigade
PO Box 20066
Seattle, WA 98102
(206) 328-8979
KEY PERSONNEL: Dennis Crosby; Office Manager
AFFILIATION: Seattle Clinic for Venereal Health
FACILITY TYPE: Support group
STAFF: Paid professional 4; Volunteers 320
YEAR FOUNDED: 1983
FUNDING: Federal government; State government; Private; Fund-raisers
NETWORKS: Northwest AIDS Foundation
SEMINARS: Provide volunteer training and meetings on third and fourth Thursday of each month
ADDITIONAL INFO: The Chicken Soup Brigade is an all-volunteer support network for people with AIDS/ARC. Services provided include "grocery shopping or pharmacy pick-ups, transportation to and from medical appointments, personal visits or just checking in with a friendly phone call, occasional outings, help with house-keeping and laundry chores, and maybe even preparing a meal"
AVAILABLE LITERATURE: *The Chicken Soup Brigade*, a brochure describing the organization; Newsletter

741. Crisis Clinic/Seattle
1515 Dexter Ave N, #300
Seattle, WA 98109
(206) 447-3222, 461-3210
FACILITY TYPE: Support group
ADDITIONAL INFO: Provides emergency emotional support 24 hours

742. Gay Men's Health Group/Seattle
2353 Minor Ave E
Seattle, WA 98102
FACILITY TYPE: Educational
ADDITIONAL INFO: Source of additional AIDS information

743. Health Information Network
PO Box 30762
Seattle, WA 98103
(206) 784-5655
KEY PERSONNEL: Kathi Knowles; Project Director
FACILITY TYPE: Educational; Advocacy
STAFF: Paid professional 2; Volunteers 6
YEAR FOUNDED: 1981
FUNDING: Federal government; Private; Fund-raisers; Fees for services or products
OUTREACH: Speakers bureau
RESEARCH: Health care costs associated with AIDS, information dissemination, educational outreach delivery
ADDITIONAL INFO: This agency began to provide AIDS education in 1982, produced an STD community resources directory in 1983, and expanded that directory in 1985 to include resources in Washington, Oregon, Idaho, and Alaska
AVAILABLE LITERATURE: *Health Information Network's Educational Outreach Service Exhibits at Conferences and Health Fairs*, a list of exhibits and conferences attended; *Health Information Network's Educational Outreach Service Invited Addresses and In-Services*, a list of presentations; *What is the Health Information Network?*, an informational pamphlet; *AIDS Services in Puget Sound*, a list of services; *AIDS Services in Washington State*, a listing of available services; *AIDS Informational Resources for Health Care Professionals*; *Please Don't Call Me a Victim*, a brochure for helping PWAs

744. Hospice of Seattle/Providence Home Care
230 Fairview Ave N, Ste 100
Seattle, WA 98109
(206) 326-5969
KEY PERSONNEL: Robert Anderson; Administrator
AFFILIATION: Sisters of Providence Health Care Corp
FACILITY TYPE: Hospice; Home care
STAFF: Paid professional 70; Volunteers 60
YEAR FOUNDED: 1976
FUNDING: Federal government; State government; Private; Fund-raisers; Fees for services or products

OUTREACH: Speakers bureau
AVAILABLE LITERATURE: *In Touch*, a quarterly community newsletter

745. In Touch, A Community Service Program
1206 E Pike
Seattle, WA 98122
(206) 328-2711
KEY PERSONNEL: Molly McCormick; Program Director
FACILITY TYPE: Educational; Support group
STAFF: Paid professional 2; Volunteers 60
YEAR FOUNDED: 1984
FUNDING: Private; Fund-raisers
OUTREACH: AIDS educationals to massage therapists needing state certification for AIDS education requirements
SEMINARS: Feb 5, Apr 12, Sep 9, Nov 12, 1989—"AIDS Certification Training"
RESEARCH: Documentation of benefits fo massage for people who have AIDS
ADDITIONAL INFO: This agency provides cost free massage therapy for PWAs by licensed massage therapists once a week on a one-on-one basis.
AVAILABLE LITERATURE: Distribute various brochures to advertise the services of the organization

746. Kitsap County AIDS Task Force
109 Austin Dr
Bremerton, WA 98312
(206) 478-5235; Toll-free: (800) 874-AIDS
KEY PERSONNEL: Stephen Smith; AIDS/STD Program Coordinator
AFFILIATION: Bremerton-Kitsap County Health Dept
FACILITY TYPE: Task force
STAFF: Volunteers 30
YEAR FOUNDED: 1987
FUNDING: Local government; Fund-raisers
SEMINARS: Nov 1988—"AIDS in the Workplace"
ADDITIONAL INFO: This task force began as a networking facilitator of community resources for PWA/ARC/HIVs and their families and friends

747. David Morgan AIDS Relief Fund
1114 Howell St
Seattle, WA 98101
(206) 624-7493
FACILITY TYPE: Support group
ADDITIONAL INFO: Provides emergency financial support for people with AIDS/ARC

748. Northwest AIDS Foundation
1818 Madison
Seattle, WA 98122
(206) 329-6963, 329-6923
KEY PERSONNEL: Jeffrey Phillips; Information and Referral Coordinator
FACILITY TYPE: Educational; Support group; Fund-raising
STAFF: Paid professional 12; Paid nonprofessional 10; Volunteers 400
YEAR FOUNDED: 1985
FUNDING: Federal government; State government; Private; Fund-raisers
OUTREACH: Educational outreach, case management and advocacy, emergency grants, low cost housing, financial support
ADDITIONAL INFO: The Northwest AIDS Foundation is committed to providing plain talk education that will prevent the spread of this disease and to ensure that people with AIDS and ARC have housing, food, medical care and personal support
AVAILABLE LITERATURE: *Northwest AIDS Foundation Report to the Community July 1987-June 1988*, a flyer of highlights *SpringBoard*, a newsletter by and for people with AIDS; *S*, safer sex button; *Journey: Catholic AIDS Spiritual Ministry*, an informational brochure; *Chicken Soup Brigade*, an informational brochure; *Be In Touch With In Touch*, an informational brochure about this massage program; *Seattle Counseling Service*, a brochure describing this community mental health service for sexual minority people; *Home Care for AIDS Patients*, a brochure describing the service of the Swedish Hospital Medical Center; *Women Do Get AIDS*, an informational flyer for women; *Seattle AIDS-Support Group*, an informational brochure about this support group; *If Your Test for Antibody to the AIDS Virus Is Positive*, an American Red Cross brochure; *Caring for the AIDS Patient at Home*, an American Red Cross brochure; *Women and AIDS*, a brochure for women;

Stonewall Recovery Services, a brochure about this addiction counseling service for the lesbian and gay community; *Shanti*, a brochure about this emotional support group; *AIDS in the Black Community*, a brochure for Blacks produced by the People of Color Against AIDS Network; *Washington State AIDS Resources*, a county by county resource list; *AIDS Drugs*, a flyer listing the various available drugs; *Variables Unique to AIDS and Grief*, a flyer of words and phrases with their meanings for partner, family and friends; *Seattle Area AIDS Resources*, a resource flyer for Seattle; *Resource Manual for People with AIDS/ARC and Their Advocates*, a manual; *Infection Control at Home*, a guideline for care givers to follow; *The Seattle Reiki/AIDS Project*, a flyer card that describes the project; *When a Friend has AIDS*, a flyer with tips on what to say and what to do; *Self-Care Guidelines*, guidelines for people with AIDS/ARC who are not in a hospital setting
LANGUAGES: Spanish, American Sign Language

749. Office of Human Rights/Seattle
PO Box 3449
Seattle, WA 98114
(206) 464-6500; 753-6770
FACILITY TYPE: Legal
ADDITIONAL INFO: Receives and investigates complaints of discrimination because of AIDS/ARC or perceived AIDS/ARC

750. Office on HIV/AIDS
FORMER NAME: AIDS Program
Airdustrial Park, Bldg 14, Mail stop LP-20
Olympia, WA 98504
(206) 586-0426; Hotline: (800) 272-2437
KEY PERSONNEL: Mimi Fields; Director
AFFILIATION: Washington State Dept of Social and Health Services
FACILITY TYPE: Health department
STAFF: Paid professional 12; Paid nonprofessional 2
YEAR FOUNDED: 1986
FUNDING: Federal government; State government
OUTREACH: Referrals to local, state or national resources related to HIV/AIDS, informational/educational materials to individuals, agencies, and organization, training of health care professionals to do HIV/AIDS counseling and testing, work with other state and local agencies on HIV/AIDS policy development, education, and coordination of delivery of services, administer federal AZT funds
RESEARCH: Participates in the family of HIV seroprevalence studies funded by the Centers for Disease Control
AVAILABLE LITERATURE: Publish pamphlets and brochures and a monthly update of state and national statistics
LANGUAGES: Spanish, American Sign Language

751. Open Worried Well Group/Seattle
1505 Broadway
Seattle, WA 98122
(206) 329-8707
FACILITY TYPE: Educational; Support group
ADDITIONAL INFO: Provides information for persons concerned about their risk of contracting AIDS. Monday evenings, 6:30-8:30

752. People of Color Against AIDS Network (POCAAN)
105 14th Ave, Ste 2E
Seattle, WA 98122
KEY PERSONNEL: P Catlin Fullwood; Executive Director
FACILITY TYPE: Educational
STAFF: Paid professional 5
YEAR FOUNDED: 1986
FUNDING: Federal government; State government; Private
OUTREACH: Educational outreach
SEMINARS: May 25-26, 1988—"People of Color and AIDS: Meeting the Challenge of the Decade"
AVAILABLE LITERATURE: *Famous Last Words*, a brochure; *Famous Last Words*, posters; brochures in Asian language; comic book

753. Seattle AIDS Action Committee
704 E Pike
Seattle, WA 98122
(206) 323-1229
KEY PERSONNEL: George Bakan, Coordinator
FACILITY TYPE: Educational; Support group
ADDITIONAL INFO: A grass roots organization dedicated to the love and support of people with AIDS

754. Seattle AIDS Assessment Clinic
610 3rd Ave
Seattle, WA 98104
FACILITY TYPE: Clinic
ADDITIONAL INFO: Source of additional AIDS information

755. Seattle AIDS Support Group (SASG)
102 15th Ave E
Seattle, WA 98112
(206) 322-AIDS
KEY PERSONNEL: Susan J Dunshee; Director
AFFILIATION: Northwest AIDS Foundation
FACILITY TYPE: Support group
STAFF: Paid professional 1.5; Volunteers 50
YEAR FOUNDED: 1984
FUNDING: Fund-raisers
NETWORKS: National AIDS Network (NAN)
ADDITIONAL INFO: This agency provides a drop-in center which is open 65 hours a week for anyone affected by the HIV virus, especially diagnosed PWAs. It also offers 19 emotional support groups a week for those with the virus, as well as family, friends, and lovers.
AVAILABLE LITERATURE: Brochure describing the agency

756. Seattle Counseling Service for Sexual Minorities (SCS)
1505 Broadway
Seattle, WA 98122
(206) 329-8737; Hotline: (206) 329-8707
KEY PERSONNEL: Arleen B Nelson; AIDS Programs Coordinator
FACILITY TYPE: Educational; Mental health agency
YEAR FOUNDED: 1969
FUNDING: Federal government; State government; Private; Fund-raisers; Fees for services or products
OUTREACH: AIDS training to health service providers, training about homosexuals, transvestites, and transgenderals
SEMINARS: Mar 26, 1987, Apr 15, 1987, Apr 27, 1987, May 7, 1987, Jun 16, 1987, Jun 26, 1987, Aug 8, 1987, Sep 17, 1987, Sep 29, 1987, Oct 19, 1987, Nov 6, 1987, Nov 12, 1987, May 17, 1988, May 20, 1988, May 25, 1988, Jul 19, 1988—"Psychosocial Issues Workshop," provided for Community Psychiatric Center staff and board, Physicians and staff in Yakima, Family Counselor Group staff, Lutheran Social Service Agencies of King, Snohomish and Kitsap counties staff, Eastside Community Mental Health staff, Journey volunteers, Olympia/Thurston County Community Mental Health Center staff, Overlake Hospital social work staff, DeWitt Group staff, Seattle Mental Health Institute staff, Western State Hospital Mental Health and Social Services staff, Counterpoint Community Mental Health Center staff, Central Area Mental Health Center staff; Jul 10, 1987, Aug 14, 1987, Sep 8, 1987, May 10, 1988, Jun 3, 1988—"Bio-Medical Issues, Psychological Issues, Resources re AIDS Seminar," provided to Kitsap Community Mental Health Conference, Bellingham Health Care Conference, Island County Mental Health Conference, Port Angeles/Clallum County Mental Health Conference, Aberdeen/Grays Harbor County Mental Health Conference; Jul 22, 1988, Aug 23, 1988, Sep 8, 1988—"AIDS Dementia and Client/Therapist Relationship Workshop," provided to the United Way Consortium, Seattle Counseling Service and Seattle Mental Health Institute
ADDITIONAL INFO: Provides information and referral, therapy, support groups, education and training, and student interns for the people of the sexual minority community, their families and friends
AVAILABLE LITERATURE: *Seattle Counseling Service: A Community Mental Health Service for Sexual Minority People*, an informational brochure; *AIDS Service*, a card outlining AIDS services provided by SCS; *Support Group for Persons with ARC*, a card indicating what the group can do
LANGUAGES: Spanish, American Sign Language

757. Seattle Gay Clinic
500 19th Ave E
Seattle, WA 98112
(206) 461-4540
KEY PERSONNEL: Lee Kramer; President
AFFILIATION: Chicken Soup Brigade
FACILITY TYPE: Clinic
STAFF: Paid professional 4
YEAR FOUNDED: 1980

FUNDING: Local government; Private; Fund-raisers
OUTREACH: Counseling and testing for HIV Antibody, health care services for HIV Positive individuals

758. Seattle Shanti Foundation
PO Box 20698
Seattle, WA 98102
(206) 322-0279
FACILITY TYPE: Educational; Support group
FUNDING: Federal government; State government; Local government; Private; Fund-raisers
ADDITIONAL INFO: Provides free emotional support and friendship for individuals and loved ones facing AIDS

759. Seattle-King County AIDS Prevention Project
1116 Summit Ave, Ste 200
Seattle, WA 98101
(206) 296-4649; Hotline: (206) 296-4999
KEY PERSONNEL: Tim Burak; Project Manager
AFFILIATION: Seattle-King County Dept of Public Health
FACILITY TYPE: Research; Educational; Clinic; Support group; Task force
STAFF: Paid professional 30; Paid nonprofessional 10; Volunteers 20
YEAR FOUNDED: 1983
FUNDING: Federal government; State government; Local government; Private; Donations
NETWORKS: National AIDS Network (NAN)
SEMINARS: 1988—"AIDS and Substance Abuse," "People of Color and AIDS," "Women and AIDS"
RESEARCH: AIDS knowledge and attitudes among gay men, risk reduction interventions for IV drug users
AVAILABLE LITERATURE: *AIDS Surveillance Report*, a quarterly newsletter
LANGUAGES: Spanish

760. Shoulders
102 15th Ave, E
Seattle, WA 98112
(206) 322-AIDS
AFFILIATION: Seattle AIDS Support Group
FACILITY TYPE: Support group
ADDITIONAL INFO: Support group for friends, lovers, and family members of persons who have AIDS

761. Southwest Washington Health District
2000 Fort Vancouver Way
Vancouver, WA 98663
(206) 695-9215
KEY PERSONNEL: Thomas L Milne; Executive Director
AFFILIATION: Washington State Government
FACILITY TYPE: Educational; Clinic; Task force
STAFF: Paid professional 7.5; Paid nonprofessional 3.5; Volunteers 4
YEAR FOUNDED: 1929
FUNDING: Federal government; State government; Local government; Private
OUTREACH: Area educational resource clearinghouse, speakers bureau, curriculum development for schools, training for health and allied professionals, general public presentations on AIDS
RESEARCH: Seroprevalence rates in the area
ADDITIONAL INFO: This is the lead agency for the region VI AIDS network and is the convening agency for task forces in Clark, Skamania, and Klickitat counties
AVAILABLE LITERATURE: *Southwest Washington Health District*, a quarterly newsletter; *Southwest Washington AIDS Resources, December 1987*, a listing of the various resources for the area
LANGUAGES: Spanish

762. Tacoma-Pierce County Gay Men's Support Group
415 North I St, Ste 204
Tacoma, WA 98403
(206) 473-3279; 383-5315
FACILITY TYPE: Support group
ADDITIONAL INFO: A support group for all gay men 18 years and older, including those who have been diagnosed with AIDS/ARC

763. Volunteer Attorneys for Persons With AIDS (VAPWA) Legal Referral Project
FORMER NAME: Volunteer Attorneys for Persons With AIDS (VAPWA)
900 4th Ave, 600 Bank of California Bldg
Seattle, WA 98164-1005
(206) 624-4772
KEY PERSONNEL: Michael Leigh; Project Coordinator
AFFILIATION: Seattle-King County Bar Association (SKCBA)
FACILITY TYPE: Legal
STAFF: Paid professional 1; Volunteers 50
YEAR FOUNDED: 1989
FUNDING: Federal government; Local government
OUTREACH: Outreach to health and support organizations
ADDITIONAL INFO: VAPWA was started with no staff in 1986. The present organization was started in 1989 as part of the Seattle-King County Bar Association. The project will move to Northwest AIDS Foundation in 1990.
LANGUAGES: Spanish, American Sign Language

764. Washington State Office on HIV/AIDS
FORMER NAME: AIDS Program
Airdustrial Park, Bldg 14, Mail stop LP-20
Olympia, WA 98504
(206) 586-0426; Hotline: (800) 272-2437
KEY PERSONNEL: Mimi Fields; Director
AFFILIATION: Washington State Dept of Social and Health Services
FACILITY TYPE: Educational
STAFF: Paid professional 14
YEAR FOUNDED: 1986
FUNDING: Federal government; State government
OUTREACH: Education through distribution of materials
RESEARCH: The epidemiology section participates in the family of HIV seroprevalence studies funded by the Centers for Disease Control
ADDITIONAL INFO: Provides referrals to local, state or national resources related to HIV/AIDS. Provides informational/educational materials to individuals, agencies, and organizations, trains health care professionals to do HIV/AIDS counseling and testing, works with other state and local agencies on HIV/AIDS policy development, education, and coordination of delivery of services, and administers federal AZT funds
AVAILABLE LITERATURE: Publishes a monthly update of state and national statistics; *What is AIDS*, an informational brochure; *Advice About AIDS*, a brochure for health, public safety, and emergency services personnel; *AIDS*, an informational card; *Surgeon General's Report on Acquired Immune Deficiency Syndrome*; *New Points to Stop AIDS*, a brochure of facts about AIDS; *AIDS and Children*, a brochure of information for parents; *AIDS: What You and Your Friends Need to Know*, a brochure of safer sex information; *What You Should Know About AIDS*, a booklet from the Centers for Disease Control; *Recommendations for Prevention of HIV Transmission in Health Care Settings*, a booklet of information for health care workers; *Coping with AIDS: Psychological and Social Considerations in Helping People with HIV Infection*, a booklet from the National Institute of Mental Health
LANGUAGES: Spanish, American Sign Language

765. Youth Help Stepps Program
W 1101 College
Spokane, WA 99202
(509) 326-9550
KEY PERSONNEL: Pat Gruis; Director
FACILITY TYPE: HIV counseling and testing; Substance abuse treatment

WEST VIRGINIA

766. AIDS Prevention Program, West Virginia State Health Dept
151 11th Ave
South Charleston, WV 25303
(304) 348-2950; (800) 642-8244 (in West Virginia only)
KEY PERSONNEL: Loretta Haddy, Acting Director, Division of Surveillance Disease Control; Ronald Bryant, AIDS Coordinator; Thomas Dobbs, AIDS Health Education Coordinator; Dave Brangan, Health Educator
FACILITY TYPE: Educational; HIV counseling and testing
FUNDING: Federal government

LIBRARY: Available to public on request
AVAILABLE LITERATURE: *AIDS Facts*, general information about AIDS

767. AIDS Task Force of the Upper Ohio Valley
PO Box 6360
Wheeling, WV 26003-6360
(304) 232-6822; Hotline: (304) 234-6181
KEY PERSONNEL: Jay Adams; President
FACILITY TYPE: Support group; Task force
STAFF: Volunteers 35
YEAR FOUNDED: 1985
FUNDING: State government; Private; Fund-raisers
OUTREACH: Speakers bureau, buddy program, support groups, counseling
SEMINARS: May 21-23, 1988—"Buddy Training Workshop"
AVAILABLE LITERATURE: A monthly newsletter

768. Charleston AIDS Network (CAN)
FORMER NAME: Mountain State AIDS Network, Charleston
PO Box 1024
Charleston, WV 25324
(304) 345-4673; Hotline: (304) 345-4673
KEY PERSONNEL: Terrie Lee; Chairperson
FACILITY TYPE: Support group
STAFF: Volunteers 20
YEAR FOUNDED: 1988
FUNDING: State government; Private
OUTREACH: Speakers bureau, workshops, distribution of pamphlets
SEMINARS: Nov 19, 1988—"Buddy Training Workshop;" Aug, Sep 1988—"Training Sessions for Hotline Volunteers"
AVAILABLE LITERATURE: *AIDS: What You Can Do*, a brochure describing services in which one can become involved

769. Mountain State AIDS Network (MSAN)
PO Box 1401
Morgantown, WV 26507
(304) 599-6726
KEY PERSONNEL: Roger Banks; Executive Director
FACILITY TYPE: Educational; Support group; Fund-raising; Task force; Client services/case management
STAFF: Volunteers 125
YEAR FOUNDED: 1986
FUNDING: State government; Private; Fund-raisers
OUTREACH: High risk behavior outreach programs, community forums, media campaigns
NETWORKS: National AIDS Network (NAN); National Association of People With AIDS (NAPWA); United Way
AVAILABLE LITERATURE: *West Virginia AIDS Resource Manual*
LANGUAGES: Spanish, American Sign Language

770. Western West Virginia Chapter of the American Red Cross
1111 Veterans Memorial Blvd
Huntington, WV 25701
(304) 522-0328
KEY PERSONNEL: Penney Hall; Public Relations Assistant
AFFILIATION: American National Red Cross
FACILITY TYPE: Educational; Task force
STAFF: Paid professional 2; Volunteers 3
FUNDING: Private; Fees for services or products
OUTREACH: AIDS education to high schools, teacher inservices, and community and civic groups
SEMINARS: Jan 1988—"Training for Working Beyond Fear," a training program for high school AIDS speakers
ADDITIONAL INFO: Provides education to the area, maintains a statewide American Red Cross AIDS network, and is planning more training for AIDS speakers bureau

WISCONSIN

771. Among Friends
PO Box 426
Madison, WI 53589
(608) 873-3147
KEY PERSONNEL: Jay Hatheway; Publisher
FACILITY TYPE: Educational
STAFF: Volunteers 10
YEAR FOUNDED: 1984
FUNDING: Private; Fund-raisers; Fees for services or products

OUTREACH: Rural AIDS educational programs
AVAILABLE LITERATURE: *Among Friends*, a newsletter; *CAIR*, a publication of Condensed AIDS Information and Resources

772. Blue Bus Clinic
1552 University Ave
Madison, WI 53705-0485
(608) 262-7330
KEY PERSONNEL: Timothy S Tillotson; STD Program Coordinator
AFFILIATION: University of Wisconsin, Madison
FACILITY TYPE: Research; Clinic
STAFF: Paid professional 4; Paid nonprofessional 2; Volunteers 24
YEAR FOUNDED: 1970
FUNDING: State government; Local government; Fees for services or products
OUTREACH: Provides community prevention programs for general and targeted high-risk audiences
NETWORKS: National Coalition of Gay Sexually Transmitted Disease Services (NCGSTDS)

773. Brady East STD Clinic
FORMER NAME: Farwell Center
1240 E Brady St
Milwaukee, WI 53202
(414) 272-2144
KEY PERSONNEL: Douglas Johnson, Board of Directors President; Dave Cadle, Vice President; Marcos Huffman, Medical Director
FACILITY TYPE: Educational; Clinic
FUNDING: Donations; Grants
SEMINARS: Feb 1983—"Great Lakes Lesbian/Gay Health Conference;" assisted in establishing HTLV III testing program in conjuction with the Wisconsin Division of Health through conferences around the state (1985)
RESEARCH: Research with Abbott Lab and Southeastern Blood Center of Wisconsin on HTLV-III and sexually transmitted diseases
ADDITIONAL INFO: Founded in 1974 as a clinic with current programs concerned with AIDS and testing
AVAILABLE LITERATURE: *Guidelines and Recommendations for Healthful Gay/Lesbian/Bi-Sexual Activity*, a 5-fold brochure from NCGSTDS discussing safer sex; *Needles, Sex, AIDS: It Could Be You*, a 2-fold brochure, also in Spanish, with general information on AIDS and drugs; *AIDS: Cable de Salvamento: La mejor defensa en contra el AIDS es la informacion, Alcohol, Drugs and AIDS* and *Women and AIDS*, three brochures from the San Francisco AIDS Foundation; *Acquired Immune Deficiency Syndrome (AIDS)*, a pocket card of AIDS facts; *Safer Sex: A Simple Guide for Gay Men*, a 3-fold brochure of safer and not-so-safe sex recommendations
LANGUAGES: Spanish

774. Center Project, Inc
PO Box 1062
Green Bay, WI 54305-1062
(414) 437-7400
FACILITY TYPE: Research

775. City of Milwaukee Health Dept
841 N Broadway
Milwaukee, WI 53202
(414) 278-3333
KEY PERSONNEL: Thomas Schlenkes; Deputy Commissioner of Health
AFFILIATION: Milwaukee City Government
FACILITY TYPE: Research; Educational; Health department
FUNDING: Local government

776. Eau Claire County Dept of Human Services
202 Eau Claire St
Eau Claire, WI 54703
(715) 833-1977
KEY PERSONNEL: Judith S Hodgson; Administrator
AFFILIATION: Eau Claire County Government
FACILITY TYPE: Support group; Health department
STAFF: Paid professional 100; Paid nonprofessional 100
YEAR FOUNDED: 1978
FUNDING: Federal government; State government; Local government
OUTREACH: Public education
NETWORKS: Eau Claire County AIDS Task Force
ADDITIONAL INFO: Provides in-home support services—housekeeping, personal care, companionship, attendant. Provides information and referral, medical services, and mental health services

777. Green Tree Hospice
FORMER NAME: Mount Sinai Hospice
6925 N Port Washington Rd
Milwaukee, WI 53217
(414) 352-3300
KEY PERSONNEL: Barbara Prasso; Administrator
FACILITY TYPE: Hospice
STAFF: Paid professional 30; Paid nonprofessional 7; Volunteers 20
YEAR FOUNDED: 1980
FUNDING: Federal government; State government; Private; Fees for services or products
RESEARCH: Symptom management in the terminally ill person with AIDS, factors influencing decisions to elect hospice care
ADDITIONAL INFO: Provides a full range of care in a home-like inpatient unit, home, or nursing home
LANGUAGES: American Sign Language, Spanish, German, Yiddish, Hebrew

778. Madison AIDS Support Network (MASN)
PO Box 731
Madison, WI 53701
(608) 255-1711
KEY PERSONNEL: Marge A Sutinen; Program Director
FACILITY TYPE: Educational; Support group; Fund-raising
STAFF: Paid professional 4; Paid nonprofessional 2; Volunteers 40
YEAR FOUNDED: 1985
FUNDING: Federal government; State government; Local government; Private; Fund-raisers
OUTREACH: Outreach to minorities, university students, and others
NETWORKS: National AIDS Network (NAN); Gay Men's Health Crisis (GMHC); AIDS Alert
AVAILABLE LITERATURE: Publishes a monthly newsletter, brochures, pamphlets, posters, and buttons
LANGUAGES: Spanish

779. Madison Dept of Public Health
City County Bldg, Rm 507, 210 Martin Luther King, Jr Blvd
Madison, WI 53710
(608) 266-4821
KEY PERSONNEL: Marjorie Hurie; Communicable Disease Control Specialist
FACILITY TYPE: HIV counseling and testing; Health department
FUNDING: Local government
OUTREACH: Educational programs for high risk women through the jail and community agencies, programs students of all ages, programs for professionals, community organizations, and occupational groups
ADDITIONAL INFO: Provides anonymous, free HIV counseling and testing. Provides education and follow-up of AIDS cases

780. Milwaukee AIDS Project (MAP)
PO Box 92505
Milwaukee, WI 53202
(414) 273-2437; Hotline: (414) 273-2437; Toll-free: (800) 344-2437
KEY PERSONNEL: Carolyn P Syverson; Acting Executive Director
AFFILIATION: AIDS Resource Center of Wisconsin, Inc (ARCW)
FACILITY TYPE: Educational; Support group; Fund-raising; Client services/case management; Legal
STAFF: Paid professional 12; Volunteers 300
YEAR FOUNDED: 1974
FUNDING: Federal government; State government; Local government; Private; Fund-raisers; Fees for services or products
OUTREACH: Professional community health educators, volunteer speakers bureau, support groups for PWAs and their significant others, individual buddy support for PWAs, social workers, state hotline, satellite project
NETWORKS: National AIDS Network (NAN); AIDS Action Council; Persons With AIDS Coalition; Society for Nonprofit Organizations; Volunteer Center of Greater Milwaukee; City of Milwaukee AIDS Coalition; Milwaukee County AIDS Task Force
SEMINARS: Jun 1988—"AIDS of a Different Color: People of Color Working Together;" Jun 1988—"Gay and Lesbian Community Education Forum"
ADDITIONAL INFO: MAP was formerly a service of the Brady East STD Clinic, Inc. (BESTD). Provides educational materials to the community and social services to PWAs, PWARCs, and HIV positive individuals

AVAILABLE LITERATURE: *MAP RAP*, a newsletter for volunteers; *AIDS Update*, a community informational newsletter; distributes pamphlets and other materials on a state-wide basis from various organizations
LANGUAGES: Spanish

781. Milwaukee Hospice Home Care, Inc (MHHC)
1022 N 9th St
Milwaukee, WI 53233
(414) 271-3686
KEY PERSONNEL: Jim Ewens, Director
FACILITY TYPE: Support group
FUNDING: Fees for services or products; Donations; Grants
LIBRARY: Contains magazine articles, pamphlets, guidelines, and other materials of interest concerning hospices. Open to any professional for in-house use
ADDITIONAL INFO: Founded in 1979 as a hospice home care agency
AVAILABLE LITERATURE: *Milwaukee Hospice Home Care Newsletter*, a monthly newsletter about the hospice, its volunteers, and its staff

782. National Coalition of Gay Sexually Transmitted Disease Services (NCGSTDS)
PO Box 239
Milwaukee, WI 53201-0239
(414) 277-7671
KEY PERSONNEL: Mark Behar; Chairperson and Editor
FACILITY TYPE: Educational; Publisher
STAFF: Volunteers 1
YEAR FOUNDED: 1979
FUNDING: Fees for services or products
NETWORKS: National Lesbian Gay Health Foundation; Computerized AIDS Information Network (CAIN)
AVAILABLE LITERATURE: *Sexual Health Reports, Spring 88*, a quarterly publication of excerpts and reprints of articles covering all aspects of STD

783. Racine Health Dept, City of Racine, HIV Antibody Counseling and Testing Site
730 Washington Ave
Racine, WI 53403
(414) 636-9498
KEY PERSONNEL: Jacquelyn Evans; Epidemiologist
FACILITY TYPE: Educational; Clinic; HIV counseling and testing
STAFF: Paid professional 1
YEAR FOUNDED: 1985
FUNDING: Federal government; State government; Local government; Fees for services or products
OUTREACH: AIDS/STDS community resource
ADDITIONAL INFO: Provide anonymous HIV antibody counseling and testing, information and referral sources to reported AIDS cases

784. Wood County Health Dept
604 E 4th St
Marshfield, WI 54449
(715) 387-8646
KEY PERSONNEL: Ann Ruesch; Deputy Director
FACILITY TYPE: HIV counseling and testing; Health department
STAFF: Paid professional 10
FUNDING: State government; Local government
OUTREACH: Education to all groups, home care, alternate HIV counseling and testing site
ADDITIONAL INFO: Another office of this agency is maintained in Wisconsin Rapids. Lucie Weeler is the administrator. The telephone number (715) 421-8525

WYOMING

785. AIDS Coalition/Caspar
Caspar Natrona County Public Health Dept, 1200 E 3rd St
Caspar, WY 82601
(307) 777-7431
KEY PERSONNEL: Dr Nelson Frissell; Director, Public Health Dept
FACILITY TYPE: Educational; HIV counseling and testing; Referral
ADDITIONAL INFO: Coalition of Caspar Natrona County Public Health Dept, Wyoming AIDS Project, and Hospice. Provides testing, counseling, educational materials, and physician referrals

786. AIDS Counseling and Testing Service/Cheyenne
Cheyenne, WY
(800) 327-3577 (in Wyoming only)
FACILITY TYPE: HIV counseling and testing
ADDITIONAL INFO: Source of AIDS information

787. Wyoming AIDS Project
FORMER NAME: Natrona County AIDS Coalition
PO Box 9353
Casper, WY 82609
(307) 237-7833
KEY PERSONNEL: Gene Ferris; President
FACILITY TYPE: Educational; Referral
STAFF: Volunteers 6
YEAR FOUNDED: 1985
FUNDING: State government; Fund-raisers; Fees for services or products
OUTREACH: Presentations to groups, distribution of printed materials, speakers bureau

PUERTO RICO

788. Centro Latinoamericano de Enfermedades de Transmision Sexual (CLETS)
Call Box STD, Caparra Heights Station
San Juan, PR 00922
(809) 754-8118; Hotline: (809) 765-1010
KEY PERSONNEL: Rafael Rivera-Castano; Director
AFFILIATION: Puerto Rico Dept of Health
FACILITY TYPE: Research; Educational; Clinic; Health department
STAFF: Paid professional 50; Paid nonprofessional 50
YEAR FOUNDED: 1980
FUNDING: Federal government; State government
OUTREACH: Outreach to local communities
RESEARCH: Epidemiologic studies, psychosocial aspects
AVAILABLE LITERATURE: Provides educational materials for specific interests
LANGUAGES: Spanish

789. Fundacion SIDA de Puerto Rico
FORMER NAME: Fundacion AIDS
GPO Box 4842
San Juan, PR 00936
(809) 751-4200
KEY PERSONNEL: Jose Toro Alfonso; Executive Director
FACILITY TYPE: Educational; Support group; Fund-raising
STAFF: Paid professional 5; Paid nonprofessional 6; Volunteers 40
YEAR FOUNDED: 1983
FUNDING: Federal government; State government; Private; Fund-raisers
OUTREACH: Education/prevention to the community at large, gay community, PWAs, HIV-positive individuals and families
NETWORKS: COSSMHO; National AIDS Network (NAN)
SEMINARS: Jun 24, 1988—"Conference on AIDS and Adolescents"
ADDITIONAL INFO: This agency also provides emotional and practical support, buddy system, financial aid, group support, and advocacy.
AVAILABLE LITERATURE: Provide a newsletter, pamphlets, and other educational materials
LANGUAGES: Spanish

790. Latin American STD Center
Centro Medico
Rio Piedras, PR 00922
FACILITY TYPE: Clinic
ADDITIONAL INFO: Source of additional AIDS information

791. Puerto Rico Community Health Center Association
Villa Nevarez Professional Center, Ste 404
Rio Piedras, PR 00927
(809) 758-3411
KEY PERSONNEL: Zenaida Fernandez; Executive Director
AFFILIATION: National Association of Community Health Centers
FACILITY TYPE: Task force
STAFF: Paid professional 4
YEAR FOUNDED: 1984
FUNDING: Federal government; State government; Fund-raisers; Fees for services or products

OUTREACH: Coordination of educational activities on administrative and clinical issues regarding primary care
NETWORKS: Puerto Rico Academy of Medical Directors; Cooperative Agreement of the Dept of Health of Commonwealth of Puerto Rico
SEMINARS: Jul 12-15, 1988—"National Health Service Corps In Service Conference," Puerto Rico
RESEARCH: AIDS and primary care services, AIDS multimedia campaigning for community education
ADDITIONAL INFO: The PRCHCA members includes 15 community and migrant health centers in Puerto Rico. Provides services to the medically underserved population
AVAILABLE LITERATURE: *Salud Comunal*, a quarterly newsletter; *AIDS Protocols for Primary Care Services*, a brochure
LANGUAGES: Spanish

CANADA

792. AIDS Committee of Cambridge, Kitchener/Waterloo and Area (ACCKWA)
PO Box 1925
Kitchener, ON N2G 4R4
FACILITY TYPE: Educational
ADDITIONAL INFO: Source of additional AIDS information

793. The AIDS Committee of Ottawa (ACO)
267 Dalhousie St, Ste 201
Ottawa, ON K1N 7E3
(613) 234-3687
KEY PERSONNEL: Gilles Melanson; Chairperson
FACILITY TYPE: Educational; Support group
STAFF: Paid professional 5; Volunteers 70
YEAR FOUNDED: 1985
FUNDING: State government; Private; Fund-raisers
OUTREACH: Speakers bureau, media contacts, community liaison
NETWORKS: Ontario AIDS Network; Canadian AIDS Society
AVAILABLE LITERATURE: *Help for Persons with AIDS or ARC*, a brochure in French and English with information for PWAs and PWARCs; *AIDS Prevention is Everyone's Responsibility*, a bilingual brochure of general AIDS information; *The Adventures of Captain Condom*, a brochure of safer sex information and the use of condoms using a cartoon format
LANGUAGES: French, American Sign Language

794. AIDS Committee of Thunder Bay (ACT-B)
PO Box 3586
Thunder Bay, ON P7B 6E2
(807) 345-1516; Hotline: (807) 345-SAFE
KEY PERSONNEL: Michael Sobota; Executive Director
FACILITY TYPE: Educational; Support group; Fund-raising
STAFF: Paid professional 2.5; Volunteers 30
YEAR FOUNDED: 1986
FUNDING: Federal government; State government
OUTREACH: Volunteer and professional staffing of the AIDS Information phoneline, support services for seropositive individuals and PWAs, speakers bureau, special outreach to Native communities, safer sex workshops
NETWORKS: Canadian AIDS Society; The Ontario AIDS Network
SEMINARS: Oct 16-22, 1988—"AIDS Awareness Week," featured 8 separate events and presentations
ADDITIONAL INFO: ACT-B was created when a group of concerned citizens realized that local health care agencies were unable to cope creatively with PWAs. The committee has developed into a fully education-oriented organization. Provides resource people to school boards, health care providers, social service agencies, etc. Much of the work is directed toward awareness of AIDS viral infection and the incorporation of safer sex techniques
AVAILABLE LITERATURE: Quarterly newsletter for physicians, social service agencies, educational institutions, news media, volunteers, and ACT-B board members; pamphlets, posters and flyers
LANGUAGES: French

795. AIDS Committee of Toronto (ACT)
PO Box 55, Station F
Toronto, ON M4Y 2L4
(416) 926-1626
KEY PERSONNEL: Stephen Manning, Executive Director
FACILITY TYPE: Educational; Clinic; Support group

FUNDING: Federal government; State government; Local government; Donations

LIBRARY: Contains selected books, periodicals, newspaper clippings, and other information about AIDS for researchers, media, and selective general public

OUTREACH: Speakers bureau, AIDS Hotline

NETWORKS: Canadian AIDS Society; Ontario Public Education Panel on AIDS

SEMINARS: Nov 14-16, 1986—"Canadian AIDS Conference;" Jun 7-13, 1987—"AIDS Awareness Week IV"

ADDITIONAL INFO: Founded in 1983 as an educational agency with clinic facilities and counseling support

AVAILABLE LITERATURE: *Safe Sex for Hookers*, a 1-fold brochure of safe sex recommendations; *AIDS: Get the Facts*, a 5-fold brochure of AIDS facts; *This Is a Test; This is Only a Test: Should You Take It?*, a 5-fold brochure with questions and answers about the HTLV III blood test; *When a Friend Has AIDS*, a 2-fold brochure of what to say and what to do; *Condom Sense*, a 4-page pamphlet on choosing the right condom; *Which of These Will Give You AIDS?*, a poster of what will not give you AIDS; *Fun With Condoms*, a poster recommending the use of condoms; *ACT Bulletin*, monthly newsletter with statistics and AIDS information; *It's Raining Men...Do You Have Your Rubbers On?*, a pocket brochure recommending the use of condoms

796. AIDS Committee of Windsor (ACW)

1586 Wyandotte St E, Ste 205
Windsor, ON N9A 3L2
(519) 973-0222; Hotline: (519) 256-AIDS
FACILITY TYPE: Educational; Support group; Fund-raising; Advocacy
STAFF: Paid nonprofessional 3.5; Volunteers varies
YEAR FOUNDED: 1985
FUNDING: Federal government; State government; Private; Fund-raisers
OUTREACH: Speakers bureau, phoneline, resource center, one-on-one counseling, referrals
NETWORKS: Ontario AIDS Network (OAN); Canadian AIDS Society (CAS)
RESEARCH: Alternative treatments and therapies for PWAs
ADDITIONAL INFO: Provides a full range of support services for PWAs, HIV positive persons, IV drug users, friends, and families. It holds numerous seminars on an ad hoc basis
AVAILABLE LITERATURE: Publishes a monthly internal and a monthly informational newsletter, safe sex pamphlets and other informational materials

797. AIDS Network of Edmonton Society

FORMER NAME: AIDS Network of Edmonton
10704 108 St, 2nd Fl
Edmonton, AB T5H 3A3
(403) 424-4767; Hotline: 429-AIDS
KEY PERSONNEL: Barry Breau, Executive Director; Marion Dempster, Chairperson of the Board of Directors
AFFILIATION: Canadian AIDS Society
FACILITY TYPE: Educational; Support group; HIV counseling and testing; Referral
STAFF: Paid professional 5; Paid nonprofessional 2; Volunteers 125
YEAR FOUNDED: 1984
FUNDING: Federal government; State government; Local government; Private; Donations; Grants
OUTREACH: Speakers bureau, support groups for PWAs, the worried well, and family and friends, volunteer support services (hospital visits, practical support and buddy program)
NETWORKS: Alberta Community Council on AIDS, Edmonton Interagency Council on AIDS, Province of Alberta Risk Reduction Committee
SEMINARS: Monthly Safer Sex workshops for gay men, participates in local health conferences
ADDITIONAL INFO: The society was founded in 1984 and incorporated in 1986 with its purpose to provide support to persons affected by HIV/AIDS and to educate the public with a view to reducing HIV infection
AVAILABLE LITERATURE: *The Ross Armstrong Memorial Fund*, a 2-fold brochure describing the memorial fund with money used for PWAs and PWARCs; *Blood Test for AIDS?*, a 3-fold brochure describing the AIDS blood test and what it does or does not tell you; *Facts About AIDS*, a 2-fold brochure with general information about AIDS; *Introducing the AIDS Network of Edmonton*, a 2-fold brochure describing the network; *AIDS in Canada: What You Should Know/Le SIDA au Canada: Ce que vous devriez savoir*, a 7-fold Canadian Health and Welfare brochure with general information about AIDS; *Newsletter: AIDS Network of Edmonton*, a monthly newsletter with information about the network, its staff, and AIDS in general; distributes six fact sheets from the Ontario Ministry of Health: *Women and AIDS*; *Information for Parents and Teachers*; *Detecting AIDS*; *Information About AIDS*; *AIDS and Health Care Workers*; and *AIDS and the Workplace*

LANGUAGES: French

798. AIDS Regina

PO Box 432
Regina, SK S4P 3A2
(306) 525-0902
KEY PERSONNEL: Nils Clausson; Executive Director
FACILITY TYPE: Educational; Support group; Fund-raising
STAFF: Paid professional 1; Paid nonprofessional .5; Volunteers 20
YEAR FOUNDED: 1985
FUNDING: Federal government; State government; Private; Fund-raisers
NETWORKS: Canadian AIDS Society; International Society for AIDS Education
SEMINARS: Jun 14, 1988—"Women and AIDS," a public forum
AVAILABLE LITERATURE: *AIDS Regina: Your Best Defense Against AIDS is Information*, an informational brochure about the agency; *There is a Blood Test That Can Detect Exposure to the AIDS Virus...Should You Take It?*, a brochure describing the HIV antibody test; *AIDS Regina: The Newsletter*

799. AIDS Saskatoon

PO Box 4062
Saskatoon, SK S7K 4E3
(306) 242-5005; Toll-free: (800) 667-6876 (SK only)
KEY PERSONNEL: Erin Shoemaker; Project Coordinator
FACILITY TYPE: Educational; Support group; Fund-raising; Task force
STAFF: Paid professional 1; Paid nonprofessional .5
YEAR FOUNDED: 1986
FUNDING: Federal government; State government; Fund-raisers
OUTREACH: Speakers bureau, distribution of materials
NETWORKS: Saskatchewan Persons with AIDS Network
ADDITIONAL INFO: Offers support groups for PWAs and PWARCs, friends and families, attitudinal healing, and HIV positive individuals
AVAILABLE LITERATURE: Publishes a newsletter and distributes information from other agencies
LANGUAGES: French

800. AIDS Vancouver Island

FORMER NAME: Vancouver Island AIDS Society
1175 Cook St, Ste 108
Victoria, BC V8V 4A1
(604) 384-2366; Hotline: (604) 384-4554
KEY PERSONNEL: Judith English; Executive Director
AFFILIATION: Canadian AIDS Society
FACILITY TYPE: Educational; Support group
STAFF: Paid professional 1; Paid nonprofessional 2; Volunteers 100
YEAR FOUNDED: 1985
FUNDING: Federal government; Fund-raisers
OUTREACH: Street program for education of street people, speakers bureau, safer sex workshops
RESEARCH: AIDS knowledge, safer sex and safe injection knowledge and behavior of street people
ADDITIONAL INFO: Provides HIV positive support groups, buddy support program, speakers, educational brochures, videos, and books
AVAILABLE LITERATURE: *Can We Talk?*, a newsletter; *Hugging is Safe Sex*, a button
LANGUAGES: French

801. APGHL AIDS Educational Committee

PO Box 6368, Station A
Saint John, NB E2L 4R8
AFFILIATION: New Brunswick Dept of Health
FACILITY TYPE: Educational
ADDITIONAL INFO: Source of additional AIDS information

802. Canadian Public Health Association (CPHA), AIDS Education and Awareness Program

1565 Carling Ave, Ste 400
Ottawa, ON K1Z 8R1

(613) 725-3769
KEY PERSONNEL: David Walters; Program Director
FACILITY TYPE: Educational
STAFF: Paid professional 2.5; Paid nonprofessional 3
YEAR FOUNDED: 1986
FUNDING: Federal government
OUTREACH: Clearinghouse, distributes information, sponsorship of seminars, meetings, workshops, and conferences
SEMINARS: 1988—"Canadian Conference on AIDS"
AVAILABLE LITERATURE: *Join the Attack on AIDS*, a poster, kit and button; *The New Facts of Life*, an informational brochure; *The New Facts of Life*, a quarterly newsletter
LANGUAGES: French

803. Comite SIDA Aide Montreal (CSAM)
3600 Hotel De Ville
Montreal, PQ H2X 3B6
(514) 282-9888
KEY PERSONNEL: Lise Lauctot; Executive Director
FACILITY TYPE: Educational; Support group; Fund-raising
STAFF: Paid professional 2; Paid nonprofessional 7; Volunteers 200
YEAR FOUNDED: 1985
FUNDING: Federal government; State government; Local government; Private
OUTREACH: Educational material distribution, support groups, home care, counseling, speakers bureau, safer sex campaigns
ADDITIONAL INFO: Networks with a wide range of individuals and organizations including health care providers and organizations, educators, professional associations, media and community-based groups
AVAILABLE LITERATURE: *Le Virulent*, a bimonthly newsletter; *Prevention Support Advocacy/Prevenir Soutenir Intervenir*, an informational brochure about the agency; posters
LANGUAGES: French

804. Gays and Lesbians in Health Care
PO Box 6973, Station A
Toronto, ON M5W 1X7
FACILITY TYPE: Educational; Clinic
ADDITIONAL INFO: Source of additional AIDS information

805. Gays of Ottawa
PO Box 2919 Stn "D"
Ottawa, ON K1P 5W9
(613) 233-0152
KEY PERSONNEL: Shelia McComb; President
FACILITY TYPE: Educational; Support group
STAFF: Volunteers 50
YEAR FOUNDED: 1971
FUNDING: Private; Fund-raisers; Fees for services or products
OUTREACH: Education and Information
NETWORKS: Coalition Lesbian and Gay Rights Ontario (CLGRO); International Lesbian and Gay Association (ILGA)
AVAILABLE LITERATURE: *GO Info*, a bimonthly newspaper
LANGUAGES: French

806. Hamilton AIDS Network for Dialogue and Support (HANDS)
PO Box 44, Station B
Hamilton, ON L8L 7T5
FACILITY TYPE: Educational
ADDITIONAL INFO: Source of additonal AIDS information

807. Hassle Free Clinic
556 Church St
Toronto, ON M4Y 2E3
Men's Clinic: (416) 922-0603; Women's Clinic: (416) 922-0566
KEY PERSONNEL: Leo Mitterni; Counselor
FACILITY TYPE: Clinic; HIV counseling and testing
STAFF: Paid professional 4; Paid nonprofessional 6; Volunteers 1
YEAR FOUNDED: 1972
FUNDING: State government; Local government
OUTREACH: Body Positive—a self-help support group for HIV positive persons, educational and testing programs at bath houses
NETWORKS: AIDS Committee of Toronto; PWA Foundation; Ministry of Health; HIV Primary Care Physicians Group; University of Toronto Epidemiology Study
SEMINARS: Sep 1987—"AIDS Update Conference For Primary Care Physicians"

ADDITIONAL INFO: Provides counseling and support to PWAs and PWARCs
AVAILABLE LITERATURE: *Body Positive*, a flyer about a self-support program for HIV positive people; *STD: A Guide for Gay Men*, a pocket booklet describing the various STDs
LANGUAGES: French, Italian, Spanish

808. Kingston AIDS Project
PO Box 120
Kingston, ON K7L 4V1
(613) 545-3698; Hotline: (613) 545-1414
KEY PERSONNEL: Robert Allan; Support Services Coordinator
FACILITY TYPE: Educational; Support group
STAFF: Paid professional 2.5
YEAR FOUNDED: 1986
FUNDING: Federal government; State government; Local government; Private; Fund-raisers
OUTREACH: Public forums, speakers bureau, eroticising safer sex workshops, outreach to prisons and rural communities, support and counseling to hospitals, prisons, rural communities, social service agencies
NETWORKS: Canadian AIDS Society; Ontario AIDS Network
ADDITIONAL INFO: This is a volunteer, non-profit, community organization established to confront and address the problems and realities raised by the AIDS virus. The project's goals are to prevent the spread of the AIDS virus, to educate the public and affected groups about AIDS, and to support those affected by the AIDS virus
AVAILABLE LITERATURE: *Eroticizing Safer Sex*, a poster advertising safer sex sessions; *Get the Facts*, a flyer announcing a public forum on AIDS; *Kingston AIDS Project: Prevention, Education, Support*, a poster advertising the agency; *Kingston AIDS Project: Confronting AIDS Through Prevention, Education and Support*, an informational brochure; *Yes I Practice Safe Sex*, a button; *AIDS*, a button with red hearts
LANGUAGES: French, American Sign Language

809. Metro Area Committee on AIDS
PO Box 1013 Station M
Halifax, NS B3J 2X1
(902) 425-4882
KEY PERSONNEL: Madeline Comeau; Executive Director
FACILITY TYPE: Educational; Support group; Fund-raising
STAFF: Paid nonprofessional 2; Volunteers 50
YEAR FOUNDED: 1985
FUNDING: Federal government; Local government; Fund-raisers
OUTREACH: Speakers bureau
SEMINARS: 1988-1989—"AIDS Awareness Week"
AVAILABLE LITERATURE: *Stopping the Spread of AIDS: Guidelines for Affected Groups*, a pamphlet outlining AIDS risk reduction; *Get It Under Cover*, safer sex information including the use of condoms; *Which of These Will Give You AIDS*, a myths poster

810. Montreal AIDS Resource Committee—Association des Resources Montrealais sur la SIDA (MARC/ARMS)
PO Box 1164, Postal Station H
Montreal, PQ H3G 2N1
(514) 937-7596
KEY PERSONNEL: Cheh Cho, Director; Jean Daou, Public Relations; Donna Rae Dubois, Assistant Director
FACILITY TYPE: Research; Educational
FUNDING: Donations; Grants
LIBRARY: Pamphlets, articles, books, and related materials on AIDS and STD. Open to the general public
OUTREACH: Seminars, speakers bureau
NETWORKS: Canadian National AIDS Society; Montreal Coalition of Gay Organizations and Affiliated Establishments; Montreal Ecumenical Council on AIDS; Ville-Marie Social Services; AHM-GMA, Inc
SEMINARS: May 10-12, 1985—"Canadian National Conference on AIDS"
RESEARCH: Psychosocial aspects of AIDS
ADDITIONAL INFO: Founded in 1983 as an agency to provide education on all aspects of AIDS, conduct research in the psychosocial aspects of AIDS, and provide counseling
AVAILABLE LITERATURE: *Acquired Immune Deficiency Syndrome*, a 12-page pamphlet with general information on AIDS and safe sex. Also available in French; *How Not To*, a 17-page pamphlet on birth control published by Julius Schmid of Canada Ltd; *Is AIDS God's Wrath?*, a 2-fold brochure produced by Dignity Montreal dispelling

the question of God's wrath. The following pamphlets and brochures produced by the Canadian government are distributed by the committee: *Sexually Transmitted Diseases; Le Test, Le Virus, La Protection Sexuelle; AIDS in Canada: What you Should Know; Information for Parents and Teachers; Renseignements a l'Intention des Parents et des Enseignants; Detecting AIDS; La Detection du SIDA; Women and AIDS; Les Femmes et le SIDA; AIDS and the Workplace; Le SIDA et le Milieu de Travail; Information About AIDS, Renseignements sur le SIDA; Montreal General Hospital Infection Committee Bulletin*; and *Hospital General de Montreal Comite pour le Controle des Infections Bulletin*
LANGUAGES: French

811. National Advisory Committee on AIDS (NAC-AIDS)
301 Elgin St
Ottawa, ON K1A 0L2
(613) 957-1772
KEY PERSONNEL: Charlotte Tremblay; Secretary
AFFILIATION: Federal Centre for AIDS (FCA)
FACILITY TYPE: Scientific committee
YEAR FOUNDED: 1983
FUNDING: Federal government

812. Newfoundland and Labrador AIDS Committee, Inc
FORMER NAME: Saint John's AIDS Information Committee
PO Box 1364 Station C
Saint John's, NF A1C 5N5
(709) 739-7975
KEY PERSONNEL: Wally Upward; Coordinator
AFFILIATION: Canadian AIDS Society
FACILITY TYPE: Educational; Support group; Fund-raising
STAFF: Paid nonprofessional 2; Volunteers 40
YEAR FOUNDED: 1987
FUNDING: Federal government; Local government; Fund-raisers
OUTREACH: Safer sex sessions, seminars, support groups for PWAs, PWARCs, HIV positive individuals, families, and friends
AVAILABLE LITERATURE: Distributes materials from other agencies
LANGUAGES: French, American Sign Language

813. Ontario Public Education Panel on AIDS
15 Overlea Blvd
Toronto, ON M4A 1H9
FACILITY TYPE: Educational
ADDITIONAL INFO: Source of additional AIDS information

814. SIDA Quebec
1001 Rue St Denis
Montreal, PQ H2X 3H9
FACILITY TYPE: Educational
ADDITIONAL INFO: A source of additional AIDS information for Quebec

815. Toronto PWA Foundation
FORMER NAME: Toronto PWA Coalition
464 Yonge St, Ste 201B
Toronto, ON M4Y 1X3
(416) 925-7112
KEY PERSONNEL: Thomas Nash; Executive Director
FACILITY TYPE: Research; Support group; Fund-raising; Client services/case management
STAFF: Paid professional 2; Paid nonprofessional 1; Volunteers 40
YEAR FOUNDED: 1987
FUNDING: Private; Fund-raisers
NETWORKS: Ontario AIDS Network; Canadian AIDS Society
LANGUAGES: French

816. Vancouver AIDS Society (AIDS Vancouver)
1033 Davie St, Ste 509
Vancouver, BC V6E 1M7
(604) 687-5220; Hotline: (604) 687-2437
KEY PERSONNEL: Brian Peel; Executive Director
FACILITY TYPE: Educational; Support group; Fund-raising
STAFF: Paid professional 10; Volunteers 300
YEAR FOUNDED: 1983
FUNDING: Federal government; Local government; Private; Fund-raisers; Fees for services or products; Donations
OUTREACH: Speakers bureau
NETWORKS: Canadian AIDS Society

SEMINARS: Oct 26, 1987—"Women and AIDS;" Dec 10, 1987—"AIDS Is a Labour Issue;" Jun 11-13, 1988—"AIDS is a Trade Union Issue"
ADDITIONAL INFO: "AIDS Vancouver provides information to the general public and to high-risk groups, provides emotional and practical support to people with AIDS and ARC, and for their lovers, families and friends. Holds seminars and forums, publishes brochures and newsletters, and provides speakers for any group wishing information
AVAILABLE LITERATURE: *Women and AIDS: What Does It Take to Be Safe?*, a brochure for women; *You're Not Alone*, a brochure describing the services of the facility; *Sex and AIDS: Can We Talk?*, a brochure of safer sex guidelines; *AIDS Update, Spring/Summer 1988*, a brochure of AIDS facts; *When a Friend Has AIDS*, a brochure outlining what one can say and do; *True Fears*, a comic book about the use of condoms; *Volunteer Newsletter; Surveillance Update: AIDS in Canada*, a flyer giving AIDS statistics for Canada
LANGUAGES: American Sign Language

817. Vancouver PWA Coalition
PO Box 136, 1215 Davie St
Vancouver, BC V6E 1N4
(604) 683-3381
KEY PERSONNEL: Jackie Hegadorn; Administrative Assistant
AFFILIATION: Canadian AIDS Society
FACILITY TYPE: Educational; Support group; Fund-raising
STAFF: Paid professional 1; Volunteers 191
YEAR FOUNDED: 1986
FUNDING: Federal government; Local government; Private; Fund-raisers
OUTREACH: Library, peer counseling, speakers bureau
RESEARCH: Alternative therapies
ADDITIONAL INFO: "The Vancouver Persons with AIDS Society is a self-help, self-care organization operated by and on behalf of those diagnosed as persons with AIDS/ARC in the Vancouver area." It provides support group meetings, peer counseling, art psychotherapy, Tai Chi, retreats, meditation, health related financial assistance, advocates of life extension and improvement of quality of life. It works to get new drugs and treatments released.
AVAILABLE LITERATURE: *An Overview*, a pamphlet describing the organization; *Vancouver PWA Society Information*, a detailed pamphlet describing the organization; *Governing Structure of the Vancouver P.W.A. Coalition; Vancouver PWA Coalition Newsletter*, a monthly newsletter; *World AIDS Day, Dec 1, 1988*, button; *Silence=Death*, pink triangle button; *S*, safer sex button; *10K for PWA*, button
LANGUAGES: French

818. Village Clinic and Winnipeg Gay Community Health Centre, Inc (WGCHC,Inc)
FORMER NAME: Winnipeg Gay Community Health Centre, Inc
709 Corydon Ave
Winnipeg, MB R3M 0W4
(204) 453-0045; Hotline: (204) 453-2114
KEY PERSONNEL: Ron Harris; Executive Director
FACILITY TYPE: Educational; Clinic; Support group; HIV counseling and testing
STAFF: Paid professional 10; Volunteers 75
YEAR FOUNDED: 1983
FUNDING: Federal government; State government
OUTREACH: Counseling, education
NETWORKS: Computerized AIDS Information Network; Canadian AIDS Society; Manitoba Association of Community Health Centres
ADDITIONAL INFO: This is a general service clinic that also offers pre- and post-test counseling
AVAILABLE LITERATURE: *Guidelines for Household Contacts of People Infected With HTLV-III*, an informational brochure; *Dental Care for Gay and Bisexual Men*, a brochure of facts about AIDS and oral care; *Safer Sex Guidelines*, a safer sex brochure; *AIDS Care*, a monthly newsletter
LANGUAGES: French

819. Ville Marie Social Service Centre/Centre de Services Sociaux Ville Marie
2155 Guy St, no 1010
Montreal, PQ H3H 2R9
(514) 989-1885

KEY PERSONNEL: David Cassidy; AIDS Liaison
FACILITY TYPE: Research; Educational; Hospital; Client services/case management; Social service agency
YEAR FOUNDED: 1973
FUNDING: State government
OUTREACH: Community outreach and education to those who request

AVAILABLE LITERATURE: *Spectrum*, newsletter
LANGUAGES: French

DIRECTORY OF ORGANIZATIONS – INDEX BY TYPE

Advocacy

AIDS Action Committee (AAC); MA, 373
AIDS Committee of Windsor (ACW); ON, 796
The Atlanta Gay Center, Inc; GA, 243
Connecticut AIDS Action Council (CAAC); CT, 160
Fund for Human Dignity; NY, 503
Health Information Network; WA, 743
LifeLink, PWA Coalition of Washington, DC; DC, 193
Michigan Organization for Human Rights (MOHR); MI, 399
Women's AIDS Network (WAN); CA, 140

Client services/case management

Action AIDS, Inc; PA, 625
AID Atlanta; GA, 240
Aid For AIDS, Inc; CA, 30
Aid for AIDS of Nevada; NV, 438
AIDS/ARC Clothing Depot; CA, 33
AIDS ARMS Network; TX, 673
AIDS Clinic, Harborview Medical Center; WA, 733
AIDS Council of Northeastern New York, Inc (ACNENY); NY, 475
AIDS Foundation Houston, Inc (AFH); TX, 676
AIDS Interfaith Network (AIN); TX, 677
AIDS Program Office (APO); DE, 178
AIDS Project, Duval County Public Health Unit; FL, 211
AIDS Project of the East Bay (APEB); CA, 43
AIDS Services Foundation for Orange County (ASF); CA, 47
AIDS Services of Austin (ASA); TX, 681
AIDS-Related Community Services (ARCS); NY, 485
Alaskan AIDS Assistance Association (4A's); AK, 6
Arizona AIDS Project, Inc (AAP); AZ, 16
Association of People Living With AIDS (APLWA); WA, 737
Cascade AIDS Project, Inc (CAP); OR, 612
Catholic Community Services Homecare ("Chore Services"); WA, 739
Center One, Anyone in Distress, Inc; FL, 216
Coastal Bend AIDS Foundation, Inc (CBAF); TX, 687
Coming Home/Coming Home Support Services; CA, 65
Community AIDS Council (CAC); AZ, 18
Cristo AIDS Ministry; AZ, 19
Damien Center; IN, 296
El Centro Human Services Organizations, Milagros AIDS Project; CA, 72
Face To Face, Sonoma County AIDS Network (SCAN); CA, 73
God's Love We Deliver, Inc (GLWD); NY, 507
Hyacinth Foundation AIDS Project; NJ, 459

Kupona; IL, 281
La Casa de Don Pedro, Inc; NJ, 461
LifeLink, PWA Coalition of Washington, DC; DC, 193
Long Island Association for AIDS Care, Inc (LIAAC); NY, 519
Malama Pono/Kauai AIDS Project; HI, 259
Milwaukee AIDS Project (MAP); WI, 780
Mobile AIDS Support Services (MASS); AL, 3
Mountain State AIDS Network (MSAN); WV, 769
National Association of People With AIDS Atlanta Chapter (NAPWA Atlanta); GA, 250
New York City Dept of Health, Division of AIDS Program Services; NY, 531
Prince George's County Health Dept, Office on AIDS; MD, 366
Project AHEAD (AIDS Health Education and Assistance Delivery); CA, 114
PWA Health Group; NY, 539
Sacramento AIDS Foundation (SAF); CA, 116
San Francisco AIDS Foundation; CA, 119
Social Security AIDS Regional Office V; IL, 288
Solano County Health Dept, AIDS Program; CA, 127
South Jersey AIDS Alliance (SJAA); NJ, 466
Southwest AIDS Committee, Inc (SWAC); TX, 719
Stanislaus Community AIDS Project (SCAP); CA, 131
Toronto PWA Foundation; ON, 815
Tucson AIDS Project, Inc (TAP); AZ, 24
Village Nursing Home AIDS Day Treatment Program (AIDS DTP); NY, 547
Ville Marie Social Service Centre/Centre de Services Sociaux Ville Marie; PQ, 819
Washington County AIDS Task Force; AR, 28
West Side AIDS Project; NY, 548
Western New York AIDS Program (WNYAP); NY, 550
Wicomico County Health Dept; MD, 372

Clinic

Adult Immunodeficiencies Clinic/San Francisco; CA, 29
AIDS Activities Coordinating Office (AACO); PA, 626
AIDS Clinic, County/University of Southern California Medical Center; CA, 35
AIDS Clinic, Harborview Medical Center; WA, 733
AIDS Committee of Toronto (ACT); ON, 795
AIDS Comprehensive Family Care Center; NY, 474
AIDS Control Program, Mobile County Health Dept; AL, 1

AIDS Epidemiology Program/Albany; NY, 478
AIDS Project, Duval County Public Health Unit; FL, 211
The AIDS Project, Inc (TAP); ME, 343
AIDS Project/Norwalk; CT, 158
AIDS Services; TX, 680
AIDS Services, County Health Care Services; CA, 46
Allegheny County Health Dept; PA, 630
Amarillo Bi-City County Health Dept; TX, 682
Arkansas Dept of Health AIDS Prevention Program (APP); AR, 27
Association for Women's AIDS Research and Education (Project AWARE); CA, 55
The Atlanta Gay Center, Inc; GA, 243
Baltimore City Health Dept, Preventive Medicine and Epidemiology Bureau of Sexually Transmitted Diseases; MD, 350
Bartholomew County Health Dept, Counseling and Testing Site; IN, 295
Bay CPHU; FL, 214
Beekman Downtown Hospital; NY, 489
Betances Health Unit, Inc; NY, 491
Blue Bus Clinic; WI, 772
Brady East STD Clinic; WI, 773
Bronx Municipal Hospital Center; NY, 494
Brown County Health Dept; SD, 658
Canton City AIDS Task Force; OH, 571
Carroll County Health Dept; TN, 664
Case Western Reserve University; OH, 573
Centro Latinoamericano de Enfermedades de Transmision Sexual (CLETS); PR, 788
Charles County Health Dept; MD, 352
Chase-Brexton Clinic; MD, 353
Chinatown Health Clinic; NY, 499
Ciaccio Memorial Clinic of the Beach Area Community Health Center; CA, 63
Cincinnati Health Dept, AIDS Program; OH, 574
Cleveland City, Dept of Health and Human Resources; OH, 577
The Clinic; ME, 344
Clinic for AIDS and Related Disorders (C.A.R.D.); CA, 64
Clinical AIDS Program/Boston City Hospital; MA, 375
Collier County AIDS Task Force; FL, 219
Columbia/Boone County Health Dept; MO, 421
Columbus Health Dept; OH, 580
Community Clinic, Inc/San Antonio; TX, 688
Community Drug Board; OH, 582
Community Health Project (CHP); NY, 500
Cook County Dept of Public Health (CCDPH); IL, 272
Cook County Hospital AIDS Service; IL, 273
Cordelia Martin Health Center, Neighborhood Health Association, Inc; OH, 583

Danbury Health Dept AIDS Program; CT, 163

DARCO, Drug Services, Inc; TX, 690

Dayton Free Clinic and Counseling Center; OH, 585

DeKalb County Board of Health; GA, 247

Denver AIDS Prevention Program; CO, 145

Desert AIDS Project; CA, 68

Division of AIDS Activities/San Francisco; CA, 69

Dodge City Family Planning Clinic, Inc; KS, 318

Dorchester County Health Dept, AIDS Health Service Coordination; MD, 355

Douglas County Health and Social Services Health Center; OR, 613

Duke University AIDS Clinical Trials Unit; NC, 554

DuPage County Health Dept; IL, 274

East Bay AIDS Center (EBAC); CA, 71

East Orange Health Dept, HIV Counseling and Testing Site; NJ, 457

Eastside Neighborhood Health Center; CO, 146

El Paso City-County Health District, Sexually Transmitted Disease Clinic, Tillman Center; TX, 691

Englewood Community Health Organization (ECHO); IL, 275

Evansville-Vanderburgh County Dept of Public Health; IN, 298

Fairbanks Health Center; AK, 9

Feminist Health Center of Portsmouth STD Clinic; NH, 444

Fenway Community Health Center (FCHC); MA, 379

Fort Worth Public Health Dept; TX, 694

Franklin-Williamson Bi-County Health Dept; IL, 276

Garfield County Health Dept; OK, 607

Gary Health Dept, Counseling and Testing Site; IN, 299

The Gay and Lesbian Community Services Center; CA, 76

Gay Men's Health Collective/Berkeley; CA, 78

Gay Men's Venereal Disease Clinic/ Washington; DC, 190

Gays and Lesbians in Health Care; ON, 804

Genesee County Health Dept; MI, 393

Grand Island/Hall County Dept of Health; NE, 435

Greater Cincinnati AIDS Task Force; OH, 587

Greenwich Dept of Health, Office of HIV Information and Services; CT, 165

Haight-Ashbury Free Clinics; CA, 79

Harbor/UCLA Medical Center; CA, 80

Harris County Health Dept; TX, 696

Hartford Gay and Lesbian Health Collective, Inc; CT, 166

Hassle Free Clinic; ON, 807

Hemophilia Center of Western Pennsylvania (HEWP); PA, 637

Hemophilia Council of California (HCC); CA, 82

Hemophilia Foundation of Illinois; IL, 278

Hemophilia Foundation of Michigan (HFM); MI, 396

Hennepin County Medical Center (HCMC); MN, 410

HIV Counseling and Testing Service, Feminist Health Center—Portsmouth; NH, 445

HIV Education and Counseling Center; OH, 589

Howard Brown Memorial Clinic (HBMC); IL, 269

Howard County Health Dept; MD, 358

HRS/Hillsbourough County Health Dept/ AIDS Program; FL, 225

Illinois Alcoholism and Drug Dependence Association (IADDA), AIDS Project; IL, 280

Institute for Immunological Disorders; TX, 701

Interfaith Medical Center; NY, 515

Iowa City Free Medical Clinic; IA, 315

Jackson County Health Dept; MI, 397

Johns Hopkins Hospital First AIDS Service; MD, 359

Kansas City Free Health Clinic; MO, 426

La Ahanza Hispana, Inc; MA, 381

La Casa de Don Pedro, Inc; NJ, 461

Latin American STD Center; PR, 790

Laurens County Health Department/South Central Health District; GA, 249

Lee County Health Dept; IL, 283

Lee County Public Health Unit, Immunology Clinic; FL, 229

Leon County Public Health Unit; FL, 230

Lexington Fayette County Health Dept (LFCHD); KY, 325

Life Foundation/Honolulu; HI, 258

Lincoln Hospital Acupuncture Clinic; NY, 518

Mahoning County Area AIDS Task Force; OH, 594

Maryland Dept of Health and Mental Hygiene, AIDS Administration; MD, 360

Massachusetts Center for Disease Control, Division of Communicable Disease Control; MA, 384

Medical College of Ohio; OH, 595

Memorial Sloan-Kettering Cancer Center; NY, 521

Metropolitan AIDS Project (MAP); NY, 522

Mission Crisis Service; CA, 100

Monroe County Health Dept, AIDS Education Project (MCPHU, AEP); FL, 231

Montgomery County (Ohio) Health Dept; OH, 596

Montrose Clinic; TX, 704

Montrose Counseling Center (MCC); TX, 705

Multnomah County Health Division AIDS Program; OR, 617

Municipality of Anchorage, Dept of Health and Human Services; AK, 11

New Mexico Public Health Div, District IV Health Office; NM, 472

New Orleans Health Dept, Delgado (STD) Clinic; LA, 337

North East Neighborhood Association (NENA); NY, 534

Norwalk Health Dept, AIDS Program; CT, 173

Oak Lawn Counseling Center; TX, 707

Ohio Dept of Health, AIDS Unit; OH, 599

Orange County Health Care Agency; CA, 111

Parkland Memorial Hospital AIDS Clinic; TX, 711

Peoria City County Health Dept (PCCHD); IL, 285

Persad Center, Inc; PA, 642

Philadelphia Community Health Alternatives/The Philadelphia AIDS Task Force (PCHA/PATF); PA, 643

Placer County Health Dept; CA, 113

Planned Parenthood Association of Southwest Florida, Naples Chapter; FL, 234

Prince George's County Health Dept, Office on AIDS; MD, 366

Racine Health Dept, City of Racine, HIV Antibody Counseling and Testing Site; WI, 783

Red Door Clinic; MN, 413

Rhode Island Dept of Health, AIDS Program; RI, 651

Riverside County Office of AIDS Coordination (COAC); CA, 115

Roosevelt Hospital and AIDS Clinic; NY, 541

Saint Joseph/Buchanan County Community Health Clinic; MO, 428

Saint Louis Effort for AIDS (EFA); MO, 429

Saint Lucie County Public Health Unit (SLCPHU); FL, 235

Saint Paul Division of Public Health; MN, 414

Saint Paul Urban Indian Health Board; MN, 415

Saline County Nursing Service; MO, 430

San Luis Obispo County AIDS Education and Prevention Project; CA, 122

Santa Clara County Health Dept AIDS Program; CA, 123

Seattle AIDS Assessment Clinic; WA, 754

Seattle Gay Clinic; WA, 757

Seattle-King County AIDS Prevention Project; WA, 759

Sexually Transmitted Disease Program, Municipality of Anchorage; AK, 13

Shasta County Public Health (SCPH); CA, 126

Solano County Health Dept, AIDS Program; CA, 127

Southwest District Health Dept (SWDHD); ID, 265

Southwest Utah District Health Dept, Health Clinic; UT, 724

Southwest Washington Health District; WA, 761

Spalding County Health Dept; GA, 253

Special Immunology Unit (SIU); OH, 603

State of Florida Dept of Health and Rehabilitative Services, AIDS Program Office, District II; FL, 236

Strafford County Prenatal and Family Planning Program (The Clinic); NH, 450

Stuyvesant Polyclinic Adult Medical Clinic; NY, 545

Tecumseh Area Planned Parenthood Association, Inc (TAPPA), AIDS Counseling and Testing Program; IN, 305

Tennessee Dept of Health and Environment, AIDS Program; TN, 668

Terrebonne Parish Health Unit; LA, 340

Toledo City Health Dept; OH, 605

Tulane-LSU AIDS Clinical Trials Unit (ACTU); LA, 341

UCLA Medical Center, Immunology Clinic; CA, 135

UCSF AIDS Clinical Research Center; CA, 136

University of California at Los Angeles AIDS Clinical Research Center (UCLA AIDS Clinical Research Center); CA, 138

University of Maryland Medical School, Infectious Disease Clinic, AIDS Patient Care Program; MD, 370

University of Miami, AIDS Clinical Research Unit (ACRU); FL, 239

University of Oregon Health Sciences Center, Division of Infectious Diseases; OR, 622

VA Cooperative Studies No. 298: Treatment of AIDS and AIDS-Related Complex; NC, 563

Village Clinic and Winnipeg Gay Community Health Centre, Inc (WGCHC,Inc); MB, 818

Waikiki Health Center (WHC); HI, 261

Washtenaw County Public Health Division, AIDS Counseling and Testing Clinic; MI, 403

Waterbury Dept of Public Health, AIDS Program; CT, 176

Wayne County Health Dept; MI, 404

Whitman-Walker Clinic, Inc; DC, 206

Wicomico County Health Dept; MD, 372

Women's AIDS Project; CA, 141

Yale University Health Services; CT, 177

Yellowstone City-County Health Dept, Deering Community Health Center; MT, 432

Educational

Action AIDS, Inc; PA, 625
Adult Immunodeficiencies Clinic/San Francisco; CA, 29
AID Atlanta; GA, 240
Aid for AIDS of Nevada; NV, 438
Aid to End AIDS Committee (ATEAC)/ Memphis; TN, 662
AIDS Action Committee (AAC); MA, 373
AIDS Action Committee/Key West; FL, 208
AIDS Action of Central Maine; ME, 342
AIDS Activities Coordinating Office (AACO); PA, 626
AIDS Advisory Council; ND, 565
AIDS/ARC Services Division of the Catholic Charities, San Francisco; CA, 34
AIDS Campaign Trust/Washington; DC, 181
AIDS Care Network; IL, 266
AIDS Center of Queens County, Inc (ACQC); NY, 473
AIDS Clinic, County/University of Southern California Medical Center; CA, 35
AIDS Clinic, Harborview Medical Center; WA, 733
AIDS Coalition/Caspar; WY, 785
AIDS Coalition of Northeast Iowa; IA, 307
AIDS Coalition of Northern Utah; UT, 722
AIDS Coastal Empire (ACE) Foundation; GA, 241
AIDS Committee of Cambridge, Kitchener/ Waterloo and Area (ACCKWA); ON, 792
The AIDS Committee of Ottawa (ACO); ON, 793
AIDS Committee of Thunder Bay (ACT-B); ON, 794
AIDS Committee of Toronto (ACT); ON, 795
AIDS Committee of Windsor (ACW); ON, 796
AIDS Comprehensive Family Care Center; NY, 474
AIDS Control Program; NC, 551
AIDS Control Program, Mobile County Health Dept; AL, 1
AIDS Council of Northeastern New York, Inc (ACNENY); NY, 475
AIDS: Counseling and Assistance Program (AIDS:CAP), Gay and Lesbian Resource Center (GLRC); CA, 36
AIDS/Denton, Inc; TX, 675
AIDS Education and Resources Center, School of Allied Health Professions; NY, 476
AIDS Education and Service Coordination Project; NY, 477
AIDS Education Programs/Jacksonville; FL, 209
AIDS Education Project/Division of Northern California Coalition for Rural Health, Inc; CA, 37
AIDS Education Project, New Jersey Lesbian and Gay Coalition; NJ, 451
AIDS Epidemiology Program/Albany; NY, 478
AIDS Foundation Houston, Inc (AFH); TX, 676
The AIDS Health Project; CA, 39
AIDS Institute; NY, 479
AIDS Interfaith Network (AIN); TX, 677
AIDS Ministries Program; CT, 152
AIDS Network of Edmonton Society; AB, 797
AIDS Positive Action League (APAL); CA, 41
AIDS Prevention Program; NM, 470
AIDS Prevention Program, West Virginia State Health Dept; WV, 766
AIDS Prevention Research Center; NY, 480

AIDS Program; AK, 5
AIDS Program, Center for Infectious Diseases, Centers for Disease Control (CDC); GA, 242
AIDS Program Office (APO); DE, 178
AIDS Project, Duval County Public Health Unit; FL, 211
AIDS Project Greater Danbury; CT, 153
AIDS Project/Greater New Britain (AP/ GNB); CT, 154
AIDS Project/Hartford (AP/H); CT, 155
The AIDS Project, Inc (TAP); ME, 343
AIDS Project Los Angeles (APLA); CA, 42
AIDS Project: Middlesex County; CT, 156
AIDS Project New Haven (APNH); CT, 157
AIDS Project/Norwalk; CT, 158
AIDS Project of the East Bay (APEB); CA, 43
AIDS Project/Seattle; WA, 734
AIDS Project/Springfield; MO, 420
AIDS Project Utah; UT, 723
AIDS Provider Education Experience (APEX); CA, 44
AIDS Regina; SK, 798
AIDS Resource Center; TX, 679
AIDS Resource, Education and Assistance (AREA); FL, 212
AIDS Resource Foundation for Children, Saint Clare's Home for Children; NJ, 452
AIDS Response Knoxville (ARK); TN, 663
AIDS Response Program of Orange County (ARP); CA, 45
AIDS Rochester, Inc (ARI); NY, 482
AIDS Saskatoon; SK, 799
AIDS Services; TX, 680
AIDS Services, County Health Care Services; CA, 46
AIDS Services Foundation for Orange County (ASF); CA, 47
AIDS Services of Austin (ASA); TX, 681
The AIDS Services Project (TASP); NC, 552
AIDS Support Group/Miami; FL, 213
AIDS Support Network of Spartanburg (ASNS); SC, 653
AIDS Support Program, Inc (ASP); OK, 606
AIDS Task Force, Inc; IN, 294
AIDS Task Force of Central New York; NY, 483
AIDS Treatment News; CA, 49
AIDS Vancouver Island; BC, 800
AIDS Volunteers of Cincinnati (AVOC); OH, 567
AIDS-Related Community Services (ARCS); NY, 485
Alaskan AIDS Assistance Association (4A's); AK, 6
The Aliveness Project Center For Living; MN, 409
Allegheny County Health Dept; PA, 630
Amarillo Bi-City County Health Dept; TX, 682
American Association of Physicians for Human Rights (AAPHR); CA, 50
American Association of Sex Educators, Counselors and Therapists (AASECT); DC, 183
American College Health Association (ACHA), Task Force on AIDS; MD, 349
American College of Obstetricians and Gynecologists (ACOG); DC, 184
American Foundation for AIDS Research (AmFAR); CA, 51
American Management Association (AMA); NY, 486
American Medical Association (AMA); IL, 268
American Red Cross AIDS Education Coalition of Nebraska (ARCAEC); NE, 433
American Red Cross, AIDS Education Program; DC, 185
American Red Cross, Columbus Area Chapter; OH, 568

American Red Cross, Erie; PA, 631
American Red Cross, Northeast Region; MA, 374
American Red Cross of Northern New Jersey; NJ, 453
American Red Cross, Roanoke Valley Chapter; VA, 728
American Red Cross, Seattle-King County Chapter; WA, 736
American Red Cross, Tanana Valley Chapter; AK, 7
American Run for the End of AIDS (AREA); NY, 487
Among Friends; WI, 771
APGHL AIDS Educational Committee; NB, 801
Arctic Gay and Lesbian Association; AK, 8
Aris Project; CA, 53
Arizona AIDS Information Line; AZ, 15
Arizona AIDS Project, Inc (AAP); AZ, 16
Arkansas A.I.D.S. Foundation; AR, 26
Arkansas Dept of Health AIDS Prevention Program (APP); AR, 27
Asian AIDS Project; CA, 54
Association for Drug Abuse Prevention and Treatment, Inc (ADAPT); NY, 488
Association for Women's AIDS Research and Education (Project AWARE); CA, 55
Association of People Living With AIDS (APLWA); WA, 737
Athens AIDS Task Force; OH, 569
The Atlanta Gay Center, Inc; GA, 243
The Austin PWA Coalition; TX, 683
Baltimore City Health Dept, Preventive Medicine and Epidemiology Bureau of Sexually Transmitted Diseases; MD, 350
Bay Area Physicians for Human Rights (BAPHR); CA, 56
Bay CPHU; FL, 214
Bayview-Hunter's Point Foundation, AIDS Education Unit; CA, 57
BEBASHI (Blacks Educating Blacks About Sexual Health Issue); PA, 633
Being Alive/People with AIDS Action Coalition, Inc, Los Angeles; CA, 58
Berks AIDS Health Crisis (BAHC); PA, 634
Betances Health Unit, Inc; NY, 491
Billings AIDS Support Network; MT, 431
Brady East STD Clinic; WI, 773
Bridgeport AIDS Advisory Committee; CT, 159
Brooklyn AIDS Task Force; NY, 495
Calhoun County AIDS Education Steering Committee; MI, 390
California Association of AIDS Agencies (CAAA); CA, 59
California Dept of Health Services, Office of AIDS; CA, 60
Canadian Public Health Association (CPHA), AIDS Education and Awareness Program; ON, 802
Canton City AIDS Task Force; OH, 571
Caribbean Haitian Council, Inc (CAHACO); NJ, 455
Cascade AIDS Project, Inc (CAP); OR, 612
Case Western Reserve University; OH, 573
Catholic Schools of Dallas; TX, 685
Center for Interdisciplinary Research in Immunology and Disease (CIRID) at UCLA; CA, 61
Center One, Anyone in Distress, Inc; FL, 216
Central Florida AIDS Unified Resources, Inc (CENTAUR); FL, 217
Central Iowa AIDS Project (CIAP); IA, 310
Central Louisiana AIDS Support Services (CLASS); LA, 330
Central Valley AIDS Team (CVAT); CA, 62
Centro Latinoamericano de Enfermedades de Transmision Sexual (CLETS); PR, 788
Charles County Health Dept; MD, 352

Fund-raising

Health department

Solano County Health Dept, AIDS Program; CA, 127

South Dakota Dept of Health, Communicable Disease Program, AIDS Surveillance and Prevention Project; SD, 660

Southwest District Health Dept (SWDHD); ID, 265

Spalding County Health Dept; GA, 253

Spartanburg County Health Dept; SC, 656

State of Nevada Health Division; NV, 441

Talbot County Health Dept, AIDS Program; MD, 368

Tazewell County Health Dept; IL, 291

Terrebonne Parish Health Unit; LA, 340

United States Conference of Local Health Officers (USCLHO); DC, 202

Vermont Dept of Health; VT, 726

Wayne County Health Dept; MI, 404

Westchester County Dept of Health; NY, 549

Wood County Health Dept; WI, 784

York City Bureau of Health; PA, 649

York Health Corp; PA, 650

HIV counseling and testing

AIDS Care Network; IL, 266

AIDS Clinic, Harborview Medical Center; WA, 733

AIDS Coalition/Caspar; WY, 785

AIDS Control Program; NC, 551

AIDS Control Program, Mobile County Health Dept; AL, 1

AIDS Counseling and Testing Service/ Cheyenne; WY, 786

AIDS Institute; NY, 479

AIDS Network of Edmonton Society; AB, 797

AIDS Prevention Program; NM, 470

AIDS Prevention Program, West Virginia State Health Dept; WV, 766

AIDS Program; AK, 5

AIDS Program Office (APO); DE, 178

AIDS Project, Duval County Public Health Unit; FL, 211

The AIDS Project, Inc (TAP); ME, 343

AIDS Project: Middlesex County; CT, 156

AIDS Project/Norwalk; CT, 158

AIDS Services; TX, 680

AIDS Services, County Health Care Services; CA, 46

AIDS Support Program, Inc (ASP); OK, 606

Alaskan AIDS Assistance Association (4A's); AK, 6

Albert Einstein College of Medicine; NY, 502

Amarillo Bi-City County Health Dept; TX, 682

American Red Cross, Columbus Area Chapter; OH, 568

ANAWIM: AIDS Pastoral Care; PA, 632

The Aquarian Effort Heroin Detox Unit; CA, 52

Arkansas A.I.D.S. Foundation; AR, 26

Arkansas Dept of Health AIDS Prevention Program (APP); AR, 27

Atlantic City Health Dept; NJ, 454

Baltimore County Health Dept; MD, 351

Bartholomew County Health Dept, Counseling and Testing Site; IN, 295

BEBASHI (Blacks Educating Blacks About Sexual Health Issue); PA, 633

Bellevue Hospital Methadone Maintenance Tretment Program; NY, 490

Beth Israel Medical Center; NY, 492

Betterway Inc 12-Step Halfway House; FL, 215

Big Island AIDS Project; HI, 254

Billings AIDS Support Network; MT, 431

Brownsville Clinic; NY, 496

Bushwick Clinic; NY, 497

Canton City Health Dept; OH, 572

Carper House, Inc; OR, 611

Central District Health Dept; ID, 262

Charles County Health Dept; MD, 352

Charles I Schwartz Chemical Dependency Treatment Center; KY, 328

Chase-Brexton Clinic; MD, 353

Chattanooga Council on AIDS Resources, Education, and Support (CARES); TN, 665

Cherry Hill Drug Abuse Rehab; MD, 354

City of Richmond Community Mental Health Center; VA, 730

Clayton County Substance Abuse Program; GA, 245

Cleveland City, Dept of Health and Human Resources; OH, 577

The Clinic; ME, 344

CODAMA Services Connection to Care; AZ, 17

Columbia/Boone County Health Dept; MO, 421

Columbus Health Dept; OH, 580

Comprehensive Alcoholism Treatment Center; NY, 501

Connecticut Counseling Centers, Inc; CT, 161

Cook County Dept of Public Health (CCDPH); IL, 272

Cook County Hospital AIDS Service; IL, 273

Counseling Associates; PA, 636

Dallas County Health Dept, AIDS Prevention Project; TX, 689

DeKalb County Board of Health; GA, 247

Delaware Lesbian and Gay Health Advocates, Inc (DLGHA); DE, 179

Desert AIDS Project; CA, 68

Desire Narcotic Rehab Center (DNRC) Inc Drug Free; LA, 332

Dimock Substance Abuse Treatment Services; MA, 378

Dodge City Family Planning Clinic, Inc; KS, 318

Dorchester County Health Dept, AIDS Health Service Coordination; MD, 355

DuPage County Health Dept; IL, 274

East Bay AIDS Center (EBAC); CA, 71

East Orange Health Dept, HIV Counseling and Testing Site; NJ, 457

El Paso City-County Health District, Sexually Transmitted Disease Clinic, Tillman Center; TX, 691

Erie County General Health District AIDS Task Force; OH, 586

Evansville-Vanderburgh County Dept of Public Health; IN, 298

Fairbanks Health Center; AK, 9

Fenway Community Health Center (FCHC); MA, 379

Fort Worth Counseling Center, AIDS Project; TX, 693

Franklin-Williamson Bi-County Health Dept; IL, 276

Garfield County Health Dept; OK, 607

Gary Health Dept, Counseling and Testing Site; IN, 299

Gay Community Center (GCC); HI, 255

Genesee County Health Dept; MI, 393

Grand Island/Hall County Dept of Health; NE, 435

Greenwich Dept of Health, Office of HIV Information and Services; CT, 165

Harris County Health Dept; TX, 696

Hartford Gay and Lesbian Health Collective, Inc; CT, 166

Hassle Free Clinic; ON, 807

Health Crisis Network, Inc (HCN); FL, 223

HIV Counseling and Testing Service, Feminist Health Center—Portsmouth; NH, 445

Horizons Community Services, Inc; IL, 279

Howard Brown Memorial Clinic (HBMC); IL, 269

Humanite Society AIDS Information and Referral Service; TX, 700

Immunological Support Program; LA, 335

Iowa City Free Medical Clinic; IA, 315

Isla Vista Medical Clinic; CA, 91

Jackson County Health Dept; MI, 397

Johns Hopkins Hospital First AIDS Service; MD, 359

Kalamazoo County AIDS Prevention Program; MI, 398

Kaleidoscope; NY, 517

Kansas City Free Health Clinic; MO, 426

Kauai District Health Office; HI, 257

Lake County Substance Abuse Program; IL, 282

Larimer County Health Dept; CO, 149

Lee County Public Health Unit, Immunology Clinic; FL, 229

Leon County Public Health Unit; FL, 230

Lexington Fayette County Health Dept (LFCHD); KY, 325

Liberation Programs, Inc; CT, 168

Madison Dept of Public Health; WI, 779

Mahoning County Area AIDS Task Force; OH, 594

Maine Dept of Human Services, Office on AIDS; ME, 345

Maricopa County Dept of Health Services; AZ, 20

Maryland Dept of Health and Mental Hygiene, AIDS Administration; MD, 360

Massachusetts Center for Disease Control, Division of Communicable Disease Control; MA, 384

Maui District Health Office, Hawaii State Dept of Health; HI, 260

Meridian House; MA, 387

Mid Cumberland Regional Health Office, Tennessee Dept of Health and Environment; TN, 666

Midway Complex Alcoholism Program; TX, 703

Mobile AIDS Support Services (MASS); AL, 3

Momentum AIDS Outreach Program; NY, 524

Montefiore MMTP Unit 2; NY, 525

Montrose Clinic; TX, 704

Montrose Counseling Center (MCC); TX, 705

Municipality of Anchorage, Dept of Health and Human Services; AK, 11

Narcotics Withdrawal Centers, Inc; TX, 706

National Association of People With AIDS Atlanta Chapter (NAPWA Atlanta); GA, 250

New Brunswick Counseling Center; NJ, 464

New London AIDS Educational, Counseling and Testing Service; CT, 171

New Orleans Health Dept, Delgado (STD) Clinic; LA, 337

New Start Residential Substance Abuse Treatment Program; GA, 251

New York City Dept of Health, Division of AIDS Program Services; NY, 531

New York State Dept of Health, HIV Counseling and Testing Program; NY, 533

North Shore University Hospital Drug Treatment and Education Center; NY, 535

Northeast Ohio Task Force on AIDS (NEOTFA); OH, 597

Northern Kentucky AIDS Task Force; KY, 327

Northern Region AIDS/STD Program; AK, 12

Norwalk Health Dept, AIDS Program; CT, 173

NUVA Inc Outpatient Alcohol and Drug Counseling; MA, 389

Office of Gay and Lesbian Health Concerns (OGLHC); NY, 537

Ohio Dept of Health, AIDS Unit; OH, 599

Olmsted County Health Dept; MN, 412

Panhandle AIDS Support Organization, Inc (PASO); TX, 710
Pennsylvania Dept of Health, Division of Acute Infectious Disease Epidemiology, AIDS Program; PA, 641
Peoria City County Health Dept (PCCHD); IL, 285
Philadelphia Community Health Alternatives/The Philadelphia AIDS Task Force (PCHA/PATF); PA, 643
Phoenix Rising; OR, 619
Phoenix Shanti Group; AZ, 22
Prince George's County Health Dept, Office on AIDS; MD, 366
Racine Health Dept, City of Racine, HIV Antibody Counseling and Testing Site; WI, 783
Rhode Island Dept of Health, AIDS Program; RI, 651
Riverside County Office of AIDS Coordination (COAC); CA, 115
Sacramento County Health Dept, AIDS Unit; CA, 117
Saint Francis Center; DC, 201
Saint Joseph/Buchanan County Community Health Clinic; MO, 428
Saint Lucie County Public Health Unit (SLCPHU); FL, 235
Saint Paul Division of Public Health; MN, 414
Saline County Nursing Service; MO, 430
San Luis Obispo County AIDS Education and Prevention Project; CA, 122
Santa Clara County Health Dept AIDS Program; CA, 123
Santa Cruz AIDS Project (SCAP); CA, 124
Sexually Transmitted Disease Program, Municipality of Anchorage; AK, 13
Sitka Health Center; AK, 14
Solano County Health Dept, AIDS Program; CA, 127
South Dakota Dept of Health, Communicable Disease Program, Pierre Area Regional Field Office; SD, 661
Southwest District Health Dept (SWDHD); ID, 265
Spalding County Health Dept; GA, 253
St Mary's Alcohol/Drug Addiction Treatment Center; IL, 287
Stamford Health Dept: AIDS Program; CT, 175
Starting Point; NY, 544
State of Florida Dept of Health and Rehabilitative Services, AIDS Program Office, District II; FL, 236
Substance Abuse and Alcoholism Treatment Center, Inc; IL, 290
Suicide Prevention Center Methadone Maintenance; CA, 134
The Sycamore Center; NC, 561
Talbot County Health Dept, AIDS Program; MD, 368
Tazewell County Health Dept; IL, 291
Tecumseh Area Planned Parenthood Association, Inc (TAPPA), AIDS Counseling and Testing Program; IN, 305
Tennessee Dept of Health and Environment, AIDS Program; TN, 668
Third Horizon; NY, 546
University of Maryland Drug Treatment Center Drug-Free Program; MD, 369
University of Miami, AIDS Clinical Research Unit (ACRU); FL, 239
VA Medical Center; NJ, 467
Vanderbilt AIDS Project (VAP); TN, 671
Vermont Dept of Health; VT, 726
Vida Latina; MI, 402
Village Clinic and Winnipeg Gay Community Health Centre, Inc (WGCHC,Inc); MB, 818
Waikiki Health Center (WHC); HI, 261

Washtenaw County Public Health Division, AIDS Counseling and Testing Clinic; MI, 403
Waterbury Dept of Public Health, AIDS Program; CT, 176
West End Drug Abuse Program; MD, 371
West Side AIDS Project; NY, 548
West Texas AIDS Foundation (WesTAF); TX, 721
WestCare Family Services Division; NV, 442
Western Health Clinics; OR, 623
Whitman-Walker Clinic, Inc; DC, 206
Wicomico County Health Dept; MD, 372
Women's AIDS Project; CA, 141
Wood County Health Dept; WI, 784
Yellowstone City-County Health Dept, Deering Community Health Center; MT, 432
York City Bureau of Health; PA, 649
York Health Corp; PA, 650
Youth Help Stepps Program; WA, 765

Home care

AIDS/ARC Home Care Program, Adult/In-Home Based Services Bureau, Social Services Div, Human Services Dept, State of New Mexico; NM, 468
AIDS Interfaith Network (AIN); TX, 677
Comprehensive AIDS Program of Palm Beach County, Inc (CAP); FL, 220
Hospice of Seattle/Providence Home Care; WA, 744
Metropolitan Visiting Nurses Association (MVNA); MN, 411
Visiting Nurses and Hospice of San Francisco (VNH); CA, 139

Hospice

AIDS Interfaith Network (AIN); TX, 677
AIDS Resource Center, Inc; NY, 481
AIDS Resource Foundation for Children, Saint Clare's Home for Children; NJ, 452
AIDS Services Foundation for Orange County (ASF); CA, 47
AIDS Task Force, Inc; IN, 294
Carper House, Inc; OR, 611
Chattanooga Council on AIDS Resources, Education, and Support (CARES); TN, 665
The Community Health Trust of Kentucky; KY, 324
Damien Center; IN, 296
Damien Ministries; DC, 186
Dorchester County Health Dept, AIDS Health Service Coordination; MD, 355
Grand Rapids AIDS Task Force (GRATF); MI, 394
Green Tree Hospice; WI, 777
Home Nursing Agency, AIDS Intravention Project of Central Pennsylvania; PA, 638
Hospice of Central Iowa (HCI); IA, 311
Hospice of Saint John; CO, 148
Hospice of Seattle/Providence Home Care; WA, 744
Metropolitan Visiting Nurses Association (MVNA); MN, 411
Mid-Missouri AIDS Project (MMAP); MO, 427
Mid-Oregon AIDS/Health/Education and Support Services, Inc (MASS); OR, 616
Norwalk Health Dept, AIDS Program; CT, 173
Omega House; TX, 708
Project Lazarus; LA, 339
Ruby House; OR, 620
San Antonio AIDS Foundation; TX, 715
San Francisco Dept of Public Health, The AIDS Office; CA, 120
Southwest AIDS Committee, Inc (SWAC); TX, 719
Topeka AIDS Project, Inc (TAP); KS, 321

Triangle AIDS Network, Inc; TX, 720
Visiting Nurses and Hospice of San Francisco (VNH); CA, 139

Hospital

AIDS Clinic, Harborview Medical Center; WA, 733
AIDS Comprehensive Family Care Center; NY, 474
AIDS Project: Middlesex County; CT, 156
Bayview-Hunter's Point Foundation, AIDS Education Unit; CA, 57
Beekman Downtown Hospital; NY, 489
Beth Israel Medical Center; NY, 492
Cabrini Medical Center; NY, 498
Case Western Reserve University; OH, 573
Clinic for AIDS and Related Disorders (C.A.R.D.); CA, 64
Clinical AIDS Program/Boston City Hospital; MA, 375
Comprehensive Pediatric AIDS Program (CPAP); MA, 376
Cook County Hospital AIDS Service; IL, 273
Danbury Health Dept AIDS Program; CT, 163
Denver AIDS Prevention Program; CO, 145
Division of AIDS Activities/San Francisco; CA, 69
Duke University AIDS Clinical Trials Unit; NC, 554
East Bay AIDS Center (EBAC); CA, 71
Good Samaritan Hospital AIDS Task Force; OR, 615
Hemophilia Council of California (HCC); CA, 82
Hemophilia Foundation of Illinois; IL, 278
Hennepin County Medical Center (HCMC); MN, 410
Immunological Support Program; LA, 335
Interfaith Medical Center; NY, 515
Jackson Memorial Hospital AIDS Center; FL, 227
Johns Hopkins Hospital First AIDS Service; MD, 359
Mobile AIDS Support Services (MASS); AL, 3
Nassau County Medical Center, AIDS Program; NY, 526
Northern Lights Alternatives, Inc; NY, 536
Parkland Memorial Hospital AIDS Clinic; TX, 711
Roosevelt Hospital and AIDS Clinic; NY, 541
Saline County Nursing Service; MO, 430
Special Immunology Unit (SIU); OH, 603
Stop AIDS Project—California; CA, 133
Tulane-LSU AIDS Clinical Trials Unit (ACTU); LA, 341
UCSF AIDS Clinical Research Center; CA, 136
University of Oregon Health Sciences Center, Division of Infectious Diseases; OR, 622
VA Cooperative Studies No. 298: Treatment of AIDS and AIDS-Related Complex; NC, 563
Ville Marie Social Service Centre/Centre de Services Sociaux Ville Marie; PQ, 819

Legal

AIDS and Employment Protection; CA, 32
AIDS Legal Hotline/Houston; TX, 678
Justice, Inc; IN, 301
Milwaukee AIDS Project (MAP); WI, 780
National Gay Rights Advocates (NGR); CA, 105
National Lawyers Guild AIDS Network; CA, 106
New York City Commission on Human Rights and Discrimination Unit; NY, 529

Office of Human Rights/Seattle; WA, 749
Volunteer Attorneys for Persons With AIDS (VAPWA) Legal Referral Project; WA, 763

Lobbying

AIDS Action Council/Washington; DC, 180
Gay Rights National Lobby/AIDS Project; DC, 191
Human Rights Campaign Fund (HRCF); DC, 192
Michigan Organization for Human Rights (MOHR); MI, 399
National Gay and Lesbian Task Force (NGLTF); DC, 198
Stanislaus Community AIDS Project (SCAP); CA, 131

Referral

AIDS Coalition/Caspar; WY, 785
AIDS/Denton, Inc; TX, 675
AIDS Network of Edmonton Society; AB, 797
Gay and Lesbian Community Center of Colorado, Inc (GLCCC); CO, 147
Malama Pono/Kauai AIDS Project; HI, 259
Wellness Networks, Inc (WNI); MI, 408
Wyoming AIDS Project; WY, 787

Religious

AIDS/ARC Services Division of the Catholic Charities, San Francisco; CA, 34
AIDS Interfaith Network (AIN); TX, 677
AIDS Ministries Program; CT, 152
Catholic Schools of Dallas; TX, 685
Cristo AIDS Ministry; AZ, 19
Jackson Metropolitan Community Church; MS, 417
Light of Love Metropolitan Community Church (MCC)—Midland/Odessa; TX, 702

Research

Adult Immunodeficiencies Clinic/San Francisco; CA, 29
AIDS Clinic, County/University of Southern California Medical Center; CA, 35
AIDS Clinic, Harborview Medical Center; WA, 733
AIDS Clinical Trials Unit (ACTU); DC, 182
AIDS Comprehensive Family Care Center; NY, 474
The AIDS Health Project; CA, 39
AIDS Institute; NY, 479
AIDS Prevention Research Center; NY, 480
AIDS Program; AK, 5
AIDS Program, Center for Infectious Diseases, Centers for Disease Control (CDC); GA, 242
AIDS Project of the Cancer Center/Baltimore; MD, 348
AIDS Project/Springfield; MO, 420
Amarillo Bi-City County Health Dept; TX, 682
American College Health Association (ACHA), Task Force on AIDS; MD, 349
American Foundation for AIDS Research (AmFAR); CA, 51
American Red Cross, AIDS Education Program; DC, 185
American Red Cross, Northeast Region; MA, 374
Arkansas Dept of Health AIDS Prevention Program (APP); AR, 27
Asian AIDS Project; CA, 54
Association for Women's AIDS Research and Education (Project AWARE); CA, 55
The Atlanta Gay Center, Inc; GA, 243
The Austin PWA Coalition; TX, 683
Blue Bus Clinic; WI, 772
Carolina AIDS Research and Education Project (CARE); SC, 654

Center for Interdisciplinary Research in Immunology and Disease (CIRID) at UCLA; CA, 61
Center Project, Inc; WI, 774
Centro Latinoamericano de Enfermedades de Transmision Sexual (CLETS); PR, 788
Children's Hospice International (CHI); VA, 729
City of Milwaukee Health Dept; WI, 775
Clinic for AIDS and Related Disorders (C.A.R.D.); CA, 64
Clinical AIDS Program/Boston City Hospital; MA, 375
Colorado Dept of Health, STD/AIDS Control; CO, 144
Cook County Hospital AIDS Service; IL, 273
Damien Center; IN, 296
DARCO, Drug Services, Inc; TX, 690
Delaware Lesbian and Gay Health Advocates, Inc (DLGHA); DE, 179
Denver AIDS Prevention Program; CO, 145
Division of AIDS Activities/San Francisco; CA, 69
Documentation of AIDS Issues and Research Foundation, Inc (DAIR); CA, 70
Duke University AIDS Clinical Trials Unit; NC, 554
Family Research Institute, Inc; DC, 189
Fenway Community Health Center (FCHC); MA, 379
Gay and Lesbian Alliance (GALA); OR, 614
Haight-Ashbury Free Clinics; CA, 79
Hawaii AIDS Task Group (HATG); HI, 256
Health Crisis Network, Inc (HCN); FL, 223
Health Education AIDS Liaison, Inc (HEAL); NY, 510
Hemophilia Center of Western Pennsylvania (HEWP); PA, 637
Hemophilia Foundation of Michigan (HFM); MI, 396
Hennepin County Medical Center (HCMC); MN, 410
Homosexual Information Center/Hollywood; CA, 83
Howard Brown Memorial Clinic (HBMC); IL, 269
Humboldt County Dept of Public Welfare; CA, 86
Institute for Advanced Study of Human Sexuality (IASHS); CA, 89
Institute for Immunological Disorders; TX, 701
International Health Research Foundation; FL, 226
Johns Hopkins Hospital First AIDS Service; MD, 359
Kansas AIDS Network, Inc (KAN); KS, 319
KS Research and Education Foundation/San Francisco; CA, 93
LaHara Steele Productions; NJ, 462
L.I.F.T., Inc, AIDS Education/Prevention Program for Minorities; NJ, 463
Lower Eastside Service Center, Inc, AIDS Prevention Program; NY, 520
Maryland Dept of Health and Mental Hygiene, AIDS Administration; MD, 360
Massachusetts Center for Disease Control, Division of Communicable Disease Control; MA, 384
Mayor's AIDS Study Group/Baltimore; MD, 361
Midwest Hispanic AIDS Coalition (MHAC)/Coalicion Hispana Sobre el SIDA del Medioeste; IL, 284
Montreal AIDS Resource Committee—Association des Resources Montrealais sur la SIDA (MARC/ARMS); PQ, 810
Multnomah County Health Division AIDS Program; OR, 617
National Association for Lesbian and Gay Gerontology (NALGG); CA, 104

National Association of Public Hospitals (NAPH); DC, 197
National Institute of Allergy and Infectious Diseases (NIAID); MD, 364
National Institute of Drug Abuse (NIDA); MD, 365
National League for Nursing, Inc (NLN); NY, 527
National Native American AIDS Prevention Center (NNAAPC); CA, 108
New York City Dept of Health, Division of AIDS Program Services; NY, 531
Ohio Dept of Health, AIDS Unit; OH, 599
Orange County Health Care Agency; CA, 111
Oregon AIDS Task Force, Research and Education Group; OR, 618
Parkland Memorial Hospital AIDS Clinic; TX, 711
The People With AIDS Coalition of Tucson (PACT); AZ, 21
Pitt Men's Study (PMS); PA, 644
The Reimer Foundation; IL, 286
Rhode Island Dept of Health, AIDS Program; RI, 651
Saint Paul Division of Public Health; MN, 414
San Antonio AIDS Medical Foundation; TX, 716
San Francisco Dept of Public Health, The AIDS Office; CA, 120
Seattle-King County AIDS Prevention Project; WA, 759
Special Immunology Unit (SIU); OH, 603
State of Florida Dept of Health and Rehabilitative Services, AIDS Program Office, District II; FL, 236
Toronto PWA Foundation; ON, 815
Tulane-LSU AIDS Clinical Trials Unit (ACTU); LA, 341
UCSF AIDS Clinical Research Center; CA, 136
University of California at Los Angeles AIDS Clinical Research Center (UCLA AIDS Clinical Research Center); CA, 138
University of Illinois at Chicago, AIDS Outreach Intervention Project; IL, 293
University of Miami, AIDS Clinical Research Unit (ACRU); FL, 239
University of Oregon Health Sciences Center, Division of Infectious Diseases; OR, 622
University of Tennessee, Memphis, The Health Science Center; TN, 670
VA Cooperative Studies No. 298: Treatment of AIDS and AIDS-Related Complex; NC, 563
Vanderbilt AIDS Project (VAP); TN, 671
Ville Marie Social Service Centre/Centre de Services Sociaux Ville Marie; PQ, 819
Whitman-Walker Clinic, Inc; DC, 206

Residential facility (adults)

AIDS/ARC Services Division of the Catholic Charities, San Francisco; CA, 34
AIDS Resource Center, Inc; NY, 481
Center One, Anyone in Distress, Inc; FL, 216
Chicago House and Social Service Agency, Inc; IL, 271
Delaware Lesbian and Gay Health Advocates, Inc (DLGHA); DE, 179
EarthTide, Inc; MD, 356
The Family Link; CA, 75
Hope House of the Palm Beaches, Inc; FL, 224
Joshua House; OH, 590
Project Lazarus; LA, 339

Residential facility (children)

The Children's Home; TX, 686

Comprehensive Pediatric AIDS Program (CPAP); MA, 376
Open Arms, Inc; TX, 709

Social service agency

AIDS Minority Health Initiative (AMHI); CA, 40
Congreso de Latinos Unidos, Inc; PA, 635
Hispanic Association of Ocean County, Inc; NJ, 458
Horizons Community Services, Inc; IL, 279
Nashville Council on AIDS Resources, Education and Services (Nashville CARES); TN, 667
Social Security Administration, El Paso; TX, 718
Social Security Administration/Upper Darby; PA, 646
Ville Marie Social Service Centre/Centre de Services Sociaux Ville Marie; PQ, 819

Substance abuse treatment

Albert Einstein College of Medicine; NY, 502
The Aquarian Effort Heroin Detox Unit; CA, 52
Association for Drug Abuse Prevention and Treatment, Inc (ADAPT); NY, 488
Bellevue Hospital Methadone Maintenance Tretment Program; NY, 490
Betterway Inc 12-Step Halfway House; FL, 215
Brownsville Clinic; NY, 496
Bushwick Clinic; NY, 497
Charles I Schwartz Chemical Dependency Treatment Center; KY, 328
Cherry Hill Drug Abuse Rehab; MD, 354
Clayton County Substance Abuse Program; GA, 245
CODAMA Services Connection to Care; AZ, 17
Comprehensive Alcoholism Treatment Center; NY, 501
Connecticut Counseling Centers, Inc; CT, 161
Counseling Associates; PA, 636
CURA (Community United for the Rehabilitation of the Addicted); NJ, 456
Desire Narcotic Rehab Center (DNRC) Inc Drug Free; LA, 332
Dimock Substance Abuse Treatment Services; MA, 378
Dorchester County Health Dept, AIDS Health Service Coordination; MD, 355
Humanite Society AIDS Information and Referral Service; TX, 700
Isla Vista Medical Clinic; CA, 91
Kaleidoscope; NY, 517
La Casa de Don Pedro, Inc; NJ, 461
LaHara Steele Productions; NJ, 462
Lake County Substance Abuse Program; IL, 282
Liberation Programs, Inc; CT, 168
Lower Eastside Service Center, Inc, AIDS Prevention Program; NY, 520
Meridian House; MA, 387
Midway Complex Alcoholism Program; TX, 703
Montefiore MMTP Unit 2; NY, 525
Narcotics Withdrawal Centers, Inc; TX, 706
New Brunswick Counseling Center; NJ, 464
New Start Residential Substance Abuse Treatment Program; GA, 251
North Shore University Hospital Drug Treatment and Education Center; NY, 535
NUVA Inc Outpatient Alcohol and Drug Counseling; MA, 389
Office of Gay and Lesbian Health Concerns (OGLHC); NY, 537
St Mary's Alcohol/Drug Addiction Treatment Center; IL, 287

Starting Point; NY, 544
Substance Abuse and Alcoholism Treatment Center, Inc; IL, 290
Suicide Prevention Center Methadone Maintenance; CA, 134
The Sycamore Center; NC, 561
Third Horizon; NY, 546
University of Maryland Drug Treatment Center Drug-Free Program; MD, 369
VA Medical Center; NJ, 467
Washington Area Council on Alcohol and Drug Abuse; DC, 205
West End Drug Abuse Program; MD, 371
WestCare Family Services Division; NV, 442
Western Health Clinics; OR, 623
Youth Help Stepps Program; WA, 765

Support group

Action AIDS, Inc; PA, 625
AID Atlanta; GA, 240
Aid For AIDS, Inc; CA, 30
Aid for AIDS of Nevada; NV, 438
Aid to End AIDS Committee (ATEAC)/ Memphis; TN, 662
AIDS Action Committee (AAC); MA, 373
AIDS/ARC Clothing Depot; CA, 33
AIDS Care Network; IL, 266
AIDS Center of Queens County, Inc (ACQC); NY, 473
AIDS Coalition of Northeast Iowa; IA, 307
AIDS Coastal Empire (ACE) Foundation; GA, 241
The AIDS Committee of Ottawa (ACO); ON, 793
AIDS Committee of Thunder Bay (ACT-B); ON, 794
AIDS Committee of Toronto (ACT); ON, 795
AIDS Committee of Windsor (ACW); ON, 796
AIDS Comprehensive Family Care Center; NY, 474
AIDS Coordinating Committee/Dallas; TX, 674
AIDS Council of Northeastern New York, Inc (ACNENY); NY, 475
AIDS: Counseling and Assistance Program (AIDS:CAP), Gay and Lesbian Resource Center (GLRC); CA, 36
AIDS Education Project/Division of Northern California Coalition for Rural Health, Inc; CA, 37
AIDS Emergency Fund (AEF); CA, 38
The AIDS Health Project; CA, 39
AIDS Help, Inc; FL, 210
AIDS Impact Drop-in Support Group/ Albuquerque; NM, 469
AIDS Interfaith Network (AIN); TX, 677
AIDS Ministries Program; CT, 152
AIDS Network of Edmonton Society; AB, 797
AIDS Program Office (APO); DE, 178
AIDS Project Greater Danbury; CT, 153
AIDS Project/Greater New Britain (AP/ GNB); CT, 154
AIDS Project/Hartford (AP/H); CT, 155
The AIDS Project, Inc (TAP); ME, 343
AIDS Project Los Angeles (APLA); CA, 42
AIDS Project: Middlesex County; CT, 156
AIDS Project New Haven (APNH); CT, 157
AIDS Project of the East Bay (APEB); CA, 43
AIDS Project/Springfield; MO, 420
AIDS Project Utah; UT, 723
AIDS Regina; SK, 798
AIDS Resource Center, Inc; NY, 481
AIDS Resource, Education and Assistance (AREA); FL, 212
AIDS Resource Foundation for Children, Saint Clare's Home for Children; NJ, 452
AIDS Response Knoxville (ARK); TN, 663

AIDS Response Program of Orange County (ARP); CA, 45
AIDS Rochester, Inc (ARI); NY, 482
AIDS Saskatoon; SK, 799
AIDS Services Foundation for Orange County (ASF); CA, 47
AIDS Services of Austin (ASA); TX, 681
The AIDS Services Project (TASP); NC, 552
AIDS Spiritual Assistance; WA, 735
AIDS Support Group; AR, 25
AIDS Support Group/West Hollywood; CA, 48
AIDS Support Network of Spartanburg (ASNS); SC, 653
AIDS Support Program, Inc (ASP); OK, 606
AIDS Task Force, Inc; IN, 294
AIDS Task Force of Central New York; NY, 483
AIDS Task Force of National Council of Churches; NY, 484
AIDS Task Force of the Upper Ohio Valley; WV, 767
AIDS Vancouver Island; BC, 800
AIDS Volunteers of Cincinnati (AVOC); OH, 567
AIDS-Related Community Services (ARCS); NY, 485
Alaskan AIDS Assistance Association (4A's); AK, 6
The Aliveness Project Center For Living; MN, 409
ANAWIM: AIDS Pastoral Care; PA, 632
Arctic Gay and Lesbian Association; AK, 8
Aris Project; CA, 53
Arizona AIDS Project, Inc (AAP); AZ, 16
Arkansas A.I.D.S. Foundation; AR, 26
Association for Drug Abuse Prevention and Treatment, Inc (ADAPT); NY, 488
Association of People Living With AIDS (APLWA); WA, 737
Athens AIDS Task Force; OH, 569
The Atlanta Gay Center, Inc; GA, 243
The Austin PWA Coalition; TX, 683
Bayview-Hunter's Point Foundation, AIDS Education Unit; CA, 57
BEBASHI (Blacks Educating Blacks About Sexual Health Issue); PA, 633
Being Alive/People with AIDS Action Coalition, Inc, Los Angeles; CA, 58
Berks AIDS Health Crisis (BAHC); PA, 634
Beth Simchat Torah; NY, 493
Big Island AIDS Project; HI, 254
Billings AIDS Support Network; MT, 431
Blood Sisters; WA, 738
Brooklyn AIDS Task Force; NY, 495
Canton City AIDS Task Force; OH, 571
Caribbean Haitian Council, Inc (CAHACO); NJ, 455
Carper House, Inc; OR, 611
Cascade AIDS Project, Inc (CAP); OR, 612
Catholic Diocese of Dallas; TX, 684
Center One, Anyone in Distress, Inc; FL, 216
Central Florida AIDS Unified Resources, Inc (CENTAUR); FL, 217
Central Louisiana AIDS Support Services (CLASS); LA, 330
Central Valley AIDS Team (CVAT); CA, 62
Charleston AIDS Network (CAN); WV, 768
Chattanooga Council on AIDS Resources, Education, and Support (CARES); TN, 665
Chicago Coalition of Black Lesbians and Gays (CCBLG); IL, 270
Chicago House and Social Service Agency, Inc; IL, 271
Chicken Soup Brigade; WA, 740
Children's Hospice International (CHI); VA, 729
Cincinnati Health Dept, AIDS Program; OH, 574
Cleveland City, Dept of Health and Human Resources; OH, 577

Clinical AIDS Program/Boston City Hospital; MA, 375

Coastal Area Support Team, Inc (CAST); GA, 246

Coastal Bend AIDS Foundation, Inc (CBAF); TX, 687

Collier County AIDS Task Force; FL, 219

Colorado AIDS Project; CO, 143

Colorado Dept of Health, STD/AIDS Control; CO, 144

Columbus AIDS Task Force; OH, 579

Columbus Health Dept; OH, 580

Comite SIDA Aide Montreal (CSAM); PQ, 803

Community AIDS Council (CAC); AZ, 18

Community Drug Board; OH, 582

Community Health Project (CHP); NY, 500

The Community Health Trust of Kentucky; KY, 324

Community Relief for People with AIDS; LA, 331

Comprehensive AIDS Program of Palm Beach County, Inc (CAP); FL, 220

Cook County Hospital AIDS Service; IL, 273

Council of Churches of Greater Springfield; MA, 377

Crisis Clinic/Seattle; WA, 741

Dallas County Health Dept, AIDS Prevention Project; TX, 689

Damien Center; IN, 296

Damien Ministries; DC, 186

Danbury Health Dept AIDS Program; CT, 163

David Morgan AIDS Relief Fund; WA, 747

Delaware Lesbian and Gay Health Advocates, Inc (DLGHA); DE, 179

Desert AIDS Project; CA, 68

Dorchester County Health Dept, AIDS Health Service Coordination; MD, 355

EarthTide, Inc; MD, 356

East Orange Health Dept, HIV Counseling and Testing Site; NJ, 457

Eastern Dakota AIDS Network (EDAN); SD, 659

Eau Claire County Dept of Human Services; WI, 776

El Centro Human Services Organizations, Milagros AIDS Project; CA, 72

Episcopal Diocese of Dallas; TX, 692

Face To Face, Sonoma County AIDS Network (SCAN); CA, 73

Families Who Care (FWC); CA, 74

Fenway Community Health Center (FCHC); MA, 379

Fort Worth Counseling Center, AIDS Project; TX, 693

Four-State Community AIDS Project (CAP); MO, 422

Fundacion SIDA de Puerto Rico; PR, 789

Gay and Lesbian Alliance (GALA); OR, 614

Gay and Lesbian Community Center of Colorado, Inc (GLCCC); CO, 147

The Gay and Lesbian Community Services Center; CA, 76

Gay Community AIDS Project (GCAP); IL, 277

Gay Community Center (GCC); HI, 255

Gay Men's Counseling Service/Sayville; NY, 505

Gays of Ottawa; ON, 805

Good Samaritan Project; MO, 424

Grand Rapids AIDS Task Force (GRATF); MI, 394

Greater Louisiana Alliance for Dignity (GLAD); LA, 334

Greenwich AIDS Task Force; CT, 164

GROW AIDS Resource Project; NC, 556

Haitian Coalition on AIDS (HCA); NY, 508

Haitian Committee on AIDS in Massachusetts; MA, 380

Health Crisis Network, Inc (HCN); FL, 223

Health Education AIDS Liaison, Inc (HEAL); NY, 510

Health Education Association, Detroit (HEAD); MI, 395

Health Education Resource Organization (HERO); MD, 357

Health Issues Taskforce of Cleveland; OH, 588

Heart of America Human Services; MO, 425

Hemophilia Center of Western Pennsylvania (HEWP); PA, 637

Hemophilia Council of California (HCC); CA, 82

Hemophilia Foundation of Illinois; IL, 278

Hemophilia Foundation of Michigan (HFM); MI, 396

Hispanic AIDS Forum; NY, 512

Hispanos Unidos Contra El SIDA/AIDS, Inc; CT, 167

Home Nursing Agency, AIDS Intravention Project of Central Pennsylvania; PA, 638

Hope and Help Center/San Francisco; CA, 84

Howard Brown Memorial Clinic (HBMC); IL, 269

Hyacinth Foundation AIDS Project; NJ, 459

Idaho AIDS Foundation; ID, 263

Immunological Support Program; LA, 335

In Touch, A Community Service Program; WA, 745

Inland AIDS Project; CA, 88

Institute for Human Identity (IHI); NY, 514

Interfaith Medical Center; NY, 515

Iowa Center for AIDS/ARC Resources and Education (ICARE); IA, 313

Iowa City Crisis Intervention Center; IA, 314

Jackson Metropolitan Community Church; MS, 417

Jefferson County Committee on AIDS Information (JCCAI); NY, 516

Johns Hopkins Hospital First AIDS Service; MD, 359

Kansas City Free Health Clinic; MO, 426

Kingston AIDS Project; ON, 808

Kupona; IL, 281

La Ahanza Hispana, Inc; MA, 381

La Casa de Don Pedro, Inc; NJ, 461

Lake County AIDS Task Force; OH, 592

Lee County AIDS Task Force (Volunteer Committee); FL, 228

Lesbian and Gay Health Project (LGHP); NC, 557

Lesbian-Gay Community Service Center of Greater Cleveland; OH, 593

Long Island Association for AIDS Care, Inc (LIAAC); NY, 519

Los Angeles Shanti Foundation; CA, 97

Madison AIDS Support Network (MASN); WI, 778

Mahoning County Area AIDS Task Force; OH, 594

Maine Health Foundation, Inc; ME, 346

Marion County AIDS Coalition; IN, 303

Maryland Dept of Health and Mental Hygiene, AIDS Administration; MD, 360

Massachusetts Center for Disease Control, Division of Communicable Disease Control; MA, 384

Medical College of Ohio; OH, 595

Metro Area Committee on AIDS; NS, 809

Metrolina AIDS Project (MAP); NC, 558

Metropolitan AIDS Project (MAP); NY, 522

Mid-Fairfield AIDS Project, Inc; CT, 170

Mid-Missouri AIDS Project (MMAP); MO, 427

Mid-Oregon AIDS/Health/Education and Support Services, Inc (MASS); OR, 616

Midwest Hispanic AIDS Coalition (MHAC)/ Coalicion Hispana Sobre el SIDA del Medioeste; IL, 284

Milwaukee AIDS Project (MAP); WI, 780

Milwaukee Hospice Home Care, Inc (MHHC); WI, 781

Minority AIDS Project/Los Angeles; CA, 99

Minority Task Force on AIDS; NY, 523

Mississippi Gay/Lesbian Alliance (MGLA); MS, 418

Mobile AIDS Support Services (MASS); AL, 3

Montgomery AIDS Outreach, Inc; AL, 4

Montgomery County (Ohio) Health Dept; OH, 596

Montrose Counseling Center (MCC); TX, 705

Mothers of AIDS Patients (MAP); CA, 101

Mountain State AIDS Network (MSAN); WV, 769

Nashville Council on AIDS Resources, Education and Services (Nashville CARES); TN, 667

National AIDS Vigil Commission; DC, 195

National Association of People With AIDS Atlanta Chapter (NAPWA Atlanta); GA, 250

National Association of People with AIDS (NAPWA); DC, 196

National Lesbian and Gay Health Foundation (NLGHF); DC, 200

Nevada AIDS Foundation; NV, 439

New Hampshire AIDS Foundation (NHAF); NH, 447

New Jersey Buddies; NJ, 465

New Mexico AIDS Services, Inc (NMAS); NM, 471

Newfoundland and Labrador AIDS Committee, Inc; NF, 812

North Central Florida AIDS Network (NCFAN); FL, 232

North State AIDS Project (NSAP); CA, 109

Northeast AIDS Council of Pennsylvania, Inc (NAC); PA, 639

Northeast Ohio Task Force on AIDS (NEOTFA); OH, 597

Northern Lights Alternatives, Inc; NY, 536

Northwest AIDS Foundation; WA, 748

Norwalk Health Dept, AIDS Program; CT, 173

Oasis Community Center, AIDS Hotline; OK, 608

Open Arms, Inc; TX, 709

Open Worried Well Group/Seattle; WA, 751

Orange County Health Care Agency; CA, 111

Panhandle AIDS Support Organization, Inc (PASO); TX, 710

Parkland Memorial Hospital AIDS Clinic; TX, 711

People with AIDS/ARC of San Francisco; CA, 112

People with AIDS Coalition Houston, Inc (PWACH, Inc); TX, 712

People with AIDS Coalition, Inc (PWA Coalition); NY, 538

People with AIDS Coalition of Dallas, Inc (PWA Coalition of Dallas, Inc); TX, 713

The People With AIDS Coalition of Tucson (PACT); AZ, 21

Persad Center, Inc; PA, 642

Philadelphia Community Health Alternatives/The Philadelphia AIDS Task Force (PCHA/PATF); PA, 643

Phoenix Rising; OR, 619

Phoenix Shanti Group; AZ, 22

Pittsburgh AIDS Task Force (PATF); PA, 645

Prince George's County Health Dept, Office on AIDS; MD, 366

Project AHEAD (AIDS Health Education and Assistance Delivery); CA, 114

Project AIDS Lafayette, Inc (PAL); IN, 304

Quad Cities AIDS Coalition (QCAC); IA, 317

Rhode Island Project/AIDS (RIP/AIDS); RI, 652

Task force

DIRECTORY OF ORGANIZATIONS –
ALPHABETICAL LIST

Abilene AIDS Task Force; TX, 672

Action AIDS, Inc; PA, 625

Adult Immunodeficiencies Clinic/San Francisco; CA, 29

AID Atlanta; GA, 240

Aid For AIDS, Inc; CA, 30

Aid for AIDS of Nevada; NV, 438

AID Jacksonville; FL, 207

Aid to End AIDS Committee (ATEAC)/ Memphis; TN, 662

AIDS Action Committee (AAC); MA, 373

AIDS Action Committee/Key West; FL, 208

AIDS Action Council/Washington; DC, 180

AIDS Action of Central Maine; ME, 342

AIDS Activities Coordinating Office (AACO); PA, 626

AIDS Advisory Committee of San Bernardino County; CA, 31

AIDS Advisory Council; ND, 565

AIDS and Employment Protection; CA, 32

AIDS/ARC Clothing Depot; CA, 33

AIDS/ARC Home Care Program, Adult/In-Home Based Services Bureau, Social Services Div, Human Services Dept, State of New Mexico; NM, 468

AIDS/ARC Services Division of the Catholic Charities, San Francisco; CA, 34

AIDS ARMS Network; TX, 673

AIDS Campaign Trust/Washington; DC, 181

AIDS Care Network; IL, 266

AIDS Center of Queens County, Inc (ACQC); NY, 473

AIDS Clinic, County/University of Southern California Medical Center; CA, 35

AIDS Clinic, Harborview Medical Center; WA, 733

AIDS Clinical Trials Unit (ACTU); DC, 182

AIDS Coalition/Caspar; WY, 785

AIDS Coalition of Northeast Iowa; IA, 307

AIDS Coalition of Northern Utah; UT, 722

AIDS Coastal Empire (ACE) Foundation; GA, 241

AIDS Committee of Cambridge, Kitchener/ Waterloo and Area (ACCKWA); ON, 792

The AIDS Committee of Ottawa (ACO); ON, 793

AIDS Committee of Thunder Bay (ACT-B); ON, 794

AIDS Committee of Toronto (ACT); ON, 795

AIDS Committee of Windsor (ACW); ON, 796

AIDS Comprehensive Family Care Center; NY, 474

AIDS Control Program; NC, 551

AIDS Control Program, Mobile County Health Dept; AL, 1

AIDS Coordinating Committee/Dallas; TX, 674

AIDS Council of Erie County, Inc; PA, 627

AIDS Council of Northeastern New York, Inc (ACNENY); NY, 475

AIDS: Counseling and Assistance Program (AIDS:CAP), Gay and Lesbian Resource Center (GLRC); CA, 36

AIDS Counseling and Testing Service/ Cheyenne; WY, 786

AIDS Crisis Taskforce/Lexington; KY, 323

AIDS/Denton, Inc; TX, 675

AIDS Education and Resources Center, School of Allied Health Professions; NY, 476

AIDS Education and Service Coordination Project; NY, 477

AIDS Education Committee, Gay Coalition of Des Moines; IA, 308

AIDS Education Programs/Jacksonville; FL, 209

AIDS Education Project/Division of Northern California Coalition for Rural Health, Inc; CA, 37

AIDS Education Project, New Jersey Lesbian and Gay Coalition; NJ, 451

AIDS Emergency Fund (AEF); CA, 38

AIDS Epidemiology Program/Albany; NY, 478

AIDS Foundation Houston, Inc (AFH); TX, 676

AIDS Foundation of Chicago (AFC); IL, 267

The AIDS Health Project; CA, 39

AIDS Help, Inc; FL, 210

AIDS Impact Drop-in Support Group/ Albuquerque; NM, 469

AIDS Institute; NY, 479

AIDS Interfaith Network (AIN); TX, 677

AIDS Intervention Project/Altoona; PA, 628

AIDS Legal Hotline/Houston; TX, 678

AIDS Ministries Program; CT, 152

AIDS Minority Health Initiative (AMHI); CA, 40

AIDS Network of Edmonton Society; AB, 797

AIDS Positive Action League (APAL); CA, 41

AIDS Prevention Program; NM, 470

AIDS Prevention Program, West Virginia State Health Dept; WV, 766

AIDS Prevention Research Center; NY, 480

AIDS Program; AK, 5

AIDS Program, Center for Infectious Diseases, Centers for Disease Control (CDC); GA, 242

AIDS Program Office (APO); DE, 178

AIDS Project, Duval County Public Health Unit; FL, 211

AIDS Project Greater Danbury; CT, 153

AIDS Project/Greater New Britain (AP/ GNB); CT, 154

AIDS Project/Hartford (AP/H); CT, 155

The AIDS Project, Inc (TAP); ME, 343

AIDS Project Los Angeles (APLA); CA, 42

AIDS Project: Middlesex County; CT, 156

AIDS Project New Haven (APNH); CT, 157

AIDS Project/Norwalk; CT, 158

AIDS Project of the Cancer Center/ Baltimore; MD, 348

AIDS Project of the East Bay (APEB); CA, 43

AIDS Project/Seattle; WA, 734

AIDS Project/Springfield; MO, 420

AIDS Project Utah; UT, 723

AIDS Provider Education Experience (APEX); CA, 44

AIDS Regina; SK, 798

AIDS Resource Center; TX, 679

AIDS Resource Center, Inc; NY, 481

AIDS Resource, Education and Assistance (AREA); FL, 212

AIDS Resource Foundation for Children, Saint Clare's Home for Children; NJ, 452

AIDS Response Knoxville (ARK); TN, 663

AIDS Response Program of Orange County (ARP); CA, 45

AIDS Rochester, Inc (ARI); NY, 482

AIDS Saskatoon; SK, 799

AIDS Services; TX, 680

AIDS Services, County Health Care Services; CA, 46

AIDS Services Foundation for Orange County (ASF); CA, 47

AIDS Services of Austin (ASA); TX, 681

The AIDS Services Project (TASP); NC, 552

AIDS Spiritual Assistance; WA, 735

AIDS Support Group; AR, 25

The AIDS Support Group/Charlottesville; VA, 727

AIDS Support Group/Miami; FL, 213

AIDS Support Group of Quad Cities; IA, 309

AIDS Support Group/West Hollywood; CA, 48

AIDS Support Network of Spartanburg (ASNS); SC, 653

AIDS Support Program, Inc (ASP); OK, 606

AIDS Task Force, Inc; IN, 294

AIDS Task Force of Central New York; NY, 483

AIDS Task Force of National Council of Churches; NY, 484

AIDS Task Force of the Lehigh Valley; PA, 629

AIDS Task Force of the Upper Ohio Valley; WV, 767

AIDS Task Force of Winston-Salem; NC, 553

AIDS Treatment News; CA, 49

AIDS Vancouver Island; BC, 800

AIDS Volunteers of Cincinnati (AVOC); OH, 567

AIDS-Related Community Services (ARCS); NY, 485

Alaskan AIDS Assistance Association (4A's); AK, 6

Albert Einstein College of Medicine; NY, 502

The Aliveness Project Center For Living; MN, 409

Allegheny County Health Dept; PA, 630

Amarillo Bi-City County Health Dept; TX, 682

American Association of Physicians for Human Rights (AAPHR); CA, 50

American Association of Sex Educators, Counselors and Therapists (AASECT); DC, 183

American College Health Association (ACHA), Task Force on AIDS; MD, 349

American College of Obstetricians and Gynecologists (ACOG); DC, 184

American Foundation for AIDS Research (AmFAR); CA, 51

American Management Association (AMA); NY, 486

American Medical Association (AMA); IL, 268

American Red Cross AIDS Education Coalition of Nebraska (ARCAEC); NE, 433

American Red Cross, AIDS Education Program; DC, 185

American Red Cross, Columbus Area Chapter; OH, 568

American Red Cross, Erie; PA, 631

American Red Cross, Northeast Region; MA, 374

American Red Cross of Northern New Jersey; NJ, 453

American Red Cross, Roanoke Valley Chapter; VA, 728

American Red Cross, Seattle-King County Chapter; WA, 736

American Red Cross, Tanana Valley Chapter; AK, 7

American Run for the End of AIDS (AREA); NY, 487

Among Friends; WI, 771

ANAWIM: AIDS Pastoral Care; PA, 632

APGHL AIDS Educational Committee; NB, 801

The Aquarian Effort Heroin Detox Unit; CA, 52

Arctic Gay and Lesbian Association; AK, 8

Aris Project; CA, 53

Arizona AIDS Information Line; AZ, 15

Arizona AIDS Project, Inc (AAP); AZ, 16

Arkansas A.I.D.S. Foundation; AR, 26

Arkansas Dept of Health AIDS Prevention Program (APP); AR, 27

Asian AIDS Project; CA, 54

Association for Drug Abuse Prevention and Treatment, Inc (ADAPT); NY, 488

Association for Women's AIDS Research and Education (Project AWARE); CA, 55

Association of People Living With AIDS (APLWA); WA, 737

Athens AIDS Task Force; OH, 569

The Atlanta Gay Center, Inc; GA, 243

Atlantic City Health Dept; NJ, 454

Auglaize County AIDS Task Force; OH, 570

The Austin PWA Coalition; TX, 683

Baltimore City Health Dept, Preventive Medicine and Epidemiology Bureau of Sexually Transmitted Diseases; MD, 350

Baltimore County Health Dept; MD, 351

Bartholomew County Health Dept, Counseling and Testing Site; IN, 295

Baton Rouge MCC/AIDS Project; LA, 329

Bay Area Physicians for Human Rights (BAPHR); CA, 56

Bay CPHU; FL, 214

Bayview-Hunter's Point Foundation, AIDS Education Unit; CA, 57

BEBASHI (Blacks Educating Blacks About Sexual Health Issue); PA, 633

Beekman Downtown Hospital; NY, 489

Being Alive/People with AIDS Action Coalition, Inc, Los Angeles; CA, 58

Bellevue Hospital Methadone Maintenance Tretment Program; NY, 490

Berks AIDS Health Crisis (BAHC); PA, 634

Betances Health Unit, Inc; NY, 491

Beth Israel Medical Center; NY, 492

Beth Simchat Torah; NY, 493

Betterway Inc 12-Step Halfway House; FL, 215

Big Island AIDS Project; HI, 254

Billings AIDS Support Network; MT, 431

Birmingham AIDS Outreach; AL, 2

Blood Sisters; WA, 738

Blue Bus Clinic; WI, 772

Brady East STD Clinic; WI, 773

Bridgeport AIDS Advisory Committee; CT, 159

Bronx Municipal Hospital Center; NY, 494

Brooklyn AIDS Task Force; NY, 495

Brown County Health Dept; SD, 658

Brownsville Clinic; NY, 496

Bushwick Clinic; NY, 497

Cabrini Medical Center; NY, 498

Calhoun County AIDS Education Steering Committee; MI, 390

California Association of AIDS Agencies (CAAA); CA, 59

California Dept of Health Services, Office of AIDS; CA, 60

Canadian Public Health Association (CPHA), AIDS Education and Awareness Program; ON, 802

Canton City AIDS Task Force; OH, 571

Canton City Health Dept; OH, 572

Caribbean Haitian Council, Inc (CAHACO); NJ, 455

Carolina AIDS Research and Education Project (CARE); SC, 654

Carper House, Inc; OR, 611

Carroll County Health Dept; TN, 664

Cascade AIDS Project, Inc (CAP); OR, 612

Case Western Reserve University; OH, 573

Catholic Community Services Homecare ("Chore Services"); WA, 739

Catholic Diocese of Dallas; TX, 684

Catholic Schools of Dallas; TX, 685

Center for Interdisciplinary Research in Immunology and Disease (CIRID) at UCLA; CA, 61

Center One, Anyone in Distress, Inc; FL, 216

Center Project, Inc; WI, 774

Central City Network/Macon; GA, 244

Central District Health Dept; ID, 262

Central Florida AIDS Unified Resources, Inc (CENTAUR); FL, 217

Central Iowa AIDS Project (CIAP); IA, 310

Central Louisiana AIDS Support Services (CLASS); LA, 330

Central Valley AIDS Team (CVAT); CA, 62

Centro Latinoamericano de Enfermedades de Transmision Sexual (CLETS); PR, 788

Charles County Health Dept; MD, 352

Charles I Schwartz Chemical Dependency Treatment Center; KY, 328

Charleston AIDS Network (CAN); WV, 768

Charlotte County AIDS Task Force; FL, 218

Chase-Brexton Clinic; MD, 353

Chattanooga Council on AIDS Resources, Education, and Support (CARES); TN, 665

Cherry Hill Drug Abuse Rehab; MD, 354

Chicago Coalition of Black Lesbians and Gays (CCBLG); IL, 270

Chicago House and Social Service Agency, Inc; IL, 271

Chicken Soup Brigade; WA, 740

The Children's Home; TX, 686

Children's Hospice International (CHI); VA, 729

Children's Immune Disorder (CID); MI, 391

Chinatown Health Clinic; NY, 499

Ciaccio Memorial Clinic of the Beach Area Community Health Center; CA, 63

Cincinnati Health Dept, AIDS Program; OH, 574

Citizen Alliance Gay/Lesbian Rights, AIDS Education; NH, 443

City of Milwaukee Health Dept; WI, 775

City of Richmond Community Mental Health Center; VA, 730

Clayton County Substance Abuse Program; GA, 245

Cleveland AIDS Foundation; OH, 575

Cleveland Area AIDS Task Force; OH, 576

Cleveland City, Dept of Health and Human Resources; OH, 577

Cleveland/Cuyahoga County AIDS Task Force; OH, 578

The Clinic; ME, 344

Clinic for AIDS and Related Disorders (C.A.R.D.); CA, 64

Clinical AIDS Program/Boston City Hospital; MA, 375

Coastal Area Support Team, Inc (CAST); GA, 246

Coastal Bend AIDS Foundation, Inc (CBAF); TX, 687

CODAMA Services Connection to Care; AZ, 17

Collier County AIDS Task Force; FL, 219

Colorado AIDS Project; CO, 143

Colorado Dept of Health, STD/AIDS Control; CO, 144

Columbia/Boone County Health Dept; MO, 421

Columbus AIDS Task Force; OH, 579

Columbus Health Dept; OH, 580

Combined Health District/Dayton; OH, 581

Coming Home/Coming Home Support Services; CA, 65

Comite SIDA Aide Montreal (CSAM); PQ, 803

Community AIDS Council (CAC); AZ, 18

Community Clinic, Inc/San Antonio; TX, 688

Community Drug Board; OH, 582

Community Health Project (CHP); NY, 500

The Community Health Trust of Kentucky; KY, 324

Community Outreach Risk/Reduction Education Program (CORE Program); CA, 66

Community Relief for People with AIDS; LA, 331

Comprehensive AIDS Program of Palm Beach County, Inc (CAP); FL, 220

Comprehensive Alcoholism Treatment Center; NY, 501

Comprehensive Pediatric AIDS Program (CPAP); MA, 376

Computerized AIDS Information Network (CAIN); CA, 67

Congreso de Latinos Unidos, Inc; PA, 635

Connecticut AIDS Action Council (CAAC); CT, 160

Connecticut Counseling Centers, Inc; CT, 161

Connecticut Dept of Health Services, AIDS Section; CT, 162

Cook County Dept of Public Health (CCDPH); IL, 272

Cook County Hospital AIDS Service; IL, 273

Cordelia Martin Health Center, Neighborhood Health Association, Inc; OH, 583

Council of Churches of Greater Springfield; MA, 377

Counseling Associates; PA, 636

Crisis Clinic/Seattle; WA, 741

Cristo AIDS Ministry; AZ, 19

CURA (Community United for the Rehabilitation of the Addicted); NJ, 456

Dallas County Health Dept, AIDS Prevention Project; TX, 689

Damien Center; IN, 296

Damien Ministries; DC, 186

Danbury Health Dept AIDS Program; CT, 163

DARCO, Drug Services, Inc; TX, 690

David Morgan AIDS Relief Fund; WA, 747

Dayton Area AIDS Task Force (DAATF); OH, 584

Dayton Free Clinic and Counseling Center; OH, 585

DeKalb County Board of Health; GA, 247

Delaware Lesbian and Gay Health Advocates, Inc (DLGHA); DE, 179

Denver AIDS Prevention Program; CO, 145

Desert AIDS Project; CA, 68

Desire Narcotic Rehab Center (DNRC) Inc Drug Free; LA, 332

Dimock Substance Abuse Treatment Services; MA, 378

Division of AIDS Activities/San Francisco; CA, 69

Documentation of AIDS Issues and Research Foundation, Inc (DAIR); CA, 70

Dodge City Family Planning Clinic, Inc; KS, 318

Dorchester County Health Dept, AIDS Health Service Coordination; MD, 355

Douglas County Health and Social Services Health Center; OR, 613

Douglas County Health Dept, Epidemiology Section/AIDS Activity; NE, 434

Duke University AIDS Clinical Trials Unit; NC, 554

DuPage County Health Dept; IL, 274

Dupont West Medical Center; DC, 187

EarthTide, Inc; MD, 356

East Bay AIDS Center (EBAC); CA, 71

East Orange Health Dept, HIV Counseling and Testing Site; NJ, 457

Eastern Dakota AIDS Network (EDAN); SD, 659

Eastside Neighborhood Health Center; CO, 146

Eau Claire County Dept of Human Services; WI, 776

El Centro Human Services Organizations, Milagros AIDS Project; CA, 72

El Paso City-County Health District, Sexually Transmitted Disease Clinic, Tillman Center; TX, 691

Englewood Community Health Organization (ECHO); IL, 275

Episcopal Diocese of Dallas; TX, 692

ERASE; NC, 555

Erie County General Health District AIDS Task Force; OH, 586

Evansville AIDS Task Force; IN, 297

Evansville-Vanderburgh County Dept of Public Health; IN, 298

Everyday Theater Youth Ensemble; DC, 188

Face To Face, Sonoma County AIDS Network (SCAN); CA, 73

Fairbanks Health Center; AK, 9

Families Who Care (FWC); CA, 74

The Family Link; CA, 75

Family Research Institute, Inc; DC, 189

Feminist Health Center of Portsmouth STD Clinic; NH, 444

Fenway Community Health Center (FCHC); MA, 379

The Fight For Life Committee, Inc; FL, 221

Florida AIDS Hotline; FL, 222

Fort Worth Counseling Center, AIDS Project; TX, 693

Fort Worth Public Health Dept; TX, 694

Foundation for Health Education; LA, 333

Foundation for Human Understanding; TX, 695

Four-State Community AIDS Project (CAP); MO, 422

Franklin-Williamson Bi-County Health Dept; IL, 276

Fund for Human Dignity; NY, 503

Fundacion SIDA de Puerto Rico; PR, 789

Garfield County Health Dept; OK, 607

Gary Health Dept, Counseling and Testing Site; IN, 299

Gay and Lesbian Alliance (GALA); OR, 614

Gay and Lesbian Community Center/ Buffalo; NY, 504

Gay and Lesbian Community Center of Colorado, Inc (GLCCC); CO, 147

Gay and Lesbian Community Information Center/Detroit; MI, 392

The Gay and Lesbian Community Services Center; CA, 76

Gay and Lesbian Resource Center/Santa Barbara; CA, 77

Gay Community AIDS Project (GCAP); IL, 277

Gay Community Center (GCC); HI, 255

Gay Men's Counseling Service/Sayville; NY, 505

Gay Men's Health Collective/Berkeley; CA, 78

Gay Men's Health Crisis, Inc (GMHC); NY, 506

Gay Men's Health Group/Seattle; WA, 742

Gay Men's Venereal Disease Clinic/ Washington; DC, 190

Gay Rights National Lobby/AIDS Project; DC, 191

Gay Services Network, Inc; MO, 423

Gays and Lesbians in Health Care; ON, 804

Gays of Ottawa; ON, 805

Genesee County Health Dept; MI, 393

Georgia Dept of Human Resources, Division of Public Health, Office of Infectious Disease, AIDS Project; GA, 248

God's Love We Deliver, Inc (GLWD); NY, 507

Good Samaritan Hospital AIDS Task Force; OR, 615

Good Samaritan Project; MO, 424

Grand Island/Hall County Dept of Health; NE, 435

Grand Rapids AIDS Task Force (GRATF); MI, 394

Greater Cincinnati AIDS Task Force; OH, 587

Greater Louisiana Alliance for Dignity (GLAD); LA, 334

Green Tree Hospice; WI, 777

Greenwich AIDS Task Force; CT, 164

Greenwich Dept of Health, Office of HIV Information and Services; CT, 165

GROW AIDS Resource Project; NC, 556

Haight-Ashbury Free Clinics; CA, 79

Haitian Coalition on AIDS (HCA); NY, 508

Haitian Committee on AIDS in Massachusetts; MA, 380

Haitian Women's Program, American Friends Services Committee; NY, 509

Hamilton AIDS Network for Dialogue and Support (HANDS); ON, 806

Harbor/UCLA Medical Center; CA, 80

Harris County Health Dept; TX, 696

Hartford Gay and Lesbian Health Collective, Inc; CT, 166

Hassle Free Clinic; ON, 807

Hawaii AIDS Task Group (HATG); HI, 256

Health Crisis Network, Inc (HCN); FL, 223

Health Education AIDS Liaison, Inc (HEAL); NY, 510

Health Education Association, Detroit (HEAD); MI, 395

Health Education Resource Organization (HERO); MD, 357

Health Information Network; WA, 743

Health Issues Taskforce of Cleveland; OH, 588

HEALTH WATCH Information and Promotion Service; NY, 511

Heart of America Human Services; MO, 425

Hemophilia Center of Western Pennsylvania (HEWP); PA, 637

Hemophilia Council of California (HCC); CA, 82

Hemophilia Foundation of Illinois; IL, 278

Hemophilia Foundation of Michigan (HFM); MI, 396

Hennepin County Medical Center (HCMC); MN, 410

Hispanic AIDS Committee for Education and Resources (HACER); TX, 697

Hispanic AIDS Forum; NY, 512

Hispanic Association of Ocean County, Inc; NJ, 458

Hispanos Unidos Contra El SIDA/AIDS, Inc; CT, 167

HIV Counseling and Testing Service, Feminist Health Center—Portsmouth; NH, 445

HIV Education and Counseling Center; OH, 589

Home Nursing Agency, AIDS Intravention Project of Central Pennsylvania; PA, 638

Homosexual Information Center/Hollywood; CA, 83

Hope and Help Center/San Francisco; CA, 84

Hope House of the Palm Beaches, Inc; FL, 224

Horizons Community Services, Inc; IL, 279

Hospice of Central Iowa (HCI); IA, 311

Hospice of Saint John; CO, 148

Hospice of Seattle/Providence Home Care; WA, 744

Houston/Harris County Panel on AIDS; TX, 698

Houston Health and Human Services Dept, Bureau of Epidemiology—AIDS Surveillance and Seroprevalence Programs; TX, 699

Howard Brown Memorial Clinic (HBMC); IL, 269

Howard County Health Dept; MD, 358

HRS/Hillsbourough County Health Dept/ AIDS Program; FL, 225

Human Health Organization (HHO); CA, 85

Human Rights Campaign Fund (HRCF); DC, 192

Human Sexuality Program, Dept of Health Education; NY, 513

Humanite Society AIDS Information and Referral Service; TX, 700

Humboldt County Dept of Public Welfare; CA, 86

Hyacinth Foundation AIDS Project; NJ, 459

ICON PWA Fund; IA, 312

Idaho AIDS Foundation; ID, 263

Idaho AIDS Program, Dept of Health and Welfare; ID, 264

Identity, Inc; AK, 10

Illinois Alcoholism and Drug Dependence Association (IADDA), AIDS Project; IL, 280

Immunological Support Program; LA, 335

Imperial AIDS Foundation; CA, 87

In Touch, A Community Service Program; WA, 745

Indiana State Board of Health AIDS Activity Office; IN, 300

Inland AIDS Project; CA, 88

Institute for Advanced Study of Human Sexuality (IASHS); CA, 89

Institute for Human Identity (IHI); NY, 514

Institute for Immunological Disorders; TX, 701

Interfaith Medical Center; NY, 515

International Gay and Lesbian Archives; CA, 90

International Health Research Foundation; FL, 226

Iowa Center for AIDS/ARC Resources and Education (ICARE); IA, 313

Iowa City Crisis Intervention Center; IA, 314

Iowa City Free Medical Clinic; IA, 315

Isla Vista Medical Clinic; CA, 91

Jackson County Health Dept; MI, 397

Jackson Memorial Hospital AIDS Center; FL, 227

Jackson Metropolitan Community Church; MS, 417

Jefferson County Committee on AIDS Information (JCCAI); NY, 516

Jersey City Mayor's AIDS Task Force; NJ, 460

Johns Hopkins Hospital First AIDS Service; MD, 359

Johnson County AIDS Project; IA, 316

Joshua House; OH, 590

Justice, Inc; IN, 301

Kalamazoo County AIDS Prevention Program; MI, 398

Kaleidoscope; NY, 517

Kansas AIDS Network, Inc (KAN); KS, 319

Kansas City Free Health Clinic; MO, 426

Kauai District Health Office; HI, 257

Kent State University AIDS Task Force; OH, 591

Kern County AIDS Task Force; CA, 92

Kingston AIDS Project; ON, 808

Kitsap County AIDS Task Force; WA, 746

KS Research and Education Foundation/San Francisco; CA, 93

Kupona; IL, 281

La Ahanza Hispana, Inc; MA, 381

La Casa de Don Pedro, Inc; NJ, 461

LaHara Steele Productions; NJ, 462

Lake County AIDS Task Force; OH, 592

Lake County Substance Abuse Program; IL, 282

Larimer County Health Dept; CO, 149

The Latin American Center; NH, 446

Latin American STD Center; PR, 790

Laurens County Health Department/South Central Health District; GA, 249

Lee County AIDS Task Force (Volunteer Committee); FL, 228

Lee County Health Dept; IL, 283

Lee County Public Health Unit, Immunology Clinic; FL, 229

Leon County Public Health Unit; FL, 230

Lesbian and Gay Health Project (LGHP); NC, 557

Lesbian and Gay Rights Chapter/Los Angeles; CA, 94

Lesbian-Gay Community Service Center of Greater Cleveland; OH, 593

Lexington Fayette County Health Dept (LFCHD); KY, 325

Lexington Gay Services Organizations; KY, 326

Liberation Programs, Inc; CT, 168

Life Foundation/Honolulu; HI, 258

Lifeline Institute, Inc; MA, 382

LifeLink, PWA Coalition of Washington, DC; DC, 193

L.I.F.T., Inc, AIDS Education/Prevention Program for Minorities; NJ, 463

Light of Love Metropolitan Community Church (MCC)—Midland/Odessa; TX, 702

Lincoln Hospital Acupuncture Clinic; NY, 518

Long Island Association for AIDS Care, Inc (LIAAC); NY, 519

Los Angeles County Dept of Health Services, AIDS Program Office; CA, 95

Los Angeles Sex Information Helpline (LASIH); CA, 96

Los Angeles Shanti Foundation; CA, 97

Louise L Hay AIDS Support Group (HAYRIDE); CA, 81

Lower Eastside Service Center, Inc, AIDS Prevention Program; NY, 520

Madison AIDS Support Network (MASN); WI, 778

Madison/Delaware County AIDS Task Force; IN, 302

Madison Dept of Public Health; WI, 779

Mahoning County Area AIDS Task Force; OH, 594

Maine Dept of Human Services, Office on AIDS; ME, 345

Maine Health Foundation, Inc; ME, 346

Maine Lesbian/Gay Political Alliance; ME, 347

Malama Pono/Kauai AIDS Project; HI, 259

Maricopa County Dept of Health Services; AZ, 20

Marion County AIDS Coalition; IN, 303

Maryland Dept of Health and Mental Hygiene, AIDS Administration; MD, 360

Massachusetts AIDS Task Force; MA, 383

Massachusetts Center for Disease Control, Division of Communicable Disease Control; MA, 384

Massachusetts Dept of Public Health, Health Resource Office; MA, 385

Maui District Health Office, Hawaii State Dept of Health; HI, 260

Mayor's AIDS Study Group/Baltimore; MD, 361

Mayor's Liaison to Lesbian and Gay Community/Boston; MA, 386

Mayor's Task Force on AIDS; CT, 169

Mayor's Task Force on AIDS/San Diego; CA, 98

Medical College of Ohio; OH, 595

Memorial Sloan-Kettering Cancer Center; NY, 521

Meridian House; MA, 387

Metro Area Committee on AIDS; NS, 809

Metrolina AIDS Project (MAP); NC, 558

Metropolitan AIDS Project (MAP); NY, 522

Metropolitan Visiting Nurses Association (MVNA); MN, 411

Michigan Organization for Human Rights (MOHR); MI, 399

Mid Cumberland Regional Health Office, Tennessee Dept of Health and Environment; TN, 666

Mid-Fairfield AIDS Project, Inc; CT, 170

Mid-Missouri AIDS Project (MMAP); MO, 427

Mid-Oregon AIDS/Health/Education and Support Services, Inc (MASS); OR, 616

Midway Complex Alcoholism Program; TX, 703

Midwest Hispanic AIDS Coalition (MHAC)/Coalicion Hispana Sobre el SIDA del Medioeste; IL, 284

Milwaukee AIDS Project (MAP); WI, 780

Milwaukee Hospice Home Care, Inc (MHHC); WI, 781

Minority AIDS Project/Los Angeles; CA, 99

Minority People AIDS Concerns/New Orleans; LA, 336

Minority Task Force on AIDS; NY, 523

Mission Crisis Service; CA, 100

Mississippi Gay/Lesbian Alliance (MGLA); MS, 418

Mississippi State Dept of Health, AIDS/HIV Prevention Program; MS, 419

Mobile AIDS Support Services (MASS); AL, 3

Momentum AIDS Outreach Program; NY, 524

Monroe County Health Dept, AIDS Education Project (MCPHU, AEP); FL, 231

Montefiore MMTP Unit 2; NY, 525

Montgomery AIDS Outreach, Inc; AL, 4

Montgomery County HERO; MD, 362

Montgomery County (Ohio) Health Dept; OH, 596

Montreal AIDS Resource Committee—Association des Resources Montrealais sur la SIDA (MARC/ARMS); PQ, 810

Montrose Clinic; TX, 704

Montrose Counseling Center (MCC); TX, 705

Mothers of AIDS Patients (MAP); CA, 101

Mountain State AIDS Network (MSAN); WV, 769

Multi-Focus, Inc; CA, 102

Multnomah County Health Division AIDS Program; OR, 617

Municipality of Anchorage, Dept of Health and Human Services; AK, 11

The Names Project, sponsors of the AIDS Memorial Quilt; CA, 103

Narcotics Withdrawal Centers, Inc; TX, 706

Nashville Council on AIDS Resources, Education and Services (Nashville CARES); TN, 667

Nassau County Medical Center, AIDS Program; NY, 526

National Advisory Committee on AIDS (NAC-AIDS); ON, 811

National AIDS Information Clearinghouse (NAIC); MD, 363

National AIDS Network (NAN); DC, 194

National AIDS Vigil Commission; DC, 195

National Association for Lesbian and Gay Gerontology (NALGG); CA, 104

National Association of People With AIDS Atlanta Chapter (NAPWA Atlanta); GA, 250

National Association of People with AIDS (NAPWA); DC, 196

National Association of Public Hospitals (NAPH); DC, 197

National Coalition of Gay Sexually Transmitted Disease Services (NCGSTDS); WI, 782

National Gay and Lesbian Task Force (NGLTF); DC, 198

National Gay Rights Advocates (NGR); CA, 105

National Institute of Allergy and Infectious Diseases (NIAID); MD, 364

National Institute of Drug Abuse (NIDA); MD, 365

National Lawyers Guild AIDS Network; CA, 106

National Leadership Coalition on AIDS; DC, 199

National League for Nursing, Inc (NLN); NY, 527

National Lesbian and Gay Health Foundation (NLGHF); DC, 200

National Mobilization Against AIDS; CA, 107

National Native American AIDS Prevention Center (NNAAPC); CA, 108

NC AIDS Control Program; NC, 559

Nebraska AIDS Education and Training Center; NE, 436

Nebraska AIDS Project; NE, 437

Nevada AIDS Foundation; NV, 439

Nevada Hispanic Services, Inc; NV, 440

New Brunswick Counseling Center; NJ, 464

New Hampshire AIDS Foundation (NHAF); NH, 447

New Hampshire Buddy System; NH, 448

New Hampshire Division of Public Health Services, Bureau of Disease Control, AIDS Program; NH, 449

New Jersey Buddies; NJ, 465

New Jewish Agenda (NJA); NY, 528

New London AIDS Educational, Counseling and Testing Service; CT, 171

New Mexico AIDS Services, Inc (NMAS); NM, 471

New Mexico Public Health Div, District IV Health Office; NM, 472

New Orleans Health Dept, Delgado (STD) Clinic; LA, 337

New Start Residential Substance Abuse Treatment Program; GA, 251

New York City Commission on Human Rights and Discrimination Unit; NY, 529

New York City Dept of Health, AIDS Education Unit; NY, 530

New York City Dept of Health, Division of AIDS Program Services; NY, 531

New York State Dept of Health, AIDS Prevention Program; NY, 532

New York State Dept of Health, HIV Counseling and Testing Program; NY, 533

Newfoundland and Labrador AIDS Committee, Inc; NF, 812

Newton Health Dept; MA, 388

NO/AIDS Task Force; LA, 338

North Central Florida AIDS Network (NCFAN); FL, 232

North Dakota State Health Dept and Consolidated Laboratories; ND, 566

North East Neighborhood Association (NENA); NY, 534

North Shore University Hospital Drug Treatment and Education Center; NY, 535

North State AIDS Project (NSAP); CA, 109

Northeast AIDS Council of Pennsylvania, Inc (NAC); PA, 639

Northeast Ohio Task Force on AIDS (NEOTFA); OH, 597

Northern Kentucky AIDS Task Force; KY, 327

Northern Lights Alternatives, Inc; NY, 536

Northern Region AIDS/STD Program; AK, 12

Northwest AIDS Foundation; WA, 748

Northwest Connecticut AIDS Project; CT, 172

Norwalk Health Dept, AIDS Program; CT, 173

NUVA Inc Outpatient Alcohol and Drug Counseling; MA, 389

Oak Lawn Counseling Center; TX, 707

Oasis Community Center, AIDS Hotline; OK, 608

Office for Civil Rights; CA, 110

Office of Gay and Lesbian Health Concerns (OGLHC); NY, 537

Office of Health and Environmental Education, Kansas Dept of Health and Environment; KS, 320

Office of Human Rights/Seattle; WA, 749

Office on HIV/AIDS; WA, 750

Ohio AIDS Coalition (OAC); OH, 598

Ohio Dept of Health, AIDS Unit; OH, 599

Ohio Dept of Health, Bureau of Preventive Medicine, Communicable Disease Division, AIDS Activities Unit; OH, 600

Okaloosa County Public Health Unit; FL, 233

Oklahoma State Health Dept, AIDS Division; OK, 609

Olmsted County Health Dept; MN, 412

Omega House; TX, 708

Ontario Public Education Panel on AIDS; ON, 813

Open Arms, Inc; TX, 709

Open Worried Well Group/Seattle; WA, 751

Orange County Health Care Agency; CA, 111

Oregon AIDS Task Force, Research and Education Group; OR, 618

Palmetto AIDS Life Support Services; SC, 655

PALS; PA, 640

Panhandle AIDS Support Organization, Inc (PASO); TX, 710

Parkland Memorial Hospital AIDS Clinic; TX, 711

Pennsylvania Dept of Health, Division of Acute Infectious Disease Epidemiology, AIDS Program; PA, 641

People of Color Against AIDS Network (POCAAN); WA, 752

People with AIDS/ARC of San Francisco; CA, 112

People with AIDS Coalition Houston, Inc (PWACH, Inc); TX, 712

People with AIDS Coalition, Inc (PWA Coalition); NY, 538

People with AIDS Coalition of Dallas, Inc (PWA Coalition of Dallas, Inc); TX, 713

The People With AIDS Coalition of Tucson (PACT); AZ, 21

Peoria City County Health Dept (PCCHD); IL, 285

Persad Center, Inc; PA, 642

Philadelphia Community Health Alternatives/The Philadelphia AIDS Task Force (PCHA/PATF); PA, 643

Phoenix Rising; OR, 619

Phoenix Shanti Group; AZ, 22

Pitt Men's Study (PMS); PA, 644

Pittsburgh AIDS Task Force (PATF); PA, 645

Placer County Health Dept; CA, 113

Planned Parenthood Association of Southwest Florida, Naples Chapter; FL, 234

Prince George's County Health Dept, Office on AIDS; MD, 366

Project AHEAD (AIDS Health Education and Assistance Delivery); CA, 114

Project AIDS Lafayette, Inc (PAL); IN, 304

Project Lazarus; LA, 339

Puerto Rico Community Health Center Association; PR, 791

PWA Health Group; NY, 539

Quad Cities AIDS Coalition (QCAC); IA, 317

Queen Anne's County Health Dept; MD, 367

Racine Health Dept, City of Racine, HIV Antibody Counseling and Testing Site; WI, 783

Red Door Clinic; MN, 413

Regional AIDS Education Training Center; NY, 540

The Reimer Foundation; IL, 286

Rhode Island Dept of Health, AIDS Program; RI, 651

Rhode Island Project/AIDS (RIP/AIDS); RI, 652

Richmond AIDS Information Network; VA, 731

Riverside County Office of AIDS Coordination (COAC); CA, 115

Roosevelt Hospital and AIDS Clinic; NY, 541

Ruby House; OR, 620

Sacramento AIDS Foundation (SAF); CA, 116

Sacramento County Health Dept, AIDS Unit; CA, 117

Saint Francis Center; DC, 201

Saint Joseph/Buchanan County Community Health Clinic; MO, 428

Saint Louis Effort for AIDS (EFA); MO, 429

Saint Lucie County Public Health Unit (SLCPHU); FL, 235

Saint Paul Division of Public Health; MN, 414

Saint Paul Urban Indian Health Board; MN, 415

Saline County Nursing Service; MO, 430

San Antonio AIDS Alliance; TX, 714

San Antonio AIDS Foundation; TX, 715

San Antonio AIDS Medical Foundation; TX, 716

San Diego AIDS Project; CA, 118

San Francisco AIDS Foundation; CA, 119

San Francisco Dept of Public Health, The AIDS Office; CA, 120

San Joaquin AIDS Foundation; CA, 121

San Luis Obispo County AIDS Education and Prevention Project; CA, 122

Santa Clara County Health Dept AIDS Program; CA, 123

Santa Cruz AIDS Project (SCAP); CA, 124

Seattle AIDS Action Committee; WA, 753

Seattle AIDS Assessment Clinic; WA, 754

Seattle AIDS Support Group (SASG); WA, 755

Seattle Counseling Service for Sexual Minorities (SCS); WA, 756

Seattle Gay Clinic; WA, 757

Seattle Shanti Foundation; WA, 758

Seattle-King County AIDS Prevention Project; WA, 759

Sexually Transmitted Disease Program, Municipality of Anchorage; AK, 13

Shanti Foundation of Tucson, Inc; AZ, 23

Shanti/Houston; TX, 717

Shanti in Oregon, Inc; OR, 621

Shanti Project; CA, 125

Shasta County Public Health (SCPH); CA, 126

Shoulders; WA, 760

SIDA Quebec; PQ, 814

Sitka Health Center; AK, 14

Social Health Association, Dayton; OH, 601

Social Security Administration, El Paso; TX, 718

Social Security Administration/Minneapolis; MN, 416

Social Security Administration/Upper Darby; PA, 646

Social Security AIDS Regional Office IV; GA, 252

Social Security AIDS Regional Office V; IL, 288

Solano County Health Dept, AIDS Program; CA, 127

South Central AIDS Assistance Network/Harrisburg; PA, 647

South Dakota Dept of Health, Communicable Disease Program, AIDS Surveillance and Prevention Project; SD, 660

South Dakota Dept of Health, Communicable Disease Program, Pierre Area Regional Field Office; SD, 661

South Jersey AIDS Alliance (SJAA); NJ, 466

Southern California Mobilization Against AIDS; CA, 128

Southern California Physicians for Human Rights (SCPHR); CA, 129

Southern Colorado AIDS Project (S-CAP); CO, 150

Southern Fairfield County AIDS Coalition; CT, 174

Southern Illinois AIDS Task Force; IL, 289

Southern Ohio AIDS Task Force; OH, 602

Southern Tier AIDS Program, Inc (STAP); NY, 542

Southwest AIDS Committee, Inc (SWAC); TX, 719

Southwest District Health Dept (SWDHD); ID, 265

Southwest Utah District Health Dept, Health Clinic; UT, 724

Southwest Washington Health District; WA, 761

Spalding County Health Dept; GA, 253

Spanish Language AIDS Hotline; CA, 130

Spartanburg County Health Dept; SC, 656

Special Immunology Unit (SIU); OH, 603

Special Office on AIDS Prevention (SOAP), Center for Health Promotion, Michigan Dept of Public Health; MI, 400

St Mary's Alcohol/Drug Addiction Treatment Center; IL, 287

Stamford Health Dept: AIDS Program; CT, 175

Stamp Out AIDS, Inc; NY, 543

Stanislaus Community AIDS Project (SCAP); CA, 131

Stanly County Task Force; NC, 560

Starting Point; NY, 544

State of Florida Dept of Health and Rehabilitative Services, AIDS Program Office, District II; FL, 236

State of Nevada Health Division; NV, 441

Stop AIDS/Los Angeles; CA, 132

Stop AIDS Project—California; CA, 133

Strafford County Prenatal and Family Planning Program (The Clinic); NH, 450

Stuyvesant Polyclinic Adult Medical Clinic; NY, 545

PART III

BIBLIOGRAPHY

ARTICLES

1. **ABC of AIDS. Being HIV antibody positive.** Grimshaw, J. British Medical Journal, v295, n6592, Jul 25, 1987, p256-57

2. **ABC of AIDS. Development of the epidemic.** Adler, M W. British Medical Journal, v294, n6579, Apr 25, 1987, p1083-85

3. **ABC of AIDS. Having AIDS.** Madeley, T. British Medical Journal, v295, n6593, Aug 1, 1987, p320-21

4. **Acquired immune deficiency syndrome in children: Medical, legal, and school related issues.** Kirkland, Martin; Ginther, Dean. School Psychology Review, v17, n2, 1988, p304-10

5. **The acquired immunodeficiency syndrome (AIDS) and infection with the human immunodeficiency virus (HIV). Health and Public Policy Committee, American College of Physicians; and the Infectious Diseases Society of America.** Annals of Internal Medicine, v108, n3, Mar 1988, p460-69

6. **Acquired immunodeficiency syndrome and adolescents: Knowledge, beliefs, attitudes, and behaviors.** Strunin, L; Hingson, R. Pediatrics, v79, n5, May 1987, p825-28

7. **Acquired immunodeficiency syndrome and Black Americans: Special psychosocial issues.** Mays, V M; Cochran, S D. Public Health Reports, v102, n2, Mar-Apr 1987, p224-31

8. **The acquired immunodeficiency syndrome: Epidemiology and risk factors for transmission.** Castro, K G; Hardy, A M; Curran, J W. Medical Clinics of North America, v70, n3, May 1986, p635-49

9. **The acquired immunodeficiency syndrome: General overview.** Friedland G. International Journal of Neuroscience, v32, n3-4, Feb 1987, p677-86

10. **Acquired immunodeficiency syndrome in low-incidence area: How safe is unsafe sex.** Fleming, Gavid W; Cochi, Stephen L; Steece, Richard S; et al. JAMA. Journal of the American Medical Association, v258, Aug 14, 1987, p785

11. **Acquired immunodeficiency syndrome. State legislative activity.** Lewis, H E. JAMA. Journal of the American Medical Association, v258, n17, Nov 6, 1987, p2410-14

12. **Activities of the Centers for Disease Control in AIDS education.** Tolsma, D D. Journal of School Health, v58, n4, Apr 1988, p133-36

13. **Adolescents and AIDS: A survey of knowledge, attitudes and beliefs about AIDS in San Francisco.** DiClemente, R J; Zorn, J; Temoshok, L. American Journal of Public Health, v76, n12, Dec 1986, p1443-45

14. **Aiding those with AIDS: A mission for the church.** Menz, Robert L. Journal of Psychology and Christianity, v6, n3, Fall 1987, p5-18

15. **AIDS: A generation of children at risk.** Bennett, K. Journal of Psychosocial Nursing and Mental Health Services, v25, n12, Dec 1987, p32-34

16. **AIDS, Africa and education.** Nunn, P. Health Education Journal, v46, n2, 1987, p63-65

17. **AIDS: An international perspective.** Piot, P; Plummer, F A; Mhalu, F S; et al. Science, v239, n4840, Feb 5, 1988, p573-79

18. **AIDS and adolescents: School health education must begin now.** Haffner, D W. Journal of School Health, v58, n4, Apr 1988, p154-55

19. **AIDS and American values.** Koop, C Everett. World Affairs Journal, v6, Fall 1987, p24-9

20. **AIDS and behavioral changes to reduce risk: A review.** Becker, M H; Joseph, J G. American Journal of Public Health, v78, n4, Apr 1988, p394-410

21. **AIDS and business: How companies deal with stricken employees; will insurers foot the bill?.** Business Week, Mar 23, 1987, p122-28

22. **AIDS and community education: NEA launches a new campaign to help communities deal effectively with the nation's number one threat to public health.** Steffens, Heidi. NEA Today, v6, Sep 1987, p14

23. **AIDS and compassion.** Friedland, G. JAMA. Journal of the American Medical Association, v259, n19, May 20, 1988, p2898-99

24. **AIDS and drug abuse: No quick fix.** Booth, William. Science, v239, n4841, Feb 12, 1988, p717

25. **AIDS and employers.** Ashton, D. Occupational Health, v39, n8, Aug 1987, p258-59

26. **AIDS and ethics: An overview.** Kelly, K. General Hospital Psychiatry, v9, n5, Sep 1987, p331-41

27. **AIDS and health insurance: Social and ethical issues.** Oppenheimer, Gerald M; Padgug, Robert A. AIDS and Public Policy Journal, v2, n1, Win 1987, p11-14

28. **AIDS and self-organization among intravenous drug users.** Friedman, S R; Des Jarlais, D C; Sotheran, J L; et al. International Journal of the Addictions, v22, n3, Mar 1987, p201-19

29. **AIDS and the traveler.** Mann, Jonathan. World Health, Dec 1987, p14

30. **AIDS and women at risk.** Buckingham, Stephan L; Rehm, Susan J. Health and Social Work, v12, n1, Win 1987, p5-11

31. **AIDS around the world: Analyzing complex patterns.** Goldsmith, Marsha F. JAMA. Journal of the American Medical Association, v259, n13, Apr 1, 1988, p1917

32. **AIDS as a handicapping condition.** Parry, J. Mental and Physical Disability Law Reporter, v9, n6, Nov-Dec, 1985, p403-06

33. **AIDS as a social phenomenon.** Bennett, F J. Social Science and Medicine, v25, n6, 1987, p529-39

34. **AIDS as a social phenomenon.** Velimirovic, B. Social Science and Medicine, v25, n6, 1987, p541-52

35. **AIDS Care in New York City: The comprehensive care alternative.** Dehovitz, Jack A; Pellegrino, Virginia. New York State Journal of Medicine, v87, n5, May 1987, p298-300

36. **AIDS, confidentiality, and the right to know.** Winston, Morton E. Public Affairs Quarterly, v2, Apr 1988, p91-104

37. **AIDS control in Uganda.** Okware, Samuel I. World Health, Mar 1988, p20

38. **The AIDS crisis: A United States health care perspective.** Shulman, Lawrence C; Mantell, Joanne E. Social Science and Medicine, v26, n10, 1988, p979-88

39. **AIDS education in black America.** Gayle, J A. Health Education Journal, v46, n2, 1987, p77-78

40. **AIDS education in school.** Yarber, W L. Sex Education Coalition News, v9, n1, Jan 1987, p1-3

41. **AIDS education in the schools: A literature review as a guide for curriculum planning.** Brown L K; Fritz, G K. Clinical Pediatrics, v27, n7, Jul 1988, p311-16

42. **AIDS: Employer concerns and options.** Ritter, David B; Turner, Ronald. Labor Law Journal, v38, Fall 1987, p67-83

43. **The AIDS epidemic: AIDS research in the life sciences.** Hersh, Evan M; Petersen, Eskild A. Life Sciences, v42, n20, 1988, p1-4

44. **The AIDS epidemic among Blacks and Hispanics.** Friedman, S R; Sotheran, J L; Abdul-Quader A; et al. Milbank Quarterly, v65, suppl 2, 1987, p455-99

45. **AIDS: Explosive growth in public awareness.** Steiber, S. Hospitals, v62, n1, Jan 5, 1987, p96

46. **AIDS: How teenagers are meeting the crisis.** Christopher, Maura; Ward, Elizabeth; Eskin, Leah. Scholastic Update, v120, n4, Oct 16, 1987, p17

47. **AIDS, HTLV-III diseases, minorities and intravenous drug abuse.** Ginzberg, Harold M; MacDonald, Mhairi G; Glass, James W. Advances in Alcohol and Substance Abuse, v6, n3, Spr 1987, p7-21

48. **AIDS in adolescents: A rationale for concern.** Hein, Karen. New York State Journal of Medicine, v87, n5, May 1987, p290-95

49. **AIDS in Africa: A public health priority.** Piot, P; Colebunders, R; Laga, M; Ndinya-Achola, J O. Journal of Virological Methods, v17, n1-2, Aug 1987, p1-10

50. **AIDS in Africa: Misinformation and disinformation.** Konotey-Ahulu, F I. Lancet, v2, n8552, Jul 25, 1987, p206-07

51. **AIDS in children and adolescents.** Belfer, M L; Krener, P K; Miller, F B. Journal of the American Academy of Child and Adolescent Psychiatry, v27, n2, Mar 1988, p147-51

52. **AIDS in children and adolescents.** Belfer, Myron L; Krener, Penelope K; Miller, Frank B. Journal of the American Academy of Child and Adolescent Psychiatry, v27, n2, Mar 1988, p147-51

53. **AIDS in historical perspective: Four lessons from the history of sexually transmitted diseases.** Brandt, A M. American Journal of Public Health, v78, n4, Apr 1988, p367-71

54. **AIDS in minority populations in the United States.** Hopkins, D R. Public Health Reports, v102, n6, Nov-Dec 1987, p677-81

55. **AIDS in prison.** Harding, T W. Lancet, v2, n8570, Nov 28, 1987, p1260-63

56. **AIDS in prison: The social construction of a reality. Annual Meeting of the American Society of Criminology 1987 Montreal, Canada.** Berg, Bruce L; Berg, Jill. International Journal of Offender Therapy and Comparative Criminology, v32, n1, Apr 1988

57. **AIDS in rural areas: Challenges to providing care.** Rounds, Kathleen A. Social Work, v33, n3, May-Jun 1988, p257-61

58. **AIDS in the developing countries.** Tinker, John. Issues in Science and Technology, v4, Win 1988, p43-8

59. **AIDS in the United States: Education and litigation.** Brahams, D. Lancet, v1, n8588, Apr 2, 1988, p779-80

60. **AIDS in the workplace.** Singer, Ira D. Nation's Business, v75, Aug 1987, p36

61. **AIDS in the workplace: How to prevent the transmission of the infection.** US Dept of Health and Human Services. International Nursing Review, v33, n4, Jul-Aug 1986, p117-22, 124

62. **AIDS in the workplace: The ethical ramifications.** Bayer, R; Oppenheimer, G. Business and Health, v3, n3, Jan-Feb 1986, p30-4

63. **AIDS instruction: A troubling test for educators.** McCormick, Kathleen. Education Digest, v53, Sep 1987, p56

64. **AIDS: Law and policy.** Law, Medicine and Health Care, v15, n1-2, Sum 1987, p3-89

65. **AIDS leads to new educational market.** McCormick, B. Hospitals, v60, n18, Sep 20, 1986, p87-88

66. **AIDS 101.** Booth, William. Science, v238, n4826, Oct 23, 1987, p477

67. **AIDS on campus: A survey of college health service priorities and policies.** Caruso, Barbara A; Haig, John R. Journal of American College Health, v36, n1, Jul 1987, p32-36

68. **The AIDS pandemic: An internationalist approach to disease control.** Chen, Lincoln C. Daedalus, v116, Spr 1987, p181

69. **AIDS phobia.** Jacob, J K; John-Jacob, K; Verghese, Abraham; John, T Jacob. British Journal of Psychiatry, v150, Mar 1987, p412-13

70. **AIDS policy in the making.** Booth, William. Science, v239, n4844, Mar 4, 1988, p1087

71. **AIDS: Politics and science.** Osborn, J E. New England Journal of Medicine, v318, n7, Feb 18, 1988, p444-47

72. **AIDS prevention and civil liberties: The false security of mandatory testing.** Hunter, Nan D. AIDS and Public Policy Journal, v2, Sum-Fall 1987, p1-10

73. **AIDS prevention: Guidelines.** Harvard Medical School Health Letter, v12, Apr 1987, p4

74. **AIDS: Psychological stresses on the family. Recommendations for counseling relatives of the AIDS patient.** Frierson, R L; Lippmann, S B; Johnson, J. Psychosomatics, v28, n2, Feb 1987, p65-68

75. **AIDS: Psychosocial aspects.** Flaskerud, J H. Journal of Psychosocial Nursing and Mental Health Services, v25, n12, Dec 1987, p8-16

76. **AIDS: Public expresses compassion for AIDS victims, but holds them responsible for contracting disease.** Gallup Report, Aug 1987, p12-19

77. **AIDS: Questions students ask.** Krim, M. Scholastic Choices, v3, n2, Oct 1987, p29-33, 42

78. **AIDS ranked as number-one US health problem.** Steiber, S R. Hospitals, v61, n9, May 5, 1987, p104

79. **AIDS: Relationship to alcohol and other drugs.** Siegel, L. Journal of Substance Abuse Treatment, v3, n4, 1986, p271-74

80. **AIDS: Resource materials for school personnel.** Fulton, G B; Metress, E; Price, J H. Journal of School Health, v57, n1, Jan 1987, 14-18

81. **AIDS risk reduction: A community health education intervention for minority high risk group members.** Williams, L S. Health Education Quarterly, v13, n4, Win 1986, p407-21

82. **AIDS risk-reduction guidelines: A review and analysis.** Siegel, K; Grodsky, P B; Herman, A. Journal of Community Health, v11, n4, Win 1986, p222-32

83. **AIDS screening, confidentiality, and the duty to warn.** Gostin, L; Curran, W J. American Journal of Public Health, v77, n3, Mar 1987, p361-65

84. **AIDS: Screening of possible carriers and human rights.** Gevers, J K M. Health Policy, v7, Fall 1987, 13-9

85. **AIDS, sex and dope: A reevaluation of ethics and morals.** Adelmann, H C. Ohio Medicine, v84, n1, Jan 1988, p7, 11

86. **AIDS, sexuality, and sexual control.** Quadland, M C; Shattls, W D. Journal of Homosexuality, v14, 1-2, 1987, 277-98

87. **AIDS: Statistics but few answers.** Barnes, Deborah M. Science, v236, n4807, Jun 12, 1987, p1423-25

88. **AIDS strains the system; the AIDS crisis is forcing a reevaluation of the country's patchwork of private and publicly financed health care, prompting clashes between victims, insurers and governments.** Kosterlitz, Julie. National Journal, v19, Jun 27, 1987, p1650-54

89. **AIDS: The legal aspects of a disease.** Birchfield, J L. Medical Law, v6, n5, 1987, p407-26

90. **AIDS: The responsibilities of health professionals.** Hastings Center Report, v18, Apr-May 1988, p25

91. **AIDS: The risks to insurers, the threat to equity.** Oppenheimer, G M; Padgug, R A. Hastings Center Report, v16, n5, Oct 1986, p18-22

92. **AIDS, the schools, and policy issues.** Price, J H. Journal of School Health, v56, n4, Apr 1986, p137-40

93. **AIDS: Update and guidelines for general dental practice.** Porter, S R; Scully, C; Cawson, R A. Dental Update, v14, n1, Jan-Feb 1987, p9-10, 12, 15-17

94. **The AIDS virus.** Gallo, Robert C. Scientific American, v256, n1, Jan 1987, p47-56

95. **AIDS: What adults should know about AIDS (and shouldn't discuss with very young children).** Skeen, Patsy; Hodson, Diane. Young Children, v42, n4, May 1987, p65-71

96. **Black male genocide: A final solution to the race problem in America.** Staples, Robert. Black Scholar, v18, n3, May-Jun 1987, p2-11

97. **Can a nurse be fired for having AIDS?.** Arbeiter, J S. RN, v50, n2, Feb 1987, p53-4

98. **Cashing in on AIDS: Turning disaster into a business proposition.** Cohen, L. Canadian Medical Association Journal, v137, n10, Nov 15, 1987, p932-33

99. **Children with AIDS: How schools are handling the crisis.** Reed, Sally. Phi Delta Kappan, v69, n5, Jan 1988, pK1

100. **Children with AIDS in the public schools: The ethical issues.** Davis, Dena S. Journal of Medical Humanities and Bioethics, v8, n2, Fall-Win 1987, p101-9

101. **Combating a deadly combination: Intravenous drug abuse, acquired immunodeficiency syndrome.** Raymond, Chris Anne. JAMA. Journal of the American Medical Association, v259, n3, Jan 15, 1988, p329

102. **Communicating the AIDS risk to college students: The problem of motivating change.** Edgar, Timothy; Freimuth, Vicki S; Hammond, Sharon L. Health Education Research, v3, n1, Apr 1988, p59-65

103. **Comparing state-only expenditures for AIDS.** Rowe, M J; Ryan, C C. American Journal of Public Health, v78, n4, Apr 1988, p424-29

104. **Compulsory premarital screening for the human immunodeficiency virus. Technical and public health considerations.** Cleary, P D; Barry, M J; Mayer, K H; et al. JAMA. Journal of the American Medical Association, v258, n13, Oct 2, 1987, p1757-62

105. **Contraception and AIDS.** World Health, Nov 1987, p23

106. **Corporate CEOs don't want to pay for AIDS.** Droste, T. Hospitals, v62, n5, Mar 5, 1988, p66

107. **The cost of AZT.** Thomas, Emily H; Fox, Daniel M. AIDS and Public Policy Journal, v2, Spr-Sum 1987, p17-21

108. **Counseling AIDS antibody-positive clients: Reactions and treatment.** Grant, D; Anne M. American Psychologist, v43, n1, Jan 1988, p72-74

109. **Critical condition: One of the nation's top AIDS labs has been crippled by internal feuds, obstructed research and staff turnover.** Blow, Richard. Rolling Stone, Mar 26, 1987, p67

110. **Cultural practices contributing to the transmission of human immunodeficiency virus in Africa.** Hardy, D B. Reviews of Infectious Diseases, v9, n6, Nov-Dec 1987, p1109-19

111. **Dealing with AIDS and fear: Would you accept cookies from an AIDS patient?.** Thompson, L M. Southern Medical Journal, v80, n2, Feb 1987, p228-32

112. **Developing an AIDS program in a juvenile detention center.** Gelder, Seymour. Children Today, v17, n1, Jan-Feb 1988, p6-9

113. **Developing policies on employees with AIDS.** Droste, T. Hospitals, v61, n20, Oct 20, 1987, p61-62

114. **Do physicians have an obligation to treat patients with AIDS?.** Emanuel, Ezekiel J. New England Journal of Medicine, v318, n25, Jun 1988, p1686-90

115. **Doctor as patient advocate.** Hotchkiss, William S. JAMA. Journal of the American Medical Association, v258, Aug 21, 1987, p947

116. **The economic impact of AIDS in the United States.** Bloom, D E; Carliner, G. Science, v239, n4840, Feb 5, 1988, p604-10

117. **The economic impact of the first 10,000 cases of acquired immunodeficiency syndrome in the United States.** Hardy, A M; Rauch, K; Echenberg, D; et al. JAMA. Journal of the American Medical Association, v255, n2, Jan 10, 1986, p209-11

118. **Educating minorities about AIDS: Challenges and strategies.** Jimenez, Richard. Family and Community Health, v10, n3, Nov 1987, p70-73

119. **Education and contact notification for AIDS prevention.** Echenberg, Dean F. New York State Journal of Medicine, v87, n5, May 1987, p296-97

120. **Education to prevent AIDS: Prospects and obstacles.** Fineberg, H V. Science, v239, n4840, Feb 5, 1988, p592-96

121. **The effect of group education in improving attitudes about AIDS risk reduction.** Valdiserri, Ronald O; Lyter, David W; Kingsley, Lawrence A. New York State Journal of Medicine, v87, n5, May 1987, p272-78

122. **The effects of the AIDS epidemic on the safety of the nation's blood supply.** Petricciani, J C; Epstein, J S. Public Health Reports, v103, n3, May-Jun 1988, p236-41

123. **An elective seminar to teach first-year students the social and medical aspects of AIDS.** Goldman, J D. Journal of Medical Education, v62, n7, Jul 1987, p557-61

124. **Emotional aspects of AIDS—implications for care providers.** Nichols, S E. Journal of Substance Abuse Treatment, v4, n3-4, 1987, p137-40

125. **Employment discrimination against AIDS victims: Rights and remedies under the Federal Rehabilitation Act of 1973.** Fagot-Diaz, Jose G. Labor Law Journal, v39, Mar 1988, p148-66

126. **Epidemic human immunodeficiency virus (HIV) infection among intravenous drug users (IVDU).** D'Aquila, R T; Williams, A B. Yale Journal of Biology and Medicine, v60, n6, Nov-Dec 1987, p545-67

127. **Epidemics and civil rights.** Koshland, Daniel E. Science, v235, n4790, Feb 1987, p729

128. **Epidemics in perspective.** Valdiserri, Ronald O. Journal of Medical Humanities and Bioethics, v8, n2, Fall-Win 1987, p95-100

129. **The epidemiology of the acquired immunodeficiency syndrome in Africa.** Imperato, P J. New York State Journal of Medicine, v86, n3, Mar 1986, p118-21

130. **Estimates of the direct and indirect costs of acquired immunodeficiency syndrome in the United States, 1985, 1986, and 1987.** Scitovsky, A A; Rice, D P. Public Health Reports, v102, n1, Jan-Feb 1987, p5-17

131. **Ethical aspects of military physicians treating servicepersons with HIV: Part III. The duty to protect third parties.** Howe, Edmund S. Military Medicine, v153, n3, Mar 1988, p140-44

132. **Ethical dilemmas about intensive care for patients with AIDS.** Lo, B; Raffin, T A; Cohen, N H; et al. Reviews of Infectious Diseases, v9, n6, Nov-Dec 1987, p1163-67

133. **Ethical dilemmas in AIDS research: Individual privacy and public health.** Melton, Gary B; Gray, Joni N. American Psychologist, v43, n1, Jan 1988, p60-64

134. **Ethical issues in the prevention and treatment of HIV infection and AIDS.** Walters, L. Science, v239, n4840, Feb 5, 1988, p597-603

135. **Ethical issues involved in the growing AIDS crisis.** JAMA. Journal of the American Medical Association, v259, n9, Mar 4, 1988, p1360

136. **The facts of life: AIDS education and the schools.** American Council of Life Insurance; Health Insurance Association of America. Teaching Topics, v34, n2, Fall 1987, p1-5

137. **Fear of AIDS.** Chodoff, P. Psychiatry, v50, n2, May 1987, p184-91

138. **Fear of AIDS.** Friedland, G. New York State Journal of Medicine, v87, n5, May 1987, p260-61

139. **The fear of AIDS: Guidelines for the counseling and HTLV-III antibody screening of adolescents.** Jaffe, Leslie R; Wortman, Richard N. Journal of Adolescent Health Care, v9, n1, Jan 1988, p84-86

140. **Financing the care of patients with the acquired immunodeficiency syndrome (AIDS).** Health and Public Policy Committee, American College of Physicians. Annals of Internal Medicine, v108, n3, Mar 1988, p470-73

141. **Financing the struggle against AIDS.** Iglehart, J K. New England Journal of Medicine, v317, n3, Jul 16, 1987, p180-84

142. **First needle-exchange program approved; other cities await results.** Raymond, Chris Anne. JAMA. Journal of the American Medical Association, v259, n9, Mar 4, 1988, p1289

143. **Foundation funding for AIDS programs.** Wells, J A. Health Affairs, v6, n3, Fall 1987, p113-23

144. **Four teens on the frontlines: Volunteers helping to educate the public and to care for people with AIDS.** Coupland, Kenneth; Ward, Elizabeth; Wohl, Alex. Scholastic Update, v120, n4, Oct 16, 1987, p15

145. **Freeing hemophiliacs from the risk of AIDS.** Rhein, Reginald Jr. Business Week, Apr 13, 1987, p38

146. **From the Surgeon General, US Public Health Service.** Koop, C Everett. Journal of Substance Abuse Treatment, v4, n1, 1987, p5-13

147. **A frustrating glimpse of the true AIDS epidemic.** Booth, William. Science, v238, n4828, Nov 6, 1987, p747

148. **The genesis of fear: AIDS and the public's response to science.** Eisenberg, L. Law, Medicine and Health Care, v14, n5-6, Dec 1986, p243-49

149. **The global struggle against AIDS: WHO's strategy.** Kay, K. International Nursing Review, v35, n2, Mar-Apr 1988, p35-40

150. **Going home to die: Developing home health care services for AIDS patients.** Droste, T. Hospitals, v61, n16, Aug 20, 1987, p54-58

151. **Guidelines for effective school health education to prevent the spread of AIDS.** Centers for Disease Control. Center for Health Promotion and Education. Journal of School Health, v58, n4, Apr 1988, p142-48

152. **Guidelines for school programs to prevent the spread of AIDS.** American Family Physician, v37, n3, Mar 1988, p419-20, 425

153. **Handicapped children and the law: Children afflicted with AIDS.** Kermani, Ebrahim J. Journal of the American Academy of Child and Adolescent Psychiatry, v27, n2, Mar 1988, p152-54

154. **Health and safety in day care.** Sells, Clifford J; Paeth, Susan T. Topics in Early Childhood Special Education, v7, n1, Spr 1987, p61-72

155. **Health care advocacy for AIDS patients.** Cecchi, R L. QRB. Quality Review Bulletin, v12, n8, Aug 1986, p297-03

156. **Health education about AIDS among seropositive blood donors.** Cleary, P D; Rogers, T F; Singer, E; et al. Health Education Quarterly, v13, n4, Win 1986, p317-29

157. **Health education. The advertising myth.** Pownall, M. Nursing Times, v82, n34, Aug 20-26, 1986, p19-20

158. **Health insurance and AIDS: The status of state regulatory activity.** Faden, R R; Kass, N E. American Journal of Public Health, v78, n4, Apr 1988, p437-38

159. **Health insurance and AIDS: The status of state regulatory activity.** Faden, R R; Kass, N E. American Journal of Public Health, v78, n4, Apr 1988, p437-38

160. **Hemophiliac patient's knowledge and educational needs concerning acquired immunodeficiency syndrome.** Hargraves, M A; Jason, J M; Chorba, T L; et al. Public Health Reports, v102, n5, Sep-Oct 1987, p468-74

161. **Heterosexual AIDS: Setting the odds.** Booth, William. Science, v240, n4852, Apr 29, 1988, p597

162. **Heterosexual contacts of intravenous drug abusers: Implications for the next spread of the AIDS epidemic.** Murphy, D L. Advances in Alcohol and Substance Abuse, v7, n2, 1987, p89-97

163. **HIV AIDS education and the Army: Unique program characteristics, components and educational opportunities.** Alexander, Linda L; Renzullo, Philip O; Bunin, Janice R. Health Education Research, v3, n1, Apr 1988, p89-96

164. **The HIV antibody test: Psychosocial issues.** Buckingham, Stephan L. Social Casework, v68, n7, Sep 1987, p387-93

165. **The HIV antibody test: Why gay and bisexual men want or do not want to know their results.** Lyter, D W; Valdiserri, R O; Kingsley, L A; et al. Public Health Reports, v102, n5, Sep-Oct 1987, p468-74

166. **HIV counselling: Some practical problems and issues.** Miller, D. Journal of the Royal Society of Medicine, v80, n5, May 1987, p278-80

167. **HIV infection among intravenous drug users: Epidemiology and risk reduction.** Des Jarlais, D C; Friedman, S R. AIDS, v1, n2, Jul 1987, p67-76

168. **HIV infection and intravenous drug use: Critical issues in transmission dynamics, infection outcomes, and prevention.** Des Jarlais, D C; Friedman, S R; Stoneburner, R L. Reviews of Infectious Diseases, v10, n1, Jan-Feb 1988, p151-58

169. **Homophobia and attitudes towards AIDS patients among medical, nursing, and paramedical students.** Royse, D; Birge, B. Psychological Reports, v61, n3, Dec 1987, p867-70

170. **Hospice care of the patient with AIDS.** Schofferman, J. Hospital Journal, v3, n4, Win 1987, p51-74

171. **Hospitalizations for AIDS, United States, 1984-1985.** Graves, E J; Moien, M. American Journal of Public Health, v77, n6, Jun 1987, p729-30

172. **Human immunodeficiency virus infection in heterosexual intravenous drug users in San Francisco.** Chaisson, R E; Moss, A R; Onishi, R; et al. American Journal of Public Health, v77, n2, Feb 1987, p169-72

173. **Human immunodeficiency virus infections in children: Public health and public policy issues.** Grossman, M. Pediatric Infectious Diseases, v6, n1, Jan 1987, p113-16

174. **Identity cards for patients infected with HIV?.** Srivastava, A C; Pinching, A J; Adler, M W; et al. British Medical Journal, v294, n6570, Feb 21, 1987, p495-96

175. **The impact of AIDS on gay male sexual behavior patterns in New York City.** Martin, J L. American Journal of Public Health, v77, n5, May 1987, p578-81

176. **The impact of AIDS on state and local health departments: Issues and a few answers.** Judson, F N; Vernon, T M Jr. American Journal of Public Health, v78, n4, Apr 1988, p387-93

177. **The impact of AIDS on the mental care system.** Cotton, D J. JAMA. Journal of the American Medical Association, v260, n4, Jul 22-29, 1988, p519-23

178. **Improving the quality and quantity of whole blood supply: Limits to voluntary arrangements.** Roberts, Russell D; Wolkoff, Michael J. Journal of Health Politics, Policy and Law, v13, Spr 1988, p169-78

179. **The incalculable cost of AIDS.** The Economist, v306, n7541, Mar 12, 1988, p44

180. **Increased risk of suicide in persons with AIDS.** Marzuk, Peter M; Tierney, Helen; Tardiff, Kenneth; et al. JAMA. Journal of the American Medical Association, v259, n9, Mar 4, 1988, p1333

181. **Inescapable problem: AIDS in prison.** Goldsmith, Marsha F. JAMA. Journal of the American Medical Association, v258, n22, Dec 11, 1987, p3215

182. **The initial impact of AIDS on public health law in the United States—1986.** Matthews, G W; Neslund, V S. JAMA. Journal of the American Medical Association, v257, n3, Jan 16, 1987, p344-52

183. **International travel restrictions and the AIDS epidemic.** Nelson, Leonard J III. American Journal of International Law, v81, Jan 1987, 230-36

184. **Intravenous drug use and AIDS prevention.** Schuster, C R. Public Health Reports, v103, n3, May-Jun 1988, p261-66

185. **Intravenous drug use and the heterosexual transmission of the human immunodeficiency virus: Current trends in New York City.** Des Jarlais, Don C; Wish, Eric; Friedman, Samuel R; et al. New York State Journal of Medicine, v87, n5, May 1987, p283-86

186. **Knowledge and attitudes of AIDS health care providers before and after education programs.** Wertz, D C; Sorenson, J R; Liebling, L; et al. Public Health Reports, v102, n3, May-Jun 1987, p248-54

187. **Knowledge, attitudes, and behavior of health professionals in relation to AIDS.** Searle, E S. Lancet, v1, n8523, Jan 3, 1987, p26-28

188. **Local policy responses to the AIDS epidemic: New York City and San Francisco.** Arno, Peter S; Hughes, Robert G. New York State Journal of Medicine, v87, n5, May 1987, p264-72

189. **Lovers of AIDS victims: A minority group experience.** Fuller, Ruth L; Geis, Sally B; Rush, Julian. Death Studies, v21, n1, 1988, p1-7

190. **Minorities and AIDS.** Evans, Patricia E. Health Education Research, v3, n1, Apr 1988, p113-15

191. **Minorities and AIDS: Knowledge, attitudes, and misconceptions among Black and Latino adolescents.** DiClemente, R J; Boyer, C B; Morales, E S. American Journal of Public Health, v78, n1, Jan 1988, p55-57

192. **Mobilizing against AIDS.** Nathan, Jean. Scholastic Update, v120, n4, Oct 16, 1987, p8

193. **The monkey's blood.** The Economist, v304, Jul 25, 1987, p76

194. **The moral challenge of AIDS.** Boyd, K M. Journal of the Royal Society of Medicine, v80, n5, May 1987, p281-83

195. **The National AIDS Information Campaign: Once upon a time in America.** Dan, B B. JAMA. Journal of the American Medical Association, v258, n14, Oct 9, 1987, p1942

196. **National health insurance: An idea whose time has come back.** Kuttner, Robert. Business Week, Aug 3, 1987, p14

197. **A new world with AIDS-health promotion as a catalyst for change.** Meyer, A J. Western Journal of Medicine, v147, n6, Dec 1987, p716-18

198. **A no-fault proposal for AIDS high risks.** Booth, William. Science, v239, n4843, Feb 26, 1988, p973

199. **The nonprofit sector's response to the AIDS epidemic.** Arno, P S. American Journal of Public Health, v76, n11, Nov 1986, p1325-30

200. **Occupational risk of HIV, HBV and HSV-2 infections in health care personnel caring for AIDS patients.** Kuhls, T L; Viker, S; Parris, N B; et al. American Journal of Public Health, v77, n10, Oct 1987, p1306-09

201. **Occupational risk of the acquired immunodeficiency syndrome among health care workers.** McCray, E. New England Journal of Medicine, v314, n17, Apr 24, 1986, p1127-32

202. **On being gay, single, and bereaved.** Oerlemans-Bunn, M. American Journal of Nursing, v88, n4, Apr 1988, p472-76

203. **Partner notification for preventing human immunodeficiency virus (HIV) infection—Colorado, Idaho, South Carolina, Virginia.** MMWR. Morbidity and Mortality Weekly Report, v37, n25, Jul 1, 1988, p393-96, 401-02

204. **Placing children with AIDS.** Hart, Graham. Adoption and Fostering, v11, n1, 1987, p41-43

205. **Plagues, history, and AIDS.** Swenson, Robert M. American Scholar, v57, n2, Spr 1988, p183

206. **Policy issues surrounding children with AIDS in schools.** Manning, D Thompson; Balson, Paul M. Clearing House, v61, n3, Nov 1987, p101

207. **The politics of AIDS: A review essay.** Queen, Carol. Insurgent Sociologist, v14, n2, Sum 1987, p103-24

208. **The polls—a report: AIDS.** Singer, Eleanor. Public Opinion Quarterly, v51, Win 1987, p580-95

209. **Power, prestige, profit: AIDS and oppression of homosexual people.** Gronfors, Martti; Stalstrom, Olli. Acta Sociologica, v30, n1, 1987, p53-66

210. **A practical guide for dealing with AIDS at work.** Waldo, William S. Personnel Journal, v66, n8, Aug 1987, p135-38

211. **Preventing the sexual transmission of AIDS during adolescence.** Remafedi, G J. Journal of Adolescent Health Care, v9, n2, Mar 1988, p139-43

212. **Prevention and control of acquired immunodeficiency syndrome: An interim report.** JAMA. Journal of the American Medical Association, v258, n15, Oct 16, 1987, p2097

213. **Prevention, not prejudice.** The Economist, v306, n7535, Jan 30, 1988, p43

214. **The prevention of acquired immunodeficiency syndrome in the United States: An objective strategy for medicine, public health, business, and the community.** Francis, D P; Chin, J. JAMA. Journal of the American Medical Association, v257, n10, Mar 13, 1987, p1357-66

215. **Prevention of AIDS among adolescents: Strategies for the development of comprehensive risk-education health education programs.** DiClemente, Ralph J; Boyer, Cherrie B; Mills, Stephen J. Health Education Research, v2, n3, Sep 1987, p287-91

216. **The prevention of HIV infection associated with drug and alcohol use during sexual activity.** Stall, R. Advances in Alcohol and Substance Abuse, v7, n2, 1987, p73-88

217. **Problems and dynamics of organizing intravenous drug users for AIDS prevention.** Friedman, Samuel R; de Jong, Wouter M; des Jarlais, Don C. Health Education Research, v3, n1, Apr 1988, p49-57

218. **Prostitutes and AIDS: A health department priority?.** Rosenberg, M J; Weiner, J M. American Journal of Public Health, v78, n4, Apr 1988, p418-23

219. **Providing empowerment to the person with AIDS.** Haney, Patrick. Social Work, v33, n3, May-Jun 1988, p251-53

220. **The provision and financing of medical care for AIDS patients in US public and private teaching hospitals.** Andrulis, D P; Beers, V S; Bentley, J D; Gage, L S. JAMA. Journal of the American Medical Association, v258, Sep 11, 1987, p1343

221. **Psychiatric aspects of AIDS.** Faulstich, Michael E. American Journal of Psychiatry, v144, n5, May 1987, p551-56

222. **Psychiatric consequences of AIDS: An overview.** Ostrow, D G. International Journal of Neuroscience, v32, n3-4, Feb 1987, p647-59

223. **Psychological implications of AIDS.** Frierson, R L; Lippmann, S B. American Family Physician, v35, n3, Mar 1987, p109-16

224. **Psychosocial aspects of AIDS.** Goldmeier, D. British Journal of Hospital Medicine, v37, n3, Mar 1987, p232-34, 238-40

225. **Psychosocial impact of the AIDS epidemic on the lives of gay men.** Stuhlberg, Ian; Smith, Margaret. Social Work, v33, n3, May-Jun 1988, p277-81

226. **Public attitudes toward the control of AIDS: The homosexual's plight.** Ottenberg, P. Transactions and Studies of the College of Physicians of Philadelphia, v8, n2, Jun 1986, p113-19

227. **Public health enemy no. 1.** Kissel, S J. Health and Social Work, v12, n3, Sum 1987, p166-68

228. **Public health measures for prevention and control of AIDS.** Hopkins, D R. Public Health Reports, v102, n5, Sep-Oct 1987, p463-67

229. **Public Health Service guidelines for counseling and antibody testing to prevent HIV infection and AIDS.** New York State Journal of Medicine, v88, n2, Feb 1988, p74-76

230. **Public perceptions regarding the AIDS epidemic: Selected results from a national poll.** Bausell, R B; Damrosch, S; Parks, P, Soeken, K. AIDS Research, v2, n3, Sum 1986, p253-58

231. **Public supports AIDS education, research.** Steiber, S. Hospitals, v61, n1, Jan 5, 1987, p67

232. **Quarantine and the problem of AIDS.** Musto, David F. Milbank Quarterly, v64, suppl 1, 1986, p97-117

233. **Quarterly report to the Domestic Policy Council on the prevalence and rate of spread of HIV and AIDS in the United States.** MMWR. Morbidity and Mortality Weekly Report, v37, n14, Apr 15, 1988, p223-26

234. **Raising the shades on sex education.** National Journal, v19, Jan 31, 1987, p274-75

235. **Recommended guidelines for dealing with AIDS in the schools from the National Education Association.** Journal of School Health, v56, n4, Apr 1986, p129-30

236. **Report on the European Community Workshop on Epidemiology of HIV Infections: Spread among intravenous drug abusers and the heterosexual population. Robert Koch Institute, Berlin, 12-14 November 1986.** Brunet, J B; Des Jarlais, D C; Koch, M A. AIDS, v1, n1, May 1987, p59-61

237. **A review of AIDS-related legislative and regulatory policy in the United States.** Gostin, L; Ziegler, A. Law, Medicine and Health Care, v15, n1-2, Sum 1987, p5-16

238. **Risk communication about AIDS in higher education.** Keeling, Richard P. Science, Technology, and Human Values, v12, n3-4, 1987, p26-36

239. **Risk factors for AIDS among Haitians residing in the United States. Evidence of heterosexual transmission. The Collaborative Study Group of AIDS in Haitian-Americans.** JAMA. Journal of the American Medical Association, v257, n5, Feb 6, 1987, p635-39

240. **Risk factors for AIDS and HIV seropositivity in homosexual men.** Moss, A R; Osmond, D; Bacchetti, P; et al. American Journal of Epidemiology, v125, n6, Jun 1987, p1035-47

241. **The risk of AIDS: Psychological impact on the hemophiliac population.** Agle, D; Gluck, H; Pierce, G F. General Hospital Psychiatry, v9, n1, Jan 1987, p11-17

242. **Risk of human immunodeficiency virus (HIV-I) infection among laboratory workers.** Weiss, S H; Goedert, J J; Gartner, S; et al. Science, v239, n4835, Jan 1, 1988, p68-71

243. **Risk of human immunodeficiency virus transmission from heterosexual adults with transfusion-associated infections.** Peterman, Thomas A; Stoneburner, Rand L; Allen, James R; et al. JAMA. Journal of the American Medical Association, v259, n1, Jan 1, 1988, p55

244. **Risks of abstinence: Sexual decision making in the AIDS era.** Gochros, Harvey L. Social Work, v33, n3, May-Jun 1988, p254-56

245. **Role of drug-abuse treatment in limiting the spread of AIDS.** Hubbard, R L; Marsden, M E; Cavanaugh, E; Rachel, J V; Ginzberg, H M. Reviews of Infectious Diseases, v10, n2, Mar-Apr 1988, p377-84

246. **The role of prostitution in AIDS and other STDs.** Adams, Reed. Medical Aspects of Human Sexuality, v21, n8, Aug 1987, p27-33

247. **Safeguard your health—and your sexual freedom.** Brown, Helen Gurley. Cosmopolitan, v202, May 1987, pA22

248. **Schools, communicable diseases, and the law.** Cole, K; Faust, T R. Journal of School Health, v57, n7, Sep 1987, p293-96

249. **Screening blood donors for human immunodeficiency virus antibody: Cost-benefit analysis.** Eisenstaedt, R S; Getzen, T E. American Journal of Public Health, v78, n4, Apr 1988, p450-54

250. **Screening for AIDS: Efficacy, cost, and consequences.** Gostin, Larry. AIDS and Public Policy Journal, v2, Fall-Win 1987, p14-24

251. **Sex, AIDS, and gay American men.** Kus, R J. Holistic Nursing Practice, v1, n4, Aug 1987, p42-51

252. **Sex education programs that work in public schools.** Barron, James. Education Digest, v53, n6, Feb 1988, p24

253. **Sex experts and medical scientists join forces against common foe: AIDS.** Goldsmith, Marsha F. JAMA. Journal of the American Medical Association, v259, n5, Feb 5, 1988, p641

254. **Sex in the age of AIDS calls for common sense and condom sense.** Goldsmith, Marsha F. JAMA. Journal of the American Medical Association, v257, May 1, 1987, p2261

255. **Sexual contacts of intravenous drug abusers: Implications for the next spread of the AIDS epidemic.** Brown, L S Jr; Primm, B J. Journal of the National Medical Association, v80, n6, Jun 1988, p613-15

256. **Significant others of I.V. drug abusers with AIDS: New challenges for drug treatment programs.** Grief, G L; Porembski, E. Journal of Substance Abuse Treatment, v4, n3-4, 1987, p151-55

257. **Social aspects of AIDS.** World Health, Mar 1988, p17

258. **The sociological study of AIDS: A critical review of the literature and suggested research agenda.** Kaplan, H B; Johnson, R J; Bailey, C A; Simon, W. Journal of Health and Social Behavior, v28, n2, Jun 1987, p140-57

259. **The staggering price of AIDS.** Lord, Lewis J. US News and World Report, v102, Jun 15, 1987, p16-18

260. **State Medicaid coverage of AZT and AIDS-related policies.** Buchanan, R J. American Journal of Public Health, v78, n4, Apr 1988, p432-36

261. **State Medicaid policies and hospital care for AIDS patients.** Andrulis, D P; Beers, V S; Bentley, J D; Gage, L S. Health Affairs, v6, n4, Win 1987, p110-18

262. **Sterile needles and the epidemic of acquired immunodeficiency syndrome: Issues for drug abuse treatment and public health.** Selwyn, P A. Advances in Alchohol and Substance Abuse, v7, n2, 1987, p99-105

263. **Stigmatization of AIDS patients by physicians.** Kelly, J A; St Lawrence, J S; Smith, S Jr; et al. American Journal of Public Health, v77, n7, Jul 1987, p789-91

264. Strategies for AIDS prevention: Motivating health behavior in drug dependent women. Mondanaro, Josette. Journal of Psychoactive Drugs, v19, n2, Apr-Jun 1987, p143-49

265. Strategies for volunteers caring for persons with AIDS. Lopez, Diego; Getzel, George S. Social Casework, v68, n1, Jan 1987, p47-53

266. The syphilis epidemic and its relations to AIDS. Brandt, Allan M. Science, v239, n4838, Jan 1988, p375-80

267. Teaching children about AIDS. Schnall, J; Harbaugh, M. Instructor, v97, n2, Sep 1987, p26-28

268. Teaching children about AIDS. Baum, S G. Sex Education Coalition News, v9, n1, Jan 1987, p5-6

269. Television's role in communicating on AIDS. Palmer, Edward L. Health Education Research, v3, n1, Apr 1988

270. Testing for HIV without permission. Gillon, R. British Medical Journal, v294, n6575, Mar 28, 1987, p821-23

271. Throwing money at AIDS: Funds for AIDS education and testing should be directed at high-risk groups, not spread around. Smith, Lee. Fortune, v116, Aug 31, 1987, p64-7

272. Transmission of the human immunodeficiency virus. Friedland, G H; Klein, R S. New England Journal of Medicine, v317, n18, Oct 29, 1987, p1125-35

273. Transmission of the human immunodeficiency virus to sexual partners of hemophiliacs. Smiley, M L; White, G C; Becherer, P; et al. American Journal of Hematology, v28, n1, May 1988, p27-32

274. Unsuspected human immunodeficiency virus in critically ill emergency patients. Baker, J L; Kelen, G D; Sivertson, K T; Quinn, T C. JAMA. Journal of the American Medical Association, v257, n21, May 15, 1987, p2609-11

275. Update: Human immunodeficiency virus infections in health-care workers exposed to blood of infected patients. MMWR. Morbidity and Mortality Weekly Reports, v36, n19, May 22, 1987, p285-89

276. Vaccination for AIDS: Legal and ethical challenges from the test tube, to the human subject, through to the marketplace. Gostin, Larry. AIDS and Public Policy Journal, v2, n2, Spr-Sum 1987, p9-16

277. The war against AIDS. Bowen, Otis R. Journal of Medical Education, v62, n7, Jul 1987, p543-48

278. What is safe sex? Suggested standards linked to testing for human immunodeficiency virus. Goedert, J J. New England Journal of Medicine, v316, n21, May 21, 1987, p1339-42

279. What is the occupational risk to emergency care providers from the human immunodeficiency virus?. Baker, J L. Annals of Emergency Medicine, v17, n7, Jul 1988, p700-03

280. When AIDS hits home. Micheli, Robin. Money, v16, n12, Nov 1987, p137

281. Women and AIDS. Reid, Elizabeth. World Health, Mar 1988, p28

282. Working together to face the AIDS epidemic. Scholastic Update, v120, n4, Oct 16, 1987, p4

283. The workplace and AIDS: A guide to services and information. Personnel Journal, v66, Oct 1987, p65-80

284. The worried well: Maximizing coping in the face of AIDS. Harowski, K J. Journal of Homosexuality, v14, n1-2, 1987, p299-306

285. Your child and children with AIDS: A parent information booklet. Santacroce, S; Wiener, L S; Schubert, W. Oncology Nursing Forum, v24, n4, Jul-Aug 1987, p83-85

BIBLIOGRAPHIES

286. Acquired Immune Deficiency Syndrome. Evans, Joanna W. Library of Congress, Science and Technology Div, Science Reference Section, Washington DC 20540 1985 8p LC 33.10:85-11
A brief AIDS bibliography

287. Acquired Immune Deficiency Syndrome (1983-May 1984). Frederick Cancer Research Center Scientific Library. Distributed by NTIS, Springfield VA 1984 48p PB84-866961
Citations from the life sciences collection database of the Scientific Library of the Frederick Cancer Research Center

288. Acquired Immunodeficiency Syndrome. Kenton, Charlotte; Abrams, Estelle J. US Dept of Health and Human Services, Public Health Service, National Institutes of Health, Bethesda MD 20209 1983- HE 20.3614/2:83-
A quarterly updated bibliography beginning with citations from January 1980

289. Acquired Immunodeficiency Syndrome (AIDS): January 1980-. National Library of Medicine. US Dept of Health and Human Services, Public Health Service, National Institutes of Health, National Library of Medicine, Superintendent of Documents, Washington DC 20402 1986 HE 20.7008:Ac 7
Bibliography series produced at the National Library of Medicine and consisting of periodical citations about AIDS primarily drawn from the medical literature

290. AIDS, 1981-1983: An Annotated Bibliography. Garoogian, Rhoda. CompuBibs, 358 Willis Ave, Mineola NY 11501 1984 92p $15.00 0-914791-05-2
An annotated AIDS bibliography

291. AIDS: A Bibliography. Reed, Robert D. R & E Publishers, PO Box 2008, Saratoga CA 95070 1987 64p 0-88247-757-9
A selected bibliography of general articles on AIDS from magazines, newspapers, and books

292. AIDS: A Bibliography from All Fields of Periodical Literature, 1982-1986. Lincoln Associates, PO Box 507, Madison WI 53701 1987 118p

293. AIDS: A Bibliography from All Fields of Periodical Literature 1982-1986. Lincoln Associates, PO Box 507, Madison WI 53701 1987 118p $40.00
A 5-year bibliography of AIDS articles arranged by name of periodical title. A list of AIDS books is included

294. AIDS: A Multimedia Bibliography. Booklist, vol 84, Oct 15, 1987, p365-68

295. AIDS: A Research and Clinical Bibliography. Pearce, Richard B; Babcock, Gary; Baun, Jim. AIDS/KS National Foundation, 54 10th St, San Francisco CA 94103 1983, 3rd ed, 43p
A bibliography stressing the clinical and research aspects of AIDS

296. AIDS: Abstracts of the Psychological and Behavioral Literature, 1983-1988. Dessaint, Alain Y; Kerby, Jody L; McLean, Barbara E. American Psychological Association, 1200 17th St NW, Washington DC 20036 1988 53p 0-55798-041-1
Includes literature citations drawn from the American Psychological Association's *PsychLIT* database

297. AIDS (Acquired Immune Deficiency Syndrome). Tyckoson, David A. Oryx Press, 2214 N Central at Encanto, Phoenix AZ 85004 1985 64p 0-89774-203-6
Contains over 200 briefly annotated entries covering articles which appeared from 1982-1985

298. AIDS (Acquired Immune Deficiency Syndrome), 2nd edition. Tyckoson, David A. Oryx Press, 2214 N Central at Encanto, Phoenix AZ 85004-1483 1986, 2nd ed 91p $16.00 0-89774-323-7
Bibliography of general AIDS articles arranged by topic

299. AIDS (Acquired Immunodeficiency Syndrome): A Bibliography from All Fields of Periodical Literature, 1982-1986. Lincoln Associates, PO Box 507, Madison WI 53701 1987 118p
A fairly comprehensive bibliography on AIDS with quarterly updates

300. AIDS Bibliography. National Library of Medicine, 8600 Rockville Pike, Bethesda MD 20894HE-20-3615-3
A periodical consisting of bibliographic citations culled from the National Library of Medicine's MEDLINE and CATLINE databases. Available from the US Government Printing Office, Superintendent of Documents, Washington, DC 20402

301. AIDS Bibliography for Nineteen Eighty-One to Nineteen Eighty-Six. Weissberg, Nancy C. Whitston Publishing Company, Incorporated, PO Box 958, Troy NY 12181 1988 643p $48.50 0-87875-356-7
A comprehensive bibliography on AIDS covering a wide range of formats, with references to both general and technical information sources

302. AIDS: Diagnosis, with Medical Subject Analysis and Reference Bibliography. Raber, Martin David. ABBE Publishers Association of Washington, 4111 Gallows Rd, Annandale VA 22003 1985 156p $29.95, $21.95 (paper) 0-88164-488-9, 0-88164-489-7 (paper)
A medical bibliography on AIDS

303. AIDS: Index of Modern Information. Bartone, John. ABBE Publishers Association of Washington, DC, 4111 Gallows Rd, Virginia Division, Annandale VA 22003 1988 150p $34.50 0-88164-804-3
A bibliography on AIDS

304. AIDS: Index of Modern Medical Reviews Compiling 7000 References. Abell, Alphonse R. ABBE Publishers Association of Washington, 4111 Gallows Rd, Virginia Division, Annandale VA 22003 1988 150p $34.50 0-88164-778-0
A medical bibliography on AIDS

305. AIDS legal bibliography. Leonard, Arthur S. AIDS and Public Policy Journal, v2, n2, Spr-Sum 1987, p54-61

306. AIDS 1987. Tyckoson, David A. Oryx Press, 2214 N Central Ave, Phoenix AZ 85004 1988 153p $16.00 0-89774-434-9
Topically arranged and annotated bibliography of 637 general AIDS articles published during the second half of 1987

307. AIDS 1988, Part 1. Tyckoson, David A. Oryx Press, 2214 N Central at Encanto, Phoenix AZ 85004 1988 144p $19.50 0-89774-504-3
Contains references to over 500 articles covering all aspects of the AIDS crisis

308. AIDS 1988, Part 2. Tyckoson, David A. Oryx Press, 2214 N Central at Encanto, Phoenix AZ 85004 1989 176p $19.50 0-89774-505-1
Contains references to over 500 articles covering all aspects of the AIDS crisis

309. AIDS 1989, Part 1. Tyckoson, David A. Oryx Press, 2214 N Central at Encanto, Phoenix AZ 85004 1989 144p $19.50 0-89774-578-7
Contains references to over 500 articles covering all aspects of the AIDS crisis

310. AIDS Resource List. Technical Information Service. US Dept of Health and Human Services, Public Health Service, Centers for Disease Control, Center for Prevention Services, Technical Information Service, Superintendent of Documents, Washington DC 20402 1987 21p HE 20.7312:Ac 7
A selected bibliography of AIDS resources

311. An Annotated Bibliography of Scientific Articles on AIDS for Policymakers. Korda, Holly. US Dept of Health and Human Services, Public Health Service, Superintendent of Documents, Washington DC 20402 1987 varies $30.00 HE 20.11/2:Ac 7
A bibliography of articles intended for AIDS public policymakers prepared by ABT Associates for the Office of the Assistant Secretary for Health

312. Citations from the Life Sciences Collection Database, Acquired Immune Deficiency Syndrome (June 84-March 86). NTIS. NTIS, Springfield VA 22161 1986 T-22, 203, S-20p PB 86-861028
Comprehensive AIDS bibliography that supersedes PB 84-866961

313. Collected Papers on AIDS Research, 1976-1986. BioScience Information Service of Biological Abstracts. BIOSIS, BioSciences Information Services, 2100 Arch St, Philadelphia PA 19103 1987 300p 0-916246-15-9
This book contains citations to papers on AIDS drawn from the BIOSIS (*Biological Abstracts*) database and is updated by the monthly publication *AIDS Research Today*

314. Consolidated Bibliography on AIDS. National Institute of Allergy and Infectious Diseases. National Institute of Allergy and Infectious Diseases, National Institutes of Health, 9000 Rockville Pike, Bethesda MD 20892 1984 92p
A comprehensive bibliography on AIDS

315. Gays and Acquired Immune Deficiency Syndrome: A Bibliography. 2nd edition. Miller, Alan V. Canadian Gay Archives, PO Box 639, Station A, Toronto ON M5W 1G2 Canada 1983, 2nd ed 67p 0-969098-10-8
A general bibliography on AIDS

316. Gays and Acquired Immune Deficiency Syndrome (AIDS): A Bibliography. Revisionist Press, PO Box 2009, Brooklyn NY 11202 1986 $79.95 0-87700-875-2
A comprehensive bibliography of information sources on AIDS

317. HTLV-III Antibody Testing: Efficacy and Impact on Public Health. January 1984 through June 1986, 420 Citations in English. Patrias, Karen; Parker, Christine. US Dept of Health and Human Services, Public Health Service, National Institutes of Health, National Library of Medicine, Superintendent of Documents, Washington DC 20402 1986 32p HE 20.3414/2:86-6
A bibliography of 420 periodical citations drawn primarily from the medical literature

318. Medical, Social and Political Aspects of the Acquired Immune Deficiency Syndrome (AIDS) Crisis: A Bibliography. McLeod, Donald W; Miller, Alan. Canadian Gay Archives, Box 639 Station A, Toronto, Ontario M5W 1G2 Canada 1985 314p 0-969081-2-X
Important though presently dated bibliography of periodical literature on AIDS

319. Reports on AIDS Published in the Morbidity and Mortality Weekly Report: June 1981 through February 1986. Centers for Disease Control. US Dept of Health and Human Services, Public Health Service, Centers for Disease Control, Superintendent of Documents, Washington DC 20402 1986 155p HE 20.7009/a:Ac 7/981-86

A compilation of reports on AIDS published in the Centers for Disease Control's *Morbidity and Mortality Weekly Report (MMWR)*, a journal of national disease occurrence statistics.

320. Subject Index to Abstracts: III International Conference on AIDS. Smith, W Hovey. Whitehall Press-Budget Publications, Rte. 1 Box 603, Sandersville GA 31082 1988 92p $10.00pbk 0-916565-12-2
A subject index to abstracts of papers and posters presented at the 1987 *Third International Conference on AIDS* held in Washington, DC

BOOKS

321. Acquired Immune Deficiency Syndrome. McHugh, Theresa. Legislative Research, Oregon Legislative Assembly, State Capitol, Salem OR 97310 1985
General information on AIDS and AIDS legislation

322. Acquired Immune Deficiency Syndrome. New Jersey State Dept of Health. New Jersey State Dept of Health, CN 360, Trenton NJ 08625 1986
General information about AIDS

323. Acquired Immune Deficiency Syndrome. Selikoff, Irving J; Teirstein, Alvin S; Hirschman, Shalom Z. New York Academy of Sciences, 2 E 63rd St, New York NY 10021 1984 622p $140.00 0-89766-268-7
Published as *Annals of the New York Academy of Sciences*, Vol. 437, 1984

324. Acquired Immune Deficiency Syndrome, 100 Questions and Answers: AIDS. New York State Dept of Health. New York State Dept of Health, Tower Bldg, Empire State Plaza, Albany NY 12237 1986
Miscellaneous information about AIDS for the general public

325. Acquired Immune Deficiency Syndrome: A Demographic Profile of New York State Inmate Mortalities, 1981-1986. Gaunay, William; Gido, Rosemary L. New York State Commission on Correction, New York State Dept of Correctional Services, State Campus, Bldg 2, Albany NY 12226 1987 35p
A statistical analysis of AIDS deaths in New York State prisons from 1981-1986

326. Acquired Immune Deficiency Syndrome (AIDS). Heller, Barbara R. Aspen Systems Corp, 1600 Research Blvd, Bethesda MD 20850 1984 86p 0-89443-756-9

327. Acquired Immune Deficiency Syndrome (AIDS), Hearing Before the Subcommittee on Health and the Environment of the Committee on Energy and Commerce, House of Representatives, Ninety-eighth Congress, Second Session, September 17, 1984. United States Congress, House Committee on Energy and Commerce, Subcommittee on Health and the Environment. Superintendent of Documents, US Government Printing Office, Washington DC 20402 1985 138p Y4.En2 3:98-185
Congressional hearing regarding AIDS prevention and the financing of AIDS research

328. Acquired Immune Deficiency Syndrome and Chemical Dependancy. Petrakis, Peter L. US Dept of Health and Human Services, Public Health Service, Alcohol, Drug Abuse, and Mental Health Administration, National Institute on Alcohol Abuse and Alcoholism, Superintendent of Documents, Washington DC 20402 1987 78p $2.50 HE 20.8302:Ac 7
Consists of papers presented at the "AIDS and Chemical Dependency Forum," held in San Francisco in 1986

329. Acquired Immune Deficiency Syndrome: Guidance Notes for Environmental Health Officers. Institution of Environmental Health Officers. Institution of Environmental Health Officers, Chadwick House, Rushworth St, London, Great Britain SE1 0QT Great Britain 1987 46p 0-900103-32-9
Information for public health officials regarding AIDS

330. Acquired Immune Deficiency Syndrome Research Funding, Hearing Before a Subcommittee of the Committee on Appropriations, United States Senate, Ninety-ninth Congress, First Session: Special Hearing, Dept of Health and Human Services, Nondepartmental Witnesses. United States Congress, Senate Committee on Appropriations, Subcommittee on Departments of Labor, Health and Human Services, Education, and Related Agencies. Superintendent of Documents, US Government Printing Office, Washington DC 20402 1986 285p Y4.Ap6.2.hrg/99-433
Congressional hearing regarding AIDS research funding requirements

331. Acquired Immunodeficiency Syndrome. Klein, Eva. S. Karger, 79 5th Ave, New York NY 10003 1986 398p 3-8055-4156-2

332. Acquired Immunodeficiency Syndrome (AIDS). Vilmer, E; Gluickman, J C. Elsevier Science Publishing Company, Inc, 62 Vanderbilt Ave, New York NY 10017 1986 299p $45.00 2-906077-01-1
Contains papers presented at the "International Conference on AIDS," held in Paris, June 1986

333. Acquired Immunodeficiency Syndrome (AIDS). Gallin, John I; Fauci, Anthony S. Raven Press, 1140 Avenue of the Americas, New York NY 10036 1985 178p 0-88167-077-4

334. Acquired Immunodeficiency Syndrome, AIDS: Recommendations and Guidelines, November 1982-November 1986. Centers for Disease Control. US Dept of Health and Human Services, Public Health Service, National Institutes of Health, Centers for Disease Control, Superintendent of Documents, Washington DC 20402 1987 74p HE 20.7009:Ac 7
A compilation of Centers for Disease Control (CDC) AIDS prevention guidelines

335. Acquired Immunodeficiency Syndrome (AIDS) Research Centers. Dept of Health and Human Services, Public Health Service, Alcohol, Drug Abuse, and Mental Health Administration, National Institute of Mental Health, National Institute on Drug Abuse, 5600 Fishers Lane, Rockville MD 20857 1986
Listing of research centers

336. Acquired Immunodeficiency Syndrome: Current Issues and Scientific Studies. Imperato, Pascal J. Human Sciences Press, 72 5th Ave, New York NY 10011 1989 0-89885-465-2
Contains reprints of journal articles previously published in the *New York State Journal of Medicine*

337. Advice for Life: A Woman's Guide to AIDS Prevention. Norwood, Chris. Pantheon Books, 201 E 50th St, New York NY 10022 1987 0-39456-238-0
AIDS prevention practices for women

338. Advocate Guide to Gay Health. Fenwick, R D. Alyson Publications, 40 Plympton St, Boston MA 02118 1982 236p 0-932870-23-6
General information on gay health concerns, including, but not limited to, AIDS

339. After the Joy...A Manual of Safe Sex. Kilby, Donald C. C V Mosby Co, 11830 Westline Industrial Dr, Saint Louis MO 63146 1986 $14.95 0-8016-2684-6
A general-audience safer sex manual, also published under the title, *Manual of Safe Sex*

340. AIDS. Hawkes, Nigel. Gloucester Press, 387 Park Ave S, New York NY 10016 1987 32p $10.90 0-531-17054-3
Information about AIDS for children and adolescents

341. AIDS. Long, Robert E. H W Wilson, 950 University Ave, Bronx NY 10452 1987 192p $10.00 0-8242-0751-3
Part of the publisher's *The Reference Shelf* series containing general information on AIDS reprinted from a variety of sources

342. AIDS. Menitove, Jay E; Kolins, Jerry. American Association of Blood Banks, 1117 N 19th St, Ste 600, Arlington VA 22209 1986 106p $17.00 0-915355-26-4
Includes papers presented at a 1986 AIDS Technical Workshop held in San Francisco covering syndrome etiology, incidence, clinical aspects, immunology and antibody testing

343. AIDS. Check, William. Chelsea House Publishers, PO Box 419, Edgemont PA 19028 1988 122p $17.95 0-7910-00540-0
Discussion of AIDS for the general public

344. AIDS. Nourse, Alan E. Watts, Sherman Tpke, Danbury CT 06816 1986 128p $11.90 0-531-10235-1

345. AIDS: A Catholic Call for Compassion. Flynn, Eileen P. Sheed and Ward, PO Box 414292, Kansas City MO 64141-0281 1985 99p $4.95 0-934134-73-1
Discussion of the concerns of Catholics about AIDS

346. AIDS: A Guide for Survival. Harris County Medical Society; Houston Academy of Medicine. Houston Academy of Medicine, 1133 M D Anderson Blvd, Houston TX 77030 1987 87p $1.95
AIDS prevention information for general audiences

347. AIDS: A Guide to Survival. Tatchell, Peter. Alyson Publications, Inc, 40 Plypton St, Boston MA 02118 1987 164p $6.95 0-946097-21-6
Advice on safer sexual practices geared to gay men

348. AIDS: A Health Care Management Response. Blanchet, Kevin D. Aspen Publications, Incorporated, 1600 Research Blvd, Rockville MD 20850 1988 319p $38.50 0-87189-877-2
An overview of AIDS-related issues for health facility administrators

349. AIDS: A Manager's Guide. Schachter, Victor; Von Seeburg, Susan. Executive Enterprises Publications, 22 W 21st St, New York, NY 10010 1986 71p 0-880575-95-6
Issues surrounding AIDS in the workplace, with emphasis on labor legislation

350. AIDS: A Manual for Pastoral Care. Sunderland, Ronald H; Shelp, Earl E. Westminster Press, 925 Chestnut St, Philadelphia PA 19107 1988 76p $6.95 0-664-24088-7
A text for people providing pastoral counseling to AIDS patients, focusing on general AIDS facts, treatments, the grieving process, and ethics

351. AIDS: A Plague in Us: A Social Perspective, The Condition and its Social Consequences. Vass, Antony A. Venus Academica, PO Box 14 Saint Ives, Huntington, Great Britain PE18 9EX Great Britain 1986 177p £7.95 0-9509676-1-0
A sociological discussion of AIDS and its consequences for society

352. AIDS: A Self-Care Manual. Moffatt, Bettyclare; Spiegal, Judith. IBS Press, 2339 28th St, Santa Monica CA 90405 1987 320p $12.95 0-9616605-1-1
A comprehensive manual for people with AIDS, caregivers and those concerned about the syndrome, including a listing of self-care resources

353. AIDS: A Status Report on Foundation Funding. Foundation Center, 79 5th Ave, New York NY 10003 1987 104p $20.00 0-879-54-236-5
A sourcebook for information on private funding for AIDS research, giving detailed data on foundations providing grant money

354. AIDS: A Status Report on Foundation Funding. Foundation Center, 79 5th Ave, New York NY 10003 1987 104p $20.00 0-879-54-236-5
A sourcebook for information on available AIDS research funding

355. A.I.D.S.: A Study. Kurban, Loretta. Libra Press, 2316 E Porter, Los Angeles CA 90021 $5.00 0-938863-23-1

356. A.I.D.S. Acquired Immune Deficiency Syndrome. Fromer, Margot J. Pinnacle Books, 1430 Broadway, New York NY 10018 1983 273p $3.95 0-523-42130-3
One of the first books written about AIDS for the general public

357. AIDS, Acquired Immune Deficiency Syndrome. Gay Men's Health Crisis, Inc. Gay Men's Health Crisis, Inc, PO Box 274, New York NY 10011 1983 62p
Educational information for gay men about AIDS

358. AIDS: Acquired Immune Deficiency Syndrome, and Other Manifestations of HIV Infection, Epidemiology, Etiology, Immunology, Clinical Manifestations, Pathology, Control, Treatment and Prevention. Wormser, Gary P; Stahl, Rosalyn; Bottone, Edward J. Noyes & Company, Incorporated, 120A Mill Rd, Park Ridge NJ 07656 1987 1103p $98.00 0-8155-1108-6
A comprehensive textbook on AIDS intended for medical professionals, but of potential interest to concerned others

359. AIDS, Acquired Immunodeficiency Syndrome: Information and Guidelines Regarding HTLV-III Infections. Dominguez, Lee B; Caldwell, Glyn G; Englander, Steven J. Arizona Dept of Health Services, Office of Infectious Disease Control, 1740 W Adams St, Phoenix AZ 85007 1986 47p
Handbook for preventing and controlling exposure to the AIDS-causing virus

360. AIDS: An Administrative Reference Manual. Massachusetts Hospital Association Task Force on AIDS. Massachusetts Hospital Association, 5 New England Executive Park, Burlington MA 01803 1987 115p
An AIDS information reference tool for hospital administrators

361. AIDS: An International Forum—Policy, Politics and AIDS. Hummel, Robert F; Leavy, William F; Rampolla, Michael; Chorost, Sherry. Plenum Publishing Corporation, 233 Spring St, New York NY 10013 1987 180p $49.50 0-306-42540-8
A review of international political and health policy activities to control the spread of AIDS

362. AIDS and Adolescents: The Time for Prevention is Now. Haffner, Debra W. Center for Population Options, 1012 14th St, NW, Washington DC 20005 1987 28p
This report features highlights from the first national AIDS and Adolescents meeting, sponsored by the Center for Population Options held April 1987. Included are recommendations for educators and policymakers on how to implement effective AIDS prevention programs geared to teens

363. **AIDS and Drug Abuse in the Workplace: Resolving the Thorny Legal-Medical Issues.** Bakaly, Charles; Kramer, Saul.' Harcourt, Brace and Javonovich, 1250 6th Ave, San Diego CA 92101 1986 309p $40.00
A discussion of the complex problems posed by AIDS and substance abuse, focusing on pertinent labor laws and industrial hygiene legislation

364. **AIDS and Drug Abuse in the Workplace: Resolving the Thorny Legal-Medical Issues.** Bakaly, Charles G; Kramer, Saul G. Harcourt Brace and Jovanovich, Inc, 1250 6th Ave, San Diego CA 92101 1986 309p
Discussion of employment issues surrounding AIDS and drug abuse

365. **AIDS and Healthful Gay Sexual Acitvity.** American Association of Physicians for Human Rights, PO Box 14366, San Francisco CA 94114 Write for information

366. **AIDS and Hemophilia Module.** National Hemophilia Foundation, 110 Greene St, Ste 406, New York NY 10012 1985 29p Free
This module was created for social workers, nurses, and physicians, and may be used for patient education about AIDS

367. **AIDS and Immune Deficiency: Macrobiotic Approach.** Kushi, Michio; Cottrell, Martha C. Japan Publications USA Incorporated, 45 Hawthorn Pl, Briarcliff Manor NY 10510 1987 320p $16.95 0-87040-680-9
Macrobiotic diet therapies for AIDS and related immunologic disorders

368. **AIDS and Immune Deficiency: Macrobiotic Approach.** Kushi, Michio; Cottrell, Martha C. Japan Publications, 45 Hawthorne Pl, Briarcliff Manor NJ 10510 1987 320p $16.95 0-87040-680-9
Alternative diet therapies for treating AIDS

369. **AIDS and its Metaphors.** Sontag, Susan. Farrar, Straus & Giroux, Inc, 19 Union Sq W, New York NY 10003 1988 $14.95 0-374-10257-0
Philosophical discussion about AIDS as it is perceived in society

370. **AIDS and IV Drug Abusers: Current Perspectives.** Galea, Robert; Lewis, Benjamin; Baker, Lori. National Health Publishing, 99 Painters Mill Rd, Owings Mills MD 21117 1987 150p $37.00 0-932500-71-4
Treatise on the interplay between intravenous drug abuse and the transmission of HIV, the AIDS-causing virus

371. **AIDS and IV Drug Abusers: Current Perspectives.** Galea, Robert P; Lewis, Benjamin F; Baker, Lori A. National Health Publishers, 99 Painters Mill Road, Owings Mill MD 21117 1988 328p $35.00 0-932500-71-4
Detailed information on the risks to intravenous drug abusers of exposure to the AIDS-causing virus

372. **AIDS and Patient Management: Legal, Ethical and Social Issues.** Witt, Michael D. National Health Publishers, 99 Painters Mill Road, Owings Mill MD 21117 1986 263p $35.00 0-932500-46-3
Consists of papers presented at the "AIDS: The Ethical, Legal, and Social Considerations" conference, sponsored by Public Responsibility in Medicine and Research

373. **AIDS and Substance Abuse.** Siegel, Larry. Haworth Press, Inc, 12 W 32nd St, New York NY 10001 1988 206p $14.95 0-86656-819-0 $16 Discussion of the relationship between drug abuse and AIDS. This publication also appreared in 1987 as vol 7, no 2, of the journal, *Advances in Alcohol and Substance Abuse*

374. **AIDS and Syphilis: The Hidden Link.** Coulter, Harris L. North Atlantic Books, 2320 Blake St, Berkeley CA 94704 1987 80p $20.00 1-55643-021-3
Discussion of the proposed theory that AIDS and syphilis are related disorders

375. **AIDS and the Blood: A Practical Guide.** Jones, Peter. Newcastle Haemophilia Reference Centre, the Haemophilia Society, and the Terence Higgins Trust, Newcastle Great Britain 1985 76p 0-951026-30-5
Information for the general public about AIDS, and particularly its spread through blood transfusion

376. **AIDS and the Church.** Shelp, Earl E; Sunderland, Ronald H. Westminster Press, 925 Chestnut St, Philadelphia PA 19107 1987 151p $8.95 0-664-24091-7
A discussion of the Christian perspective on AIDS and ministering to those with the syndrome

377. **AIDS and the Doctors of Death: An Inquiry into the Origins of the AIDS Epidemic.** Cantwell, Alan. Aries Rising Press, 2132 Alcyona Dr, Los Angeles CA 90065 1988 239p $18.95 0-917211-00-6
Controversial discussion of the cause and epidemiology of AIDS

378. **AIDS and the Employer: Guidelines on the Management of AIDS in the Workplace.** Warshaw, Leon J. New York Business Group on Health, 622 Third Ave, 34th Fl, New York NY 10017 1986 86p
The topics of health services to HIV-infected employees and personnel management issues related to AIDS in the workplace are discussed in this volume, the proceedings from the "NYBGH Forum on AIDS and the Employer," held December 1985 in New York

379. **AIDS and the Healer Within.** Bamforth, Nick. Amethyst Books, 160 W 71st St, No 17D, New York NY 10023 1988 144p $6.95 0-944256-00-7
A discussion of alternative, self-care methods for treating AIDS

380. **AIDS and The Law.** Dornette, William H L. John Wiley and Sons, Inc, 605 3rd Ave, New York NY 10158 1987 375p 0-471-85740-8
This book explains the medical context of infections with the AIDS-causing virus and associated legal issues

381. **AIDS and the Law: A Guide for the Public.** Dalton, Harlon L; Burris, Scott. Yale University Press, 302 Temple St, New Haven CT 06520 1987 382p $22.50 0-300-04077-6
A thorough analysis of school, workplace, housing, civil rights, insurance, military and prison AIDS-related legal issues

382. **AIDS and the New Puritanism.** Altman, Dennis. Pluto Press, 105A Torriano Ave, London England NW5 2RX Great Britain 1986 228p 0-7453-0012-X
Discussion of the implications of AIDS during current conditions of social and economic conservativism

383. **AIDS and the Public Schools.** Hooper, Susan; Gregory, Gwendolyn H. National School Boards Association, 1680 Duke St, Alexandria VA 22314 1986 55p $15.00
This report was written for parents of school-age children and includes factual information about AIDS in an attempt to dispel misunderstandings and myths parents may have regarding HIV infection

384. **AIDS and the Third World.** Sabatier, Renee; Panos Institute Staff. New Society Publishers, 4527 Springfield Ave, Philadelphia PA 19143 1988 192p $34.95 0-86571-143-7
A discussion about the impact of the AIDS pandemic on Third World nations, particularly countries in Africa

385. **AIDS and You.** Balch, James F; Balch, Phyllis. Good Things Naturally, 610 W Main St, Greenfield IN 46140 1988 250p $10.95 0-942023-01-3
A general-audience discussion of AIDS

386. **AIDS. Blunt Talk on How to Avoid It.** Norman, Randolph. ARSoft Publishers, PO Box 132, Woodsboro MD 21798 $5.95 0-86668-057-8
Guidelines for avoiding AIDS

387. **The AIDS Book: Creating A Positive Approach.** Hay, Louise L.. Hay House, 3029 Wilshire Blvd, Ste 206, Santa Monica CA 90404 1987 $16.95
Health maintenance techniques for people with AIDS using positive thinking

388. **The AIDS Book: Information for Workers with Supplement. 2nd ed.** Service Employees International Union, Health and Safety Dept, 1313 L St, NW, Washington DC 20005 1987 64p $3.00
Discussion of AIDS workplace issues presented in question-and-answer format

389. **The AIDS Bureaucracy.** Panem, Sandra. Harvard University Press, 79 Garden St, Cambridge MA 02138 1988 194 p $22.50 0-674-01270-4
A critical analysis of the national research efforts and health care delivery systems established for dealing with AIDS

390. **AIDS, Cancer and the Medical Establishment.** Brown, Raymond Keith. Robert Speller & Sons, Publishers, Inc, 30 E 23rd St, New York NY 10108 1986 185p $16.95 0-8315-0196-0

391. **The AIDS Caregiver's Handbook.** Edison, Ted. Saint Martin's Press, 175 5th Ave, New York NY 10010 1988 272p $19.95 0-312-02151-6
Support information for those providing care to people with AIDS

392. **The AIDS Connection.** Vandeman, George E. Pacific Press Publishing Association, PO Box 7000, Boise ID 83704 1986 48p 0-816306-59-1

393. **AIDS Conspiracy.** Barrrus, Emery. John Daniel Publisher, PO Box 21922, Santa Barbara CA $9 93121 1988 176p $8.95 0-936784-44-X
A controversial analysis of the cause of the AIDS epidemic

394. **AIDS Cover-Up? The Real and Alarming Facts About AIDS.** Antonio, Gene. Ignatius Press, PO Box 18990, San Francisco CA 94118 1986 237p $9.95 0-89870-129-5

395. The AIDS Crisis. Social Issues Resources Series, Inc, PO Box 2348, Boca Raton FL 33427 1987 100 articles $80.00 0-89777-840-5

This is an annually-updated publication containing reprints of key articles about AIDS. The original volume included approximately 60 articles, with each update adding about 20 additional items

396. The AIDS Crisis: Conflicting Social Values. McCuen, Gary E. Gary E McCuen Publications, 411 Mailalieu Dr, Hudson WI 54016 1987 176p $11.95 0-86596-061-5

Reviews the history of the AIDS epidemic, the federal government's response, religious and moral questions raised by the crisis, and political implications

397. AIDS Crisis: Impact on the Gay Subculture. Michaels, Kevin. MLP Enterprises, 236 E Durham St, Philadelphia PA 19119 1986 $11.95 0-939020-77-7

Discourse on the effect AIDS has had on gay lifestyles

398. AIDS Crisis: Impact on the Gay Subculture. Part 2. Michaels, Kevin. MLP Enterprises, 236 E Durham St, Philadelphia PA 19119 1987 110p $12.95 0-939020-79-3

A review of the impact AIDS has had on gays

399. AIDS: Cultural Analysis-Cultural Activism. Crimp, Douglas. MIT Press, 55 Hayward St, Cambridge MA 02142 1988 275p $20.00 0-262-03140-X

A discussion of the cultural impact of AIDS, focusing on the reactions of various subcultures to the crisis

400. AIDS: Deadly Threat. Silverstein, Alvin; Silverstein, Virginia B. Enslow Publishers, Inc, Bloy St and Ramsey Ave, Box 777, Hillside NJ 07205 1986 96p $12.95 0-89490-128-1

Information about AIDS for the general public

401. AIDS, Defining the Legal Issues: A Legal Symposium. Suffolk Univ Law School Center for Continuing Professional Development; Boston Bar Association, Young Lawyers Section. Suffolk Univ Law School, 41 Temple St, Boston MA 02114 1985 150p

Discussion of the legal implications of AIDS

402. AIDS Education: The Public Health Challenge. Siegel, Karolyn. John Wiley & Sons, 605 3rd Ave, New York NY 10158 1986 164p $25.95 0-471-62400-4

This is a reprint of the journal *Health Education Quarterly,* volume 1 number 4, discussing public health issues surrounding AIDS

403. AIDS: Employer Rights and Responsibilities. Commerce Clearing House, 4025 W Peterson Ave, Chicago IL 60646 1985 95p $10.00 0-317-47587-8

Employment and management issues related to AIDS

404. AIDS. Ending the Fear Plague. Do It Now Foundation, PO Box 21126, Phoenix AZ 85036 1986 $0.25 0-89230-166-X

405. The AIDS Epidemic. Cahill, Kevin M. St. Martin's Press, Inc, 175 5th Ave, New York NY 10010 1983 173p $12.95 0-312-01498-8

One of the first books to be published about AIDS for the general public

406. The AIDS Epidemic: A Citizen's Guide to Protecting Your Family and Community from the Gay Plague. Lockman, Lawrence E. Vic Lockman, PO Box 1916, Ramona CA 92065 1986 107p $6.95 0-936175-04-4

407. The AIDS Epidemic: How You Can Protect Your Family—Why You Must. Slaff, James I. Warner Books, Inc, 666 5th Ave, New York NY 10103 1985 285p $3.95 0-446-30143-4

408. AIDS: Ethics and Public Policy. Pierce, Christine; VanDeVeer, Donald. Wadsworth Publishing Company, 10 Davis Dr, Belmont CA 94002 1988 241p 0-534-08286-6

Ethical issues relative to public policy options regarding HIV testing and the treatment of AIDS patients are discussed

409. AIDS: Everything You Must Know About Acquired Immune Deficiency Syndrome, The Killer Epidemic of the 80s. Baker, Janet. R & E Publishers, PO Box 2008, Saratoga CA 95070 1983 109p 7.95 0-88247-700-5

A general account for the layperson on what AIDS is, its symptoms, how it is transmitted, and where to go for help

410. The AIDS Fact Book. Mayer, Kenneth H; Pizer, H F. Bantam Books, 666 5th Ave, New York NY 10019 1983 135p 0-553-23870-1

411. AIDS Fact Book. North Dakota State Dept of Health. North Dakota State Dept of Health, State Capitol, Bismarck ND 58505 1986 4 loose-leaf pages

412. AIDS Facts and Issues, Revised and Updated. Gong, Victor; Rudnick, Norman. Rutgers University Press, 109 Church St, New Brunswick NJ 08901 1986 388p $25.00 0-8135-1201-8

Revised and updated edition of a popular, comprehensive review of AIDS issues

413. AIDS: Fears and Facts. Irwin, Michael H K. Public Affairs Committee, 381 Park Ave S, New York NY 10016 1986 28p $1.00 0-88291-064-7

414. The AIDS File: What We Need to Know About AIDS Now. Jacobs, George; Kerrins, Joseph. Cromlech Books, Nobska Rd, Box 145, Woods Hole MA 02543 1987 128p $7.95 0-9618059-0-0

AIDS information for adolescents and adults

415. AIDS: From Fear to Hope, Channeled Teachings Offering Insight and Inspiration. Spirit Speaks Staff. New Age Publishing, PO Box 011549, Miami FL 33101 1987 269p $9.95 0-934619-02-6

Alternative, inspirational coping techniques for dealing with AIDS

416. AIDS, From the Beginning. Cole, Helene M; Lundberg, George D. American Medical Association, 535 N Dearborn St, Chicago IL 60610 1986 441p 0-89970-207-4

This is a detailed account of the history of the AIDS epidemic

417. The AIDS Health Crisis: Psychological and Social Interventions. Kelly, Jeffrey A; Saint Lawrence, Janet S. Plenum Publishing Corporation, 233 Spring St, New York NY 10013 1988 0-30642-896-2

Discussion of psychological and social interventions for the prevention and control of AIDS

418. AIDS, Herpes and Everything You Should Know About VD in Australia. 2nd ed. Bradford, David. International Specialized Book Services, 5602 NE Massalo St, Portland OR 97213 Australia 1985 300p $6.95 0-522-84311-5

Information for general audiences about sexually transmitted diseases, with emphasis on AIDS

419. AIDS Home Care and Hospice Manual. Visiting Nurses and Hospice of San Francisco, 401 Duboce Ave, San Francisco CA 94117 1987 196p $95.00

A comprehensive manual for home and hospice care, providing educational guidelines and resources for administrators, staff and volunteers responsible for the care of people with AIDS

420. AIDS Hysteria. Ide, Arthur F. Monument Press, 513 S Rosemont, Dallas TX 75208 1986 117p $5.95 0-930383-08-7

421. AIDS Hysteria. 2nd ed. Ide, Arthur F. Monument Press, PO Box 160361, Los Colinas TX 75016 1988 154p $6.00 0-930383-12-5

General narrative about the AIDS crisis

422. AIDS, Impact on Public Policy: An International Forum. Hummel, Robert F; Leavy, William F; Rampolla, Michael; Chorost, Sherry. Plenum Press, 233 Spring St, New York NY 10013 1986 169p $49.50 0-306-42540-8

Proceedings of a New York conference co-sponsored by the New York State Dept of Health and the Milbank Memorial Fund, May 1986

423. AIDS: Impact on Schools. Weiner, Roberta. A.I.D.S. International/Information Distribution Service, PO Box 2008, Saratoga CA 95070 1986 274p $65.00 0-93792-502-0

How AIDS has and will effect our schools is discussed in this general treatise, which features two case studies and recommendations for developing local school AIDS policies

424. AIDS in Africa. Gunn, Albert E. Foundation for Africa's Future, 2300 N St NW, Washington DC 20037 1988 49p

Discussion of the AIDS crisis in Africa

425. AIDS in America: Our Chances, Our Choices. Lee, Robert E. Whitston Publishing Company, Incorporated, PO Box 958, Troy NY 12181 1987 208p $18.50 0-87875-355-9

An historical review of how AIDS has impacted on American society and government

426. AIDS in Children, Adolescents and Heterosexual Adults: An Interdisciplinary Approach to Prevention. Schinazi, R F; Nahmias, A J. Elsevier Science Publishing Company, 52 Vanderbilt Ave, New York NY 10017 1988 433p $34.95 0-444-01316-4

A thorough treatise on AIDS prevention within the general heterosexual population

427. AIDS in Correctional Facilities: Issues and Options. 3rd ed. Hammett, Theodore M. US Dept of Justice, National Institute of Justice, Office of Communication and Research Utilization, Superintendent of Documents, Washington DC 20402 1988 296p $11.00 J 28.23:Ai 2/988

A report on AIDS for public policy, legal service, and public safety personnel

428. AIDS in Michigan: A Report to Gov. James J. Blanchard. Michigan Dept of Public Health. Michigan Dept of Public Health, 3500 N Logan St, Lansing MI 48909 1986
This is a state document concerning the impact of the AIDS epidemic on Michigan

429. AIDS in Prisons and Jails: Issues and Options. Hammett, Theodore M; US Dept of Justice, National Institute of Justice. Superintendent of Documents, US Government Printing Office, Washington DC 20402 1986 J 28.24:A:2
This US government document focuses on the complex problems posed by AIDS care and transmission in prisons and jails

430. AIDS: In Search of a Killer. LeVert, Suzanne. Julian Messner, 1230 Ave of the Americas, New York NY 10020 1987 147p $11.95 0-671-62840-2
General discussion of the origins of AIDS, how it has affected specific populations, civil rights issues for those with the syndrome, and future implications of the epidemic

431. AIDS in the Mind of America. Altman, Dennis. Anchor Press, 245 Park Ave, New York NY 10017 1986 228p $16.96 0-385-19523-0
A social history of the AIDS epidemic in America

432. AIDS in the Workplace: Legal Questions and Practical Answers. Banta, William F. Lexington Books, 125 Spring St, Lexington MA 02173 1988 257p $27.95 0-669-15334-6
A discussion of the legal implications of AIDS in the workplace, with references to relevent federal, state and local laws

433. AIDS in the Workplace: Resource Material. Bureau of National Affairs, 1231 25th St NW, Washington DC 20037 1986 322p
Discussion of AIDS and employment issues

434. AIDS: Information for the General Public. Illinois Dept of Public Health. Illinois Dept of Public Health, 535 W Jefferson St, Springfield IL 62761 1985
This is a state document with general AIDS information

435. AIDS Issues. Hearings Before the Subcommittee on Health and the Environment of the Committee on Energy and Commerce, House of Representatives, Ninety-ninth Congress, First Session, on Research and Treatment for Acquired Immune Deficiency Syndrome, July 22, 1985; Protection of Confidentiality of Records of Research Subjects and Blood Donors, July 29, 1985; Cost of AIDS Care and Who is Going to Pay, November 1, 1985. United States Congress, House Committee on Energy and Commerce, Subcommittee on Health and the Environment. Superintendent of Documents, US Government Printing Office, Washington DC 20402 1985 357p Y4.En2 3:00-45
AIDS issues, including the status of research and patient care, confidentiality and privacy concerns, and the costs of medical care, were discussed and documented in this Congressional hearings transcription

436. AIDS, Law and Policy. Gostin, Larry; Curran, William J. American Society of Law and Medicine, 765 Commonwealth Ave, Boston MA 02215 1987 96p
Discussion of the legal aspects of medical practice and AIDS, also published as volume 15 numbers 1-2, 1987 of the journal *Law, Medicine and Health Care*

437. AIDS: Legal and Human Resource Issues for the Employer. Schachter, Victor. Executive Enterprises, 22 W 21st St, New York NY 10010 1986 varies 0-880575-07-7
Contains information for employers regarding their legal rights and obligations in response to AIDS

438. AIDS: Legal Aspects of a Medical Crisis. Alter, Eleanor B. Law Journal Seminars Press, 111 8th Ave, New York NY 10011 1986 760p
Discussion of public health legislation and AIDS

439. AIDS Legal Guide. 2nd ed. Lambda Legal Defense and Education Fund, Inc, 132 W 43rd St, New York NY 10036 1987 various pagings $35.00
A manual about legal concerns related to AIDS for jurisprudence professionals

440. AIDS Literature. University Publishing Group, 107 E Church St, Frederick MD 21701 1986 650p $95.00 1-55572-005-6
This book is also published under the title *AIDS Reference and Research Collection*

441. AIDS: Meeting the Community Challenge. Cosstick, Vicky. Saint Paul Publications, Saint Pauls House, Middlegreen Slough, Great Britain SL3 6BT Great Britain 1987 190p £5.95 0-854392-64-5
A review of how British communities are dealing with the AIDS crisis

442. AIDS, Minorities and the Law. Harrington, Eugene. University Publishing Group, 107 E Church St, Frederick MD 21701 1988 325p $45.00
A review of AIDS-related legal issues for minority groups, women and children taken from a national conference held in September 1987

443. AIDS: Myths and Realities. Whitham, Neil. PPI Press, Inc, 940 E 149th St, Bronx NY 10455 1985 79p
Discussion of social aspects of AIDS, including public opinion and prevention

444. AIDS Network Manual. National Lawyers Guild, 853 Broadway, Ste 1705, New York NY 10003 1986

445. AIDS on Campus: Emerging Issues for College and Univ Administrators. Steinbach, Sheldon E. American Council on Education, 1 Dupont Circle, Washington DC 20036 1985 16p
Discussion of the impact of AIDS on America's college campuses

446. AIDS on the College Campus: ACHA Special Report. Keeling, Richard P. American College Health Association, 15879 Crabbs Branch Way, Rockville MD 20855 1986 65p
A discussion of AIDS and safer sex for college and university students

447. AIDS: Opposing Viewpoints. Modl, Tom; Hall, Lynn. Greenhaven Press, 577 Shoreview Park Rd, Saint Paul MN 55126 1987 223p $13.95 0-89908-427-3
A variety of sometimes conflicting points of view regarding AIDS are presented

448. AIDS: Origins, Prevention and Cure. Gordon Press, PO Box 459 Bowling Green Station, New York NY 10004 1987 4 vols $79.95 0-8490-3958-4
A fairly comprehensive account of the history of AIDS with additional discussion of prevention measures and potential for a cure

449. AIDS Package. Locklear, Edmond Jr. Carlton Press, Incorporated, 11 W 32nd St, New York NY 10001 1987 192p $11.95 0-8062-3077-0
Basic AIDS information packet

450. AIDS: Papers from *Science*, 1982-1985. Kulstad, Ruth. Westview Press, 5500 Central Ave, Boulder CO 80301 1986 653p $32.85 0-87168-313-X
Included are 108 papers from the journal *Science* on AIDS, including many of the original articles documenting the identification of the AIDS-causing virus, HIV

451. AIDS: Passageway to Transformation. Shealy, C Norman; Myss, Caroline. Stillpoint Publishing, PO Box 640, Walpole NH 03608 1987 105p $10.95 0-913299-47-2
A presentation of alternative therapies for AIDS

452. The AIDS Patient: An Action Agenda. Rogers, David E; Ginzberg, Eli. Westview Press, 5500 Central Ave, Boulder CO 80301 1988 $26.95 0-8133-7678-5
Contains papers taken from the fourth Cornell University Medical College Conference on Health Policy, held February 1988 in New York

453. AIDS. Personal Stories in Pastoral Perspective. Shelp, Earl E. Pilgrim Press, the United Church Press, 132 W 31st St, New York NY 10001 1986 205p $7.95 0-8298-0739-X

454. The AIDS Plague. Gordon Press Publishers, PO Box 459 Bowling Green Station, New York NY 10004 1987 $79.95 0-8490-3923-1
A general discourse on the AIDS epidemic

455. The AIDS Plague. McKeever, James M. Omega Publications, PO Box 4130, Medford OR 97501 1986 191p $16.95, $5.95 (paper); 0-86694-105-3, 0-86694-104-5 (paper)

456. AIDS: Plague or Panic. Trager, Oliver. Facts on File, 460 Park Ave S, New York NY 10016 1988 218p 0-816019-38-X
A compilation of editorials and columns about AIDS from American newspapers

457. AIDS Practice Manual: A Legal and Educational Guide. Paul, Albert; Graff, Leonard; Schatz, Benjamin. National Gay Rights Advocates and National Lawyers Guild, 540 Castro St, San Francisco CA 94114 1988 varies $35.00 0-960218-80-7
Information for public policy and legal service personnel

458. AIDS Prevention and Control: Invited Presentations and Papers from the World Summit of Ministers of Health on "Programmes for AIDS Prevention". World Health Organization. Pergamon Press, Maxwell House, Fairview Park, Elmsford New York 10523 1988 $100.00 0-08-036142-0
Papers and presentations were drawn from a meeting jointly organized by the World Health Organization and the government of the United Kingdom, held January 26-28, 1988

459. AIDS: Principles, Practice and Politics. Corless, Inge B; Pitman-Lindeman, Mary. Hemisphere Publishing Corporation, 79 Madison Ave, Ste 1110, New York NY 10016 1988 252p $15.95 0-89116-772-2

A discussion and the public policy and political issues surrounding AIDS

460. AIDS: Psychiatric and Psychosocial Perspectives. Paine, Leslie. Methuen, Inc, 29 W 35th St, New York NY 10001 1987 92p 0-7099-5605-5

Includes papers on the psychiatric and psychosocial aspects of AIDS drawn from an Association of Directors of Social Services co-sponsored conference held at the Institute of Psychiatry, London, February 1987

461. AIDS: Psychosocial Factors in the Acquired Immune Deficiency Syndrome. Baumgartner, Gail H. Charles C Thomas, 2600 S First St, Springfield IL 62717 1985 113p $18.50 0-398-05188-7

462. AIDS: Public Health and Legal Dimensions. Jayasuria, D C. Kluwer Academic Publishers, 101 Philip Dr, Assinippi Park, Norwell MA 02061 1988 9-0247-3686-2

Legal considerations relative to the public health context of the AIDS crisis

463. AIDS: Public Policy Dimensions. Griggs, John. United Hospital Fund of New York, 55 5th Ave, New York NY 10003 1987 308p $30.00pbk 0-934459-35-5

A collection of papers and excerpts based on a two-day conference on AIDS held in New York in 1986, including appendixes with world AIDS statistics and lists of resources and organizations

464. AIDS: Questions and Answers About Acquired Immune Deficiency Syndrome. Ostrow, David G. Irvington Publishers, 740 Broadway, New York NY 10003

465. The AIDS Reader: Documentary History of a Modern Epidemic. Clarke, Lauren K; Potts, Malcolm. Branden Publishing, Box 843 Brookline Village, Boston MA 02147 1988 350p $14.95 0-8283-1918-9

Reprints of articles documenting the history of AIDS

466. AIDS Reference and Research Collection. University Publishing Group, 107 E Church St, Frederick MD 21701 1988 various pagings $245.00 1-55572-002-1

This publication includes reprints of federal government hearings and reports, bibliographic references to various literature formats and lists of informational resources on AIDS

467. AIDS Reference and Research Collection: Hearings and Agency Reports. University Publishing Group, 107 E Church St, Frederick MD 21701 1988 various paging $115.00 1-55572-006-4

Reprints of various governmental hearings and reports pertaining to AIDS

468. AIDS Reference Guide: A Sourcebook for Planners and Decision Makers. Atlantic Information Services, Inc, 1050 17th St NW, Ste 480, Washington DC 20036 1988 various pagings $398.00

This guide culls from a wide range of sources information pertinent to the financial, social and economic impact of the AIDS epidemic, and is aimed at policy makers, community leaders, researchers and employers

469. AIDS Resource Manual. New York State Dept of Social Services; Rockefeller College of Public Affairs and Policy, Professional Development Program. New York State Dept of Social Services, 10 Eyck Bldg, 40 N Pearl St, 16th Fl, Albany NY 12243 1987 varies

A manual of resources for social agencies in New York State

470. AIDS, Sex and Protection. Bertacchi, Gloria M. National Medical Seminars, PO Box 2570, Fair Oaks CA 95628 1988 64p $4.95 0-945753-00-4

An overview of AIDS prevention and sexuality issues

471. AIDS: Spirits Share Understanding and Comfort from the Other Side. Nickell, Molli. Spirit Speaks, PO Box 84304, Los Angeles CA 90073 1986 110p $9.95 0-938283-99-5

AIDS coping techniques utilizing meditation

472. AIDS: Testing and Privacy. Gunderson, Martin; Mayo, David; Rhame, Frank S. University of Utah Press, 101 University Services Bldg, Salt Lake City UT 84112 1989 0-87480-317-9

A general discussion of the ethical issues surrounding HIV antibody test result confidentiality

473. AIDS: The Acquired Immune Deficiency Syndrome. 2nd ed. Daniels, Victor G. Kluwer Academic, 101 Philip Dr, Assinippi Park, Norwell MA 02061 1987 208p $19.95 0-7462-0035-8

Second edition of a popular general information resource about AIDS

474. AIDS: The Burdens of History. Fee, Elizabeth; Fox, Daniel. University of California Press, 2120 Berkeley Way, Berkeley CA 94720 1988 340p $25.00 0-520-06395-3

An historial review of the AIDS epidemic, focusing on the process of medical research and research methodologies

475. AIDS: The Deadly Epidemic. Hancock, Graham; Carim, Enver. David & Charles, Incorporated, PO Box 257, North Pomfret VT 05053 1987 192p $23.95 0-575-03836-5

A history of the AIDS crisis for general readers

476. AIDS: The Emerging Ethical Dilemmas. Levine, Carol; Bermel, Joyce. Hastings Center, Institute of Society, Ethics and Life Sciences, 360 Broadway, Hastings-on-Hudson NY 10706 1985 32p

477. AIDS: The Facts. Langone, John. Little, Brown and Company, 34 Beacon St, Boston MA 02108 1988 247p $17.95 0-316-51412-8

A history of the AIDS epidemic with additional information on the sydrome, its cause, prevention and control

478. AIDS: The Legal Complexities of a National Crisis. Alter, Eleanor B. Law Journal Seminars Press, 111 8th Ave, New York NY 10011 1987 272p

Collected works focusing on the legal implications of AIDS

479. AIDS: The Medical Mystery. Siegal, Frederick P. Grove Press, 196 W Houston St, New York NY 10014 1983 269p $19.50 0-394-53505-7

An early history of the AIDS epidemic

480. AIDS: The Moral Degeneration of Our Contemporary Society and the Future of Humanity. Blackmore, James G. American Classical College Press, PO Box 4526, Albuquerque NM 87196 1987 137p $88.85 0-961781-80-7

481. AIDS: The Mystery and the Solution. Gordon Press, PO Box 459 Bowling Green Station, New York NY 10004 1987 $79.95 0-8490-3924-X

A general account of the AIDS epidemic

482. AIDS: The Mystery and the Solution. 2nd ed. Cantwell, Alan. Aries Rising Press, 2132 Alcyona Dr, Los Angeles CA 90068 1986 210p $14.95, $9.95 (paper); 0-917211-08-1, 0-917211-16-2 (paper)

483. AIDS: The Public Context of an Epidemic. Bayer, Ronald; Fox, Daniel M; Willis, David P. Cambridge University Press, 32 E 57th St, New York NY 10022 1986 182p 0887-378X

Also published by the Milbank Memorial Fund in the journal, *The Milbank Quarterly*, vol 64 sup 1

484. AIDS: The Safety of Blood and Blood Products. Petricciani, John C. John Wiley and Sons, 605 3rd Ave, New York NY 10158 1987 $33.00 0-471-91338-3

Published by Wiley on behalf of the World Health Organization

485. AIDS: The Social Impact. Life Skills Education, 541 Columbia St, Weymouth MA 02190 1986 14p

486. AIDS: The Spiritual Dilemma. Fortunato, John E. Harper & Row, 10 E 53rd St, New York NY 10022 1987 156p $7.95 0-062503-38-3

A text for religious/spiritual counselors of people facing AIDS

487. AIDS: The Story of a Disease. Green, John; Miller, David. Grafton Books, 8 Grafton St, London, Great Britain W1X 3LA Great Britain 1986 151p 0-246-12982-4

A readable history of the AIDS crisis

488. AIDS: The Ultimate Challenge. Kubler-Ross, Elisabeth. Macmillan Publishing Co Inc, 866 3rd Ave, New York NY 10022 1987 320p $18.95 0-02-567170-7

Bestseller about AIDS and other chronic, debilitating illnesses by a controversial and insightful author

489. AIDS: The Women. Rieder, Ines; Ruppelt, Patricia. Cleis Press, PO Box 8933, Pittsburgh PA 15221 1988 300p $9.95 0-939416-21-2

A general discussion of the problem of women with AIDS

490. AIDS: The Workplace Issues. American Management Association, Membership Publications Division. American Management Association, Fulfillment Dept, Trudeau Rd, Saranac Lake NY 12983 1985 81p $10.00 0-814423-21-3

Employment and management issues surrounding AIDS in the workplace

491. AIDS: Therapeutics in HIV Disease. Youle, Michael. Churchill Livingstone, 1560 Broadway, New York NY 10031 1988 0-443-04029-X

492. AIDS—What a Woman Needs to Know/El SIDS—Lo Que Toda Mujer Necesita Saber. Hispanic AIDS Committee for Education and Resources Inc (HACER), 301 S Frio, San Antonio TX 78207 $1.25

A bilingual book for women presenting basic information about AIDS including how it is transmitted, risks to women and their children, symptoms, testing, treatment, and protection

493. AIDS: What Does It Mean to You? Revised Edition. Walker & Company, 720 5th Ave, New York NY 10019 1987 128p $14.95 0-8027-6699-4

AIDS information for young adults grades 7 and up, discussing medical progress, avoiding exposure, and the Surgeon General's report on the syndrome

494. AIDS: What is Now Known. Selwyn, Peter A. H P Publishing Co, 575 Lexington Ave, New York NY 10022 1986 72p

Contains articles previously published in the journal *Hospital Practice*

495. AIDS: You Can't Catch it Holding Hands. de SaintPhalle, Niki; Barandun, Silvio. Lapis Press, 1850 Union St, Ste 466, San Francisco CA 94123 1986 $5.95

This book, in the format of an illustrated letter from mother to son, gives advice in explicit language on how AIDS is and is not transmitted

496. AIDS: You Just Think You're Safe. Adams, Moody. Global Publishers, PO Box 21788, Chattanooga TN 37421 1986 246p $7.95

A general discussion of AIDS from a religious perspective

497. A.I.D.S.: Your Child and the School. Reed, Robert D; Kaus, Danek S. R & E Publishers, PO Box 2008, Saratoga CA 95070 1986 24p $3.00 0-88247-756-0

This book is a resource guide for parents and teachers concerning AIDS-related issues in schools, and includes listings of regional information centers, hotlines, educational organizations, and a bibliography

498. AIDS: Your Questions Answered. Fisher, Richard B. Alyson Publications, 40 Plympton St, Boston MA 02118 1984 126p $3.95 0-907040-29-2

General information about AIDS

499. The AIDS-Related Diet: How the Food We Eat Builds or Destroys Immunity Against Infectious and Contagious Diseases. Muramoto, Noboru. George Ohsawa Macrobiotic Foundation, 1511 Robinson St, Oroville CA 95965 1988 $12.95 0-918860-48-2

500. AIDS-Related Services. University Publishing Group, 107 E Church St, Frederick MD 21701 1986 25p $20.00

Included are listings of both government and volunteer-sponsored AIDS-related services at the federal, state, and local levels

501. AIDS-Zits: A Sextionary for Kids. Marsh, Carole. Gallopade, Main St, Bath NC 27808 1987 48p $7.95 1-55609-210-5

A dictionary of sex terminology for children

502. Alternative and Holistic Health Care for AIDS and its Prevention: A Sourcebook of Descriptions, Bibliography, and Practitioners in the Washington, DC-Baltimore, MD Area. Van Ness, Paul N. Whitman-Walker Clinic, Inc, 2335 18th St NW, Washington DC 20009 1985 25p

503. And the Band Played On: Politics, People, & the AIDS Epidemic. Shilts, Randy. St Martin's Press, Inc, 175 5th Ave, New York NY 10010 1987 $24.95 0-312009-94-1

Shilts, a journalist with the *San Francisco Chronicle* and the author of *The Mayor of Castro Street: The Life and Times of Harvey Milk*, examines the first five years of the AIDS epidemic, including the political and sociological factors which may have contributed to its spread

504. Answers About AIDS. American Council on Science and Health. American Council on Science and Health, 1995 Broadway, New York NY 10023 1988 60p $2.00

This book answers questions about AIDS regarding symptoms, risk factors, at-risk groups, fatality rates, causes and modes of virus transmission, and clinical manifestations

505. The Anti-AIDS Pill ZPG-1: Available Over the Counter. Sergio, William. Sergio Publishing, 132 W 24th St, Ste 747, New York NY 10011 1985 200p $14.95 0-936003-00-6

Discussion of an alternative drug therapy for AIDS

506. Beyond the AIDS Crisis: Christian Ministry to the Gay Community. Reid, Greg. Larksdale, 1706 Seamist, No 575, Houston TX 77008 1988 192p $9.95 0-89896-166-1

An analysis of the problems endemic to providing religious ministrations to gay men and women in light of AIDS

507. Biobehavioral Control of AIDS. Ostrow, David G. Irvington, 740 Broadway, Ste 905, New York NY 10003 1987 255p $29.50 0-8290-1779-8

Includes papers presented at a workshop organized by the American Association of Physicians for Human Rights, the National Coalition of Gay STD Services and the National Gay and Lesbian Health Education Foundation at the First International AIDS Conference, Atlanta 1985

508. Blood, Blood Products, and AIDS. Madhok, R; Forbes, C D; Evatt, B. Johns Hopkins University Press, 615 N Wolfe St, Baltimore MD 21205 1987 244p $45.00 0-8018-3608-5

This book includes discussion of the impact of AIDS on the nation's blood supply and blood collection system and is a volume in the *Johns Hopkins Series in Contemporary Medicine and Public Health*

509. Borrowed Time: An AIDS Memoir. Monette, Paul. Harcourt, Brace & Jovanovich, 1250 6th Ave, San Diego CA 92101 1988 342p $18.95 0-151135-98-3

Monette chronicles the death of a friend from AIDS

510. Third BMA Statement on AIDS. British Medical Association Working Party on AIDS. British Medical Association, BMA House, Tavistock Square London WC1H 9JR UK 1987 26p

511. Candida, Silver (Mercury) Fillings and the Immune System, 3rd revised ed. Russell-Manning, Betsy. Greensward Press, PO Box 640472, San Francisco CA 94164 1986 239p $15.95 0-930165-10-1

This third, revised edition includes information about the oral condition Candida albicans, frequently linked with AIDS

512. Caring for Persons with AIDS and Cancer: Ethical Reflections on Palliative Care for the Terminally Ill. Tuohey, John F. Catholic Health Association of the United States, 4455 Woodson Rd, Saint Louis MO 63134 1988 0-87125-150-7

Discussion of ethical issues related to the care of terminally-ill people, including those with AIDS

513. CDC Reports on Acquired Immunodeficiency Syndrome (AIDS). Centers for Disease Control. Superintendent of Government Documents, US Government Printing Office, Washington DC 20402 1984 32p HE 20.7009/a:ac 7

A compilation of Centers for Disease Control reports on AIDS as published in *Morbidity and Mortality Weekly Reports*, current as of 1984

514. Changing Bodies, Changing Lives: A Book for Teens on Sex and Relationships. Revised Edition. Bell, Ruth. Random House, Incorporated, 201 E 50th St, New York NY 10022 1987 254p $17.45 0-394-50304-X

This new, revised edition of the popular 1980 book on the physical and emotional changes wrought by puberty has been updated to include important information for teens about AIDS

515. Choose to Live: An AIDS Healing Companion. Badgley, Laurence E. Human Energy Press, 370 W San Bruno, Ste D, San Bruno CA 94066 1987 70p $7.95 0-941523-01-2

Alternative therapeutic techniques for managing AIDS

516. Chronicle: The Human Side of AIDS. Greenly, Mike. Irvington Publishers, 740 Broadway, New York NY 10003 1986 422p $17.95 0-8290-1800-X

517. The Color of Light: Meditations for All of Us Living with AIDS. Tilleraas, Peter. Harper/Hazelden Press, Box 176, Center City MN 55012 1988 350p $7.95 0-06255-490-5

Inspirational ruminations for those with AIDS and their loved ones

518. Communicable Diseases. Metos, Thomas H. Franklin Watts, 387 Park Ave S, New York NY 10016 1987 96p

Information for secondary school children about communicable diseases, including AIDS

519. Communicable Diseases and the Enrolled Student: A Model Policy and Rules. Iowa Dept of Public Instruction. Iowa Dept of Health, E 12th and Walnut Sts, Des Moines IA 50319 1986 7p

520. A Community Resource Guide for Assisting People With AIDS. Massachusetts Dept of Public Health, Health Resource Office. Massachusetts Dept of Public Health, 150 Tremont St, Boston MA 02111 1987 168p

This guide for people working with AIDS patients includes community and social support resource information. The guide is also published under the title *AIDS, Acquired Immune Deficiency Syndrome: Community Resource Guide*

521. The Complete Guide to Safe Sex. McIlvenna, Ted; Lourea, David; Moser, Charles; Rubenstein, Maggi; Taylor, Clark. Multifocus, Inco, 1525 Franklin St, San Francisco CA 94109 1987 216p $6.95 0-930846-05-2

This safer sex manual, produced by the Institute for Advanced Study of Human Sexuality, is intended to "turn people on to safe sex." Included are discussions of sexual practice risk levels, HIV transmission and exposure prevention

522. The Condom Book: The Essential Guide for Men and Women. Everett, Jane; Glanz, Walter D. NAL Penguin, Inc, 1633 Broadway, New York NY 10019 1987 139p $3.95 0-45115-173-9

The authors evaluate 100 brands of condoms and offer advice on safer sex

523. Confronting AIDS: Directions for Public Health, Health Care, and Research. Institute of Medicine, Committee on a National Strategy for AIDS. National Academy Press, 2101 Constitution Ave, Washington DC 20418 1986 374p 0-309-03699-2

524. Confronting AIDS: Update 1988. Institute of Medicine Oversight Committee. National Academy Press, 2101 Constitution Ave NW, Washington DC 20418 1988 239p $15.95 0-309-03879-0

A review of recent progress in research, public health and health care relevant to AIDS

525. Conquering AIDS Now: With Natural Treatment, a Non-Drug Approach. Gregory, Scott J. Warner Books, 666 5th Ave, New York NY 10103 1987 190p $15.95 0-446-38733-9

This book contains a variety of alternative, natural treatments for AIDS and was originally published in 1986 under the title, *Conquering a Modern Plague*, by Tree of Life Publications, Santa Monica, CA

526. Conquering AIDS Now! With Natural Treatment, A Non-Drug Approach. 3rd ed. Gregory, Scott J; Leonardo, Bianca. Tree of Life Publications, PO Box 126, Joshua Tree CA 92252 1986 224p $12.95 0-93085-202-8

Holistic, alternative treatment recommendations for persons with AIDS

527. Coping with AIDS: Facts and Fears. Kurland, Morton L. Rosen Publishing Group, 29 E 21st St, New York NY 10010 1987 118p $9.97 0-8239-0687-6

528. Coping with AIDS: Psychological and Social Considerations in Helping People with HTLV-III Infections. National Institute of Mental Health. Superintendent of Documents, US Government Printing Office, Washington DC 20402 1986 19p HE 20.8102 Ac 7

Discussion of social and psychological considerations for people diagnosed as having been exposed to the AIDS-causing virus

529. Counseling in HIV Infection and AIDS. Green, John; McCreaner, Alana. Blackwell Scientific Publications, 52 Beacon St, Boston MA 02108 1988 352p $15.95 0-632-01924-7

Contains information for counselors of people with AIDS or those that are HIV-positive

530. Crisis: Heterosexual Behavior in the Age of AIDS. Masters, William. Grove Press, 920 Broadway, New York NY 10010 1988 243p $15.95 0-8021-1049-5

Controversial Masters & Johnson report about AIDS, focusing on HIV transmission, safer sex and disease epidemiology

531. Current Information on Acquired Immune Deficiency Syndrome. United States Public Health Service, Office of Public Affairs. Public Health Service, Office of Public Affairs, 200 Independence Ave SW, Washington DC 20201 1983 14p

532. Current Medical-Legal Issues—AIDS: Program Material: San Francisco, Friday and Saturday, July 25 and 26, 1986: Los Angeles, Friday and Saturday, August 8 and 9, 1986. California Continuing Education of the Bar, 2300 Shattuck Ave, Berkeley CA 94704 1986 384p

533. The Current Status of HTLV-III Testing. Otter, Jean. American Association of Blood Banks, 1117 N 19th St, Ste 600, Arlington VA 22209 1986 46p $5.50pbk 0-915355-34-5

The proceedings of a teleconference workshop held July 30, 1986 in Boston presenting views on HIV testing

534. Death Rush: Poppers and AIDS. Lauritsen, John; Wilson, Hank. Pagan Press, 26 St Mark's Place, New York NY 10003 1986 64p $3.00 0-943742-05-6

The authors draw links between the use of amyl nitrate and the occurrence of AIDS

535. The Deepening Shade: Psychological Aspects of Life-Threatening Illness. Sourkes, Barbara M. University of Pittsburgh Press, 127 N Bellefield Ave, Pittsburgh PA 15260 1982 126p $6.95 0-822934-56-6

This book discussed the impact of life-threatening illnesses on families, friends and caregivers

536. Disease and Representation: Images of Illness from Madness to AIDS. Gilman, Sander L. Cornell University Press, 124 Roberts Place, PO Box 250, Ithaca NY 14851 1988 320p 0-8014-2119-5

Discussion of the history of attitudes towards illness and the "sick role" as depicted in the arts

537. El SIDA no Descrimina (AIDS Does Not Discriminate). AIDS Community Education Project. Orange County Health Care Agency, 1725 W 17th St, Rm 116-C, Santa Ana CA 92706 1987 20p

A booklet in Spanish using a fictional story of a Latino family to present information about AIDS transmission, antibody testing, risk behaviors, and risk reduction

538. An Emergency War Plan to Fight AIDS and Other Pandemics. Hamerman, Warren J. Executive Intelligence Review, PO Box 17557, Washington DC 20041 1986 138p

539. Emergency Workers and the AIDS Epidemic: A Guide book for Law Enforcement, Fire Service, and Ambulance Service Personnel. California Firefighter Foundation, 300 T St, Sacramento CA 95814

540. Employment Testing: A National Reporter on Polygram, Drug, AIDS and Genetic Testing. Hurd, Sandra N. University Publications of America, 44 N Market St, Frederick MD 21701 1987 0-890939-38-1

Review of the controversies surrounding employment testing for AIDS, drug use, and other "bio-detectable" conditions

541. Epidemic of Courage: Facing AIDS in America. Nungesser, Lon. Saint Martin's Press, 175 5th Ave, New York NY 10010 1988 255p $7.95 0-312-01560-7

Discussion of the psychological ramifications of the AIDS epidemic

542. The Epidemiology and Health Economics of Acquired Immunodeficiency Syndrome in Minnesota: Current Status and Future Projections. AIDS Unit, Acute Disease Epidemiology Section. Minnesota Dept of Health, 717 Delaware St SE, Minneapolis MN 55440 1986 121p

This state document considers the occurrence and costs of AIDS

543. Epidemiology of the Acquired Immunodeficiency Syndrome (AIDS). Peterman, Thomas A; Drotman, Peter; Curran, James W. Superintendent of Documents, US Government Printing Office, Washington DC 20402 1986 21p HE 20.7031:Ac 7

Report for the Public Health Service, US Dept of Health and Human Services, on the occurrence of AIDS in America

544. Eroticizing Safer Sex. Palacios-Jimenez, Luis; Shernoff, Michael. Gay Men's Health Crisis, Box 264, 132 W 24th St, New York NY 10011 1986 33p $8.00 0-917833-08-5

A safer sex guide, this book also goes by the title *Facilitator's Guide to Eroticizing Safer Sex*

545. The Essential AIDS Fact Book: What You Need to Know to Protect Yourself, Your Family, All Your Loved Ones. Douglas, Paul H; Pinsky, Laura. Pocket Books, 1230 Ave of the Americas, New York NY 10020 1987 63p $3.95 0-671-64772-5

A book for general audiences outlining basic facts about AIDS including cause, risk and prevention

546. Ethical Response to AIDS. America Press, 106 W 56th St, New York NY 10019 1988 174p

A general discussion of ethical issues surrounding the AIDS epidemic

547. Evangelical Terrorism, Censorship, Falwell, Robertson, and the Seamy Side of Christian Fundamentalism. Ide, Arthur Frederick. Scholars Books, PO Box 160361, Irving TX 75016 1986 193p $12.95 0-93865-901-4

According to Dr Ide, many opinions expressed by various religious and new-right leaders about AIDS have hindered educational efforts to combat the epidemic

548. Everything You Need to Know About AIDS. Taylor, Barbara. Rosen Publishing Group, 29 E 31st St, New York NY 10010 1988 64p $10.95 0-8239-0809-7

Part of the *Need to Know Library* containing AIDS information for young adults

549. Exposing the AIDS Coverup: What You Don't Know Can Kill You. Cameron, Paul. Huntington House, Incorporated, PO Box 53788, Lafayette LA 70505 1988 $6.95 0-919311-52-8

A controversial account of what has reportedly not been made public to the American people about AIDS

550. Facilitator's Guide to Eroticizing Safer Sex: A Psychoeducational Workshop Approach to Safer Sex Education. Palacios-Jimenez, Luis; Shernoff, Michael. Gay Men's Health Crisis, Box 274, 132 W 24th St, New York NY 10011 1986 33p $8.00 0-917833-01-5

This book is an instructional guide for presenting safer sex workshops, and is also called *Eroticizing Safer Sex*

551. **Facts About AIDS.** United States Public Health Service. Superintendent of Documents, US Government Printing Office, Washington DC 20402 1987 10p HE 20.2: ac 7/987
Information about AIDS for the general public

552. **Facts About AIDS and Other Sexually Transmitted Diseases: Sexual Decisions of Responsible Adults.** Bogner, Jerry L. Bogner's Limited, PO Drawer KK, Santa Barbara CA 93102 1987 108p $14.95 0-943323-00-2
A general book for adults about sexually transmitted diseases, including AIDS

553. **Family Protection Scoreboard, No. 2: Special Edition on AIDS.** Balsiger, David W. Biblical News Service Publications, PO Box 10428, Costa Mesa CA 92627 1987 48p $2.95
General information for families about AIDS

554. **The Federal Response to AIDS.** United States Congress, House Committee on Government Operations, Ninety-eighth Congress, First Session. Superintendent of Documents, US Government Printing Office, Washington DC 20402 1983 36p Y1.1/8:98-582
Report by the Committee on Government Operations on AIDS, with dissenting and additional views

555. **First AIDS: Frank Facts for Kids.** Marsh, Carole S. Gallopade: Publishing Group, Main St, Bath NC 27808 1987 25p $7.95 1-55609-205-9
Information about AIDS for young children

556. **Focus: AIDS in the Workplace.** Wexler, Richard H. Prentice Hall, Inc, Rte 9 W, Englewood Cliffs NJ 07633 1986 32p $3.75 0-13-020785-3
Consideration of social and legal aspects of AIDS for employers and employees

557. **Gay Men's Health: A Guide to the AID Syndrome and Other Sexually Transmitted Diseases.** Kassler, Jeanne. Harper and Row Publishers, Inc, 10 E 53rd St, New York NY 10022 1983 166p $13.95, $5.95 (paper); 0-06-015146-3, 0-06-091057-7 (paper)

558. **Gay: What Teenagers Should Know About Homosexuality and the AIDS Crisis.** Hunt, Morton. Farrar, Straus & Giroux, 19 Union Square W, New York NY 10003 1987 244p $12.95 0-371325-25-1
Included are discussions of safer sex and why AIDS in America has been linked with a gay lifestyle

559. **Gays, AIDS and You.** Rueda, Enrique T; Schwartz, Michael. Davin-Adair Publishers, 6 N Water St, Greenwich CT 06830 1987 117p $5.95 0-8159-5624-X
General information for gay men about AIDS prevention and HIV antibody testing

560. **The Global Impact of AIDS.** Fleming, Alan F; Carballo, Manuel; FitzSimons, David W; et al. Alan R Liss, Inc, 41 E 11th St, New York NY 10003 1988 460p $69.50 0-8451-4271-2
Documentation of the proceedings of the First International Conference on the Global Impact of AIDS, co- sponsored by the World Health Organization and the London School of Hygiene and Tropical Medicine, held in London, March 1988

561. **Guide to Public Health Practice: HTLV-III Screening in the Community.** Gebbie, Kristine M. Association of State and Territorial Health Officials Foundation, 1311A Dolley Madison Blvd, Ste 3A, McLean VA 22101 1985 20p
Discussion of medical screening for the AIDS-causing virus

562. **Guidelines for Preventing the Transmission of Human T-Cell Lymphotropic Virus Type III in the Prison Setting.** Wisconsin Dept of Health and Social Services, PO Box 309, 1 W Wilson St, Madison WI 53701 1986 34p
This state document presents guidelines for preventing the spread of the AIDS-causing virus in prison populations

563. **Guidelines on AIDS in Europe.** Regional Office for Europe, World Health Organization. World Health Organization 1986 42p 9-289-01039-8

564. **Healing AIDS Naturally: Natural Therapies for the Immune System.** Badgley, Laurence E. Human Energy Press, 370 W San Bruno, Ste D, San Bruno CA 94066 1987 411p $14.95 0-941523-00-4
Detailed discussion of alternative, natural therapies for AIDS and other diseases

565. **Heroin Addiction: Theory, Research and Treatment. 2nd ed.** Platt, James J. Krieger Publishing, PO Box 9542, Melbourne FL 32902 1988 462p $34.50 0-89464-325-8
Detailed discussion about heroin addiction, with chapters focusing on AIDS

566. **Herpes, AIDS, and Other Sexually Transmitted Diseases.** Llewellyn-Jones, Derek. Faber and Faber, Inc, 50 Cross St, Winchester MA 01890 1985 200p 0-571-13434-3, 0-571-13435-1

567. **Heterosexual AIDS: Myth or Fact?.** Matsumura, Kenneth. Alin Foundation Press, 2107 Dwight Way, Berkeley CA 94704 1988 78p $6.95 0-9606924-3-6
A review of the epidemiology or occurrence of AIDS and the transmission of HIV within the heterosexual community

568. **The Heterosexual Transmission of AIDS in Africa.** Vanderschmidt, Hennelore; Koch-Weser, Dieter. ABT Books, Incorporated, 146 Mount Auburn St, Cambridge MA 02138 1988 300p $39.50 0-89011-603-2
An analysis of HIV transmission in Africa

569. **History of AIDS.** University Publishing Group, 107 E Church St, Frederick MD 21701 1988 345p $55.00 1-55572-004-8
A thorough history of the AIDS epidemic

570. **How to Fortify Your Immune System.** Dickenson, Donald E. Arlington Books Ltd, 15-17 King St, London England SW 1Y 6QU Great Britain 1984 101p 0-85140-633-5

571. **How to Have Sex in an Epidemic: One Approach.** Berkowitz, Richard. News From the Front, PO Box 106, 70 Greenwich Ave, New York NY 10011 1983 40p

572. **How to Persuade Your Lover to Use a Condom...and Why You Should.** Breitman, Patti; Knutson, Kim; Reed, Paul. Prima Publishing and Communications, PO Box 1260C, Rocklin CA 95677 1987 83p $4.95pbk 0-914629-43-3
A book on why one should use a condom, intended for both heterosexual and gay individuals

573. **How to Protect Your Family from AIDS.** Rowe, Edward. National AIDS Prevention Institute, PO Box 2500, Culpeper VA 22701 1987 60p $6.00 0-944373-01-1
Information on how to safeguard the family from AIDS

574. **Illness as Metaphor.** Sontag, Susan. Farrar, Straus & Giroux, 19 Union Square W, New York NY 10003 1988 $15.95 0-374204-24-1
This new, revised edition includes a postscript relating the author's themes to AIDS

575. **I'm Looking for Mr. Right, But I'll Settle for Mr. Right Away: AIDS, True Love, the Perils of Safe Sex, and Other Spiritual Concerns of the Gay Male. 2nd ed.** Flood, Gregory. Brob House Books, PO Box 7829, Atlanta GA 30309 1987 115p $7.95 0-938407-00-7
Spiritual guidance for the gay male in the age of AIDS

576. **In Self-Defense: The Human Immune System.** Mizel, Steven B; Jaret, Peter. Simon and Schuster, 1230 Avenue of the Americas, New York NY 10020 1986 240p $8.95 0-671-62332-X
Discussion on how the body's immune system works, geared to the general public

577. **In the Matter of AIDS: Implications for Health, Treatment and Long-Term Care. Hearing.** California Legislature, Senate, Committee on Health and Human Services. Joint Publications Office, California Legislature, Senate, Health and Human Services Committee, State Capitol, Sacramento CA 95814 1985
This state document concerns a hearing before the California Legislature on AIDS-related issues

578. **Indiana AIDS Prevention Plan, 1986.** Indiana State Board of Health. Indiana State Board of Health, Health Bldg, 1330 W Michigan St, PO Box 1964, Indianapolis IN 46206 1986
A plan developed by the state of Indiana for confronting AIDS through promoting prevention

579. **Know About AIDS.** Hyde, Margaret O; Forsyth, Elizabeth. Walker & Company, 720 5th Ave, New York NY 10019 1987 68p $10.95 0-8027-6738-9
Information about AIDS ranging from how it is contracted to testing for HIV, geared for children grades 3 through 8

580. **Legacy of Love: How to Make Life Easier for the Ones You Leave Behind.** Petterle, Elmo A; Kahn, Robert C. San Francisco AIDS Foundation, 333 Valencia St, San Francisco CA 94101 1988 208p $12.95 0-679-73950-5
A workbook giving practical advice for getting one's affairs in order for the terminally ill and their friends, families and lovers

581. **Legal Issues in Transfusion Medicine.** Clark, Gilbert M. American Association of Blood Banks, 1117 N 19th St, Ste 600, Arlington VA 22209 1986 $20.00 0-915355-22-1
Confidentiality, negligence and liability issues are covered in this transcribed "Landmark Conference" proceeding held in 1985

582. **Living With AIDS: A Self Care Manual.** Lang, Jennifer M. AIDS Project Los Angeles, Inc, 7362 Santa Monica Blvd, Los Angeles CA 90046 1984 95p

583. Living With AIDS and HIV. Miller, David. Sheridan House, Inc, 145 Palisade St, Dobbs Ferry NY 10522 1987 144p $40.00 0-333-43243-6

Advice to those who have tested positive for exposure to the AIDS-causing virus, offering practical suggestions for making important psychological, interpersonal and lifestyle adjustments

584. Living With AIDS: How Gay Men Confront the Crisis. Severance, Lori J. California State Univ, Sacramento, 6000 J St, Sacramento CA 95819 1985 154p

585. Living With AIDS: Reaching Out. O'Connor, Tom. Corwin Publishers, Inc, PO Box 2806, San Francisco CA 94126 1986 0-938569-00-7

586. Local Government and AIDS: A Special Report with Case Studies. Lockwood, Melanie J. Public Technology, Incorporated, 1301 Pennsylvania Ave NW, Washington DC 20004 1988 93p $10.00 1-556570-05-8

A survey of community health services established to meet the AIDS challenge

587. Local Policies in Response to Acquired Immune Deficiency Syndrome (AIDS) and HLTV-III/LAV Infection. United States Conference of Mayors, AIDS Information Exchange Program. United States Conference of Mayors, 1620 I St, NW, Washington DC 20006 1986 128p

A survey of local AIDS policies throughout the US

588. The Lonely Voyage: Support or Isolation for Gay Men with AIDS. Shands, Nancy. Wide World Publishing/Tetra, PO Box 476, San Carlos CA 94070 1988 175p $9.95 0-933174-54-3

This published masters thesis discusses the sociological implications of AIDS for gay men, and was submitted to the Virginia Polytechnical Institute and State University in 1987

589. Love, Medicine and Miracles: Lessons Learned About Self-healing from a Surgeon's Experience with Exceptional Patients. Siegel, Bernie S. Harper & Row, 10 E 53rd St, New York NY 10022 1986 256p $15.95 0-06-015496-9

Popular and inspirational bestseller about courageous patients in a doctor's practice, including those with AIDS

590. Lovers, Doctors and the Law: Your Legal Rights and Responsibilities in Today's Sex-Health Crisis. Davis, Margaret; Scott, Robert S. Harper & Row, 10 E 53rd St, New York NY 10022 1988 248p $16.95 0-06-055111-9

Presentation of the legal rights and responsibilities of doctors during the current AIDS crisis

591. Making It: A Woman's Guide to Sex in the Age of AIDS. Patton, Cindy; Kelly, Janis. Firebrand Books, 141 The Commons, Ithaca NY 14850 1987 $3.95 0-932379-32-X

This book, in both English and Spanish, includes information about AIDS, safer sex practices, and health care for heterosexual and lesbian women

592. The Management of AIDS Patients. Miller, David; Weber, Jonathan; Green, John. Canadian Hospital Association, 17 York St, Ste 100, Ottawa, Ontario K1N 9J6 Canada 1988 $34.95 0-919100-74-0

593. Managing AIDS in the Workplace. Emery, Alan R; Puckett, Sam B. Addison-Wesley Publishing Company, 1 Jacob Way, Reading MA 01867 1988 191p $19.95 0-201-08058-3

A guide for employers concerned about managing AIDS-related concerns in the workplace

594. Manual of Safe Sex. Kilby, Don. B.C. Decker, Inc, PO Box 30246, Philadelphia PA 19103 1986 213p $14.95 1-55009-016-X

595. The Many Faces of AIDS: A Gospel Response. A Statement of the Administrative Board, United States Catholic Conference. United States Catholic Conference Administrative Board. United States Catholic Conference, 1312 Massachusetts Ave, Washington DC 20005 1987 30p $1.00 1-55586-195-4

A spiritual response to the provision of AIDS care

596. Maximum Immunity. Weiner, Michael A. Pocket Books, 1230 Ave of the Americas, New York NY 10020 1987 416p $4.50 0-671-63447-X

Describes the body's immune defenses, how to strengthen them, and includes a chapter on AIDS

597. Medical Answers About AIDS. Gay Men's Health Crisis Inc, 132 W 24th St, PO Box 274, New York NY 10011 1987 70p $1.00

Medical information about AIDS written for the general public, persons with AIDS, those at risk for AIDS and their families and friends, and health care providers

598. Meeting the Challenge: Foundation Responses to Acquired Immune Deficiency Syndrome. Seltzer, Michael; Allee, Susan; Ringel, Betsy; Taylor, Robert. The Foundation Center, 79th 5th Ave Dept HX, New York NY 10003 1987 35p

A summary of foundation support for AIDS research

599. Mental Health Aspects of AIDS (Acquired Immune Deficiency Syndrome): A Guide for Health Caregivers. Kay, R. National Technical Information Service (NTIS), Springfield VA 22161 1985

Available in microfiche format from NTIS, item number PB85-199909

600. Mobilizing Against AIDS: The Unfinished Story of a Virus. Nichols, Eve K. Harvard Univ Press, 79 Garden St, Cambridge MA 02138 1986 212p $15.00, $7.95 (paper); 0-674-57760-4, 0-674-57761-2 (paper)

601. Mortal Fear: Meditations on Death and AIDS. Snow, John. Cowley Publications, 980 Memorial Dr, Cambridge MA 02138 1987 92p $6.95 0-936384-49-2

A book for pastoral counselors including five meditations on AIDS, death, dying and pain

602. Needle Sharing Among Intravenous Drug Abusers: National and International Perspectives. Battjes, Robert J; Pickens, Roy W. US Deparment of Health and Human Services, Public Health Service, Alcohol, Drug Abuse, and Mental Health Administration, National Institute on Drug Abuse, Superintendent of Documents, Washington DC 20402 1988 183p $51.00 HE 20:8216.80

This book presents papers on the transmission of the AIDS-causing virus HIV through needle-sharing by intravenous drug abusers presented at a technical conference sponsored by the Division of Clinical Research, National Institute on Drug Abuse, May 1987

603. No Magic Bullet: A Social History of Venereal Disease in the United States Since 1880. 2nd ed.. Brandt, Allan M. Oxford Univ Press, 200 Madison Ave, New York NY 10016 1987 266p 0-19-504237-9

The second edition contains a chapter on AIDS

604. Notes on Living Until We Say Goodbye: A Personal Guide. Nungesser, Lon; Bullock, William D. Saint Martin's Press, 175 Fifth Ave, New York NY 10010 1988 156p $14.95 0-31201-517-8

Advice for the terminally ill on how to confront death

605. Office of Technology Assessment's Findings on the Public Health Service's Response to AIDS. Joint Hearing Before a Subcommittee of the Committee on Government Operations and the Committee on Energy and Commerce, House of Representatives, Ninety-ninth Congress, First Session, February 21, 1985. United States Congress, House, Committee on Government Operations, Intergovernmental Relations and Human Resources Subcommittee; United States Congress, House, Committee on Energy and Commerce. Superintendent of Documents, US Government Printing Office, Washington DC 20402 1985 Y4 G 74/7/T 22 3

Congressional hearings regarding the US government's response to the AIDS crisis

606. One Day at a Time: A Personal Guide to Coping with a Terminal Diagnosis. Nungesser, Lon. Saint Martin's Press, 175 Fifth Ave, New York NY 10010 1988

Advice on how to manage your life after being diagnosed with AIDS

607. Panic: The Story of AIDS. McKie, Robin. Thorsons Publishers, Ltd, Denington Estate, Wellingborough, Northants England NN8 2RQ Great Britain 1986 128p

608. The Plague in Our Midst: Sexuality, AIDS and the Christian Family. Albers, Gres. Huntington House, Incorporated, PO Box 53788, Lafayette LA 70505 1988 $6.95 0-910311051-X

Christian perspectives on sexuality, AIDS and the family

609. The Plague Years: A Chronicle of AIDS, the Epidemic of Our Times. Black, David. Simon and Schuster, 1230 Avenue of the Americas, New York NY 10020 1986 224p $16.95 0-671-61224-7

A history of AIDS

610. Plain Words About AIDS: With a Glossary of Related Terms. 3rd ed. Smith, William Hovey. Whitehall Press-Budget Publications, Whitehall, Rte 1, Box 603, Sandersville GA 31082 1988 200p $19.50 0-916565-11-4

Contains articles about AIDS drawn from the *National Wire Service,*through January 1988, in addition to excerpts from papers presented at the 1"International Conference on AIDS," 1987 Washington, 1986 Paris, and 1985 Atlanta meetings

611. Play Safe: How to Avoid Getting Sexually Transmitted Diseases. Mandel, Bea; Mandel, Byron. Center for Health Information, PO Box 4636, Foster City CA 94404 1986 98p $4.95 0-932567-01-0

612. Pleasure and Danger: Exploring Female Sexuality. Vance, Carol. Routledge and Kegan Paul, 14 Leicester Square, London England WC 2H 7PH Great Britain 1984 462p $28.00, $14.00 (paper); 0-7100-9974-6, 0-7102-0248-2 (paper)

613. Policing Desire: Pornography, AIDS and the Media. Watney, Simon. University of Minnesota Press, 2037 University Ave, SE, Minneapolis MN 55414 1987 159p $35.00 0-8166-1643-4
Watney discusses the often perjorative manner in which gays and AIDS are depicted in the media, including the press, movies and television

614. Poppers and AIDS: With Annotated Bibliography. 2nd ed. Lauritsen, John; Wilson, Hank. Committee to Monitor Poppers, 55 Mason St, San Francisco CA 94102 1985 21p

615. Preliminary Report of the Commission on the Human Immunodeficiency Virus (HIV) Epidemic. Presidential Commission on the Human Immunodeficiency Virus Epidemic; Watkins, James D. Presidential Commission on the Human Immunodeficiency Virus Epidemic, 655 15th St NW, Ste 901, Washington DC 20005 1987
The commission was chaired by retired Admiral James D Watkins, and this report sketches out preliminaries for national AIDS prevention activities

616. Presenting AIDS: A Resource Guide for Inservice Education on Acquired Immune Deficiency Syndrome and Educational Implications. Minnesota Pupil Personnel Services Section, Minnesota Dept of Education; School Nurse Organization of Minnesota. Minnesota Dept of Education, 550 Cedar St, St Paul MN 55101 1985
This state document is a guide for health education about AIDS

617. Preventing AIDS: A Practical Guide for Everyone. Benza, Joseph F Jr; Zumwalde, Ralph D. Jalsco Incorporated, PO Box 30226, Cincinnati OH 45230 1987 85p $18.95 0-9617818-0-7
General information about AIDS for all audience levels

618. Preventing AIDS: Facts and Myths. Potter, Gregory C; Pritchard, Robert E. Univ Information Associates, PO Box 209, Wenonah NJ 08090 1986 43p
General information on how to prevent and control AIDS

619. Prevention of Disease Transmission in Schools: Acquired Immune Deficiency Syndrome (AIDS). Connecticut State Dept of Education; Connecticut State Dept of Health Services; Connecticut Joint Task Force on Educating Children with Pediatric Acquired Immune Deficiency Syndrome (AIDS) and AIDS-Related Complex (ARC). Connecticut Dept of Education, PO Box 2219, 165 Capitol Ave, Hartford CT 06106 1985
Handbook on preventing the transmission of AIDS in schools

620. Private Acts, Social Consequences: AIDS and the Politics of Health Care. Bayer, Ronald. Free Press, 866 3rd Ave, New York NY 10022 1988 $22.07 0-02901-961-3
An analysis of the political and social implications of national AIDS public health policies

621. Psychiatric Implications of Acquired Immune Deficiency Syndrome. Nichols, Stuart E; Ostrow, David G. American Psychiatric Press, Inc, 1400 K St NW, Washington DC 20005 1984 137p $12.00 0-88048-063-7

622. Psychoimmunity and the Healing Process: A Holistic Approach to Immunity and AIDS. 2nd ed. Serinus, Jason. Celestial Arts Publishing Company, PO Box 7327, Berkeley CA 94707 1987 377p
Alternative, holistic medical advice for improving and sustaining the body's immune system, and for coping with AIDS

623. A Quantitative Analysis of AIDS in California. Kizer, Kenneth W. California Dept of Health, 714 P St, Sacramento CA 95814 1986 26p

624. The Question of AIDS. Liebmann, Smith R. New York Academy of Sciences, 2 E 63rd St, New York NY 10021 1985 89p

625. Questions and Answers on AIDS. Frumkin, Lyn Robert; Leonard, John Martin. Medical Economics Books, 680 Kinderkamack Rd, Oradell NJ 07649 1987 190p $21.95pbk 0-87489-461-1
One hundred eighty nine questions about various aspects of AIDS are answered by health professionals

626. The Real Truth About Women and AIDS: How to Eliminate the Risks Without Giving Up Love and Sex. Kaplan, Helen Singer. Simon & Schuster, Incorporated, 1230 Ave of the Americas, New York NY 10020 1987 192p $4.95 0-671-65743-7
A safer sex guide written for women

627. Recommendations and Guidelines Concerning AIDS: Published in the Morbidity and Mortality Weekly Report. Dept of Health and Human Services, Public Health Service, Centers for Disease Control. Superintendent of Documents, US Government Printing Office, Washington DC 20402 1986 50p HE 20.7009/a: AC 7/2/982-86
A compilation of the Centers for Disease Control guidelines and recommendations concerning AIDS originally published in the journal *Morbidity and Mortality Weekly Report*

628. References: More About AIDS. Minnesota Dept of Education, 55 Cedar St, St Paul MN 55101 1985 29p
State document regarding general AIDS information

629. Report of the Governor's Task Force on AIDS. Florida Governor's Task Force on AIDS. Florida Dept of Health and Rehabilitative Services, Health Program Office, 1323 Winewood Blvd, Tallahassee FL 32301 1986 50p
Task force report regarding Florida state government policy on AIDS

630. Respect Yourself. AIDS Education Program. Los Angeles County Department of Health Services, 313 N Figueroa St, Los Angeles CA 90012 1987 32p
This comic-book format book for black teens covers essential AIDS facts and includes discussion of safer sex practices

631. Responding to AIDS: Psychosocial Initiatives. Leukefeld, Carl G; Fimbres, Manuel. National Association of Social Workers, 7981 Eastern Ave, Silver Spring MD 20910 1987 95p $12.95 0-97101-148-4
This book reviews the psychosocial aspects surrounding AIDS and the roles health professionals need to play in order to meet the AIDS challenge

632. A Review of State and Local Government Initiatives Affecting AIDS. George Washington Univ Intergovernmental Health Policy Project; United States Office of the Assistant Secretary for Health; Association of State and Territorial Health Officials; National Governors Association; United States Conference of Mayors. George Washington Univ, Intergovernmental Health Policy Project, Washington DC 20052 1985
Discussion of state and local government reactions to the AIDS crisis

633. Rock Hudson: His Own Story. Hudson, Rock; Davidson, Sara. William Morrow and Co, Inc, 105 Madison Ave, New York NY 10016 1986 311p 0-688-06472-8

634. Roger's Recovery from AIDS. Owen, Bob. Datar Publishing, PO Box 31, Sulphur Springs MO 63083 1987 210p $19.95 0-937831-01-8
An account of someone who has "recovered" from AIDS

635. Safe Sex: How Safe is Safe?. Do It Now Foundation, PO Box 21126, Phoenix AZ 85036 1987 $.25 0-89230-221-6
Safer sex dos amd don'ts

636. Safe Sex in a Dangerous World: Understanding and Coping with the Threat of AIDS. Ulene, Art. Vintage Books, 201 E 50th St NY 10022 1987 108p $3.95 0-394-75625-8
Safer sex instruction manual for the general public

637. Safe Sex in the Age of AIDS. Institute for Advanced Study of Human Sexuality. Citadel Press, 120 Enterprise Ave, Secaucus NJ 07094 1986 88p $3.95 0-8065-0996-1
Manual of safe sexual practices

638. Safe Sex: The Pleasure Without the Pitfalls. Philipp, Elliot. Columbus Books, Limited, 19-23 Ludgate Hill, London, Great Britain EC4M 7PD Great Britain 1987 96p £ 1.95 0-862873-52-5
Safer sex manual

639. Safe Sex: The Ultimate Erotic Guide. Preston, John; Swann, Glenn. New American Library, 1633 Broadway, New York NY 10019 1986 224p $8.95 0-452-25896-0
Safer sex instruction manual for gay men

640. Safe Sex: What Everyone Should Know About Sexually Transmitted Diseases. Scotti, Angelo M; Moore, Thomas A. PaperJacks, 210 5th Ave, New York NY 10010 1987 216p $3.95 0-7701-0641-2
A safer sex manual for the prevention of sexually transmitted diseases, including AIDS

641. Safe Sex Workbook. Preston, John. Alyson Publications, Incorporated, 40 Plympton St, Boston MA 02118 1988 64p $10.00 1-55583-131-1
A safer sex manual and guide

642. The Screaming Room: A Mother's Journal of Her Son's Struggle With AIDS. Peabody, Barbara. Oak Tree Publications, Inc, 9601 Aero Dr, San Diego CA 92123 1986 254p $15.95 0-86679-030-6

643. The Search for the Virus: The Scientific Discovery of AIDS and the Quest for a Cure. Connor, Steve; Kingman, Sharon. Penguin Books, Incorporated, Bath Road, Harmonsdworth, West Drayton, Middlesex, Great Britain UB7 0DA Great Britain 1988 230p 0-140109-09-9
A history of the search for HIV, the virus family responsible for AIDS

644. Self-Treatment for AIDS: Oxygen Therapies. Russell-Manning, Betsy. Celestial Arts, PO Box 7327, Berkeley CA 94707 1987 $10.00

Alternative therapy guide for people with AIDS, addressing specifically oxygen treatments

645. Serenity: Challenging the Fears of AIDS; From Despair to Hope. Reed, Paul. Celestial Arts Publishing Company, PO Box 7327, Berkeley CA 94707 1987 97p $5.95 0-89087-506-5

Inspirational essays about coming to terms with death and reaching a state of peace

646. The Settlement of AIDS Disputes: A Report for the National Center for Health Services Research. Stein, Robert E. Environmental Mediation International, 1775 Pennsylvania Ave, NW, Ste 1000, Washington DC 20006 1987 39p

Legal advice for people with AIDS

647. Sex and Germs: The Politics of AIDS. Patton, Cindy. South End Press, 116 St. Botolph St, Boston MA 02115 1986 182p $25.00, $9.00 (paper); 0-89608-260-1, 0-89608-259-8 (paper)

648. Sex care: The Complete Guide to Safe and Healthy Sex. Covington, Timothy R; McClendon, J Frank. Pocket Books, 1230 Ave of the Americas, New York NY 10020 1987 402p $8.95 0-671-52398-8

A safer sex manual

649. Sex, Drugs, and AIDS. Kresden, Brad. Bantam Books, Inc, 666 5th Ave, New York NY 10019 1987 0-553-34454-4

Based on the film of the same title, produced by Oralee Wachter and Lynne Smilow, written by Brad Kreden

650. Sexual Orientation and the Law. Actenberg, Roberta. Clark Boardman, 435 Hudson St, New York NY 10014 1985 $75.00 0-87632-454-5

This book was written under the auspices of the National Lawyers Guild Anti-Sexism Committee, San Francisco Bay Area Chapter, and provides a guide to legal concerns for lesbians and gay men, including AIDS-related topics

651. Sexually Transmitted Diseases: A Handbook of Protection, Prevention and Treatment. Tseng, C Howard; Villanueva, T Guilas; Powell, Alvin. R & E Publishers, PO Box 2008, Saratoga CA 95070 1987 154p $9.95pbk 0-88247-770-6

This book, intended for a general audience, discusses a variety of sexually transmitted diseases, including AIDS, herpes, gonorrhea, syphilis, and chlamydia

652. Social Aspects of AIDS. Aggleton, Peter; Homans, Hilary. Taylor & Francis, Incorporated, 3 E 44th St, New York NY 10017 1988 $18.00 1-85000-364-5

Select papers on the sociology of AIDS drawn from the first "UK Conference on the Social Aspects of AIDS," held in 1986

653. The Social Dimensions of AIDS: Method and Theory. Feldman, Douglas A; Johnson, Thomas M. Praeger Publishers, PO Box 5007, Westport CT 06881 1986 274p $37.50 0-275-92110-7

Discussion of social aspects of the AIDS crisis

654. Someone Was Here: Profiles in the AIDS Epidemic. Whitmore, George. New American Library, 1633 Broadway, New York NY 10019 1988 211p $17.95 0-453-00601-9

A selection of articles about AIDS for general readers

655. Sourcebook on Lesbian/Gay Health Care. Schwaber, Fern H; Shernoff, Michael. National Gay Health Education Foundation, PO Box 65472, Washington DC 20035 1984 282p

Information drawn from the Sixth National Lesbian/Gay Health Conference, which also included the Third AIDS Forum under the auspices of the Federation of AIDS Related Organizations (FARO)

656. Special Release: US Public Health Service Guidelines on AIDS in the Workplace. Mason, James O. Research Institute of America, 111 Radio Circle, Mount Kisco NY 10549 1985

657. A Strange Virus of Unknown Origin. Leibowitch, Jacques. Ballantine Books, 201 E 50th St, New York NY 10026 1985 172p $4.95 0-345-32117-0

A history of the research into the cause of AIDS written for the general public

658. Strategies for Survival: A Gay Men's Health Manual for the Age of AIDS. Delaney, Martin; Goldblum, Peter. St Martin's Press, 175 5th Ave, New York NY 10010 1987 $9.95 0-312-00558-X

Safe sex and general health manual for gay men

659. Superimmunity: Master Your Emotions and Improve Your Health. Pearsall, Paul. Fawcett Book Group, 201 E 50th St, New York NY 10022 1988 304p $4.95 0-449-13396-6

General recommendations for improving the body's immune system using alternative, hoslitic health techniques

660. Surviving and Thriving with AIDS: Hints for the Newly Diagnosed. Callen, Michael. People with AIDS Coalition, 263A W 19th St, New York NY 10011 1987 143p

General information for those who have been recently diagnosed as having AIDS

661. A Synopsis of State AIDS Related Legislation (through Feb. 1988). Thomas, Constance. George Washington University, Intergovernmental Health Policy Project, 2011 I St NW, Ste 200, Washington DC 20006 1988 149p

Summarizes states' legislation on AIDS

662. Talking with Teens About AIDS. Quinn, Kaye. R & E Publishers, PO Box 2008, Saratoga CA 95070 1987 30p $3.95 0-88247-775-7

Advice on how to talk with teenagers about AIDS, and what to say

663. Talking with Young Children About AIDS: A Guide for Parents and Teachers. Quackenbush, Marcia; Villareal, Sylvia. Network Publications, PO Box 1830, Santa Cruz CA 95061 1988 0-941816-52-4

Practical advice for teaching kids about AIDS

664. Terrific Sex in Fearful Times. Peters, Brooks. Saint Martin's Press, 175 5th Ave, New York NY 10010 1988 205 $14.95 0-312-01519-4

A safer sex guide

665. Thinking AIDS. Bateson, Mary Catherine; Goldsby, Richard. Addison-Wesley Publishing Company Inc, 1 Jacob Way, Reading MA 01867 1988 176p $12.95 0-201-15594-X

According to the authors, while AIDS is certainly a social calamity, the epidemic also offers opportunity for "cultural evolution"

666. Third International Conference on AIDS: Abstracts. US Public Health Service & World Health Organization. University Publishing Group, 107 E Church St, Frederick MD 21701 1988 236p $35.00 1-555-7200-80

Abstracts from the third international conference on AIDS, Washington, DC

667. The Truth About AIDS: Evolution of an Epidemic. Fettner, Ann Giudicu; Check, William A. Henry Holt and Co, 521 5th Ave, New York NY 10175 1986 306p 0-8050-0198-0

This is a revised and updated edition of one of the earliest histories of the AIDS crisis

668. The Truth About the AIDS Panic. Fitzpatrick, Michael; Milligan, Don. Junius Publications, BCM JPLtd., London, Great Britain WC1N 3XX Great Britain 1987 66p 0-948392-07-X

A general statement about AIDS and its impact on society

669. Understanding AIDS. Bakerman, Seymour. Interpretive Laboratory Data, PO Box 7066, Greenvile NC 27835 1988 187p 0-945577-00-X

A general discussion of AIDS

670. Understanding AIDS. Lerner, Ethan A. Lerner Publications, 241 1st Ave N, Minneapolis MN 55401 1987 64p $9.95 0-8225-0024-8

A book for secondary school children covering all aspects of AIDS, including stories of individuals who have had the syndrome

671. Understanding AIDS. Bakerman, Seymour. Interpretive Laboratory Data, Incorporated, PO Box 7066, Greenville NC 27834 1988 187p $19.50 0-945577-01-X

A review of basic AIDS facts, geared to adults

672. Understanding AIDS: A Comprehensive Guide. Gong, Victor. Rutgers Univ Press, 109 Church St, New Brunswick NJ 08901 1986 310p $9.95 0-8135-1178-X

673. Understanding and Preventing AIDS. Colman, Warren. Childrens Press, 1224 W Van Buren St, Chicago IL 60607 1988 123p $14.60 0-516-60592-8

AIDS information for children and adolescents featuring a survey of the syndrome's history, how it is spread, prevention measures, and how AIDS may eventually be cured

674. Understanding and Preventing AIDS: A Book for Everyone. 2nd ed. Jennings, Chris. Health Alert Press, PO Box 2060, Cambridge MA 02238 1988 96p $24.95 0-936571-01-2

A gerneral account of what AIDS is and how it can be prevented

675. Understanding and Preventing AIDS: A Guide for Young People. Coleman, Warren. Children's Press, 5440 N Cumberland Ave, Chicago IL 60656 1988 $6.95 0-516-40592-6

AIDS information for adolescents grade 6 and up

676. Understanding and Preventing AIDS: The Wellness Way. Krames Communications, 312 9th St, Daly City CA 94015 1987 1p

677. Voices of Strength and Hope for a Friend With AIDS. Gallagher, Joseph. Sheed & Ward, PO Box 414292, Kansas City MO 64141 1987 53p $2.95 1-55612-073-7

Advice to the friends of people with AIDS on how to be supportive

678. A Way to Survive the AIDS Epidemic: Based on the Metaphysical Teachings of the Ancient Masters. Berg, Thomas A. Palm Publications, 2654 Gough St, No 102, San Francisco CA 94123 1983 84p $4.95 0-9613110-0-2

This small book contains alternative coping techniques for confronting AIDS

679. What Every Drug Counselor Should Know About AIDS. Sulima, John P. Manisses Communications Group, PO Box 3357, Providence RI 02906 1987 73p $24.95

A manual for drug counselors discussing essential facts about AIDS including virus transmission, at-risk groups, and current treatments

680. What Gay and Bisexual Men Should Know About AIDS. Channing L Bete Co, 200 State Rd, South Deerfield MA 01373 1984 15p

681. What is AIDS: A Manual for Health Workers. World Council of Churches. Christian Medical Commission, 150 Route de Ferney, Boite Postale 66, Geneva, Switzerland CH-1211 Switzerland 1987 28p

A general informational manual for health care workers providing care for people with AIDS

682. What to Do About AIDS: Physicians and Mental Health Professionals Discuss the Issues. McKusick, Leon. University of California Press, 2120 Berkeley Way, Berkeley CA 94720 1986 202p $25.00 1-520-05935-2

Includes papers drawn from a 1985 San Francisco conference sponsored by the AIDS Clinical Research Center, University of California, San Francisco

683. What We Need to Know About AIDS Now! The AIDS File. Jacobs, George; Kerrins, Joseph. Cromlech Books, Nobska Rd Box 145, Woods Hole MA 02543 1987 128p $7.95 0-9618059-0-0

General information about AIDS directed to adults

684. What We Told Our Kids About Sex. Weisman, Betsy A; Weisman, Michael H. Harcourt, Brace & Jovanovich/Harvest, 1250 6th Ave, San Diego CA 92101 1987 84p $4.95 0-156960-50-8

Recommendations to parents on how to talk to kids about AIDS

685. When Someone You Know Has AIDS: A Practical Guide. Martelli, Leonard J; Peltz, Fran D; Messina, William. Crown Publishers, Inc, 225 Park Ave S, New York NY 10003 1987 0-517-56555-2, 0-517-56556-0

686. When Someone You Love Has AIDS: A Book of Hope for Family and Friends. Moffatt, Betty Clare. Borgo Press, PO Box 2845, San Bernardino CA 92406 1986 $19.95 0-8095-6661-X

A self-help book for friends and family of persons with AIDS

687. Why You Should Be Informed About AIDS: Information for Health-Care Personnel and Other Care Providers. Channing L Bete Co, 200 State Rd, South Deerfield MA 01373 1984 15p

688. Winning the War Within: Understanding, Protecting, and Building Your Body's Immunity. Friedlander, Mark P Jr; Phillips, Terry M. Rodale Press, 33 E Minor St, Emmaus PA 18098 1986 204p $18.95 0-878576-48-7

Included in this general discussion of the body's immune system is a chapter on AIDS

689. Women and AIDS. Richardson, Diana. Methuen Inc, 29 W 35th St, New York NY 10001 1987 186p $25.00 0-41601-741-X

The author addresses both medical and social concerns relative to women and AIDS, including rape, risk of HIV exposure for lesbians, and how government AIDS policy affects women

690. The Works: Drugs, Sex and AIDS. San Francisco AIDS Foundation. San Francisco AIDS Foundation, 333 Valencia St 4th Fl, San Francisco CA 94103 1987 35p $1.00

An AIDS education comic book for IV drug users discussing HIV transmission, risk behaviors, and risk reduction

691. You Can Do Something About AIDS. Alyson, Sasha. Viking Penguin, Incorporated, 40 W 23rd St, New York NY 10010 1988 126p Free

This book features statements from a variety of celebrities on what can be done to stop AIDS, and was produced by the Stop AIDS Project of Boston. It is being distributed free by the publisher

692. You Can Heal Your Life. Hay, Louise L. Hay House, 3029 Wilshire Blvd, Ste 206, Santa Monica CA 90404 1984 224p $16.95 0-317-52419-4

Techniques for developing positive coping techniques for people with AIDS

693. You Can Protect Yourself and Your Family from AIDS. Cartland, Clif. H. Fleming Revel Company, 184 Central Ave, Old Tappan NJ 07675 1987 191p $8.85 0-8007-5262-7

Advice for parents on how to discuss AIDS, sex in general, and safer sex practices with their children

BROCHURES/PAMPHLETS

694. About AIDS in the Workplace. Channing L Bete Company, Incorporated. Channing L Bete Company, Incorporated, 200 State Rd, South Deerfield MA 01373 1987 16p $.78

A pamphlet providing information about AIDS and the workplace, including advice on how to react if a co-worker has AIDS

695. Acquired Immune Deficiency Syndrome. Colvin, Tom. National Conference of State Legislatures, 1050 17th St, Ste 2100, Denver CO 80265 1987 8p

A small brochure containing state and federal legal issue briefs

696. Acquired Immune Deficiency Syndrome: 100 Questions and Answers. National Sheriff's Assn. National Sheriff's Assn, 1450 Duke St, Alexandria VA 22314 1987 19p

This is an adaptation on a publication by the same title produced by the New York State Dept of Health giving brief answers to a variety of frequently-asked questions about AIDS

697. Acquired Immune Deficiency Syndrome: 100 Questions and Answers. AIDS Institute. New York State Dept of Health, 1408 Corning Tower, Empire State Plaza, Albany NY 12237 1987 19p

General AIDS information presented in question-and-answer format

698. AIDS. Hawkes, Nigel. Glousester Press, 387 Park Ave S, New York NY 10016 1987 32p $10.90 0-531-17054-3

Information about AIDS for children and adolescents

699. AIDS: Am I at Risk? A Checklist for Modern Lovers. ETR Associates. ETR Associates, 4 Carbonero Way, Scotts Valley CA 95061 1988 3-panel page $11.00 for 50

A brochure outlining sexual behaviors that may put one at risk for contracting AIDS

700. AIDS, An Epidemic of Fear. Life Skills Education, 280 Broad St, Weymouth MA 02189 1987 14p

General informational brochure about AIDS

701. AIDS and Drugs. Good Samaritan Project. Good Samaritan Project, 3940 Walnut, Kansas City MO 64111 1987 3-panel page Free

A brochure showing IV drug users how to clean their "works" to reduce the risk of AIDS

702. AIDS and HIV Counseling and Testing. AIDS Institute. New York State Department of Health, Corning Tower, Room 372, Albany NY 12237 1987 3-panel page Free

This brochure describes the HIV antibody test and what it means to be negative or positive

703. AIDS and People of Color. Massachusetts Office of Health Resources AIDS Program. Massachusetts Department of Public Health, 150 Tremont St, Boston MA 02111 1987 3 folded panels Free

This brochure presents statistics on the incidence and prevalence of AIDS in minority communities

704. AIDS and Safer Sex. AIDS Foundation Houston Inc, 3927 Essex Lane, Houston TX 77027 1987 1p Free

This brochure presents information on what AIDS is, how it is transmitted, and includes 11 risk-reduction guidelines. Also available in Spanish

705. AIDS and the Black Community. Revised ed. Texas Dept of Health, 1100 W 49th St, Austin TX 78756 1987 6p Free

General AIDS information targeted to gay Blacks

706. AIDS and the Healthcare Worker. Service Employees International Union (SEIU). Service Employees International Union (SEIU), AFL-CIO, 1313 L St NW, Washington DC 20005 1987 4-panel page $.25

A brochure providing general information about AIDS, precautions for health care workers, and details concerning the patient's right to privacy

707. AIDS and the Heterosexual Community. Life Skills Education, 280 Broad St, Weymouth MA 02189 1987 13p

General information about AIDS targeted to heterosexual readers

708. AIDS and the Ministry of the Church. Castro, R Michael. Discipleship Resources, PO Box 189, 1908 Grand Ave, Nashville TN 37202 1987 22p

A United Methodist Church General Board of Discipleship statement on AIDS

709. AIDS and the Safety of the Nation's Blood Supply. American Red Cross, 1730 E St NW, Washington DC 20006 1987 6-panel page

General information on AIDS and the safety of blood transfusions

710. AIDS and the Workplace. Texas Dept of Health, 1100 W 49th St, Austin TX 78756 1987 1p Free

This general-audience brochure focuses on AIDS transmission issues, antibody testing and counseling

711. AIDS and Women. Revised 5/88. Texas Dept of Health, 1100 W 49th St, Austin TX 78756 1988 6p Free

A straightforward brochure covering AIDS and HIV transmission, drug use, blood transfusions, antibody testing, pregnancy, artificial insemination, and fetal protection. A Spanish-language version is also available

712. AIDS and Your Legal Rights: What Everyone Needs to Know. National Gay Rights Advocates. National Gay Rights Advocates, 540 Castro St, San Francisco CA 94114 1987 8p $1.00

Outlines the legal rights of persons with AIDS

713. The AIDS Crisis. Do It Now Foundation, PO Box 21126, Phoenix AZ 85036 1987 $1.00 0-89230-227-5

A brief brochure about the current AIDS crisis

714. AIDS Does Not Discriminate. The AIDS Institute. New York State Department of Health, Corning Tower Rm 372, Albany NY 12237 1987 3-panel page Free

A general brochure giving an overview of AIDS

715. AIDS' Effects on the Brain. AIDS Health Project. University of California, San Francisco, PO Box 0834, San Francisco CA 94143 1987 2-panel page $.65

A brochure for family members and health caregivers describing how AIDS can effect the brain and nervous system

716. AIDS: Ethical Guidelines for Healthcare Providers. Bader, Diana; McMillan, Elizabeth. Catholic Health Association of the United States, 4455 Woodson Rd, Saint Louis MO 63134 1987 26p $2.50 0-87125-141-8

Brief discussion for healthcare professionals of the ethical issues surrounding the provision of care to AIDS patients

717. AIDS: Everything You Must Know. Whelan, Elizabeth M. Society for the Advancement of Education, 99 W Hawthorne Ave, No 518, Valley Stream NY 11580 1987 15p

AIDS information geared to a general audience

718. AIDS: Facts about AIDS Young Black Men Need to Know. Bebashi Inc, 1319 Locust St, Philadelphia PA 19107 no date 1 folded page

Presents a brief overview about AIDS and information about safer sex geared to Black men

719. AIDS: Facts about AIDS Young Black Women Need to Know. Bebashi Inc, 1319 Locust St, Philadelphia PA 19107 no date 1 folded page

Presents a brief overview about AIDS with information on safer sex geared to Black women

720. AIDS: Facts for Life. Illinois Dept of Public Health, 100 W Randolph St, No 6-600, Chicago IL 60601 1987 6p Free

A brief manual for health educators covering AIDS and HIV-related disorders, focusing on immunology and viral transmission

721. AIDS: How You Can Prevent its Spread, Why You Need to be Concerned but Not Afraid. Krames Communications, 312 90th St, Daly City CA 94015 1987 7p

Brief, general information about AIDS and how to prevent exposure to it

722. AIDS: If Your Antibody Test Results Are Positive. Office of AIDS. Maine Department of Human Services, State House Station 11, 157 Capitol St, Augusta ME 04333 1987 5-panel page

A brochure providing answers, advice, and a list of resources in the State of Maine for those testing positive for the HIV antibody

723. AIDS in the Black Community: The Facts. National Coalition of Black Lesbians and Gays, PO Box 2420, Washington DC 20013 1987 1 folded page

This AIDS prevention brochure written for the Black community recommends safer sex and the elimination of drug use

724. AIDS in the Black Community: When in Doubt...Pull the Condom Out. Kupona Network, 4611 S Ellis Ave, Chicago IL 60653 no date 4-panel folded page Free, $1.75 postage and handling

Basic AIDS information including discussions of related issues as they pertain to the Black community

725. AIDS Information for Inmates. AIDS Education Training Unit. New York City Department of Health AIDS Education Training Unit, 311 Broadway 4th Fl, New York NY 10007 1987 4-panel page Free

This brochure for prison inmates explains how AIDS is spread and how inmates can protect themselves

726. AIDS: Legal Implications for Health Care Providers. Radzielski, Mark A. Catholic Health Association of the United States, 4455 Woodson Rd, Saint Louis MO 63134 1987 $1.75

Topics covered in this brief pamphlet include confidentiality, personnel and workplace issues and discrimination

727. AIDS Lifeline: The Best Defense Against AIDS is Information. San Francisco AIDS Foundation. San Francisco AIDS Foundation, 333 Valencia St 4th Fl, San Francisco CA 94103 1987 3-panel page Free

A general information brochure giving basic facts about AIDS including prevention, causes, risks, modes of transmission, symptoms, treatment, and diagnosis. Also available in Spanish and Chinese

728. AIDS Prevention: Views of the Administration's Budget Proposals. Briefing Report to the Chairman, Subcommittee on Labor, Health and Human Services, Education and Related Agencies, Committee on Appropriations, United States Senate. United States General Accounting Office. US General Accounting Office, Superintendent of Documents, Washington DC 20402 1987 33p GA 1.13:HRD-87126-BR

Congressional comments regarding the Reagan Administration's budgeted appropriations for AIDS prevention activities

729. AIDS: Risk Prevention Understanding. National Leadership Coalition on AIDS, 1150 17th St NW, Ste 202, Washington DC 20036 1987 8p

A pamphlet for the workplace with information on how AIDS is spread and recommended precautions to prevent HIV infection

730. AIDS: Safer sex. Denver Disease Control Service, 605 Bannock St, Denver CO 80204 1987 3-panel page Free

Guidelines for safer sex

731. AIDS: Shooting Up and Your Health. New Mexico AIDS Services Inc, 124 Quincy Northeast, Santa Fe NM 87501 no date 2-panel page

Basic information on the health hazards of IV drug use as it relates to AIDS, hepatitis-B, and endocarditis

732. AIDS, The Law and You. AIDS Action Committee of Massachusetts Inc, 661 Boylston St, Boston MA 02116 1987 4-panel page $.15

An overview of legal provisions against AIDS-related discrimination in housing or in the workplace, including Massachusetts and federal policies on AIDS

733. AIDS: The Sexually Active Heterosexual. Denver Disease Control Service, 605 Bannock St, Denver CO 80204 1987 3-panel page

This brochure for heterosexuals presents general information on the causes and transmission of AIDS, and outlines safer and unsafe sex practices

734. AIDS: The Straight Facts/El SIDA Informacion para Heterosexuales. AIDS Education Training Unit. New York City Department of Health AIDS Education Training Unit, 311 Broadway 4th Fl, New York NY 10007 1987 4-panel page Free

A bilingual brochure about AIDS for heterosexuals, discussing methods of virus transmission, symptoms, and prevention techniques including condom use

735. AIDS—Think About It/SIDA o AIDS—Pienselo. ETR Associates, 4 Carbonero Way, Scotts Valley CA 95061 1987 3-panel page Free

A bilingual brochure providing basic AIDS facts

736. AIDS: What Every Woman Needs to Know. National Women's Health Network, 1325 G St NW, Lower Level, Washington DC 20005 1987 3-panel page $10.00 for 100

A pocket-size brochure providing safer sex guidelines for women

737. AIDS: What Everyone Should Know. American College Health Association, 15879 Crabbs Branch Way, Rockville MD 20855 1987 5-panel page $.45

A brochure covering AIDS risk behaviors, virus transmission, antibody testing, and protection techniques. Included are lists of symptoms and the risk of AIDS for men, women, and people of color

738. AIDS: What Workers Should Know. National Safety Council, 444 N Michigan Ave, Chicago IL 60611 1987 9p $.57

Workplace AIDS guidelines for employers and employees

739. AIDS, Your Child and You: Anwers About Children and AIDS. AID Atlanta Inc, 1132 W Peachtree St NW, Atlanta GA 30309 1987 3-panel page Free

An informative brochure with advice for parents about children and their risk for AIDS, including information about virus transmission, exposure, and protection

740. Andrea and Lisa. Health Education Resource Organization (HERO), 101 W Read St, Ste 812, Baltimore MD 21201 1987 10p $.50

A comic book for teenage girls discussing AIDS and safer sex practices

741. Are You Man Enough?. Community Outreach Risk Reduction Education Program (CORE), 6570 Santa Monica Blvd, Los Angeles CA 90038 1987 8p $.35
A pamphlet using frank language to inform sexually active men about HIV transmission and practices for reducing the risk of AIDS. Also available in Spanish

742. Asian Americans and AIDS. Multicultural Prevention Resource Center (MPRC), 1540 Market St, Ste 320, San Francisco CA 94102 no date 3-panel page $.25
Multilingual brochure emphasizing that Asians are not immune to AIDS, though incidence among Asians is relatively low. Available in Japanese, Korean, Tagalog, Chinese, and Vietnamese

743. The Best Way to "Score"! (or How to Use a Rubber). Neon Street Center for Youth, 3227 N Sheffield, Chicago IL 60657 1987 4-panel folded page Free
Clear and explicit instructions on how to use a condom

744. Children and AIDS. AIDS Control Program. Rhode Island Department of Health, 75 Davis St, Cannon Bldg, Rm 105, Providence RI 02908 1987 2-panel page Free
A brochure answering frequently-asked questions concerning children and AIDS

745. Children and AIDS: The Challenge for Child Welfare. Anderson, Gary R. Child Welfare League of America, 440 1st St NW, Washington DC 20001 1986 38p 0-87868-265-1
Analysis of social and welfare issues related to AIDS and children

746. Children Can Get AIDS, Too: Questions and Answers. Pediatric AIDS Team of the Division of Immunology. Albert Einstein College of Medicine, 1300 Morris Park Ave, Rm F-401, New York NY 10461 1987 3-panel page Free
General information about AIDS with an emphasis on children. Also available in Spanish

747. The Christian Attitude Toward AIDS. Cromie, Richard M. Desert Ministries, PO Box 13235, Pittsburgh PA 15243 1987 18p $1.00 0-914733-09-5
Christian perspectives on the AIDS epidemic

748. Condom Sense. Saint Louis Effort for AIDS, 4050 Lindell Blvd, Saint Louis MO 63108 1986 3-panel page $15.00 for 100
Discusses reasons for using condoms, types available, and their effectiveness in preventing the spread of AIDS

749. Condoms for Couples. San Francisco AIDS Foundation, 333 Valencia St 4th Fl, San Franciso CA 94103 1988 3-panel page
Promotes the use of condoms by sexually active heterosexuals

750. Condoms, Safer Sex and AIDS. AIDS Education Unit, New York City Department of Health AIDS Education Training Unit, 311 Broadway 4th Fl, New York NY 10007 1987 4-panel page Free
A general information brochure about AIDS, emphasizing safer sex practices with explicitly illustrated instructions

751. Coping With AIDS. San Francisco AIDS Foundation, 333 Valencia St 4th Fl, San Francisco CA 94103 1987 4-panel page Free
Contains general AIDS/ARC information and takes a compassionate look at living with AIDS

752. Coping with ARC. San Francisco AIDS Foundation, 333 Valencia St 4th Fl, San Francisco CA 94103 1987 18p Free
A booklet that discusses various aspects of the AIDS-related complex (ARC), including symptoms, treatments, sexuality, and stress

753. Correctional Information Bulletin: Acquired Immune Deficiency Syndrome (AIDS). American Correctional Health Services Administration, 4321 Hartwick Rd, Ste L-208, College Park MD 20740 1987 28p
An analysis of AIDS and HIV transmission within America's correctional facilities

754. Could I Get AIDS?. AIDS Administration. Maryland Department of Health and Mental Hygiene, 201 W Preston St, Baltimore MD 21201 1987 3-panel page Free
A general brochure on AIDS with questions to ask yourself to determine if you have been exposed to the AIDS-causing virus

755. Could Your Kid Die Laughing?: AIDS and Today's Adolescent. Marsh, Carole S. Gallopade Publishing Group, Main St, Bath NC 27808 1987 30p $7.95 1-55609-225-3
AIDS information for adolescents, including discussion of condom use during sex

756. Disease Does Not Discriminate: You Don't Have to be White or Gay to Get AIDS. Good Samaritan Project, 3940 Walnut, Kansas City MO 64111 1987 3-panel folded page Free
This brochure warns members of minority groups about the risk of AIDS through needle-sharing and promotes safer sex practices

757. Drugs and AIDS. Do It Now Foundation, PO Box 21126, Phoenix AZ 85036 1987 8p $.25 0-89230-220-8
Brief information about AIDS and substance abuse

758. Eating Right and AIDS. AIDS Education Training Unit. New York City Department of Health AIDS Education Training Unit, 311 Broadway 4th Fl, New York NY 10007 1987 3-panel page Free
A brochure in English and Spanish discussing proper nutrition for people with AIDS, listing types of foods to eat and those to avoid

759. El Despertar de Ramon (Awakening of Ramon). Novela Health Foundation. Multi-Cultural Health Education Programs, 2524 16th Ave S, Seattle WA 98144 1988 4p $.30
A photo-novela about how a Latino father comes to terms with AIDS when his son is diagnosed with the syndrome

760. Face AIDS with Facts. Gay and Lesbian Community Servcies Center. Gay and Lesbian Community Services Center, 1213 N Highland Ave, Los Angeles CA 90038 1987 16p Free
General AIDS information and ways to lessen the risk of HIV infection

761. Face It: Safer Sex Is a Decision You Can Live With. Saint Louis Effort for AIDS, 4050 Lindell Blvd, Saint Louis MO 63108 1986 3-panel page $15.00 for 100
This brochure aimed at high-risk groups stresses the need to practice safer sex

762. The Facts About AIDS and How Not to Get It. American Foundation for AIDS Research (AmFAR), 40 W 57th St, Ste 406, New York NY 10019 1987 10p Free
A brochure that answers questions about AIDS for the general public

763. The Facts: AIDS and Adolescents. Center For Population Options, 1012 14th St NE, Ste 1200, Washington DC 20005 1987 1p $.17
A fact-list of information on AIDS with references to other publications for more information

764. Facts on AIDS: A Law Enforcement Guide. New Jersey Department of Health, Health & Agriculture Bldg, John Fitch Plz, CN 360, Trenton NJ 08625
A brochure featuring essential AIDS facts for police personnel, including workplace guidelines for avoiding exposure to HIV

765. Facts on AIDS: A Law Enforcement Guide. Utah Division of Peace Officer Standards and Training. Utah Dept of Public Safety, 4501 S 27th West St, Salt Lake City UT 84119 1988 8p
This small brochure, intended for law enforcement officers, outlines the facts about AIDS

766. Foreign Policy Implications of AIDS. Whitehead, John C. US Dept of State, Bureau of Public Affairs, Superintendent of Documents, Washington DC 20402 1988 2p S 1.71/4:1-26
Discussion of the foreign policy implications of the AIDS pandemic

767. Gay Health and STD Guide. Gay Men's Health Project, 74 Grove St, No RW, New York NY 10014 $3.00
A guide for gay men on sexually transmitted diseases

768. Here's What Teenagers are Saying About Condoms. Planned Parenthood of Alameda County/San Francisco, 815 Eddy St, San Francisco CA 94109 1988 4-panel folded page $20.00 per 100
This brochure, written by and for teenagers, discusses reasons for using condoms

769. HIV Antibody Testing. AIDS Foundation Houston Inc, 3927 Essex Lane, Houston TX 77027 1987 4-panel page Free
A general brochure on the HIV antibody test stressing the related issues of anonymity, confidentiality, and counseling

770. HIV III Antibody: Information for Individuals with a Positive Test Result for Antibody Against the HIV Virus. American Red Cross, 1730 E St NW, Washington DC 20006 1988 3-panel page
A brochure for those that test HIV-positive, explaining what the test and results means

771. HIV-III Antibody: Information for Individuals Interested in Being Tested for Antibody Against HIV Virus. American Red Cross, 1730 E St NW, Washington DC 20006 1988 3-panel page
A brochure describing the HIV antibody test, explaining the significance of positive and negative results

772. How to Talk to Your Teens and Children About AIDS. National Parents and Teachers Association, 700 N Rush St, Chicago IL 60611 1988 6-panel page $.20
General information about AIDS for parents, with advice on how to lead discussions on the topic with preschoolers, young children, preteens, and teenagers

773. How to Use a Condom (Rubber). Health Education Resource Organization (HERO), 202 W Read St, Ste 812, Baltimore MD 21201 no date 4-panel page $.30
Contains drawings with text describing the proper way to use a condom. Also available in Spanish

774. If You Know About AIDS You Don't Have to Panic—Get the Facts...Not AIDS. New York City Department of Health, AIDS Education Training Unit, 311 Broadway, 4th Fl, New York NY 10007 1987 3-panel folded page Free
This brochure written by teens explains what AIDS is and the need to practice safer sex

775. Imagine...What If Sex Could Be Better...and Safer. AIDS Administration. Maryland Department of Health and Mental Hygiene, 201 W Preston St, Baltimore MD 21201 1987 4-panel page Free
Explains how to choose and use a condom, including the use of lubricants

776. Infection Control and AIDS. Waldron, Theresa. American Health Consultants, 67 Peachtree Park Dr, Altanta GA 30309 1988 18p
A reprint from *Hospital Infection Control* outlining methods for controling exposure to the AIDS-causing virus

777. Information and Recommendations for Prevention of HIV Infections Through Counseling and Contact Notification. Wisconsin AIDS/HIV Program. Wisconsin Dept of Health and Social Services, 234 Wilson St State Office Bldg, 1 W Wilson St, PO Box 309, Madison WI 53701 1986 16p Free
A general AIDS education brochure stressing prevention

778. Information for People of Color—Asians, Blacks, Latinos, Native Americans. San Francisco AIDS Foundation, 333 Valencia St 4th Fl, San Francisco CA 94103 1985 3-panel page Free
Provides information about AIDS as it pertains to minority groups

779. Information for Persons With a Positive HIV Antibody Test Result. North Carolina Division of Health Services. North Carolina Dept of Human Resources, Cooper Memorial Health Bldg, 225 N McDowell St, PO Box 2091, Raleigh NC 27602 1987 8p
General information and guidance for those who have tested positive for exposure to the AIDS-causing virus

780. Legal Answers About AIDS. Gay Men's Health Crisis Inc, 132 W 24th St, PO Box 274, New York NY 10011 1988 16p $.50
A legal guide for persons with AIDS living in the New York City area, in question-and-answer format

781. Lesbians and AIDS: What's the Connection?. San Francisco AIDS Foundation, 333 Valencia St 4th Fl, San Francisco CA 94103 1987 3-panel page Free
An informative brochure discussing possible AIDS risk factors for lesbians, as well as the emotional and political impact of AIDS on the lesbian community

782. Let's Talk About Sex. National Hemophilia Foundation, 110 Green St, Soho Bldg No 406, New York NY 10012 1988 8p Free
A pamphlet for teenagers with hemophilia that discusses AIDS and sex

783. Making Sex Safer. American College Health Association, 15879 Crabbs Branch Way, Rockville MD 20855 1987 4-panel page $.50
A safer sex brochure covering various sexually transmitted diseases including chlamydia, herpes, crab lice, genital warts, gonorrhea, syphilis, and AIDS, and recommending the use of condoms

784. Microscopic Monster: The Tricky Devastating AIDS Virus!. Rowe, Edward. National AIDS Prevention Institute, PO Box 2500, Culpeper VA 22701 1987 32p $2.00 0-944373-00-3
Discussion for general audiences about the AIDS-causing virus, HIV

785. Myths and Facts about AIDS. Cascade AIDS Project, 408 SW 2nd, Ste 420, Portland OR 97204 no date 2-panel page
This brochure counters several of the most common AIDS myths with facts

786. Nature as a Basis of Medical Ethics. Ashley, Benedict. Pope John XXIII Center, 186 Forbes Rd, Braintree MA 02184 1988 4p
This statement is volume 13 number 1 of *Ethics and Medicine* and contains "AIDS Update: An Expanding Challenge"

787. Needles, Drugs and AIDS. AIDS Task Force of Central New York. AIDS Task Force of Central New York, PO Box 1911, Syracuse NY 13201 1986 3-panel page
An informational brochure for IV drug users on ways to protect themselves and others from becoming infected or reinfected with the AIDS-causing virus

788. An Ounce of Prevention: AIDS Risk Reduction Guidelines for Healthier Sex. AIDS Prevention Project. Seattle-King County Department of Public Health, 1116 Summit Ave, Ste 200, Seattle WA 98101 1987 4-panel page $.15
Presents the basic facts about AIDS transmission, incidence and prevention

789. Pregnancy and AIDS. San Francisco AIDS Foundation, 333 Valencia St 4th Fl, San Francisco CA 94103 1988 1p $.30
Specific information for women considering pregnancy or already pregnant, including discussions about AIDS transmission, needle and condom use, antibody testing, casual contagion, and risks to unborn children. Also available in Spanish

790. Problems Associated With AIDS: Response by the Government to the Third Report from the Social Services Committee Session 1986-87. Department of Health and Social Security, Great Britain. Her Majesty's Stationery Office, Publications Centre, 51 Nine Elms Lane, London, Great Britain SW9 5DR Great Britain 1988 33p 0-101029-72-1
A statement by the British government in response to questions raised concerning care for AIDS patients

791. Protejase Contra AIDS/SIDA! Tambien es un Problema Hispano (Protect Yourself Against AIDS! It is also an Hispanic Problem. AIDS Foundation Houston Inc, 3927 Essex Lane, Houston TX 77027 1987 3-panel page Free
A brochure in Spanish giving essential information about AIDS

792. Questions and Answers About Acquired Immune Deficiency Syndrome. Maine Bureau of Health Division of Disease Control. Maine Bureau of Health, State House, Station 11, Augusta ME 04333 1987 21p
A general AIDS information brochure in question-and-answer format

793. Questions and Answers About AIDS. City of Chicago Dept of Health, Daley Center 50 W Washington St, 2nd Fl, Chicago IL 60602 1987 4p
A brief brochure with general AIDS information

794. Questions and Answers About the HIV Antibody Test. Health Education Resource Organization (HERO), 101 W Read St, Ste 812, Baltimore MD 21201 1987 8p $.50
This brochure discusses the HIV antibody test in question-and-answer format

795. Rappin'—Teens, Sex and AIDS. Multicultural Prevention Resource Center (MPRC), 1540 Market St, Ste 320, San Francisco CA 94102 1987 4p $1.00
A comic book for urban teenage Black and Latina women discussing safer sex, pregnancy prevention, and AIDS

796. Reaching Ethnic Communities in the Fight Against AIDS. Communication Technologies; Research and Decisions Corporation. San Francisco AIDS Foundation, 333 Valencia St, San Francisco CA 94101 1986 16p Free
Advice, based on attitudinal research of the Black, Asian and Latino communities, regarding the most effective means of communicating about AIDS to minority audiences

797. Recommendations for Children and Employees With Acquired Immune Deficiency Syndrome—HIV Infection in the Synagogue Setting. Union of American Hebrew Congregations, 838 5th Ave, New York NY 10021 1987 4p
A statement regarding AIDS infection control

798. Recommended Precautions for Caregivers of Children with AIDS. Pediatric AIDS Team of the Division of Immunology. Albert Einstein College of Medicine, 1300 Morris Park Ave, Rm F-401, New York NY 10461 1987 3-panel page Free
This brochure gives specific instructions for the care of children with AIDS or HIV infection

799. Safe Sex for Men and Women Concerned about AIDS. Health Education Resource Organization (HERO), 202 W Read St, Ste 812, Baltimore MD 21201 1987 3-panel page $.30
A safer sex brochure outling safe, maybe safe, and dangerous sexual practices

800. Safer Sex Can Be Sensuous. Tidewater AIDS Crisis Taskforce, 814 W 41st St, Norfolk VA 23508 1987 4-panel page $.15
A frank brochure explaining how to have safer sex and techniques for enhancing the experience

801. The Safer Sex Condom Guide for Men and Women. Gay Men's Health Crisis Inc, 132 W 24th St, PO Box 274, New York NY 10011 1987 6-panel page Free
An illustrated brochure showing how to use a condom, including information on types and lubricants

802. Safer Sex, Condoms and AIDS. Planned Parenthood of Central Ohio, 206 East State St, Columbus OH 43266 1987 3-panel page Free
This bluntly-worded brochure stresses the use of condoms as protection against AIDS

803. Safer Sex—Your Responsibility—Your Choice. Good Samaritan Project, 3940 Walnut, Kansas City MO 64111 1987 3-panel page Free
This brochure, using slang terminology, explains which sexual activities put one at risk for AIDS

804. Seven Out of Ten Women with AIDS Are Women of Color. Maryland Department of Health and Mental Hygiene. AIDS Administration, 201 West Preston St, Baltimore MD 21201 1987 3-panel folded page Free
This brochure geared to Black and Hispanic women discusses the spread of AIDS through sexual contact, the sharing of IV drug "works," and pregnancy

805. Sex and AIDS. AIDS Control Program. Rhode Island Department of Health, 75 Davis St, Cannon Bldg, Rm 105, Providence RI 02908 1987 2-panel page Free
Briefly describes the sexual transmission of AIDS and categorizes various activities as either low- moderate- or high-risk behaviors

806. Sex Talk for a Safe Child. American Medical Association, 525 N Dearborn St, Chicago IL 60610 1985 34p $5.00 0-89970-199-X
Suggestions on how to talk to children about sex

807. Should I Take the Test?. Bay Area Physicians for Human Rights, PO Box 14546, San Francisco CA 94114 1986 3-panel page Free
This brochure discusses the pros and cons of taking the HIV antibody test

808. Sindrome de Immunodeficiencia Adquirida: 100 Preguntas y Respuestas, SIDA (AIDS). Estado de Nueva York, Depto de Salud. New York State Dept of Health, 1408 Corning Tower, Empire State Plaza, Albany NY 12237 1987 22p
A Spanish-language general information guide about AIDS

809. Some Things You Should Know About AIDS. Planned Parenthood of Central Oklahoma, 619 NW 23rd St, Oklahoma City OK 73103 1987 1p $.25
Contains general information about AIDS, safer sexual practices, and antibody testing

810. Statement on Acquired Immune Deficiency Syndrome and Education: Report of the Board of Science and Education. British Medical Association, Tavistock Square, London WC1H 9JR Great Britain 1986 11p
A statement from the British Medical Association regarding AIDS education

811. Survey of Company Practices and Policies: AIDS and Benefit Plans. Johnson & Higgins, 95 Wall St, New York NY 10005 1988 12p
A review of corporate responses to AIDS in the workplace

812. Talking to Your Family About AIDS. Lutheran Church of America, Division for Parish Services, 8765 W Higgins Rd, Chicago IL 60631 1987 7p
A brochure for parishoners about AIDS and how it may affect the family

813. Talking with Your Child About AIDS. ETR Associates, 4 Carbonero Way, Scotts Valley CA 95061 1988 3-panel page $11.00 per 50
A brochure helping parents broach the topic of AIDS with their children, with sensitivity to the apprehensions parents may have discussing AIDS or sex with their children

814. Talking with Your Partner About Safer Sex. ETR Associates, 4 Carbonero Way, Scotts Valley CA 95061 1987 3-panel page $11.00 for 50
A brochure with advice on how to talk to your partner about safer sex

815. Talking with Your Teenager About AIDS. ETR Associates, 4 Carbonero Way, Scotts Valley CA 95061 1988 4-panel page $11.00 per 50
A brochure containing comprehensive guidelines to help parents approach the subject of AIDS with their teenage children

816. Teens and AIDS: Basic Information About Acquired Immunodeficiency Syndrome for Teens, Parents, and School Personnel. Mississippi State Department of Health, 2423 N State St, PO Box 1700, Jackson MS 39215 1987 4-panel folded page Free
A brochure presenting basic facts about AIDS for teenagers, their parents, and teachers

817. Teens and AIDS: Playing It Safe. American Council of Life Insurance/Health Insurance Association of America, 1001 Pennsylvania Ave NW, Washington DC 20004 1987 6p $10.00 per 100
Discusses basic facts about transmission and prevention of AIDS for teenagers

818. Teens and AIDS!—Why Risk It?. ETR Associates, 4 Carbonero Way, Scotts Valley CA 95061 1987 2-panel folded page $11.00 per 50
A brochure for teenagers discussing how you can and cannot get AIDS, and condom use

819. Third BMA Statement on AIDS. British Medical Association Working Party on AIDS. British Medical Association, Professional Scientific and International Affairs Divisions, Tavistock Square, London WC1H 9JR Great Britain 1987 26p
A reprint of the British Medical Association's statement on AIDS

820. Understanding and Preventing AIDS: The Wellness Way. Krames Communications, 312 9th St, Daly City CA 94015 1987 1p Free
Alternative therapy techniques for people with AIDS

821. Using a Condom. AIDS Education of the Oregon Health Division. Oregon Department of Human Resources, PO Box 231, Portland OR 97207 1987 3-panel page $.10
This cartoon-format brochure discusses reasons for using a condom, with how-to guidelines

822. Usted y Su Familia—Pueden Protegerse del SIDA. Es facil! (You and Your Family Can Protect Yourselves from AIDS. It's Easy!). Minority AIDS Project. Unity Fellowship Church of Christ, 5882 W Pico Blvd, Ste 210, Los Angeles CA 90019 1987 2-panel page
A brochure in Spanish giving basic information about AIDS, geared to an Hispanic audience

823. What Do You Know About AIDS? The National AIDS Awareness Test. Metropolitan Life Insurance Company, One Madison Ave, New York NY 10010 1987 12p Free
A 55-question true/false and multiple choice test about AIDS, with correct answers

824. What Every Woman Should Know About AIDS. AIDS Control Program. North Carolina Department of Human Resources, PO Box 2091, Raleigh NC 27602 1987 4-panel page Free
Contains information on AIDS as it pertains specifically to women

825. What Everyone Should Know About AIDS. North Carolina AIDS Control Program. North Carolina Dept of Human Resources, Cooper Memorial Health Bldg, 225 N McDowell St, PO Box 2091, Raleigh NC 27602 1987 8p Free
A general brochure focusing on routes of AIDS transmission, directly addressing safer sex and substance abuse issues

826. What is Safer Sex?. ETR Associates, 4 Carbonero Way, Scotts Valley CA 95061 1987 3-panel page $11.00 for 50
Discusses safer sex methods, recommending the use of condoms

827. What is "The Test"?. AID Atlanta Inc, 1132 W Peachtree St NW, Atlanta GA 30309 1987 4-panel page Free
An informational brochure describing the antibody test for detecting exposure to the AIDS-causing virus, HIV

828. What Parents Need to Tell Children About AIDS. The AIDS Institute. New York State Department of Health, Corning Tower, Rm 372, Albany NY 12237 1987 6p Free
A pamphlet encouraging parents to talk to their children about AIDS, also available in Spanish

829. What Women Should Know about HIV Infections, AIDS and Hemophilia. National Hemophilia Foundation, 110 Greene St, Soho Bldg, No 406, New York NY 10012 1988 10p Free
A pamphlet for women providing information on HIV infection, including causes, symptoms, and prevention

830. What You Should Know About the AIDS Virus but Were Afraid to Ask. Tidewater AIDS Crisis Taskforce, 814 W 41st St, Norfolk VA 23508 1987 3-panel page $.10
General information about AIDS

831. While You Are Waiting. Mississippi State Department of Health, 2423 N State St, PO Box 1700, Jackson MS 39215 1987 2-panel page Free
A brochure intended for those who have had the AIDS antibody test but have not received the results. It outlines the meaning and limitations of positive and negative results

832. Who to Tell...When You Are Positive on the HIV Antibody Test and How to Tell Them!. Wellness Networks, Incorporated, PO Box 438, Flint MI 48501 no date 4-panel page Free
A brochure about who one should tell after testing positive for the HIV antibody

833. Women and AIDS. North Central Florida AIDS Network, 1103 SW 2nd Ave, Gainesville FL 32601 1987 4-panel page Free
Explains why AIDS should be a concern to all women, emphasizing safer sex practices

834. Women and AIDS. Saint Louis Effort for AIDS, 4050 Lindell Blvd, Saint Louis MO 63108 1987 5-panel page $15.00 for 100
Provides essential information about AIDS for women in question-and-answer format

835. Women and AIDS. The AIDS Institute. New York State Department of Health, Corning Tower Rm 372, Albany NY 12237 1987 3-panel page Free

Includes information about how women contract AIDS and how to protect yourself. Also available in Spanish

836. Women and AIDS. San Francisco AIDS Foundation, 333 Valencia St 4th Fl, San Francisco CA 94103 1987 4-panel page Free

Outlines current guidelines for AIDS prevention geared to women. Also available in Spanish

837. Women and AIDS Clinical Resource Guide. 2nd ed. Women's Health Outreach. San Francisco AIDS Foundation, 333 Valencia St, San Francisco CA 94101 1987

A manual for women containing information on AIDS risk, transmission, diagnosis, prevention and control, and psychosocial considerations

838. Women and AIDS: What You Know About It May Save Your Life. AID Atlanta, Incorporated, 1132 W Peachtree St NW, Atlanta GA 30309 1987 4-panel page Free

Discusses the transmission of AIDS from men to women, women to men, and women to unborn children

839. You and Your Family: You Can Protect Yourselves from AIDS, It's Easy. Office of Health Resources AIDS Program. Massachusetts Department of Public Health, 150 Tremont St, Boston MA 02111 1987 2-panel page Free

A general brochure giving basic facts about AIDS, including what the syndrome is, how it is transmitted, and how to protect yourself and your family

840. You Don't Have to Be White or Gay to Get AIDS. Health Education Resource Organization (HERO), 101 W Read St, Ste 812, Baltimore MD 21201 1987 3-panel folded page $.30

The cause and transmission of AIDS, with emphasis on the risks of needle-sharing, are the focus of this brochure aimed at the Black community

841. Your Test is Negative. Mississippi State Department of Health, 2423 N State St, PO Box 1700, Jackson MS 39215 1987 1p Free

This brochure addresses what a negative HIV antibody test result means

CURRICULUM/EDUCATION PROGRAMS

842. Acquired Immune Deficiency Syndrome. Taff, Mark L; Siegal, Frederick P. Medcom, Inc, PO Box 3225, Garden Grove CA 92641 1983 54 slides with 2 sound cassettes 30 min each $105.00

A teaching module on AIDS

843. Acquired Immune Deficiency Syndrome. Klein, Robert S. Network for Continuing Medical Education, 15 Columbus Circle, New York NY 10023 1985 47 min videocassette with booklet

A telecourse on AIDS

844. Acquired Immune Deficiency Syndrome, AIDS: An Adult Education Program. Health EduTech, Inc. ZTEK Co, PO Box 1968, Lexington KY 40593 1987 40 min videodisc

An general presentation about AIDS for adult audiences in an interactive videodisc format

845. AIDS. Greenwood, J R. Medcom, Inc, PO Box 3225, Garden Grove CA 92641 1986 Slides with audio cassettes $122.00 per part

This is a course on AIDS and published in two parts, each available separately

846. AIDS: A Resource Guide. Upper Elementary AIDS Curriculum; Middle School-Junior High AIDS Curriculum; Senior High AIDS Curriculum. Nebraska Department of Education, 301 Centennial Mall South, Lincoln NE 68509 no date 3v Free

Guides outlining information on AIDS with lesson plans, questions, and worksheets for use with a variety of student groups

847. AIDS and Substance Abuse: A Training Manual for Health Care Professionals. AIDS Health Project. University of California, San Francisco, PO Box 0834, San Francisco CA 94143 1987 75p $25.00

A training guide and self-paced text for health care workers covering substance abuse and its relationship to AIDS

848. An AIDS Curriculum for Adult Audiences. Arizona Department of Health Services, Office of Health Promotion and Education, 3008 N Third St, Rm 103, Phoenix AZ 85102 1987 108p

A curriculum designed for training professionals to give AIDS presentations in the community or at worksites

849. AIDS Education Activities Workshop. National Women's Health Network, 1325 G St NW, Lower Level, Washington DC 20005 1987 31p $20.00

This packet contains guidelines and support materials for leaders and participants in workshops about AIDS for young, sexually active women

850. AIDS Facts for Life (Multi-Component Public Service Campaign Kit). AIDS Activity Section. Illinois Department of Public Health, 100 W Randolph St, Chicago IL 60601 1987 Free

This AIDS awareness public service kit includes poster, fact sheet, wallet-size card and brochures presenting essential AIDS facts and is targeted to residents of Illinois

851. AIDS in the Workplace 1987. San Francisco AIDS Foundation, 333 Valencia St, San Francisco CA 94103 1987

This multi-component AIDS awareness package includes the video, *An Epidemic of Fear: AIDS in the Workplace,* along with a variety of brochures, guides and manuals for mangers and employees, including information on alternative HIV antibody test sites. The video addresses real-life AIDS-related work situations and provides examples of how to deal with them. The manager's guide provides specific information for supervisory staff, and the employee's guide addresses co-worker concerns and reinforces the message of the video. Each component in this package is individually priced

852. AIDS in the Workplace: An Employee Education Program. Dartnell Corporation, 4660 Ravenswood Ave, Chicago IL 60640 1987 $565.00

This is an integrated employee AIDS education program consisting of the video program, *One of Our Own* and a variety of complimenting print brochures, guides, and poster. The overall package is a comprehensive review of measures management should take when confronted with an employee with AIDS

853. AIDS Prevention Program for Youth. American Red Cross. American Red Cross, 1730 E St NW, Washington DC 20006 1987-1988

This multi-component family and school-based AIDS awareness program features three videocassette programs, student workbook, parent's guide, and curriculum/teacher's guide. The videos, *Answers About AIDS, A Letter from Brian,* and *Don't Forget Sherrie* address a wide range of AIDS-related concerns for teens. The teacher's guide presents instruction suggestions, and the parent's guide advises parents of the curriculum's content and answers basic questions about AIDS. Each component is individually priced

854. AIDS Update. Globe Book Company, 50 W 23rd St, New York NY 10010 1988 43p $3.79

Contains 5 lesson plans for high school AIDS-prevention instruction

855. AIDS: What Are the Risks?. Carolina Biological Supply Co, 2700 York Rd, Burlington NC 27215 1986 Two filmstrips with narrative cassettes and teacher's guide $115.00

A two-part program for PWAs, family, and friends that provides a clear, step-by-step explanation of AIDS and its various methods of transmission

856. AIDS: What We Need to Know. PRO-ED Publishing. PRO-ED Publishing, 5341 Industrial Oaks Blvd, Austin TX 78735 1988 various pagings

This is a multi-component, two-level curriculum package for junior and senior high school students consisting of level 1 and 2 instructional programs, student workbooks for both levels, and parents' guide. Each component is priced separately. The instructional program package for teachers includes lesson plans, tests, and role-play exercises. The student workbooks include homework assignments, worksheets and glossary. Topical coverage includes discussions of basic AIDS facts, routes of transmission, who's at risk, and for older students, risky sexual behaviors, pregnancy issues, and the role substance abuse plays in the spread of AIDS

857. AIDS: What You and Your Friends Need to Know. AIDS Prevention Project. Seattle—King County Department of Public Health, 1116 Summit Ave, Ste 200, Seattle WA 98101 1987 29p $15.00

A lesson plan for high school use that includes slides and a brochure presenting facts about AIDS and its prevention

858. AIDS, what you and your friends need to know: A lesson plan for adolescents. Miller, L; Downer, A. Journal of School Health, v58, n3, Apr 1988, p137-41

859. AIDS: What Young Adults Should Know. Instructor's Guide. Yarber, William L. American Alliance for Health, Physical Education, Recreation and Dance, 1900 Association Dr, Reston VA 22009 1987 44p 0-883143-53-4

This AIDS education instructor's guide includes statements of objectives, lesson plans, outlines, test questions, worksheets, handouts and answers to questions

860. AIDS: What Young Adults Should Know. Student's Guide. Yarber, William. American Alliance for Health, Physical Education, Recreation and Dance, 1900 Association Dr, Reston VA 22009 1987 20p 0-883143-52-6

This guide includes discussion of AIDS symptoms, prevention measures, sexual practices, condom use and substance abuse issues

861. AIDS: What Young People Should Know. Yarber, William L. Douglas & McIntyre, 1615 Venables St, Vancouver, British Columbia V5L 2H1 Canada 1987 42p $11.95 0-920841-43-0
AIDS information for children and adolescents. Published in the United States as *AIDS: What Young Adults Should Know*

862. Does AIDS Hurt? Educating Young Children About AIDS. Quackenbush, Marcia; Villarreal, Sylvia. Network Publications, PO Box 1830, Santa Cruz CA 95061 1988 148p $19.95 0-941816-52-4
General recommendations for instructing children about AIDS

863. Educator's Guide to AIDS and Other STDs. Health Education Consultants, 1284 Manor Park, Lakewood OH 44107 1988 various pagings $25.00
A thorough guide presenting AIDS in the context of other sexually transmitted and communicable diseases

864. Facts, Choices, Prevention: An Educational Package on AIDS. National Safety Council, 444 N Michigan Ave, Chicago IL 60611 1988
This multi-format curriculum package for teens features the video, *Choices: Learning About AIDS,* administrator's and teacher's guides, and student's and parent's booklets. The administrator's guide addresses establishing a school-based AIDS education program, and the teacher's guide provides instruction suggestions. The video and student's booklet discuss basic facts about AIDS using some slang. The parent's booklet advises parents of what their children will be learning, and addresses the issue of AIDS transmission in the school. Each item in the package is individually priced

865. Learn and Live: A Teaching Guide on AIDS Prevention. Massachusetts Department of Public Health, 150 Tremont St, Boston MA 02111 1987 17p $6.95
This AIDS prevention curriculum program features eight lesson plans geared for junior and senior high school student instruction. The program addresses sexuality issues, the AIDS-causing virus, basic facts about the syndrome, routes of transmission and prevention techniques including refraining from drug abuse and using condoms during sexual intercourse

866. Learning About AIDS. Silverstein, Alvin; Silverstein, Virginia. Enslow Publishers, Bloy St & Ramsey Ave, Hillside NJ 07205 1989 64p $12.95 0-89490-176-1
AIDS information for children grades 4 through 6

867. Managing AIDS in the Workplace—1987. Workplace Health Communications Corporation, 4 Madison Pl, Albany NY 12202 1987 various pagings
This is a multi-component training package for both executives and employees consisting of training manual for administrators, slides and guidebooks for employees, and general information brochures for all. The components are individually priced. The training manual provides managers with comprehensive information on work-related AIDS issues including civil rights, employee screening, antibody testing, discrimination, and insurance considerations. The slide/guidebook materials focus on interpreting and quelling employee fears about AIDS

868. New York State Dept of Social Services AIDS Trainer's Guide. Rockefeller College of Public Affairs and Policy, Professional Development Program. New York State Dept of Social Services, 10 Eyck Bldg, 40 W Pearl St, 16th Fl, Albany NY 12243 1987 varies
A training manual for instructors who teach social workers how to cope when managing patients with AIDS

869. Preventing Transmission of Infectious Diseases in the Workplace. Resource Technical Services, Incorporated, PO Box 295, Morgan Hill CA 95037 1987 various pagings $124.50
This multi-component AIDS education package features a 20 minute videocassette, slide/audiocassette program and script, and focuses on the workplace use of Centers for Disease Control guidelines for infection control

870. Special Topic Curriculum Resources Packet: Acquired Immune Deficiency Syndrome (AIDS). Connecticut Department of Health Services, 150 Washington St, Hartford CT 06106 1987 50p Free
This curriculum kit for junior and senior high school students covers essential AIDS information, and includes objective and goal statements, tests, transparency masters, glossary of terms and references to other related materials

871. STD: Sexually Transmitted Diseases. Teacher's Guide. Abbott Laboratories, Dept 383 Abbott Park, N Chicago IL 60064 1987 16p $5.00
Included in this high school curriculum package are six lesson plans discussing sexually transmitted diseases, including AIDS

872. Teaching About AIDS. Flynn, Eileen P. Sheed & Ward, PO Box 414292, Kansas City MO 64141 1988 88p $8.95 1-55612113-X
A guide to teaching about AIDS for schools

873. Teaching About AIDS: A Teachers Guide. Kaus, Danek S; Reed, Robert D. R & E Publishers, PO Box 2008, Saratoga CA 95070 1987 75p $6.50 0-88247-766-8
AIDS information instruction manual for school teachers

874. Teaching AIDS. Revised ed. Quackenbush, Marcia; Sargent, Pamela. Network Publications, PO Box 1830, Santa Cruz CA 95061 1988 150p $14.95 0-941816-41-9
A teacher's guide for AIDS information instruction in the classroom

875. Truth About AIDS. Educational Dimensions Group, PO Box 126, Stamford CT 06904-9981 1985 2 film strips, 2 audio cassettes, and a teacher's guide $77.00
An educational kit that addresses AIDS in a simple, direct manner

DIRECTORIES

876. AIDS: A Resource Guide for New York City. New York City Dept of Health. New York City Dept of Health, 125 Worth St, New York NY 10013 1985
Directory of metropolitan New York City AIDS support resources

877. AIDS: A Resource Guide for the Cornell Community. Amelkin, Amy; Caron, Sandra L; Coons, Bill. Albert R. Mann Library, Cornell University, Ithaca NY 14853 1988 18p
This resource directory covers materials available in the Mann Library and services available at Cornell University

878. AIDS/HIV Experimental Treatment Directory. Abrams, Donald. American Foundation for AIDS Research (AmFAR), 40 W 57th St, Ste 406, New York NY 10019 1988 119p $10.00
A directory for health care professionals and service providers listing various experimental AIDS/HIV infection treatments

879. AIDS: How and Where to Find Facts and Do Research. Reed, Robert D. R & E Publishers, PO Box 2008, Saratoga CA 95070 1986 40p $4.00 0-88247-758-7
A directory of resources for general information on AIDS, particularly suited for school use

880. AIDS Information Resources Directory. Halleran, Trish A; Pisaneschi, Janet I. American Foundation for AIDS Research (AmFAR), 40 W 57th St, Ste 406, New York NY 10019 1988 192p $10.00
A thorough source of information about various brochures, pamphlets, posters, educational materials, and films pertaining to AIDS. The text is arranged by topic and includes annotations for each entry and indexes

881. AmFAR Directory of Experimental Treatments for AIDS and ARC. American Foundation for AIDS Research. Mary Ann Liebert Inc, 1651 Third Ave, New York NY 10128 1987 125p $50.00; $69.00 (foreign)
For each entry the following information is included: Chemical name of the drug, its manufacturer, a contact person, the status of the drug with the Food and Drug Administration, and a general description of the drug's mechanism of action, clinical trial results, and side effects. Purchase of the volume includes six bimonthly supplements

882. DAITA: The Directory of Antiviral and Immunomodulatory Therapies for AIDS. Charles Henderson, PO Box 830409, Birmingham AL 35283-0409 1989— varies $26 US, $30 international
This directory is the print version of DAITA, available online through AIDSQUEST. It contains information from the Pharmaceutical Manufacturers Association file on AIDS medicines in development and is revised every 120 days

883. Directory of AIDS-Related Services. National Gay Task Force; United States Conference of Mayors. United States Conference of Mayors, 1620 I St NW, Washington DC 20006 1985 103p
A listing of AIDS-related community health and social service organizations for every state

884. How to Find Information About AIDS. Lingle, Virginia A; Wood, Sandra M. Harrington Park Press, Inc, 12 W 32nd St, New York NY 10001 1988 130p $6.95 0-918393-52-3
A handy directory of resources for AIDS information

FICTION

885. Boy's Town. Bosch, Art. Alyson Publications, Inc, 40 Plympton St, Boston MA 02118 1987 151p $7.95 1-55583-126-5
Novel about gay life in West Hollywood in which a character is diagnosed with AIDS

886. A Cry in the Desert. Bryan, Jed A. Banned Books, PO Box 33280, No 231, Austin TX 78764 1987 236p $9.95 0-934411-04-2
Fictional account of efforts to control the spread of AIDS by the quarantining of HIV-positive people in a small Nevada town

887. Facing It: A Novel of AIDS. Reed, Paul. Gay Sunshine Press, Box 40397, San Francisco CA 94140 1984 217p $35.00, $7.95 (paper); 0-917342-42-7, 0-917342-44-5 (paper)

888. Good-Bye, I Love You. Pearson, Carol L. Random House, Inc, 201 E 50th St, New York NY 10022 1986 227p $15.95 0-394-55032-3

889. Good-Bye, Tomorrow. Miklowitz, Gloria D. Delacorte Press, 1 Dag Hammarskjold Plaza, New York NY 10017 1987 150p $13.95 0-385295-62-6
A novel for young adults about a high-school senior who is diagnosed with the AIDS-related complex after receiving a blood transfusion

890. Hot Living: Erotic Stories About Safe Sex. Preston, John. Alyson Publications, Inc, 40 Plympton St, Boston MA 02118 1985 195p 0-932870-85-6
Fictional stories about safe sex written primarily for a gay audience

891. June Mail. Warmbold, Jean. Permanent Press, RD 2 Noyac Rd, Sag Harbor NY 11963 1986 224p $17.95 0-932966-67-5
Fiction with an AIDS theme

892. Night Kites. Kerr, M E. Harper & Row, 10 E 53rd St, New York NY 10022 1986 216p $11.50 0-060232-53-6
A novel about a family's reactions when a son is diagnosed with AIDS

893. Safestud: The Safesex Chronicles of Max Exander. Exander, Max. Alyson Publications, 40 Plympton St, Boston MA 02118 1985 127p 0-932870-98-0
Safe sex stories written primarily for a gay audience

FILMS/VIDEO/AUDIO RESOURCES

894. A is for AIDS. Peregrine Productions. Perennial Education, Incorporated, 930 Pitner Ave, Evanston IL 60202 1987 videocassette
Animated presentation on AIDS for students grades 4 through 6

895. About A.I.D.S.. Rosenthal, A Ralph (Producer); Kightley, Russell D J (Director). Pyramid Film and Video, PO Box 1048, Santa Monica CA 90406 1986 18 min videocassette $195.00 (video); $125.00 (1/2 inch video); $325 (16mm film); $55.00 (rental)
A general presentation for adults about AIDS

896. Acquired Immune Deficiency Syndrome. Department of Pediatrics, Emory Univ, School of Medicine. A.W. Calhoun Medical Library, Woodruff Memorial Bldg, Atlanta GA 30322 1983 48 min videocassette $135.00; $41.00 (rental)
A general presentation on AIDS produced by the Emory Medical Television Network

897. Acquired Immune Deficiency Syndrome: A New, Mysterious, and Fatal Disorder. Hill, Harry R. Univ of Utah, School of Medicine, Continuing Medical Education, 50 N Medical Dr, Salt Lake City UT 84132 1983 45 min videocassette
A general presentation about AIDS

898. Acquired Immune Deficiency Syndrome (AIDS): Information and Precautions for Laboratory Personnel. Lipscomb, Helen L. Univ of Nebraska Medical Center, 42nd St and Dewey Ave, Omaha NB 68105 1984 35 min audiocassette
Contains information and precautions of interest to laboratory personnel

899. Acquired Immune Deficiency Syndrome: Current Status and Concerns. Thorup, Oscar A. Univ of Virginia Medical Center, PO Box 395, Medical Center, Charlottesville VA 22908 1983 60 min videocassette
A general presentation on AIDS

900. Acquired Immunodeficiencies in Adults. Goodman, Jesse L. Symposiums International, 130 El Camino Dr, Beverly Hills CA 90212 1983 60 min audiocassette
A discussion of acquired immunodeficiences in adults

901. AIDS. Hathaway, Bruce. Marshfield Regional Video Network, 1000 N Oak Ave, Marshfield WI 54449 1985 32 min videocassette $35.00 loan fee
A taped lecture about AIDS for medical professionals produced by the Marshfield Medical Foundation

902. AIDS. Audio-Stats Educational Services, Inc, 924 N Market St, Ingelwood CA 90302 1983 Three 90 min audio cassettes
A general presentation on AIDS

903. AIDS. Hicks, Mary Jane; Huestis, Douglas W; Petersen, Eskild A; Porter, Bruce; Rifkind, David. Univ of Arizona Biomedical Communications, 1501 N Campbell Ave, Tucson AZ 85724 1984 Two 90 min videocassettes
A general presentation on AIDS

904. AIDS. Armstrong, Donald; Head, J J. Carolina Biological Supply Company, 2700 York Rd, Burlington NC 27215 1986 28 min videocassette $49.95
This video for health professionals focuses on the AIDS-causing virus, how it disables the body's immune system, and which opportunistic infections are most commonly seen in people infected with the virus

905. A.I.D.S.: A Challenge to Health Care Professionals. Univ of Toronto, Faculty of Medicine, Division of Instructional Services, 121 St George, Toronto ON M5S 1A1 Canada 1983 29 min videocassette $290.00
A presentation for health care professionals

906. AIDS: A Family Experience. Weatherstone Productions. Carle Medical Communications, 110 W Main St, Urbana IL 61801 1987 35 min videocassette $395.00; rental fee $$75.00
This award-winning video documents the experiences of a family in their attempts to cope when a member is diagnosed with AIDS

907. AIDS: A Model for Care. Contra Costa County Hospice, 2500 Alhambra Ave, Martinez CA 94553 1984 60 min videocassette
A training film to promote understanding and sensitivity in caring for patients who have AIDS

908. AIDS: A Story. Mierendorf, Michael. WCCO Television, Inc, 90 S 11th St, Minneapolis MN 55413 1986 60 min videocassette
A general discussion of AIDS, including a biography of Fabian Calvin Bridges

909. AIDS: Acquired Immune Deficiency Syndrome. Parrent, Joanne; Bricknell/Parrent Films. Walt Disney Educational Media Co, 500 S Buena Vista St, Burbank CA 91521 1986 18 min $341.00 videocassette; $455.00 film
This video for adolescents and adults uses animation and computer-generated graphics to tell the story of AIDS, how it is transmitted and can be prevented, and includes discussion of condom use during sexual intercourse

910. AIDS: Acquired Immune Deficiency Syndrome. San Diego County Office of Education. Media Services, San Diego County Office of Education, 210 Broadway St W, San Diego CA 92101 1986 Videocassette
A general presentation on AIDS

911. AIDS: After the Fear. Ontario Ministry of Health. Univ of Toronto, Faculty of Medicine, Division of Instructional Media Services, 121 St George St, Toronto ON M5S 1A1 Canada 1984 20 min videocassette $200.00; $30.00 (rental)
A presentation that documents the fear that AIDS has created

912. AIDS Alert. Thompson, Chic. MultiFocus, 1525 Franklin St, San Francisco CA 94109 1986 23-min videocassette $150.00; rental cost $25.00
A program for adolescents about AIDS transmission and prevention, using cartoon illustrations and featuring an introduction by Dr. Richard Keeling, head of the Task Force on AIDS for the American College Health Assn

913. AIDS Alert. Creative Media Group, Health Alert Division. Medical Electronic Educational Services, 123 4th St NW, Charlottesville VA 22901 1986 23-min videocassette $125.00; $50.00 (rental)
An educational film on AIDS

914. AIDS: An ABC News Special Assignment. ABC Video Enterprises, 1330 Ave of the Americas, New York NY 10019 1986 12 min $350.00 videocassette or 16mm film
This award-winning ABC documentary feature includes discussions about AIDS with medical experts and people with the syndrome

915. AIDS: An Enemy Among Us. Halios Productions; White, Dale; Maurer, Joseph; Seidelman, Arthur A. Churchill Films, 662 N Robertson Blvd, Los Angeles CA 90069 1987 45 min videocassette
In this production, a scenario is presented where a teenage boy with AIDS is asked to leave school, but is later readmitted after a local medical authority dispells community fears about how AIDS is spread

916. AIDS: An Old or New Acquaintance?. Emory Medical Television Network; Emory Univ School of Medicine. A.W. Calhoun Medical Library, Woodruff Memorial Bldg, Atlanta GA 30322 1985 42 min videocassette $150.00; $45.00 (rental)
A general historical discussion on AIDS

917. AIDS and Ethics. Burck, Russell. Rush Presbyterian St Luke's Medical Center, Biomedical Communications, 600 S Paulina, Chicago IL 60612 1984 Three 72-min videocassettes
A comprehensive presentation on all aspects of AIDS including the ethical issues

918. AIDS and Hepatitis-B Precautions. Criss, Elizabeth A. MedFilms, Incorporated, 6841 N Cassim Pl, Tucson AZ 85704 1988 8 min videocassette $190.00

Discussion for health care providers of the risks for infection with HIV or hepatitis-B with four key precautionary measures to take to avoid this occurrence

919. AIDS and the Arts. Films for the Humanities and Sciences, Incorportaed, 21 Highland Circle, PO Box 2053, Princeton NJ 08543 1987 20 min videocassette $149.00

This documentary featuring Elizabeth Taylor and writer Harvey Fierstein draws attention to the effect AIDS has had on the arts in America

920. AIDS and the Health Care Provider. Advanced Imaging, Inc. Carevideo Productions, PO Box 45132, Westlake OH 44145 1986 22 min videocassette $195.00; $45.00 (rental)

A presentation on AIDS and its impact on the health care provider

921. AIDS and the Health Care Worker. MTI Teleprograms, Inc; AMI Television. Coronet, 65E S Water St, Chicago IL 60601 1985 27 min videocassette $425.00; $85.00 (rental)

An educational presentation for health care workers discussing AIDS

922. AIDS and the Immune System. Churchill Films, 662 N Robertson Blvd, Los Angeles CA 90069 1986 12 min videocassette $225.00; rental fee $60.00

This film uses animation and live action to describe how AIDS effects the body's immune system, and is geared to students grades 4 through 6

923. AIDS and the Law. Univ of Pennsylvania Law School. American Law Institute, American Bar Association Committee on Continuing Professional Education, 4025 Chestnut St, Philadelphia PA 19104 1986 Two videocassettes

A presentation for the legal profession on AIDS and the law

924. AIDS and the San Francisco Women's Community. Horen, Debi; Roser, Jan; Shaw, Nancy. San Francisco AIDS Foundation, 333 Valencia St, San Francisco CA 94101 1986 44 min videocassette

A video covering the impact of AIDS on women , drawn from the sping 1986 Bay Area Career Women Conference on AIDS

925. AIDS and Your Job: What Everyone Should Know About AIDS. Audiovisual Services, Laboratory Program Office; Centers for Disease Control. National Audiovisual Center, 8700 Edgeworth Dr, Capitol Heights MD 20743 1984 20 min videocassette $80.00

A general presentation on AIDS in the workplace

926. The AIDS Antibody Test. Adair/Armstrong Production. San Francisco AIDS Foundation, 333 Valencia St, 4th Fl, San Francisco CA 94103 1987 15 min videocassette $45.00

This video includes discussion of the HIV virus and how it attacks the immune system, what the HIV antibody test is and what positive and negative test results mean

927. AIDS Antibody Test Counseling. Cappello, Dominic. MultiFocus, 1525 Franklin St, San Francisco CA 94109 1987 19 $150.00; Rental cost $25.00

A program featuring three counseling "roleplay" sessions focusing on the various considerations that must be addressed when clients consider taking the AIDS antibody test

928. AIDS Anxiety. Truax, A Brad. Abbott Laboratories, Diagnostics Division, Abbott Park, North Chicago IL 60064 1985 45 min videocassette

A presentation on the psychosocial aspects of AIDS, especially anxiety

929. AIDS Awareness Week, 1986. Austin Community College Learning Resources Services, 900 N Grand Ave, Sherman TX 75090 1986 Videocassette

A public relations videorecording on AIDS Awareness Week at the Austin Community College

930. AIDS: Beyond Fear. Center for Learning Technologies, Cultural Education Center, Rm C-7, Albany NY 12230 1987 30 min videocassette

A general discussion of who is at risk for contracting AIDS, how the AIDS-causing virus is transmitted, and how presence of the virus is detected (the AIDS antibody test)

931. AIDS: Can I Get It?. Shane, Michael; Keyworth, George A; Baltimore, David. Light VideoTelevision, 21 Highland Circle, Needham Heights MA 02194 1987 50 min videocassette

A discussion for general audiences of how AIDS is transmitted

932. AIDS: Care Beyond the Hospital. Schietinger, Helen; Reynolds, Bobby. San Francisco AIDS Foundation, 333 Valencia St, San Francisco CA 94103 1984 42 min videocassette

A presentation on the home care of AIDS patients and the psychological aspects of home care

933. AIDS Carriers in My Practice?. Taylor, Robert H; Nahmias, Brigitte B. Medical Video Productions, 450 N New Ballas Rd, Ste 205, Saint Louis MO 63141 1987 28 min videocassette $149.00

A discussion of AIDS antibody-positive people in the practices of family or general practitioners (doctors)

934. AIDS: Changing the Rules. Getchell, Franklin; Hoffman, John; MacMurphy; AIDSFILMS, Inc. WETA-TV (Television station), PO Box 2626, Washington DC 20013 1987 58 min videocassette

A documentary on AIDS and its spread among heterosexuals, featuring the music of Liz Swados, and hosts Ron Reagan, Beverly Johnson and Ruben Blades

935. AIDS: Chapter I. WGBH Television. WGBH Television, 125 Western Ave, Boston MA 02134 1985 Videocassette

An historical presentation on AIDS

936. The AIDS Crisis and the Church. United Methodist Communications, 810 12th Ave S, Nashville TN 37203 1987 60 min videocassette

A video on pastoral responses to AIDS, focusing on working with the sick

937. AIDS Encounters: Can the Doctor Make a Difference?. Kaiser Permanente, 825 Colorado Blvd, Rm 319, Los Angeles CA 90041 1986 25 min videocassette $59.00

This video attempts to sensitive physicians to the cultural and/or lifestyle considerations of gay and Asian clients, and uses a roleplay example to demonstrate techniques for eliciting a medical history without being judgemental

938. The AIDS Epidemic. Assn of American Law Schools (AALS), Section on Employment Discrimination; AALS Section on Gay and Lesbian Legal Issues; AALS Section on Law and Medicine. Recorded Resources Corp, 1468 Crofton Pkwy, Crofton MD 21114 1987

A recording of the Joint Mini Workshop of the Employment Discrimination Law, Gay and Lesbian Issues, and Law and Medicine Sections of the Association of American Law Schools, held during the association's 1987 Los Angeles Meeting

939. AIDS epidemic and the HTLV-III Antibody Test. Polk, B Frank. Johns Hopkins Univ School of Medicine, 720 Rutland Ave, Baltimore MD 21205 1986 Four 46 min sound cassettes

A presentation on the diagnosis, prevention, and control of AIDS with special reference to the human T-cell leukemia virus and C-type viruses as they pertain to the HTLV-III antibody test

940. The AIDS Epidemic: Dollars vs. Delivery. Miller, Steve. Hospital Satellite Network, 2020 Ave of the Stars, Ste 550, Los Angeles CA 90067 1988 74 min videocassette

Financial discussion of AIDS patient management, including third-party payment issues and the impact of the epidemic on commerical insurers

941. The AIDS Epidemic: Is Anyone Safe?. Guidance Associates, Communications Park, Box 3000, Mount Kisco NY 10545 1988 50 min videocassette

How an AIDS diagnosis impacts on patients and their families, including discussions of medical costs, and psychosocial and physiological aspects of the syndrome

942. AIDS: Everything You and Your Family Need to Know But Were Afraid to Ask. Stafford, Vincent; Monet, Gaby. Home Box Office (HBO) Studio Productions, 1370 Ave of the Americas, New York NY 10019 1987 40 min videocassette

US Surgeon General C Everett Koop answers a wide range of frequently-asked questions about AIDS and its transmission

943. AIDS: Face to Face. Donahue, Phil. Films for the Humanities, PO Box 2053, Princeton NJ 08543 1987 30 min videocassette

Television personality and talk-show host Phil Donahue interviews patients with AIDS about how they cope with the syndrome, their attitudes about death, and their lifestyles

944. AIDS: Facts, Fictions, Decisions. Random House/Educational Enrichment Materials. Random House, Incorporated, 201 E 50th St, New York NY 10022 1987 20 min filmstrip with audiotape $32,00 0-537-81387-X

General discussion of AIDS facts focusing on prevention techniques geared to an adolescent audience

945. AIDS: Facts Over Fears. Walters, Barbara. ABC Video Enterprises, 1330 Ave of the Americas, New York NY 10019 1985 10 min $200.00 videocassette; $250.00 16mm film

This presentation, produced for the ABC *20/20* television program, features Barbara Walters as host and focuses on how AIDS is transmitted

946. AIDS: Fears and Facts. United States Public Health Service. National Audio Visual Center, 8700 Edgeworth Dr, Capitol Heights MD 20743-3701 1986 videocassette

Presents questions and answers about AIDS as to what causes it, who can get it, how it is transmitted, risk reduction, and finding a cure

947. AIDS: Fight Fear with Fact. Connecticut Department of Health Services, 150 Washington St, Hartford CT 06106 1987 19 min videocassette

This video features two state health educators explaining essential facts about AIDS incidence and HIV transmission, with some included discussion specifically geared to residents of Connecticut

948. AIDS Hits Home. CBS, Incorporated. Carousel Films, 241 E 34th St, Rm 304, New York NY 10016 1986? 48 min videocassette $330.00

CBS newsperson Dan Rather hosts this general discussion about AIDS geared to teenagers and adults. Topical coverage focuses on the social and moral ramifications of the syndrome's spread in America

949. AIDS: How to Better Protect Yourself. Levy, Philip H; Samowitz, Perry M; Deckelbaum, Sheldon. Young Adult Institute, 460 W 34th St, New York NY 10001 1987 12 min videocassette $145.00

A video for the disabled on what AIDS is and how to avoid contracting it

950. AIDS/HTLV-III in the Public Health Environment. Grady, George F. Abbott Laboratories, Diagnostics Division, Abbott Park, North Chicago IL 60064 1985 Videocassette

A presentation for public health workers covering prevention and control

951. AIDS in the Hospital. Neu, Harold C; Bissinger, Janet M. Network for Continuing Medical Education, 15 Columbus Circle, New York NY 10023 1986 30 min videocassette

A presentation on the fears and facts of AIDS with an emphasis on preventing stroke and treating vertebrobasilar insufficiency

952. AIDS in the Hospital: The Fears and the Facts; Parts 1 and 2. Howrey, Sara; Mendelson, R; Columbia University College of Physicians and Surgeons. Visual Information Systems, 1 Harmon Plaza, Secaucus NJ 07091 1986 30 min videocassette $175.00

A hospital "plan of action" for patient care delivery is presented, focusing on facts about AIDS and Centers for Disease Control (CDC) AIDS prevention guidelines

953. AIDS in the Pediatric Age Group. Oleske, James M; Emory Univ School of Medicine. Emory Univ School of Medicine Production Co, Emory Medical Television Network, Woodruff Memorial Bldg, Atlanta GA 30322 1986 44 min videocassette

A presentation of AIDS as it affects children

954. AIDS in the Workplace. Public Broadcasting Service Video, 1320 Braddock Pl, Alexandria VA 22314 1986 180 min videocassette $345.00

A taped teleconference first aired March 26, 1986 featuring a wide variety of medical, policy and legal experts in a discussion for business and government administrators about the workplace implications of AIDS. Topics covered include: AIDS testing prior to employment; legal, privacy and handicap status of people with AIDS; the impact of AIDS on commercial insurers; and the legal rights of co-workers of people with AIDS

955. AIDS in Your School. Perennial Education, Inc. Altschul Group, 920 Pitner St, Evanston IL 60202 1987 23 min videocassette

Two students interview medical experts in a general discussion about AIDS. As well, three people with AIDS discuss how they are dealing with their illness

956. AIDS: Issues for Health Care Workers. Clover, Thomas. Churchill Films, 662 N Robertson Blvd, Los Angeles CA 90069 1988 20 min videocassette $295.00; Loan fee $60.00

Information for health care providers on the risks of exposure to HIV during the course of work

957. AIDS Media Campaign. Special Office on AIDS Prevention. Michigan Department of Public Health, 3500 N Logan St, PO Box 30035, Lansing MI 48909 1988

This package consists of posters, print ads, eight television and twelve radio commercials. The TV and radio "spots" focus on public fear of AIDS, the dangers associated with intravenous substance abuse, and risky umprotected sexual practices. The campaign stresses education and prevention measures, including avoidance of drugs and practicing monogamy

958. AIDS: Medical Education for the Community. Palance, Jack. Medical Electronic Educational Services, Inc, PO Box 50700, Tucson AZ 85703 1986 30 min videocassette $125.00

An AIDS documentary for the general public and health professionals

959. AIDS Movie. Durrin, Ginny. New Day Films, 22 Riverview Dr, Wayne NJ 07470 1986 26 min film or videocassette $450.00 (film); $385.00 (videocassette); $57.00 (rental)

A presentation of AIDS facts for ages 14 to adult

960. AIDS: Myths vs Realities. Christmas, William A; Schepp, Kay Frances; Mead, Philip B; Oliaro, Paul Michael. Univ of Vermont Instructional Development Center, Video Unit, Burlington VT 05405 1986 Videocassette

A presentation that answers many of the questions surrounding AIDS including the many myths that have been created

961. AIDS Overview. Fairview General Audio Visuals. Fairview General Hospital, Audio Visual Communication, 18101 Loraine Ave, Rm AU1, Cleveland OH 44111 1985 14 min videocassette $295.00

A general overview of the AIDS crisis and how attempts are being made to control the spread of the disease

962. AIDS: Parts 1 and 2, The New Mexico Story. Kruzic, Dale; Rhodes, Hal; KNME TV; Illustrated Daily. KNME TV, 1130 Univ NE, Albuquerque NM 87102 1985 60 min videocassette

A general presentation on AIDS aired in New Mexico. Part one is the anatomy of the disease and part two is the human response

963. AIDS: Payment, Treatment and Liability. Phair, John P; Schurgin, William P; Yezzo, Richard; American Hospital Assn Medical Center. American Hospital Assn, 840 N Lake Shore Dr, Chicago IL 60611 1987 180 min videocassette

This video focuses on the financing of care for AIDS patients, and the legal and financial liabilities of hospitals caring for people with AIDS and administering the AIDS antibody test

964. AIDS Prevention: Choice not Chance. Educational Activities, Incorporated., PO Box 392, Freeport NY 11520 1987? 13 min videocassette $129.00

A general discussion about AIDS for adolescents stressing healthy lifestyle choices

965. AIDS Prevention on a College Campus. Cappello, Dominick. MultiFocus, 1525 Franklin St, San Francisco CA 94109 1987 19 min videocassette $150.00; rental cost $25.00

AIDS prevention techniques, including the use of condoms, are discussed by a university health educator with six college students

966. AIDS: Prevention Through Education. Hush Hush Productions, 1841 Hicks Rd, Ste D, Rolling Meadows IL 60008 1987 30 min videocassette $39.95

A straightforward discussion of what AIDS is, how it is transmitted, and how it can be prevented

967. AIDS: Profile of an Epidemic. WNET New York. Indiana Univ, Bloomington, Audio Visual Center, Bryan Hall, Bloomington IN 47405 1986 58 min videocassette $180.00; $35.00 (rental)

An historical narrative of the AIDS epidemic

968. AIDS: Profile of an Epidemic Update. WNET Television, New York. MPI Home Video, 356 W 58th St, New York NY 10019 1986 60 min videocassette

A general profile of the AIDS epidemic for the general public

969. AIDS: Protect Yourself. Harris County Medical Society. Houston Academy of Medicine, 1133 MD Anderson Blvd, Ste 400, Houston TX 77030 1987 16 min videocassette

This video for teens features dramatizations of AIDS prevention measures set to rock music

970. AIDS: Protecting Hospital Employees. American Hospital Assn Media Center; Molter, Rich; Machin, James; Mitchell, Al. American Hospital Assn, 840 N Lake Shore Dr, Chicago IL 60611 1987 120 min videocassette

A panel discussion about recommended employee infection-control guidelines for the prevention of HIV exposure in the health care setting

971. AIDS: Psychosocial Interventions. Norman Baxley and Associates. Carle Medical Communications, 110 W Main St, Urbana IL 61801 1987 25 min videocassette $385.00; Loan cost $65.00

This video for mental health and allied professionals discusses various psychosocial techniques for dealing with AIDS diagnoses

972. AIDS: Public Health and Private Rights. Keeling, Richard P; Rein, Michael F. Univ of Virginia Medical Center, Medical Television Services, PO Box 395, Charlottesville VA 22908 1985 Two 60 min videocassettes

A presentation for public health workers outlining the private rights of AIDS patients

973. AIDS: Public Health and Public Policy. Finberg, Robert; Rosen, Mel; Silverman, Mervyn. John F Kennedy School of Government, Harvard Univ, Cambridge MA 02138 1984 Two 60 min videocassettes

A presentation for public health administrators and workers discussing public health and policy as it relates to AIDS

974. AIDS Public Service Announcments-1987. AIDS Education Training Unit. New York City Department of Health, 311 Broadway, 4th Fl, New York NY 10007 1987 Nine 30 sec videotaped messages Free

Nine brief AIDS awareness messages are included on this videotape, focusing primarily on the risks to mothers (and indirectly their babies) through intravenous substance abuse or having sexual contact with drug-abusing partners. Three of the nine announcements are available in Spanish

975. AIDS: Questions and Concerns for Us All. Maki, Dennis. University of Wisconsin, Stevens Point, University Telecommunications, University Center, Stevens Point WI 54481 1987 40 min videocassette

Dr Dennis Maki, University of Wisconsin, Stevens Point, discusses how AIDS is spread

976. AIDS Radio Public Service Announcements. AIDS Education Training Unit. New York City Department of Health, 311 Broadway, 4th Fl, New York NY 10007 1987 Seven 60 sec audiotaped messages Free

Included on this audiotape are seven AIDS prevention announcements recommending safer sex, and in particular the use of condoms, during sexual intercourse

977. AIDS Scare: Fact and Fiction. London Weekend Television, Ltd, South Bank TV Centre, Kent House Upper Ground, London SE1 9LT Great Britain 1985 Videocassette

A general presentation that answers many of the questions about AIDS

978. AIDS: Social Response to a Medical Crisis. Bayer, Ronald. State Univ of New York, Upstate Medical Center, 155 Elizabeth Blackwell St, Syracuse NY 13210 1984 48 min videocassette

A presentation that addresses the social problems connected with AIDS

979. AIDS: Suddenly Sex is Very Dangerous. Goodday Video. Cuero Educational Media, 115 N Esplanade, Cuero TX 77954 1987 3 videocassettes

Doctors and adolescents discuss the dangers of AIDS in this program available in three versions—for young people, teachers, and parents

980. AIDS: The Legacy. Johnson, Frances; Miles-Lawrence, Robert. Educational Productions, 4925 SW Humphrey Park Crest, Portland OR 97221 1987 4 videocassettes, 30 min each

The course of hospital care for an AIDS patient is traced from the perspectives of the patient, his physician, nurse and social worker, focusing on the impact AIDS has on the health care team

981. AIDS: The Need for Awareness. Denver, Colorado Dept of Health and Hospital Services; Cohn, David L; Schwiesow, Mark; Ralin, Peter; Corbett Productions. Media Design Associates, PO Box 3189, Boulder CO 80307 1987 28 min videocassette

A frank look at AIDS featuring discussions with students and medical professionals

982. AIDS: The Surgeon General's Update. Consultants International. Pyramid Film & Video, PO Box 1048, Santa Monica CA 90406 1988 32 min videocassette $95.00

Surgeon General Everett Koop delivers a personal message about education as the best defense against AIDS

983. AIDS: Threats to the Individual and Threats to the Public. Towers, Bernard; Stiehm, E Richard; Krasnow, Robert. UCLA Office of Instructional Development, 405 Hilgard Ave, Los Angeles CA 90024 1983 audio cassette

A presentation on AIDS in general and specifically the psychological problems associated with the disease

984. AIDS: Tracking the Mystery. United States Public Health Service; Frost Media Associates, Inc. National Audiovisual Center, 8700 Edgeworth Dr, Capitol Heights MD 20743-3701 1984 20 min videocassette $80.00

An historical narrative on AIDS research

985. AIDS Update. Bartlett, John G. Johns Hopkins Univ, School of Medicine, Office of Continuing Education, 720 Rutland Ave, Baltimore MD 21205 1985 Four 34-min audio cassettes

An updated presentation of the progress of AIDS research

986. AIDS Virus. Mazza, Joseph. Marshfield Regional Video Network, 1000 N Oak Ave, Marshfield WI 54449 1987 60 min videocassette

A taped lecture for medical professioanls focusing on the immunological aspects of AIDS and HIV infection

987. AIDS: What Do We Tell Our Children. Teich, Larry; Iwatak, Joel; Longo, Joe; Shorr, Richard. Walt Disney Educational Media Company, 500 S Buena Vista St, Burbank CA 91521 1987 22 min videocassette $345.00

Narrator Carol Burnett interviews and questions physicians and health educators about how to teach children about AIDS

988. AIDS: What Every Kid Should Know. Barr Films, 12801 Schabarum Ave, PO Box 7878, Irwindale CA 91706-7878 1987 15 min videocassette or 16 mm film

This production geared to adolescents features basic facts about AIDS, its transmission and prevention. The first segment focuses on the essentials and includes discussion of risky sexual practices, the use of condoms and spermicides during intercourse, and avoiding the use of unclean syringes. The second segment stresses abstinence from sex and drugs as the best prevention against AIDS. The program's format allows for stopping the tape or fast-forwarding through portions some communities may find inappropriate for younger viewers

989. AIDS: What Everyone Needs to Know. Renan, Sheldon. Churchill Films, 662 N Robertson Blvd, Los Angeles CA 90069 1987 20 min videocassette

A general introduction for teens and adults to the body's immune system and AIDS, using dramatization, animation and cinemamicography

990. AIDS: What Is It?. Health and Life, Southfield MI 48037 1985 Videocassette

A general presentation that discusses the disease in general terms

991. AIDS: What is Practical to Rule Out. Weiss, Geoffrey R. Univ of Texas Health Science Center at San Antonio, Teleconference Network of Texas, 7703 Floyd Curl Dr, San Antonio TX 78284-7790 1986 60 min sound cassette

A general presentation on AIDS discussing methods of transmission that can be ruled out

992. AIDS: Where Are We?. Voeller, Bruce; Coulson, Anne; Gottlieb, Michael. InfoMedix, 12800 Garden Grove Blvd, Garden Grove CA 92643 1987 87 min audiotape

A recording of both presentations and panel discussions held at the Society for the Scientific Study of Sex, Western Region annual conference, held in March 1987. Included are discussions of AIDS incidence, medical treatments, vaccines, and prevention techniques

993. AIDS, Women and Sexuality. Exodus Trust, 1523 Franklin St, San Francisco CA 94109 1986 17 min videocassette $150.00

Seven sexually-active women discuss how the AIDS crisis has altered their perceptions of key issues including sexual identity and decision-making, womens' roles, safer sex practices, and communicating with sex partners

994. Ally and AIDS. Sheedy, Ally. Walt Disney Educational Media Co, 500 S Buena Vista, Burbank CA 91521 1986 18 min film or videocassette

A film for teenagers explaining how the disease is and is not transmitted and what precautions to take to avoid its spread

995. At the Gym. Mach, Henry. MultiFocus, 1525 Franklin St, San Francisco CA 94109 1987 8 min videocassette $150.00; rental cost $25.00

An explicit safer-sex video for gay men

996. Avoiding AIDS: What You Can Do. Yarber, William. Marsh Film Enterprises, PO Box 8082, Shawnee Mission KS 66208 1988 12 min filmstrip with audiotape $42.95

Brief AIDS overview for junior and senior high school students

997. Battle Against AIDS: Testing for HTLV-III. Considine, Bob; Gingold, Howard. Lifetime Medical Television, 1211 Avenue of the Americas, New York NY 10036 1985 Two 60 min videocassettes

A general presentation about the human T-cell leukemia virus and testing program

998. Beyond Fear. Allen, John Seldon; Vaughn, Robert. American Red Cross, 2025 E St NW, Washington DC 20006 1986 30 min videocassette

A general presentation on AIDS made in conjunction with the American Council of Life Insurance and the Health Insurance Association of America

999. Black People Get AIDS, Too. Pounds, Cedrick. Multicultural Prevention Resource Center (MPRC), 1540 Market St, Ste 320, San Francisco CA 94102 1987 22 min videocassette $350.00

This AIDS awareness video discusses the impact of the syndrome on the Black community, and includes discussions of high-risk behaviors, the HIV antibody test, needle-cleaning techniques, and the use of condoms and spermicides during sexual intercourse

1000. Blood Banks in the Age of AIDS. American Assn of Blood Banks, 1117 N 19th St, Ste 600, Arlington VA 2209 1987 10 min videocassette $99.00

A video for blood bank donation recruiters on how to quell donors' fears about AIDS transmssion

1001. Can AIDS be Stopped?. Dugan, David; Whitby, Max. Coronet Film & Video, 108 Wilmot Rd, Deerfield IL 60015 1986 58 min videocassette

This program was a BBC-Television production for the Public Broadcasting Service's television series *NOVA*, and includes discussions of how the AIDS-causing virus attacks the body's immune system, how the virus is transmitted, methods of prevention, and current areas of research

1002. Caring for the Latino AIDS Patient: Lessons from a Case History. Novela Health Foundation. Multi-Cultural Health Education Programs, 2524 16th Ave S, Seattle WA 98144 1988 28 min videocassette $55.00; loan fee $15.00

A discussion of the care given a Latino AIDS patient by a multidisciplinary health care team focusing on diagnosis, in- and outpatient care, support systems, and death and dying issues

1003. Caring for the Latino AIDS Patient: Lessons from a Case History. San Francisco AIDS Foundation, 333 Valencia St, San Francisco CA 94101 1987 28 min videocassette

Culturally-appropriate advice for health care workers providing care to the Latino AIDS patient

1004. Condom Sense. Perennial Education, Incorporated, 930 Pitner Ave, Evanston IL 60202 1987 25 min $450.00 videocassette or 16mm film; rental cost $45.00

This film, first produced in 1983, features two San Francisco comics in a variety of skits dramatizing the message that condoms are an effective contraceptive. This film does not discuss condoms as a shield against sexually transmitted diseases, including AIDS

1005. Counseling the HIV Antibody Positive Patient. Niemack/Hassett Productions. Los Angeles County Medical Association, 1925 Wilshire Blvd, Los Angeles CA 90011 1987 15 min videocassette $35.00

This video for medical professionals features a physician counseling a bisexual male patient after the patient tests positive for exposure to HIV. The doctor explains what the positive result means and recommends safer sexual practices

1006. A Death in the Family. Main, Stewart; Wells, Peter; New Zealand Film Commission. Wombat Film and Video, 250 W 57th St, Ste 916, New York NY 10019 1988 48 min videocassette

An award-winning dramatization of the life of Andrew Boyd, the fourth person in New Zealand to die of AIDS

1007. Discussing Health Care and AIDS. Exodus Trust, 1523 Franklin St, San Francisco CA 94109 1986 25 min videocassette $150.00

This video includes a roleplay session between a health care provider and a women with a negative HIV antibody test result, and features frank discussion of sexuality issues

1008. Doctor Talks to You About Acquired Immune Deficiency Syndrome (AIDS): A Discussion. Enlow, Roger W. Soundwords, 56-11 217 St, Bayside NY 11364 1984 50 min sound cassette

A doctor's presentation for the general public

1009. Donor Notification. Tomasulo, Peter. Abbott Laboratories, Diagnostics Division, Abbott Park, North Chicago IL 60064 1985 60 min videocassette

A presentation about AIDS and blood donors

1010. An Early Frost. Cowen, Ronald; Lipman, Daniel; Erman, John; NBC Production. NBC Productions, 30 Rockefeller Plaza, New York NY 10020 1985 120 min videocassette

A made-for-TV drama concerning the emotional effects of AIDS on a PWA, his lover, and family

1011. An Educational Awareness Presentation on AIDS. Maki, Dennis. University of Wisconsin, Stevens Point, University Telecommunications, University Center, Stevens Point WI 54481 1987 120 min videocassette

Dr. Dennis Maki of the University of Wisconsin, Stevens Point, talks about AIDS and takes questions from a campus audience

1012. Epidemiology of AIDS. Mazza, Joseph. Marshfield Regional Video Network, 1000 N Oak, Marshfield WI 54449 1987 59 min videocassette

A taped lecture on the incidence of AIDS, geared for health professionals

1013. Ethical Issues in Ministry to Persons with AIDS. Vaux, Kenneth. College of Chaplains, 840 N Lake Shore Dr, Chicago IL 60611 1987 audiotape

A discussion of pastoral counseling and care for the AIDS patient

1014. Facing the Challenge Together: The Impact of AIDS. Rutland, Jack; Slade, Eric. Cascade AIDS Project, 408 SW 2nd St, Ste 412, Portland OR 97204 1987 32 min videocassette

A discussion of AIDS and the AIDS-related complex

1015. Fear of AIDS and the Future. Educational Dimensions Group, Box 126, Stamford CT 06904 1988 28 min videocassette $89.95

This film focuses on projections for the spread of AIDS, particularly among heterosexuals, and is geared to junior and senior high school students

1016. Fear of Caring: The AIDS Dilemma. American Hospital Association, 840 N Lake Shore Dr, Chicago IL 60611 1986 videocassette

A psychosocial presentation concerning the care of PWAs

1017. For Our Lives. Gay/Lesbian Community Services Center; Modern Media Firm. Multifocus, 333 W 52nd St, New York NY 10019 1984 25 min videocassette

A presentation on AIDS in general and its social aspects

1018. General Series on AIDS. Centers for Disease Control, 1600 Clifton Rd, Bldg 3, Rm 5B-1, Atlanta GA 30333 1983 23 slides

General information on AIDS for classroom use

1019. Heroism: A Community Responds. John Canalli, 182-B Castro St, San Francisco CA 94114 1987 30 min videocassette

Representatives from a variety of volunteer and support groups for people with AIDS and ARC discuss their efforts, and people with AIDS comment on how this support from the community has helped them

1020. Institutional Response to AIDS. Younkin, Scott; Carle Foundation; Norman Baxley and Associates, Inc. Carle Medical Communications, 510 W Maine St, Urbana IL 61801 1986 17 min videocassette $385.00; $65.00 (rental)

A presentation that depicts a day in the life of a hospital after the admittance of its first confirmed AIDS patient

1021. International Impact of AIDS. Quinn, Thomas C. Johns Hopkins Univ School of Medicine, 34th and Charles St, Baltimore MD 21218 1986 Four 33 min sound cassettes

A presentation for the international scene that covers the occurrence, etiology, prevention, control, and transmission of AIDS

1022. Is it Worth the Risk: Safe Handling of Blood and Body Fluids. American Hospital Association Media Center. American Hospital Association, 840 N Lake Shore Dr, Chicago IL 60611 1987 20 min videocassettes $300.00

This video, geared to health care workers, discusses the need to observe universal precaution guidelines for avoiding exposure to blood and other potentially dangerous bodily fluids

1023. Killer in the Village. BBC TV. Texture Films, Inc, 80 Wood Lane, London Great Britain WL2 0TT 1983 56 min videocassette $ 480.00

An historical presentation on AIDS

1024. A Letter from Brian. Warren, Michael. American Red Cross, 17th and D St NW, Washington DC 20006 1987 29 min videocassette

A teenage girl receives a letter from a former boyfriend telling her he has been diagnosed with AIDS

1025. Life, Death, AIDS. Farinet, Gene; Brokaw, Tom; NBC. Films Incorporated, 440 Park Ave S, New York NY 10016 1986 52 min videocassette $198.00

A TV documentary on AIDS

1026. The Limits of Confidentiality: The Test Case of AIDS. Rein, Michael F; Abraham, Kenneth; Childress, James F; Thorup, Oscar A. University of Virginia Medical Television Services, Charlottesville VA 22903 1987 59 min videocassette

A panel discussion of when doctors may be legally and/or morally obligated to breach the confidentiality of an AIDS diagnosis

1027. Living with AIDS. DiFeliciantonio, Tina; Coleman, Todd. Carle Medical Communications, 110 W Main St, Urbana IL 61801 1986 24 min videocassette $385.00

This video, produced by the Stanford University Dept of Communications, features the personal narrative of a person living with AIDS

1028. Men, Women, Sex and AIDS. Brokaw, Tom; Greenberg, Paul W; Feders, S; Pepper, Guy. Films Inc, 5547 N Ravenswood Ave, Chicago IL 60640 1987 60 min videocassette

A video for general audiences discussing human sexuality and AIDS

1029. Minnesota Aidlines Public Service Announcements on AIDS. Hennepin County Administration, 2308 Government Center, Minneapolis MN 55487 1987 Three 30 sec videotaped messages $75.00
Included on this videocassette are three AIDS awareness announcements geared to teens, one focusing on the need to practice safer sex, one on the harm of sharing needles, and the other dramatizing the social ostracism of a person with AIDS

1030. Needle Talk. AIDS Education Training Unit. New York City Department of Health, 311 Broadway, 4th Fl, New York NY 10007 1987 27 min videocassette Free
This documentary features physicians and educators discussing in frank language essential facts about AIDS transmission, drug use and risky sexual practices. Also available in Spanish

1031. Nightcap: HERO Condom Public Service Announcement. Health Education Resource Organization (HERO), 101 W Reed St, Ste 812, Baltimore MD 21201 1987 30 sec audio public service message $75.00
This is a thirty-second public service announcement promoting condom use, featuring an intimate conversation between a young heterosexual couple

1032. Nightline: A National Town Meeting on AIDS. ABC Video Enterprises, 1330 Ave of the Americas, New York NY 10019 1987 120 min videocassette $250.00
A 2-hour ABC *Nightline* special presentation on the social aspects of AIDS including discussions of sexuality, vaccines, substance abuse, euthanasia, attitudes of health care workers towards AIDS patients, the availability of AIDS "medicines" in Mexico, and education for children and adolescents about HIV transmission

1033. No Sad Songs: A Film. Sheehan, Nick. AIDS Committee of Toronto, PO Box 55, Station F, Toronto Ontario M44 2L4 Canada 1985 30 min $500.00 videocassette; loan cost $55.00
A film on AIDS, attitudes about death, and the family (available in a variety of formats, including video)

1034. Not Ready to Die of AIDS. WBZ-TV (Television station); Ahrendt, Barry; Cronan, Paul; Blake, Jeanne. Films for the Humanities, PO Box 2053, Princeton NJ 08543 1987 52 min videocassette
A documentary about how one man comes to terms with an AIDS diagnosis

1035. Ojos Que No Ven. Instituto Familiar de la Raza. Latino AIDS Project, 2512 24th St, No 2, San Francisco CA 94110 1987 52 min videocassette $350.00
An AIDS awareness video for Hispanics in soap-opera format with a plot that addresses a wide range of AIDS-related issues in a culturally-sensitive manner

1036. On Guard: Infection Control for Safety and Health Care Professionals. Focal Point Production. Pyramid Film & Video, PO Box 1048, Santa Monica CA 90406 1988 23 min videocassette $295.00
This video presents a variety of case examples to promote Centers for Disease Control guidelines for preventing the spread of contagious diseases through exposure to bodily fluids, and is geared to police officers, ambulance drivers, paramedics, and emergency room staff

1037. On the Brink: An AIDS Chronicle. Centre Productions, 12801 Schabarum Ave, Irwindale CA 91706 1988 38 min videocassette $485; $50 rental fee
This video for adults features interviews with various international health care experts and focuses on global considerations of the AIDS epidemic

1038. One of Our Own. Dartnell, 4660 Ravenswood Ave, Chicago IL 60640 1987 30 min $565.00 videocassette
A high-impact general discussion of workplace AIDS issues for both administrators and their employees, featuring dramatization and narration

1039. Oprah Winfrey Show. Winfrey, Oprah; DiMaio, Debra; ABC. American Broadcasting Co; dist by Electronic News Services, Inc, 1330 Avenue of the Americas, New York NY 10019 1987 46 min videocassette
Videorecording of the ABC-TV program which aired Feb 18, 1987, concerning acquired immune deficiency syndrome and the far-reaching implications of this viral disease

1040. The Other Crisis: AIDS Mental Health. AIDS Health Project. University of California, San Francisco, PO Box 0834, San Francisco CA 94143 1987 45 min videocassette $175.00
A discussion of the concerns mental health professionals have when providing care to patients with AIDS, with particular focus on problems associated with counseling HIV antibody-positive clients

1041. Our Worst Fears: The AIDS Epidemic. Saslow, Nancy; Hartnett, Robert. Films for the Humanities, PO Box 2053, Princeton NJ 08543 1987 57 min videocassette
A general review of those at-risk for AIDS and how to prevent the spread of the syndrome

1042. Overcoming AIDS: Hypno-Sleep Tape. Massari, Tom. Seth Hermes Foundation, PO Box 4111, Simi Valley CA 93063 1987 90 min audiotape $12.95
Positive-attitude suggestions for people with AIDS to listen to as they go to sleep

1043. Overcoming AIDS: Subliminal Motivation. Massari, Tom. Seth Hermes Foundation, PO Box 4111, Simi Valley CA 93063 1987 60 min audiotape $12.95
Positive-attitude healing suggestions set to music for people with AIDS

1044. Overcoming Irrational Fear of AIDS: A Coping Strategy for Health Care Providers. Lange, Arthur J; Carle Foundation; Norman Baxley and Associates, Inc. Carle Medical Communications, 510 W Maine St, Urbana IL 61801 1987 22 min videocassette $385.00; $65.00 (rental)
A presentation explaining why many health care providers approach AIDS patients with conflicting emotions and, in some cases, anxiety and fear

1045. Parting Glances. Mandel, Yoram; Silverman, Arthur; Kaplan, Paul A; Sherwood, Bill; Laskus, Jacek. CBS/Fox, 51 W 52nd St, New York NY 10019 1986 90 min videocassette
An "R" rated commercially released film in which one of the major characters is suffering from AIDS

1046. Politics of AIDS. Novick, Alvin. Fairfield Univ Media Center, N Benson Rd, Fairfield CT 06430 1986 videocassette
A presentation on the political issues surrounding AIDS

1047. Psychosocial Interventions in AIDS. Tross, Susan; Carle Foundation; Norman Baxley and Associates, Inc. Carle Medical Communications, 510 W Main St, Urbana IL 61801 1987 22 min videocassette $385.00; $65.00 (rental)
A presentation that clarifies the complex interrelationship among medical, psychological, and social challenges that contribute to the full picture of psychological distress experienced by PWAs

1048. Safe Sex for Men and Women. Cinema Group Home Video, 1875 Century Park E, Ste 300, Los Angeles CA 90067 1987 60 min videocassette $29.95
Actress Morgan Fairchild interviews AIDS researcher Dr Michael Gottlieb and marriage and family therapist Laura Schlessinger in this discussion of heterosexual concerns and AIDS transmission

1049. Safe Sex: With American Health. Warner Audio, 599 Broadway, 12th Fl, New York NY 10012 1987 45 min audiotape $9.95
The editors of *American Health* discuss safer sex issues including AIDS, other sexually transmittted diseases, contraception, and abortion

1050. Sex, Drugs and AIDS. Kesden, Bradley; Getchell, Franklin; Wachter, Oralee; Smilow, Lynn; Chong, Rae Dawn. ODN Productions, 74 Varick St, Ste 304, New York NY 10013 1987 18 min videocassette
A video for teens using narration and dramatization to discuss how AIDS is transmitted, high-risk groups and how to avoid HIV exposure

1051. Sex Education and AIDS. KQED, Inc, 500 Eighth St, San Francisco CA 94103 1987 30 min videocassette $200.00; Rental cost $95.00
The Director of Information and Education for the Center for Population Options, Washington, DC presents the case for sex education including discussions about AIDS in schools, and is debated by Phyllis Schlafly, well-known opponent of school sex education, in this video for education professionals and concerned others

1052. Sixty Minutes to Smart Sex. Edell, Dean. Audio Renaissance Tapes, 9110 Sunset Blvd, Los Angeles CA 90069 1987 60 min audiotape $9.95
A how-to tape about safer sex that additionally answers a variety of questions about AIDS and other sexually transmitted diseases

1053. Sixty Minutes to Smart Sex. Edell, Dean. A.I.D.S. International/ Information Distribution Service, PO Box 2008, Saratoga CA 95070 1987 60 min audiocassette $9.95
Safer sex instructions for adults, featuring twenty commonly-asked questions about AIDS and other sexually transmitted diseases

1054. The Subject is AIDS. ODN Productions, Incorporated, 74 Varick St, Ste 304, New York NY 10013 1987 18 min videocassette $325.00
This video with actress Rae Dawn Chong is geared to teens and features a discussion of basic AIDS facts, with an introduction by Surgeon General C Everett Koop

1055. Those People: AIDS in the Public Mind. KQED (Television station) Current Affairs Dept. PBS Video, 1320 Braddock Pl, Alexandria VA 23314 1986 30 min videocassette $200.00; loan cost $95.00

This video considers the psychosocial ramifications of the AIDS epidemic and is geared for a general audience

1056. 'Til Death Do Us Part. Durrin Films/New Day Films, 1748 Kalorama Rd NW, Washington DC 20009 1988 16 min videocassette $355.00

This AIDS awareness video documents a play produced by the Everyday Theatre Youth Ensemble of Washington DC. The production utilizes rap, music and dance to convey basic facts about AIDS to Black urban teens

1057. Too Little, Too Late. Pickoff, Micki. Fanlight Productions, 47 Halifax St, Boston MA 02130 1987 48 min videocassette $280.00

A documentary featuring families in which a member has died of AIDS. This video focuses on the issues of prejudice, rejection and grief, and is geared to the families and friends of people with AIDS or ARC

1058. Treating the Gay Patient. Audio Video Digest Foundation, 1577 E Chevy Chase Dr, Glendale CA 91206 1983 57 min videocassette $75.00; $29.95 (rental)

A videotape postgraduate course for the primary care physician

1059. Understanding AIDS. Cygnus Corp, Edina MN 55416 1985 25 min videocassette

A general presentation on AIDS

1060. Update on Acquired Immune Deficiency Syndrome, Moral Problems Surrounding AIDS: The Patient, the Health Professional, and the Public Good. Purtilo, Ruth Bryant; Creighton Univ Biomedical Communications. Creighton Biomedical Television, 2500 California St, Omaha NE 68178 1986 35 min videocassette

A general presentation on AIDS for the health professional and the general public

1061. Update on AIDS: Social and Clinical Significance. Thorup, Oscar A. Univ of Virginia Medical Center, PO Box 395, Charlottesville VA 22908 1983 Videocassette

A general presentation on AIDS stressing the social and clinical aspects

1062. VD: More Bugs, More Problems. Wallen, Stephen; Higgins, Alfred; Girioux, Con. Alfred Higgins Productions, 9100 Sunset Blvd, Los Angeles CA 90069 1986 20 min videocassette

A general presentation on VD including AIDS, herpes, and chlamydia

1063. What If the Patient Has AIDS: What Everyone Should Know About AIDS. United States Public Health Service; Frost Media Associates, Inc. National Audiovisual Center, 8700 Edgeworth Dr, Capitol Heights MD 20743 1984 20 min videocassette $80.00

A general presentation on AIDS

1064. What is AIDS?. J Gary Mitchell Film Co, Mitchell Gebhardt Film Co, San Francisco CA 94109 1988 16 min $335.00 videocassette; $435.00 16mm film

An AIDS-education film for youngsters, focusing on how AIDS is transmitted, and how the immune system works and is compromised by the AIDS-causing virus

1065. What You Should Know Video: About AIDS. Channing L Bete Company, Incorporated, 200 State Rd, S Deerfield MA 01373 1988 20 min videocassette $300.00

This video uses cartoons, advice from experts, and "people on the street" interviews to present basic facts about AIDS and pratical information for preventing the spread of HIV

1066. What Young People Should Know Video: Young People and AIDS. Channing L Bete Company, Incorporated, 200 State Rd, South Deerfield MA 01373 1988 18 min videocassette $300.00

This video for teens features cartoons, "people-on-the-street" interviews and statements from physicians in a presentation of basic AIDS facts, focusing on AIDS awareness and prevention

1067. When Facts are Not Enough: Managing AIDS in the Workplace. American Hospital Assn Media Center; American Society for Healthcare, Human Resources Administration of the American Hospital Assn; American Hospital Assn Dept of Infection Control and Environmental Health. American Hospital Assn, 840 N Lake Shore Dr, Chicago IL 60611 1986 24 min videocassette

This video focuses on the education needs of people who provide care for people with AIDS (PWA) and coworkers of PWAs, and guidelines for establishing workplace AIDS policies

ONLINE DATABASES

1068. Acquired Immune Deficiency Syndrome Database (AIDD). Bureau of Hygiene and Tropical Diseases. BRS Information Technologies, 555 E Lancaster Ave, Saint Davids PA 19087

The AIDD database is produced by the non-profit Bureau of Hygiene and Tropical Diseases, Great Britain, and includes bibliographic citations to articles, conferences, books and reports on a wide variety of AIDS-related topics including incidence, transmission, clinical aspects, immunology, public health and safety, and pathology. Despite its British origin, over half of the database's literature references were published in the US. English-language abstracts are available for most citations and have been critically evaluated. AIDD is available from BRS Information Technologies

1069. AIDS Information and Education Worldwide. Libraries-To-Go. CD Resources, Incorporated, 35 E Wacker Dr, Ste 2150, Chicago IL 60601-2204 1988 $795.00

This CD-ROM format database includes the full-text of core source materials on AIDS drawn from the World Health Organization, the US Centers for Disease Control, and international sources from West and Central Africa, Europe, Asia, South America and Australia. The collection includes technical reports, case studies, articles, bibliographic references, and the complete text of over 200 publications. Nearly all aspects of the AIDS crisis are represented, both social and scientific. Access is through subscription; updates are available at an additional cost

1070. AIDS Information Clearinghouse. Health Information Network. Information Companies of America, Incorporated, 1500 Walnut St, Philadelphia PA 19102

The Health Information Network (HIN) is a database and electronic communication network providing health care professionals with access to constantly-updated health information. The *AIDS Information Clearinghouse,* a part of HIN, includes: news items; releases from various federal agencies such as the Centers for Disease Control, the Surgeon General's office and the Food and Drug Administration; and data regarding conferences, meetings, and important legal decisions. Access is available directly from Information Companies of America, Inc. or through AT&T's ACCUNET communication system

1071. AIDS Knowledge Base (ASFG). Massachusetts Medical Society; San Francisco General Hospital, Dept of Internal Medicine. BRS Information Technologies, 555 E Lancaster Ave, Saint Davids PA 19087

The *AIDS Knowledge Base i*s an electronic "textbook" developed at the San Francisco General Hospital, and includes monthly-updated information on AIDS covering incidence, psychosocial issues, diagnosis, treatment, education, prevention and control. The database is a primary information source arranged like a text, with a table of contents, and is geared to health care professionals. Access is through BRS Information technologies, a major database vendor. The *AIDS Knowledge Base* is also available as part of *Compact Library: AIDS,* a CD-ROM (compact disk digital data) product

1072. AIDSLINE. National Library of Medicine, 8600 Rockville Pike, Bethesda MD 20894

AIDSLINE is a computerized bibliographic database of citations to scientific articles about AIDS covering current research, clinical aspects, epidemiology and health policy issues. Included references are drawn from the National Library of Medicine's *MEDLINE* database and date from 1980 to the present. The entire file is updated twice monthly. In early 1989, additional citations from NLM's *CANCER-LINE* and *Health Planning and Administration* databases will be added. Many of the article references have abstracts in English. *AIDSLINE* is available by applying for a password from the National Library of Medicine

1073. AIDSQUEST. Charles Henderson, PO Box 830409, Birmingham AL 35283-0409 1989—

Contains articles covering all areas of AIDS research and development. Also available in print format as *CDC AIDS Weekly*

1074. AMA/NET AIDS Information Service. AMA/NET; American Medical Association. SoftSearch, Incorporated, 1560 Broadway, Ste 900, Denver CO 80202

The *AIDS Information Service* is available on the American Medical Association's computerized information network, AMA/NET. The service includes current news, a selection of both clinical and general literature searches, and references to AIDS information sources available through other AMA/NET services. The network is geared to health professionals, and access is made available by signing a subscription agreement

1075. BRS/Colleague. BRS Technologies, 555 E Lancaster Ave, Saint Davids PA 19087

BRS/Colleague is a computerized information search system developed for health professionals providing access to information from a wide range of bibliographic and full-text databases. AIDS information is available from *MEDLINE*, the *Health Planning and Administration* database, the *Acquired Immune Deficiency Syndrome Database*, the *AIDS Knowledge Base* from the San Francisco General Hospital, as well as many other topically-arranged sources. Passwords to BRS/Colleague are available from BRS Technologies

1076. Compact Library: AIDS. Medical Publishing Group. Massachusetts Medical Society, 1440 Main St, Waltham MA 02154-1649 1988 $875.00

Included on this CD-ROM product are references culled from the databases of the Bureau of Hygiene and Tropical Diseases and National Library of Medicine (MEDLINE), the full-text of journal articles from seven premier medical journals, and the entire contents of the San Francisco General Hospital's *AIDS Knowledge Base. Compact Library: AIDS* is available as a subscription, and is updated quarterly

1077. Computerized AIDS Information Network (CAIN). California Department of Health Services Office of AIDS. Gay and Lesbian Community Service Center in Los Angeles, 1213 N Highland Ave, Los Angeles CA 90038

CAIN is an electronic database and community "bulletin board" intended to facilitate networking and resource-sharing among agencies, community groups and individuals interested in AIDS. Included in the database are news items, educational materials, questionnaires, and informational sources. Access is through the Delphi communication service, or directly from the Gay and Lesbian Community Service Center

1078. Health Planning and Administration. American Hospital Association. National Library of Medicine, 8600 Rockville Pike, Bethesda MD 20894 1975-

The National Library of Medicine (NLM) and the American Hospital Association have jointly sponsored the *Health Planning and Administration* database, a computerized source for bibliographic citations to literature on the administrative and managerial aspects of the delivery of health care. The database dates from 1975. Included information on AIDS focuses on economic, insurance, legislation, liability, policy, and operational aspects. Access is available through the database vendors BRS Technologies, DIALOG Information Services, Inc, or the National Library of Medicine. Arrangements for passwords must be made through the vendors or NLM

1079. MEDLINE. MEDLARS Management. National Library of Medicine, 8600 Rockville Pike, Bethesda MD 20894 1966-

MEDLINE is one of several computerized databases developed by the National Library of Medicine (NLM) as a repository for accessing the world's biomedical literature. *MEDLINE* includes bibliographic references to journal articles from over 3000 publications representing all fields of biomedical study. The database dates from 1966, and is updated twice monthly. Literature about AIDS as both a medical and social phenomenon is included, and currently there are in excess of 5000 citations about the topic in the database. Access to *MEDLINE* is available through the database vendors BRS Technologies and DIALOG Information Services, Inc, or directly from the National Library of Medicine. Arrangements for passwords must be made through the vendors or NLM

1080. PaperChase. Beth Israel Hospital, 330 Brookline Ave, Boston MA 02215

PaperChase is a service providing access to the National Library of Medicine's *MEDLINE*, a bibliographic database containing references to biomedical literature drawn from over 3000 journals published all over the globe. The entire *MEDLINE* database dates from 1966 and contains in excess of 5 million records. References to AIDS-related journal literature are part of the database, and topically include clinical, social and research areas of study. PaperChase is a "user-friendly" system for accessing the database, and is available directly from Beth Israel Hospital

1081. Understanding AIDS. SAE Software, Incorporated, 670 S 4th St, Edwardsville KS 66113 1988 $49.95

This unique program is a computer-assisted instruction (CAI) interactive tool for self-paced, programmed instruction about AIDS. Included are discussions of; the history of AIDS, at-risk groups, transmission of HIV, how HIV cripples the immune system, a glossary of terms, and periodic self-assessment tests with feedback. The program can be run on both Apple and IBM personal computers and network systems.

PERIODICALS

1082. AAPHR Letter. American Association of Physicians for Human Rights, PO Box 14366, San Francisco CA 94114

A quarterly newsletter of the American Association of Physicians for Human Rights with information of interest to members of the association about seminars, resources, and position statements dealing with human rights, including AIDS

1083. ACT Bulletin. AIDS Committee of Toronto, PO Box 55, Station F, Toronto ON M4Y 2L4 Canada

An irregularly published newsletter containing local, organizational, and national news on AIDS including fund-raising events and statistics on AIDS in the Toronto area

1084. Advocate. Liberation Publications, Inc, 6922 Hollywood Blvd, 10th Fl, Hollywood CA 90028

A biweekly gay and lesbian news magazine with a regular feature on AIDS

1085. AIDS. Gower Academic Journals, Gower House, Croft Rd, Aldershot, Great Britain G011 3HR UK

General AIDS information periodical

1086. AIDS: A Quarterly Bibliography from All Fields of Periodical Literature. Lincoln Associates, PO Box 507, Madison WI 53701

A quarterly bibliography covering non-gay periodicals, arranged by name of periodical

1087. AIDS Action Committee Update. AIDS Action Committee, 661 Boylston St, Boston MA 02116

A monthly newsletter with news of the committee's activities and general news of AIDS research

1088. AIDS Action Update. AIDS Action Council, 729 8th St SE, Ste 200, Washington DC 20003

A monthly newsletter with information on lobbying as it pertains to legislation directed at AIDS, research, and human rights

1089. AIDS Alert. Pacific Center AIDS Project, PO Box 908, Berkeley CA 94701

A monthly newsletter containing information by and about the Pacific Center AIDS Project including outreach, services, and people behind the AIDS effort

1090. AIDS and ARC News. Belmont Publishing Co, 1059 Alameda, Belmont CA 94002

A newsletter for health professionals about AIDS and the AIDS-related complex (ARC)

1091. AIDS and Public Policy Journal. University Publishing Group, Inc, 107 E Church St, Frederick MD 21701

A quarterly journal providing a forum for in-depth analysis, discussion, and debate of controversial issues surrounding the AIDS epidemic

1092. AIDS Business. International Resource Development, Inc, 6 Prowitt St, Norwalk CT 06855

A newsletter of AIDS information

1093. AIDS Era Newsletter., PO Box 42511, Philadelphia PA 19101

A newsletter of information about AIDS

1094. AIDS Forum: Diverse Views About Acquired Immune Deficiency Syndrome. Significant Other, Inc, PO Box 1545, Canal St Sta, New York NY 10013 1989

Premier issue includes a critique of the original multicenter AZT trial; a discussion of the ethical and scientific issues which should govern AIDS treatment research; and excerpts from a speech by editor and publisher Michael Callen about what it's like to live with AIDS in America. To be published a minimum of 6 times per year

1095. AIDS Information Bulletin. US Dept of Health and Human Services, Public Health Service, National Institutes of Health, GPO, Washington DC 20402HE 20.2:Ac

A bulletin of the Public Health Service

1096. AIDS Information Exchange. United States Conference of Mayors, 1620 Eye St NW, Washington DC 20006

A monthly newsletter containing national information on AIDS research, programs, and grants

1097. AIDS Information Update. AIDS Surveillance Program, 1115 N MacGregor, Rm 203, Houston TX 77030

A monthly newsletter that presents the latest statistics pertaining to AIDS in the state of Texas

1098. AIDS Law and Litigation Reporter. Univ Publishing Group, Inc, 107 E Church St, Frederick MD 21701

An annual publication that provides complete retrospective, full-text coverage of all court cases, summaries of AIDS-related cases, surveys of proposed and enacted legislation and statutes, and an in-depth analysis of current thinking on critical areas of AIDS law and litigation

1099. The AIDS Letter. Royal Society of Medicine, 1 Wimpole St, London, Great Britain W2 2LT UK
A medical journal about AIDS

1100. AIDS Literature and News Review. University Publishing Group, Inc, 107 E Church St, Frederick MD 21701
A monthly bibliography that summarizes the latest and most influential literature on AIDS from prominent periodicals and national newspapers

1101. AIDS Medical Update. Center for Interdisciplinary Research in Immunology and Diseases at UCLA, UCLA Dept of Medicine, Rm 37-068 CHS, Los Angeles CA 90024
A monthly newsletter with updated statistics and information on AIDS

1102. AIDS Newsletter. Monroe County Health Dept, AIDS Education Project, 901-B Duval St, Key West FL 33040
A bimonthly newsletter with information about AIDS in the Key West area

1103. AIDS Newsletter. Bureau of Hygiene and Tropical Diseases, Keppel St, London, Great Britain WC1E 7HT UK
A newsletter covering a wide range of AIDS-related topics

1104. AIDS Nursing Update. UCLA AIDS Clinical Research Center, UCLA Dept of Medicine, Rm 37-068 CHS, Los Angeles CA 90024
A newsletter of AIDS information of interest to the nursing profession and other individuals giving care to AIDS patients

1105. AIDS Patient Care. Mary Anne Liebert, Inc, 1651 Third Ave, No 301, New York NY 10128
This journal, primarily for health professionals, focuses on patient care issues, including care planning

1106. AIDS Policy and Law. Buraff Publications, 2445 M St NW, Ste 275, Washington DC 20037
A biweekly journal reporting on AIDS-related legislation, regulations, public policy issues and litigation

1107. The AIDS Record. Bio-Data Publishers, PO Box 66020, Washington DC 20035
A current-awareness journal about AIDS

1108. AIDS Research and Human Retroviruses. Mary Anne Liebert, Inc, 16151 Third Ave, No 301, New York NY 10128
A periodical for health professionals and researchers on AIDS, HIV, and related retroviruses

1109. AIDS Research Today. BIOSIS, 2100 Arch St, Philadelphia PA 19103
A loose-leaf journal and companion to *Collected Papers on AIDS* including abstracts on current research from the publishers of *Biological Abstracts*

1110. AIDS Treatment News. James, John S, PO Box 411256, San Francisco CA 94141 $25.00
Bi-weekly newsletter with the latest information about alternative treatments for HIV infection

1111. AIDS Update. Medical Data Exchange, 445 S San Antonio Rd, Los Altos CA 94022
This journal is issued in three versions: *AIDS Update: Clinical Management, AIDS Update: Social and Psychological Issues,* and *AIDS Update: Public, Economic and Legal Issues*

1112. AIDS Update (Lansing). Michigan Dept of Public Health, PO Box 30035, Lansing MI 48909
A newsletter of current information about AIDS research and education

1113. AIDS Update (Memphis). Aid to End AIDS Committee, PO Box 40389, Memphis TN 38174
A quarterly newspaper presenting information on AIDS, statistics, and education including safe sex

1114. Angles. West Coast Angles Publishing Society, PO Box 3287 Main Post Office, Vancouver BC V6B 3W2 Canada
A monthly gay and lesbian magazine with AIDS news

1115. Another Voice. Out Publishing Services, Inc., PO Box 729, Huntington NY 11743
A biweekly gay and lesbian magazine with a regular feature on AIDS

1116. Archives of AIDS Research. Reproductive Health Center, 78 Surfsong Rd, Kiawah Island SC 29455
A periodical issued jointly by the World Federation of Contraception and Health, World Academy of Population and Health Sciences, and IVF/Andrology International, Inc

1117. A.T.I.N. AIDS-Targeted Information Newsletter. Williams & Wilkins, 428 E Preston St, Baltimore MD 21202
A periodical sponsored by the American Federation for AIDS Research (AmFAR), including abstracts of current research studies

1118. Baltimore Gay Paper. Baltimore Gay Paper, PO Box 22575, Baltimore MD 21203
A monthly gay and lesbian newspaper with regular features on AIDS

1119. BAPHRON. Bay Area Physicians for Human Rights, PO Box 14546, San Francisco CA 94114
A bimonthly newsletter with human rights articles, some of which pertain to AIDS

1120. Bay Windows. Bay Windows, Inc, 1515 Washington St, Boston MA 02118
A weekly gay and lesbian newspaper with regular features and news on AIDS

1121. Being Alive., 4222 Santa Monica Blvd, Los Angeles CA 90029
Medical information about AIDS with current analysis of legal trends

1122. BETA. Bulletin of Experimental Treatments for AIDS. San Francisco AIDS Foundation, Box 6182, San Francisco CA 94101 Free, donations accepted
Periodical updates on current, experimental HIV infection treatments

1123. Body Positive., 263 W 19th St, New York NY 10011 Free, donations accepted
Newsletter for people testing positive for HIV

1124. Body Positive. Being Alive/People With AIDS Action Coalition, Inc, 8235 Santa Monica Blvd, Ste 210, West Hollywood CA 90046
A newsletter of general information on resources and services for people with AIDS

1125. Campaign Fund Report. Human Rights Campaign Fund, 1012 14th St NW, Washington DC 20005
A monthly newsletter with general information about the agency, its programs, and activities

1126. CARE Notes. Nashville CARES, PO Box 25107, Nashville TN 37202
A newsletter of news and activities of the Nashville Council on AIDS Resources, Education and Services (Nashville CARES)

1127. CDC AIDS Weekly. Charles Henderson, 1409 Fairview Rd, Atlanta GA 30306-4611
A weekly newsletter containing national and international news on AIDS, abstracts of AIDS articles, and a comprehensive listing of upcoming AIDS meetings, symposia, and conferences throughout the world

1128. Center News. Gay and Lesbian Community Center of Colorado, Drawer E, Denver CO 80218
A monthly newsletter of the center with news of its activities, calendar of events and general AIDS information

1129. Clinical Trials—Talking it Over. National Institute of Allergy and Infectious Diseases, Office of Communications, National Institutes of Health, Bldg 31, Rm 7A32, Bethesda MD 20892 Free
Information for people considering participating in AIDS/HIV clinical trials

1130. Columbus AIDS Task Force Newsletter. Columbus AIDS Task Force, PO Box 8393, Columbus OH 43201
A monthly newsletter presenting CATF news and national AIDS updates

1131. Current Topics in AIDS. John Wiley & Sons, Inc, 605 Third Ave, New York NY 10158
A current-awareness journal about AIDS and the AIDS-causing virus, HIV

1132. DAIR Update. Documentation of AIDS Issues and Research Foundation, Inc, 2336 Market St, Ste 33, San Francisco CA 94114
A bimonthly newsletter with the latest information on AIDS treatments and research

1133. Edge. Edge Publishing, Inc, 6900 Melrose Ave, Los Angeles CA 90038
A biweekly gay and lesbian magazine with regular features on AIDS

1134. Employment Testing: A National Reporter on Polygraph, Drug, AIDS and Genetic Testing. University Publications of America, 44 N Market St, Frederick MD 21701
A periodical reporting on employment testing, including information on a variety of "biodetectable" conditions such as substance abuse, exposure to the AIDS-causing virus, and genetic potential for illness

1135. Epidemiology Notes. Houston Bureau of Epidemiology, 1115 N MacGregor, Houston TX 77030
A monthly newsletter containing epidemiological statistics in the Houston area

1136. Equal Time. Star of the North Publishing Co, 711 W Lake St, Ste 504, Minneapolis MN 55408
A biweekly gay and lesbian newspaper with regular features on AIDS

1137. ETC. Etcetera, PO Box 8916, Atlanta GA 30306
A weekly gay and lesbian magazine with a regular feature on AIDS

1138. Executive AIDS Watch. DJM Publishers, 111 3rd Ave, Seattle WA 98101
A newsletter of AIDS information

1139. Focus: A Review of AIDS Research. UCSF AIDS Health Project, PO Box 0884, San Francisco CA 94103-0884
A monthly newsletter reporting on AIDS research with a feature article each month

1140. Frontiers. Frontiers Publishing Corp, 7985 Santa Monica Blvd, Ste 109, West Hollywood CA 90046
A biweekly gay and lesbian magazine with regular feature articles on AIDS

1141. Gay News-Telegraph. Piasa Publishing Co, PO Box 14229A, St Louis MO 63178-1229
A monthly gay and lesbian newspaper with regular features on AIDS

1142. Gay Scene. Regiment Publications, PO Box 247, Grand Central Station, New York NY 10163
A monthly gay newspaper with regular features on AIDS

1143. GLAD News. Gay and Lesbian Alliance of Greater Danbury, PO Box 2045, Danbury CT 06813
A monthly gay and lesbian newsletter with regular features on AIDS

1144. Healing AIDS., 3835 20th St, San Francisco CA 94114 $15.00
Monthly periodical focusing on alternative, holistic therapies for HIV infection

1145. Health Letter. Gay Men's Health Crisis, PO Box 274, New York NY 20011
A bimonthly newsletter with information about AIDS and safe sex practices

1146. Heartspace. Los Angeles Shanti Foundation, 9060 Santa Monica Blvd, Ste 301, West Hollywood CA 90069
A quarterly publication for friends, volunteers, and staff of the foundation with foundation news and notes. Shanti is a support group for PWAs

1147. Hemophilia World. World Hemophilia AIDS Center, 2400 S Flower St, Los Angeles CA 90007-2697
A quarterly newsletter with information and statistics on AIDS and hemophilia

1148. HERO News. Health Education Resource Organization, 101 W Read St, Ste 812, Baltimore MD 21201
A monthly newsletter with news about activities of HERO and its educational programs

1149. Hope and Help Center Newsletter. Hope and Help Center, PO Box 14286, San Francisco CA 94114
A bimonthly newsletter with information about the center's activities

1150. Impetus. San Francisco AIDS Foundation, 333 Valencia St, 4th Fl, San Francisco CA 94103
A quarterly newsletter of news about new programs and services of the foundation

1151. Journal of AID Atlanta. AID Atlanta, 1132 W Peachtree St NW, Atlanta GA 30309
A journal that focuses on the true emotions and experiences of persons affected in any way by AIDS

1152. Just Out. Out Media, Inc, PO Box 15117, Portland OR 97215
A monthly gay and lesbian newspaper with regular features on AIDS

1153. Lavender Health. Office of Gay and Lesbian Health Concerns, 125 Worth St, Box 67, New York NY 10013
A quarterly newsletter on health, AIDS, and safe sex

1154. Le Virulent. C-SAM Comite SIDA-Aide Montreal, CP 98 Depot N, Montreal PQ H2X 3M2 Canada
A bimonthly bulletin with information about the Montreal AIDS Support Committee and AIDS in general

1155. Lifeline. AIDS Foundation Houston, Inc, PO Box 66973, Houston TX 77006
A monthly newsletter with local and national AIDS information

1156. Media Action. AIDS Committee of Toronto, PO Box 55, Station F, Toronto ON M4Y 2L4 Canada
A general informational newsletter of ACT

1157. MGW. MGW Publications, 1400 S St, Ste 100B, Sacramento CA 95814
A monthly gay and lesbian newspaper with a regular feature on AIDS

1158. Milwaukee Hospice Home Care Newsletter. Milwaukee Hospice Home Care, Inc, 1022 N 9th St, Milwaukee WI 53233
A monthly newsletter with information about the hospice, its volunteers, and staff

1159. Monthly Update (AIDS Vancouver). AIDS Vancouver, 1033 Davie St, Ste 509, Vancouver BC V6E 1M7 Canada
A monthly newsletter with Canadian AIDS statistics and annotations of articles on AIDS

1160. NAN Monitor. National AIDS Network, 1012 14th St NW, Ste 601, Washington DC 20005
A quarterly newsletter providing reviews and overviews on AIDS topics

1161. NAN News. National AIDS Network, 1012 14th St NW, Ste 601, Washington DC 20005
A biweekly newsletter for members of NAN providing technical assistance

1162. National Coalition of Gay STD Services Newsletter. National Coalition of Gay STD Services, PO Box 239, Milwaukee WI 53201
A quarterly newsletter providing a forum for communication among the nation's gay STD services and providers with contributions, letters, and reviews on all aspects of STD and AIDS

1163. New York Native. That New Magazine, Inc, PO Box 1475, Church St Station, New York NY 10008
A biweekly gay and lesbian newspaper with a regular feature on AIDS

1164. Newsletter: AIDS Network of Edmonton. AIDS Network of Edmonton Society, 10233 98th St, Edmonton AB T5J 0M7 Canada
A monthly newsletter with information for network members about AIDS

1165. Out!. Out!, PO Box 148, Madison WI 53701
A monthly gay and lesbian newspaper with a regular feature on AIDS

1166. Paper. E.L. Poole, PO Box 629, Guerneville CA 95446
A weekly gay and lesbian newspaper with a regular feature on AIDS

1167. Pittsburgh's Out. OPC, Inc, 640 Allenby Ave, Ste 201, Pittsburgh PA 15218
A monthly gay and lesbian newspaper with a regular feature on AIDS

1168. Preventive Medicine Monthly. Ohio Dept of Health, 246 N High St, 8th Fl, Columbus OH 43266-5480
A monthly newsletter for AIDS educators

1169. Progress Report. Arizona AIDS Project, 736 E Flynn Lane, Phoenix AZ 85014
A bimonthly newsletter with local and national AIDS news

1170. PWA Coalition Newsline., 31 W 26th St, New York NY 10010
Free, donations accepted
Newsletter featuring information on alternative and experimental treatments for HIV infection, community-based research activities, and outreach services

1171. PWA Coalition Newsline. People With AIDS Coalition, 263A W 19th St, New York NY 10011
A newsletter published by, for, and about PWAs and PWARCs

1172. San Francisco AIDS Foundation News. San Francisco AIDS Foundation, 333 Valencia St, 4th Fl, San Francisco CA 94103
A newsletter of foundation news

1173. Seattle Gay News. JT and A, Inc, 704 E Pike St, Seattle WA 98122
A weekly gay and lesbian newspaper with a regular feature on AIDS

1174. Texas Preventable Disease News. Texas Bureau of Epidemiology, 1100 W 49th St, Austin TX 78756-3180
A weekly publication covering all preventable diseases in Texas

1175. Treatment Issues: The GMHC Newletter of Experimental AIDS Therapies. Gay Men's Health Crisis, Department of Medical Information, 129 W 20th St, New York NY 10011 Free
Newsletter about current, experimental medical treatments for HIV infection

1176. TWN. The Weekly News, Inc, 901 NE 79th St, Miami FL 33138
A weekly gay and lesbian newspaper with a regular feature on AIDS

1177. Update. Topeka AIDS Project, PO Box 2655, Topeka KS 66601
A newsletter of AIDS information for Kansas

1178. Update: AIDS Products in Development. Pharmaceutical Manufacturers Association, Communications Division, 1100 15th St NW, Washington DC 20005 Write for information
Quarterly updates on diagnostic and treatment interventions for HIV infections

1179. Vancouver PWA Coalition Newsletter. Vancouver PWA Coalition, PO Box 136, Vancouver BC V6E 1N4 Canada
A monthly newsletter by, for, and about persons with AIDS or ARC

1180. Virology and AIDS Abstracts. Cambridge Scientific Abstracts, 7200 Wisconsin Ave, Bethesda MD 20814 1988
This journal, formerly titled *Virology Abstracts,* summarizes important international research publications in the field of virology, including the study of HIV, the AIDS-causing virus

1181. Wellness News. Wellness News, PO Box 1046, Royal Oak MI 48068
A newsletter of health news and safe sex information

1182. Wellspring. Colorado AIDS Project, PO Box 18529, Denver CO 80218
A bimonthly newsletter of information about the project, national news on AIDS, calendar of events, and statistics

1183. Whitman-Walker Clinic AIDS Program Newsletter. Whitman-Walker Clinic, Inc, 2335 18th St NW, Washington DC 20009
A newsletter of information about the AIDS program of the clinic

1184. Windy City Times. Sentry Publications, Inc, 3223 N Sheffield, Chicago IL 60657
A weekly gay and lesbian newspaper with regular features on AIDS

PLAYS

1185. As Is: A Play. Hoffman, William M. Random House, 201 E 50th St, New York NY 10022 1985 97p 0-394-55096-X

1186. Normal Heart. Kramer, Larry. New American Library, 1633 Broadway, New York NY 10019 1985 123p 0-453-00506-3
A play about the gay community's reaction to the AIDS crisis in New York City at the beginning of the epidemic

1187. Safe Sex. Fierstein, Harvey. Atheneum Publishers, 866 3rd Ave, New York NY 10022 1987 112p $12.95 0-689119-53-4
Three one-act plays about AIDS by the author of Torch Song Triology

POSTERS

1188. AIDS and Adolescents: Resources for Educators. Young, Rebecca. Center for Population Options, 1012 14th St NW, Washington DC 20005 1987
A list of curriculum materials about AIDS for educators of teens

1189. How to Get High and Get AIDS in One Shot—Don't Share the Works and You Won't Share AIDS. Long Island Association for AIDS Care, Incorportaed (LIAAC), PO Box 2859, Huntington Station NY 11746
This black-and-white poster includes the title message with a picture of a man's forearm readied for "shooting-up"

1190. Ignore AIDS and It Will Bury the Rest of You. Oregon Department of Human Resources, 711 State Office Bldg, 1400 SW 5th Ave, PO Box 231, Portland OR 97201 1985
This poster features the title message coupled with modernistic depictions of people with their heads stuck in the ground

1191. No One Can Afford to Ignore AIDS—You Owe it to Yourself to Get the Facts. Idaho Department of Health and Welfare, State Capitol Bldg, 700 W Jefferson St, Boise ID 83720
Featured on this poster is a group photograph representing a cross-section of Idahoans, stressing the idea that AIDS is an indiscriminatory community concern

1192. Psst...Esuchen! Tecatos! No Jueguen Con Et AIDS...Estan Jugando Contra Baraja Marcadas. Multicultural Prevention Resource Center (MPRC), 1540 Market St, Ste 320, San Francisco CA 94102 1987 $2.50
This poster aimed at intravenous substance abusers features the message, "Don't gamble with AIDS—it's a stacked deck," and features a hand holding four playing cards depicting a syringe, a pirate face, a skull and joker card labelled AIDS. Instructions for cleaning needles with bleach are included. An English version is also available

1193. Talk About AIDS Before It Hits Home. AIDS Education Training Unit. New York City Department of Health, 311 Broadway, 4th Fl, New York NY 10007 Free
This poster encourages parents to talk to their teenage children about AIDS. Also available in Spanish

1194. We Didn't Think We Could Get AIDS!. Health Education Resource Organization (HERO), 101 Reed St, Ste 812, Baltimore MD 21201 1987 $1.50
This poster features a young Black couple and the title message, stressing that AIDS is indiscriminate

BIBLIOGRAPHY – SUBJECT INDEX

Haitians

Health care

PART IV

APPENDIX A:
SELECTED STATISTICAL TABLES

Table 1. AIDS cases and annual incidence rates per 100,000 population, by state, reported May 1987 through April 1988 and May 1988 through April 1989; and cumulative totals, by state and age group, through April 1989

State of residence	May 1987-April 1988 No.	Rate	May 1988-April 1989 No.	Rate	Cumulative totals Adults/ adolescents	Children < 13 years old	Total
Alabama	180	4.4	221	5.4	502	13	515
Alaska	16	2.8	16	2.7	60	1	61
Arizona	314	9.2	259	7.4	749	4	753
Arkansas	62	2.6	77	3.2	192	3	195
California	5,238	19.0	5,865	20.9	18,793	126	18,919
Colorado	280	8.4	347	10.2	979	5	984
Connecticut	331	10.3	425	13.2	1,123	37	1,160
Delaware	44	6.9	82	12.8	172	4	176
District of Columbia	510	81.7	526	84.5	1,659	19	1,678
Florida	1,898	15.9	2,987	24.4	7,242	200	7,442
Georgia	549	8.8	968	15.3	2,217	30	2,247
Hawaii	96	8.7	92	8.2	316	2	318
Idaho	10	1.0	16	1.6	34	2	36
Illinois	797	6.9	1,002	8.6	2,632	35	2,667
Indiana	150	2.7	196	3.6	503	4	507
Iowa	34	1.2	55	1.9	127	3	130
Kansas	73	2.9	89	3.6	227	3	230
Kentucky	64	1.7	100	2.7	241	2	243
Louisiana	382	8.4	405	8.8	1,199	15	1,214
Maine	30	2.5	37	3.1	110	2	112
Maryland	459	10.3	633	14.0	1,629	36	1,665
Massachusetts	529	9.0	771	13.1	1,978	33	2,011
Michigan	270	3.0	474	5.2	1,055	19	1,074
Minnesota	134	3.2	181	4.2	504	4	508
Mississippi	79	3.0	154	5.8	277	5	282
Missouri	305	6.0	407	8.0	935	8	943
Montana	10	1.2	12	1.4	27	—	27
Nebraska	34	2.1	45	2.8	106	—	106
Nevada	116	11.8	137	13.6	331	3	334
New Hampshire	36	3.5	39	3.7	99	4	103
New Jersey	1,933	25.3	2,441	31.7	6,262	192	6,454
New Mexico	47	3.1	67	4.4	167	1	168
New York	5,057	28.3	6,613	36.9	21,754	476	22,230
North Carolina	270	4.2	341	5.3	802	18	820
North Dakota	—	—	6	0.9	13	—	13
Ohio	413	3.8	506	4.7	1,278	20	1,298
Oklahoma	120	3.6	177	5.2	395	9	404
Oregon	193	7.1	183	6.7	530	3	533
Pennsylvania	778	6.6	965	8.2	2,512	45	2,557
Rhode Island	62	6.3	94	9.6	222	6	228
South Carolina	113	3.3	200	5.7	444	14	458
South Dakota	4	0.6	7	1.0	15	—	15
Tennessee	192	4.0	307	6.3	588	10	598
Texas	1,851	10.9	2,353	13.5	6,403	51	6,454
Utah	56	3.3	77	4.5	184	5	189
Vermont	14	2.6	12	2.2	38	1	39
Virginia	297	5.1	423	7.1	1,105	22	1,127
Washington	373	8.2	453	9.9	1,230	8	1,238
West Virginia	18	0.9	29	1.5	72	2	74
Wisconsin	96	2.0	114	2.4	320	1	321
Wyoming	1	0.2	13	2.5	19	—	19
U.S. total	**24,918**	**10.3**	**31,999**	**13.0**	**90,371**	**1,506**	**91,877**
Guam	3	2.3	1	0.8	5	—	5
Pacific Islands, Trust Territory	—	—	1	0.7	1	—	1
Puerto Rico	597	18.2	1,415	42.9	2,290	53	2,343
Virgin Islands, U.S.	9	8.1	38	33.6	52	2	54
Total	**25,527**	**10.3**	**33,454**	**13.4**	**92,719**	**1,561**	**94,280**

Tables 1, 3–4, 6–9 and Technical notes are taken from: Centers for Disease Control. *HIV/AIDS Surveillance Report,* May 1989: 1–16

Table 3. AIDS cases by age group, exposure category, and sex, reported May 1987 through April 1988 and May 1988 through April 1989; and cumulative totals, by age group and exposure category, through April 1989, United States

Adult/adolescent exposure category	Males May 1987-Apr. 1988 No. (%)	Males May 1988-Apr. 1989 No. (%)	Females May 1987-Apr. 1988 No. (%)	Females May 1988-Apr. 1989 No. (%)	Totals May 1987-Apr. 1988 No. (%)	Totals May 1988-Apr. 1989 No. (%)	Cumulative total No. (%)
Male homosexual/bisexual contact	15,206 (67)	18,676 (63)	—	—	15,206 (61)	18,676 (57)	56,783 (61)
Intravenous (IV) drug use (female and heterosexual male)	3,964 (17)	5,918 (20)	1,228 (53)	1,776 (52)	5,192 (21)	7,694 (23)	18,819 (20)
Male homosexual/bisexual contact and IV drug use	1,818 (8)	2,084 (7)	—	—	1,818 (7)	2,084 (6)	6,620 (7)
Hemophilia/coagulation disorder	248 (1)	308 (1)	6 (0)	6 (0)	254 (1)	314 (1)	888 (1)
Heterosexual contact:	440 (2)	635 (2)	656 (28)	1,005 (30)	1,096 (4)	1,640 (5)	4,128 (4)
Sex with IV drug user	*136*	*282*	*411*	*636*	*547*	*918*	*1,980*
Sex with bisexual male	*—*	*—*	*75*	*88*	*75*	*88*	*270*
Sex with person with hemophilia	*1*	*2*	*11*	*14*	*12*	*16*	*37*
Born in Pattern-II[1] country	*249*	*244*	*79*	*125*	*328*	*369*	*1,370*
Sex with person born in Pattern-II country	*13*	*15*	*6*	*6*	*19*	*21*	*60*
Sex with transfusion recipient with HIV infection	*2*	*11*	*16*	*18*	*18*	*29*	*60*
Sex with person with HIV infection, risk not specified	*39*	*81*	*58*	*118*	*97*	*199*	*351*
Receipt of transfusion of blood, blood components, or tissue[2]	491 (2)	477 (2)	261 (11)	333 (10)	752 (3)	810 (2)	2,294 (2)
Other/undetermined[3]	607 (3)	1,366 (5)	152 (7)	282 (8)	759 (3)	1,648 (5)	3,187 (3)
Adult/adolescent subtotal	22,774 (100)	29,464 (100)	2,303 (100)	3,402 (100)	25,077 (100)	32,866 (100)	92,719 (100)
Pediatric (<13 years old) exposure category							
Hemophilia/coagulation disorder	27 (11)	32 (10)	—	1 (0)	27 (6)	33 (6)	89 (6)
Mother with/at risk for AIDS/HIV infection:	175 (72)	232 (73)	172 (83)	240 (88)	347 (77)	472 (80)	1,233 (79)
IV drug use	*89*	*115*	*91*	*110*	*180*	*225*	*637*
Sex with IV drug user	*36*	*52*	*33*	*46*	*69*	*98*	*243*
Sex with bisexual male	*1*	*7*	*9*	*5*	*10*	*12*	*31*
Sex with person with hemophilia	*3*	*—*	*2*	*1*	*5*	*1*	*7*
Born in Pattern-II country	*19*	*25*	*15*	*23*	*34*	*48*	*141*
Sex with person born in Pattern-II country	*1*	*1*	*1*	*—*	*2*	*1*	*4*
Sex with transfusion recipient with HIV infection	*—*	*2*	*1*	*3*	*1*	*5*	*6*
Sex with person with HIV infection, risk not specified	*7*	*11*	*2*	*13*	*9*	*24*	*47*
Receipt of transfusion of blood, blood components, or tissue	*3*	*2*	*7*	*8*	*10*	*10*	*27*
Has HIV infection, risk not specified	*16*	*17*	*11*	*31*	*27*	*48*	*90*
Receipt of transfusion of blood, blood components, or tissue	35 (14)	36 (11)	26 (13)	18 (7)	61 (14)	54 (9)	184 (12)
Undetermined	6 (2)	16 (5)	9 (4)	13 (5)	15 (3)	29 (5)	55 (4)
Pediatric subtotal	243 (100)	316 (100)	207 (100)	272 (100)	450 (100)	588 (100)	1,561 (100)
Total	**23,017**	**29,780**	**2,510**	**3,674**	**25,527**	**33,454**	**94,280**

[1] See technical notes.

[2] Includes 1 tissue recipient and 2 transfusion recipients who received blood screened for HIV antibody.

[3] "Other" is 1 health-care worker who seroconverted to HIV and developed AIDS after needlestick exposure to HIV-infected blood. "Undetermined" includes 2,234 adults/adolescents (49 children) under investigation; 552 adults/adolescents (6 children) who died, were lost to follow-up, or refused interview; and 370 adults/adolescents (0 children) whose mode of exposure to HIV remains undetermined after investigation.

Table 4. AIDS cases by age group, exposure category, and race/ethnicity, reported through April 1989, United States

Adult/adolescent exposure category	White, not Hispanic No. (%)	Black, not Hispanic No. (%)	Hispanic No. (%)	Asian/Pacific Islander No. (%)	American Indian/ Alaskan Native No. (%)	Total[4] No. (%)
Male homosexual/bisexual contact	41,235 (77)	9,084 (37)	5,888 (42)	411 (75)	55 (51)	56,783 (61)
Intravenous (IV) drug use (female and heterosexual male)	3,764 (7)	9,391 (38)	5,579 (40)	20 (4)	17 (16)	18,819 (20)
Male homosexual/bisexual contact and IV drug use	3,947 (7)	1,681 (7)	960 (7)	8 (1)	15 (14)	6,620 (7)
Hemophilia/coagulation disorder	740 (1)	55 (0)	72 (1)	11 (2)	6 (6)	888 (1)
Heterosexual contact:	811 (2)	2,641 (11)	643 (5)	18 (3)	7 (6)	4,128 (4)
Sex with IV drug user	*445*	*997*	*525*	*7*	*3*	*1,980*
Sex with bisexual male	*144*	*86*	*37*	*3*	*—*	*270*
Sex with person with hemophilia	*32*	*3*	*1*	*1*	*—*	*37*
Born in Pattern-II[1] country	*5*	*1,351*	*9*	*2*	*—*	*1,370*
Sex with person born in Pattern-II country	*17*	*40*	*3*	*—*	*—*	*60*
Sex with transfusion recipient with AIDS/HIV infection	*45*	*7*	*5*	*2*	*—*	*60*
Sex with person with HIV infection, risk not specified	*123*	*157*	*63*	*3*	*4*	*351*
Receipt of transfusion of blood, blood components, or tissue[2]	1,693 (3)	352 (1)	197 (1)	44 (8)	3 (3)	2,294 (2)
Other/undetermined[3]	1,207 (2)	1,237 (5)	673 (5)	36 (7)	5 (5)	3,187 (3)
Adult/adolescent subtotal	53,397 (100)	24,441 (100)	14,012 (100)	548 (100)	108 (100)	92,719 (100)

Pediatric (<13 years old) exposure category						
Hemophilia/coagulation disorder	63 (17)	11 (1)	12 (3)	3 (33)	—	89 (6)
Mother with/at risk for AIDS/HIV infection:	190 (52)	749 (90)	282 (82)	3 (33)	3 (100)	1,233 (79)
IV drug use	*87*	*379*	*167*	*1*	*2*	*637*
Sex with IV drug user	*40*	*123*	*78*	*—*	*—*	*243*
Sex with bisexual male	*11*	*16*	*4*	*—*	*—*	*31*
Sex with person with hemophilia	*5*	*1*	*1*	*—*	*—*	*7*
Born in Pattern-II country	*2*	*137*	*1*	*—*	*—*	*141*
Sex with person born in Pattern-II country	*—*	*3*	*—*	*—*	*—*	*4*
Sex with transfusion recipient with HIV infection	*5*	*1*	*—*	*—*	*—*	*6*
Sex with person with HIV infection, risk not specified	*9*	*23*	*13*	*1*	*—*	*47*
Receipt of transfusion of blood, blood components, or tissue	*10*	*11*	*6*	*—*	*—*	*27*
Has HIV infection, risk not specified	*21*	*55*	*12*	*1*	*1*	*90*
Receipt of transfusion of blood, blood components, or tissue	99 (27)	43 (5)	39 (11)	3 (33)	—	184 (12)
Undetermined	10 (3)	32 (4)	13 (4)	—	—	55 (4)
Pediatric subtotal	362 (100)	835 (100)	346 (100)	9 (100)	3 (100)	1,561 (100)
Total	**53,759**	**25,276**	**14,358**	**557**	**111**	**94,280**

[1] See technical notes.

[2] Includes 1 tissue recipient and 2 transfusion recipients who received blood screened for HIV antibody.

[3] "Other" is 1 health-care worker who seroconverted to HIV and developed AIDS after needlestick exposure to HIV-infected blood. "Undetermined" includes 2,234 adults/adolescents (49 children) under investigation; 552 adults/adolescents (6 children) who died, were lost to follow-up, or refused interview; and 370 adults/adolescents (0 children) whose mode of exposure to HIV remains undetermined after investigation.

[4] Includes 219 persons whose race/ethnicity is unknown.

Table 6. AIDS cases by sex, age at diagnosis, and race/ethnicity, reported through April 1989, United States

Males Age at diagnosis (years)	White, not Hispanic		Black, not Hispanic		Hispanic		Asian/Pacific Islander		American Indian/ Alaskan Native		Total[1]	
	No.	(%)	No.	(%)	No.	(%)	No.	(%)	No.	(%)	No.	(%)
Under 5	124	(0)	374	(2)	162	(1)	3	(1)	1	(1)	667	(1)
5-12	99	(0)	51	(0)	27	(0)	3	(1)	—		180	(0)
13-19	154	(0)	85	(0)	55	(0)	5	(1)	2	(2)	302	(0)
20-24	1,914	(4)	1,021	(5)	601	(5)	22	(4)	8	(9)	3,573	(4)
25-29	7,836	(15)	3,438	(17)	2,168	(17)	60	(12)	12	(13)	13,534	(16)
30-34	12,127	(24)	5,301	(26)	3,311	(26)	109	(22)	26	(29)	20,917	(24)
35-39	11,215	(22)	4,691	(23)	2,688	(21)	113	(22)	17	(19)	18,770	(22)
40-44	7,511	(15)	2,558	(12)	1,725	(14)	69	(14)	10	(11)	11,908	(14)
45-49	4,418	(9)	1,443	(7)	861	(7)	60	(12)	7	(8)	6,803	(8)
50-54	2,545	(5)	845	(4)	498	(4)	26	(5)	3	(3)	3,928	(5)
55-59	1,664	(3)	482	(2)	303	(2)	17	(3)	3	(3)	2,478	(3)
60-64	907	(2)	239	(1)	126	(1)	5	(1)	2	(2)	1,283	(2)
65 or older	842	(2)	131	(1)	86	(1)	14	(3)	—		1,075	(1)
Male subtotal	51,356	(100)	20,659	(100)	12,611	(100)	506	(100)	91	(100)	85,418	(100)

Females Age at diagnosis (years)	White, not Hispanic		Black, not Hispanic		Hispanic		Asian/Pacific Islander		American Indian/ Alaskan Native		Total[1]	
Under 5	117	(5)	362	(8)	136	(8)	1	(2)	2	(10)	621	(7)
5-12	22	(1)	48	(1)	21	(1)	2	(4)	—		93	(1)
13-19	15	(1)	41	(1)	12	(1)	1	(2)	1	(5)	70	(1)
20-24	155	(6)	265	(6)	139	(8)	2	(4)	—		564	(6)
25-29	455	(19)	894	(19)	405	(23)	4	(8)	3	(15)	1,769	(20)
30-34	508	(21)	1,313	(28)	445	(25)	14	(27)	8	(40)	2,294	(26)
35-39	325	(14)	880	(19)	306	(18)	5	(10)	2	(10)	1,520	(17)
40-44	182	(8)	394	(9)	141	(8)	8	(16)	1	(5)	726	(8)
45-49	95	(4)	179	(4)	61	(3)	4	(8)	—		341	(4)
50-54	86	(4)	100	(2)	30	(2)	3	(6)	1	(5)	220	(2)
55-59	95	(4)	59	(1)	22	(1)	1	(2)	—		177	(2)
60-64	93	(4)	38	(1)	15	(1)	3	(6)	1	(5)	150	(2)
65 or older	255	(11)	44	(1)	14	(1)	3	(6)	1	(5)	317	(4)
Female subtotal	2,403	(100)	4,617	(100)	1,747	(100)	51	(100)	20	(100)	8,862	(100)
Total	**53,759**		**25,276**		**14,358**		**557**		**111**		**94,280**	

[1] Includes 219 persons whose race/ethnicity is unknown.

Table 7. AIDS deaths and case-fatality rates, by half-year of diagnosis and age group, diagnosed through April 1989, United States

Half-year of diagnosis	Adults/adolescents			Children <13 years old		
	Cases	Deaths	Case-fatality rate	Cases	Deaths	Case-fatality rate
Before 1981	75	61	81.3	7	5	71.4
1981 Jan.-June	87	80	92.0	6	4	66.7
July-Dec.	190	174	91.6	5	5	100.0
1982 Jan.-June	329	292	88.8	13	10	76.9
July-Dec.	648	581	89.7	14	11	78.6
1983 Jan.-June	1,247	1,135	91.0	33	30	90.9
July-Dec.	1,597	1,448	90.7	41	29	70.7
1984 Jan.-June	2,492	2,142	86.0	50	42	84.0
July-Dec.	3,276	2,844	86.8	61	44	72.1
1985 Jan.-June	4,658	3,967	85.2	89	59	66.3
July-Dec.	6,017	4,970	82.6	124	88	71.0
1986 Jan.-June	7,822	6,152	78.6	123	82	66.7
July-Dec.	9,364	6,713	71.7	155	97	62.6
1987 Jan.-June	11,671	7,459	63.9	195	109	55.9
July-Dec.	12,794	6,382	49.9	213	109	51.2
1988 Jan.-June	13,573	5,120	37.7	183	72	39.3
July-Dec.	12,517	3,375	27.0	195	49	25.1
1989 Jan.-Apr.	4,362	649	14.9	54	13	24.1
Total	**92,719**	**53,544**	**57.7**	**1,561**	**858**	**55.0**

Table 8. AIDS cases by year of diagnosis and definition category, diagnosed through April 1989, United States

Definition category[1]	Year of diagnosis					
	Before May 1985	May 1985-Apr. 1986	May 1986-Apr. 1987	May 1987-Apr. 1988	May 1988-Apr. 1989	Cumulative total
	No. (%)	No. (%)	No. (%)	No. (%)	No. (%)	No. (%)
Pre-1987 definition	12,992 (98)	11,985 (93)	17,918 (89)	19,973 (76)	15,161 (70)	78,029 (83)
1987 definition:	199 (2)	931 (7)	2,195 (11)	6,305 (24)	6,621 (30)	16,251 (17)
Specific disease presumptively diagnosed	*89*	*500*	*1,186*	*3,434*	*3,696*	*8,905*
Specific disease definitively diagnosed	*66*	*157*	*305*	*541*	*431*	*1,500*
HIV encephalopathy	*15*	*77*	*243*	*802*	*797*	*1,934*
HIV wasting syndrome	*29*	*197*	*461*	*1,528*	*1,697*	*3,912*
Total	**13,191 (100)**	**12,916 (100)**	**20,113 (100)**	**26,278 (100)**	**21,782 (100)**	**94,280 (100)**

[1] Persons who meet the criteria for more than one definition category are classified in the definition category listed first.

Table 9. Adult/adolescent AIDS cases by single and multiple exposure categories, reported through April 1989, United States

Exposure category	AIDS cases	
	No.	(%)
Single mode of exposure		
Male homosexual/bisexual contact	54,564	(59)
Intravenous (IV) drug use (female and heterosexual male)	16,242	(18)
Hemophilia/coagulation disorder	523	(1)
Heterosexual contact	3,912	(4)
Receipt of transfusion of blood, blood component, or tissue	2,294	(2)
Other/undetermined	3,187	(3)
Single mode of exposure subtotal	**80,722**	**(87)**
Multiple modes of exposure		
Male homosexual/bisexual contact; IV drug use	6,008	(6)
Male homosexual/bisexual contact; hemophilia	39	(0)
Male homosexual/bisexual contact; heterosexual contact	1,012	(1)
Male homosexual/bisexual contact; receipt of transfusion	1,083	(1)
IV drug use; hemophilia	24	(0)
IV drug use; heterosexual contact	1,928	(2)
IV drug use; receipt of transfusion	475	(1)
Hemophilia; heterosexual contact	4	(0)
Hemophilia; receipt of transfusion	357	(0)
Heterosexual contact; receipt of transfusion	216	(0)
Male homosexual/bisexual contact; IV drug use; hemophilia	12	(0)
Male homosexual/bisexual contact; IV drug use; heterosexual contact	389	(0)
Male homosexual/bisexual contact; IV drug use; receipt of transfusion	184	(0)
Male homosexual/bisexual contact; hemophilia; heterosexual contact	2	(0)
Male homosexual/bisexual contact; hemophilia; receipt of transfusion	28	(0)
Male homosexual/bisexual contact; heterosexual contact; receipt of transfusion	54	(0)
IV drug use; hemophilia; heterosexual contact	8	(0)
IV drug use; hemophilia; receipt of transfusion	17	(0)
IV drug use; heterosexual contact; receipt of transfusion	122	(0)
Hemophilia; heterosexual contact; receipt of transfusion	4	(0)
Male homosexual/bisexual contact; IV drug use; hemophilia; receipt of transfusion	8	(0)
Male homosexual/bisexual contact; IV drug use; heterosexual contact; receipt of transfusion	19	(0)
Male homosexual/bisexual contact; hemophilia; heterosexual contact; receipt of transfusion	1	(0)
IV drug use; hemophilia; heterosexual contact; receipt of transfusion	3	(0)
Multiple modes of exposure subtotal	**11,997**	**(13)**
Total	**92,719**	**(100)**

Technical notes

Surveillance and reporting of AIDS

All 50 states, the District of Columbia, and U.S. dependencies and possessions report AIDS cases to CDC using a uniform case definition and case report form. The original definition was modified in 1985 (*MMWR* 1985;34:373-5) and again in 1987 (*MMWR* 1987;36 [suppl. no. 1S]:1S-15S). The revisions incorporated a broader range of AIDS-indicator diseases and conditions and used human immunodeficiency virus (HIV) diagnostic tests to improve the sensitivity and specificity of the definition. For persons with laboratory-confirmed HIV infection, the 1987 revision incorporated HIV encephalopathy, wasting syndrome, and other indicator diseases that are diagnosed presumptively (i.e., without confirmatory laboratory evidence of the opportunistic disease). AIDS cases that meet the criteria of both the pre-1987 and 1987 definitions are classified in the pre-1987 definition category. The CDC case report form includes demographic, clinical, laboratory, and exposure information.

Each issue of this update includes information received by CDC through the last day of the reporting month. Data are tabulated by date of report to CDC unless otherwise noted. Data for U.S. dependencies and possessions are included in the totals unless otherwise noted.

Reporting by age is based on the person's age at the time of diagnosis of AIDS: adult/adolescent cases include persons 13 years of age and older; pediatric cases include children under 13 years of age.

Metropolitan areas are defined as the Metropolitan Statistical Areas (MSA) for all areas except the 6 New England states. For these states, the New England County Metropolitan Areas (NECMA) are used. Metropolitan areas are named for a central city in the MSA or NECMA and may include several counties. For example, AIDS cases and incidence rates presented for the District of Columbia in Table 1 include only persons residing within the geographic boundaries of the District. AIDS cases and incidence rates for Washington, D.C., in Table 2 include persons residing within several counties in the MSA. State or metropolitan area data tabulations are based on the person's residence at the time of onset of HIV-related symptoms.

Data in this report are provisional; completeness of reporting to state and local health departments varies. In addition, multiple routes of exposure, opportunistic diseases diagnosed after the initial case report was submitted to CDC, and vital status may not be determined or reported for all cases. Caution should be used in interpreting case-fatality rates because reporting of deaths is known to be incomplete.

Exposure categories

For surveillance purposes, AIDS cases are counted only once in a hierarchy of exposure categories. Persons with more than one reported mode of exposure to HIV are classified in the exposure category listed first in the hierarchy, except for persons with a history of both homosexual/bisexual contact and intravenous drug use. They make up a separate exposure category.

"Heterosexual contact" cases include persons who report either specific heterosexual contact with a person with, or at increased risk for, HIV infection (e.g., an intravenous drug user), or persons presumed to have acquired HIV infection through heterosexual contact because they were born in countries with a distinctive pattern of transmission termed "Pattern II" by the World Health Organization (*MMWR* 1988;37:286-8,293-5). Pattern II is observed in areas of central, eastern, and southern Africa and in some Caribbean countries. In these countries, most of the reported cases occur in heterosexuals; the male-to-female ratio is approximately 1:1; and perinatal transmission is more common than in other areas. Intravenous drug use and homosexual transmission either do not occur or occur at a low level.

"Undetermined" cases are in persons with no reported history of exposure to HIV through any of the routes listed in the hierarchy of exposure categories. Undetermined cases include persons who are currently under investigation by local health department officials; persons whose exposure history is incomplete because of death, refusal to be interviewed, or loss to follow-up; and persons who were interviewed or for whom other follow-up information was available and no exposure mode was identified. Persons who have an exposure mode identified at the time of follow-up are reclassified into the appropriate exposure category.

Rates

Rates are on an annual basis per 100,000 population. The denominator for computing the rates is based on population estimates derived from 1980 census data and post-census population estimates. Each 12-month rate is the number of cases for a 12-month period divided by the estimated midyear 1987 or 1988 population multiplied by 100,000.

Case-fatality rates are on a semiannual basis by date of diagnosis. Each 6-month case-fatality rate is the sum of fatal cases reported per number of cases diagnosed in that period. Deaths reported for cases diagnosed in a particular half-year period may have occurred after that period.

—————IN DEVELOPMENT—————
—AIDS MEDICINES—
——————DRUGS AND VACCINES——————

Presented by the Pharmaceutical Manufacturers Association
In cooperation with the Food and Drug Administration

February 1989

13 More Medicines Listed
2 New Drug Approvals, 2 Treatment INDs Granted Since November

Since our last survey in November 1988, 2 drugs have been approved and 2 others given Treatment IND status. 13 drugs and vaccines also have been added to our list of medicines in development.

Two immuno-modulators—INTRON A by Schering-Plough and Roferon-A by Hoffmann-La Roche—have received new drug approvals by the U.S. Food and Drug Administration for the treatment of Kaposi's sarcoma, a malignant skin tumor condition common to AIDS patients. (The two drugs already have been approved for marketing to treat other diseases.)

Two other medicines—Cytovene and Pentam 300 (aerosol)— have received Treatment IND approvals. The FDA's Treatment IND status allows for expanded distribution of experimental therapies for immediately life-threatening or serious conditions before marketing approval has been granted, after safety and some degree of efficacy have been demonstrated in clinical testing.

Cytovene, an anti-viral being developed by Syntex, was given a Treatment IND for patients with sight-threatening CMV (cytomegalovirus). The drug is also in Phase III clinical trials—advanced human tests—for peripheral CMV retinitis (not immediately sight-threatening).

The anti-infective Pentam 300 (aerosol) by LyphoMed received its Treatment IND approval for the prevention of *Pneumocystis carinii* pneumonia (PCP). PCP is found in about 80 percent of all AIDS patients at some time during the course of the disease and is a major cause of death. Pentam 300 (aerosol) is also in Phase III testing for the treatment of PCP.

The quarter since November 1988 has been an active one for AIDS research. The latest survey by the Pharmaceutical Manufacturers Association shows that

Changes in Totals

	November 1988	February 1989
COMPANIES	47	58
MEDICINES	55	67

67 medicines and vaccines are being or have been developed, up from 55 last quarter. 58 companies are involved, up from 47 in November.

Since last quarter, 13 medicines have been added to the chart and 1 deleted, for a net gain of 12 over the three-month period. 13 new companies also were added to the chart, while 2 were deleted.

Every category of our survey has shown an increase since last quarter:

• **Anti-virals.** 16 companies are involved with 17 anti-virals, 4 more than in November. Carrisyn by Carrington Laboratories, Inc., d4T by Bristol-Myers, EL10 by Elan Corp. PLC and Novapren by Novaferon Labs, Inc. (Diapren, Inc., marketer) have been added.

• **Immuno-modulators.** 27 immuno-modulators in development by 25 companies are now listed on our chart. 2 of the 4 products added this quarter—Carrisyn and EL10—are also being tested as anti-virals. HIV core particle immunostimulant by Rorer and SK&F106528 by Smith, Kline & French Laboratories are also new to our chart. One product, Isoprinosine by Newport Pharmaceuticals, was deleted this quarter. Another—EPREX by Ortho Pharmaceutical Corp.—has been reclassified and is now listed in the new "Other" category.

• **Anti-infectives.** 10 companies have developed or are developing 11 medicines in this category, up from 7 in November. 4 products have been added this quarter. The new listings are clindamycin with primaquine by Upjohn, Mycostatin Pastille by Squibb Corp., spiramycin by Rhone-Poulenc Pharmaceuticals and Sporanox by Janssen Pharmaceutica.

• **Vaccines.** 11 vaccines now are being developed by 12 companies. One more vaccine—VaxSyn HIV-1 (p24) by MicroGeneSys—has been added to our list and is also being tested as a therapeutic. Another vaccine by MicroGeneSys— VaxSyn HIV-1 (gp160)—has progressed to Phase 1 testing as both a vaccine and a therapeutic.

• **Other.** This is a new category to our survey, listing 3 products in development by 3 companies. One product, EPREX, was previously classified as an immuno-modulator. The two other products— Megace by Bristol-Myers and Vivonex P.E.N. by Norwich Eaton Pharmaceuticals —are new to the chart. Megace is already approved for the treatment of breast cancer but is being tested to see if it can help AIDS patients regain their appetites and body weight.

Nine medicines—2 anti-virals and 7 immuno-modulators—are still being tested in combination therapy with Retrovir by Burroughs Wellcome, still the only drug approved for the treatment of AIDS itself.

Three of the immuno-modulators—a granulocyte macrophage colony stimulating factor and INTRON A by Schering-Plough, and Neupogen by Amgen—have begun Phase II trials.

Genentech is continuing its combination therapy research with gamma interferon and tumor necrosis factor to treat AIDS-related complex (ARC).

Currently, there are no New Drug Applications on file at the FDA. 9 drugs are now in Phase III clinical trials, up from 5 in November.

The results of this quarter's survey indicate that the nation's research-based pharmaceutical industry continues to expand its effort against AIDS.

[signature]

Gerald J. Mossinghoff, *President*
Pharmaceutical Manufacturers Association

AIDS Medicines In Development

Anti-virals

DRUG NAME	MANUFACTURER	INDICATION	U.S. DEVELOPMENT STATUS
AL–721®	Ethigen (Los Angeles, CA)	ARC, PGL	Phase I/II
		HIV positive, AIDS	Phase II
Betaseron® Recombinant Human Interferon Beta	Triton Biosciences (Alameda, CA)	AIDS, Kaposi's sarcoma, ARC	Phase III
Carrisyn® Acemannan	Carrington Laboratories, Inc. (Irving, TX)	AIDS, ARC (See also immuno-modulators)	Phase I
Cytovene Ganciclovir	Syntex (Palo Alto, CA)	sight-threatening CMV	Treatment IND
		peripheral CMV retinitis	Phase III
d4T Didehydrodeoxy-thymidine	Bristol-Myers (New York, NY)	AIDS, ARC	Phase I
ddI Dideoxyinosine	Bristol-Myers (New York, NY)	AIDS, ARC	Phase I
EL10	Elan Corp. PLC (Gainesville, GA)	HIV infection (See also immuno-modulators)	IND approved
Foscarnet Trisodium Phosphonoformate	Astra Pharmaceutical Products, Inc. (Westborough, MA)	CMV retinitis, HIV infection, other CMV infections	Phase I/II
HIVCID™ Dideoxycytidine; ddc	Hoffmann-La Roche (Nutley, NJ)	AIDS, ARC	Phase II/III (Orphan Drug)
Novapren®	Novaferon Labs, Inc. (Akron, OH) Diapren, Inc. (Roseville, MN, marketer)	HIV inhibitor	Phase I
Peptide T Octapeptide Sequence	Peninsula Labs (Belmont, CA)	AIDS	Phase I
Retrovir Zidovudine; AZT	Burroughs Wellcome (Rsch. Triangle Park, NC)	AIDS, adv. ARC	NDA approved
		pediatric AIDS, Kaposi's sarcoma, asymptomatic HIV infection, less severe HIV disease, neurological involvement, in combination w/other therapies, post-exposure prophylaxis in health care workers	Phase I/II
Rifabutin Ansamycin LM 427	Adria Laboratories (Dublin, OH) Erbamont (Stamford, CT)	ARC	Phase II
Uendex® Dextran Sulfate	Ueno Fine Chem. Industry Ltd. (Osaka, Japan)	AIDS, ARC, HIV positive asymptomatic	Phase II (NIAID Trials)
Virazole Ribavirin	Viratek/ICN (Costa Mesa, CA)	asymptomatic HIV positive, LAS, ARC	Phase II/III
Wellferon Alpha Interferon	Burroughs Wellcome (Rsch. Triangle Park, NC)	Kaposi's sarcoma, HIV, in combination w/Retrovir	Phase I
Zovirax Acyclovir	Burroughs Wellcome (Rsch. Triangle Park, NC)	AIDS, ARC, asymptomatic HIV positive, in combination w/Retrovir	Phase I/II

Immuno-modulators

DRUG NAME	MANUFACTURER	INDICATION	U.S. DEVELOPMENT STATUS
Antibody which neutralizes pH labile Alpha aberrant Interferon in an immuno-adsorption column	Advanced Biotherapy Concepts (Rockville, MD)	AIDS, ARC	Phase I

Provided as a Public Service by the Pharmaceutical Manufacturers Association.

Immuno-modulators

DRUG NAME	MANUFACTURER	INDICATION	U.S. DEVELOPMENT STATUS
AS–101	Wyeth-Ayerst Laboratories (Philadelphia, PA)	AIDS	Phase II
Bropirimine	Upjohn (Kalamazoo, MI)	advanced AIDS	Phase II
Carrisyn® Acemannan	Carrington Laboratories, Inc. (Irving, TX)	AIDS, ARC (See also anti-virals)	Phase I
CL246,738	American Cyanamid (Pearl River, NY) Lederle Laboratories (Wayne, NJ)	AIDS, Kaposi's sarcoma	Phase I/II
EL10	Elan Corp. PLC (Gainesville, GA)	HIV infection (See also anti-virals)	IND approved
Gamma Interferon	Genentech (S. San Francisco, CA)	ARC, in combination w/TNF (tumor necrosis factor)	Phase I
Granulocyte Macrophage Colony Stimulating Factor	Genetics Institute (Cambridge, MA) Sandoz (East Hanover, NJ)	AIDS	Phase II
Granulocyte Macrophage Colony Stimulating Factor	Hoechst-Roussel (Somerville, NJ) Immunex (Seattle, WA)	AIDS	Phase II
Granulocyte Macrophage Colony Stimulating Factor	Schering-Plough (Madison, NJ)	AIDS	Phase II
		AIDS, in combination w/Retrovir	Phase II
HIV Core Particle Immunostimulant	Rorer (Ft. Washington, PA)	seropositive HIV	Phase II
IL–2 Interleukin-2	Cetus (Emeryville, CA)	AIDS, in combination w/Retrovir	Phase I/II
IL–2 Interleukin-2	Hoffmann-La Roche (Nutley, NJ) Immunex (Seattle, WA)	AIDS, ARC, HIV, in combination w/Retrovir	Phase I
Immune Globulin Intravenous (human)	Cutter Biological (Berkeley, CA)	pediatric AIDS, in combination w/Retrovir	Phase II/III
IMREG®–1	Imreg (New Orleans, LA)	AIDS, Kaposi's sarcoma, ARC, PGL	Phase III
IMREG®–2	Imreg (New Orleans, LA)	AIDS, Kaposi's sarcoma, ARC, PGL	Phase II
Imuthiol Diethyl Dithio Carbamate	Merieux Institute (Miami, FL)	AIDS, ARC	Phase II/III
INTRON A Alpha–2 Interferon	Schering-Plough (Madison, NJ)	Kaposi's sarcoma	NDA approved
		w/Retrovir: AIDS	Phase II
Methionine-Enkephalin	TNI Pharmaceuticals (Chicago, IL)	AIDS, ARC	Phase I/II
MTP–PE Muramyl-Tripeptide	Ciba-Geigy Corp. (Summit, NJ)	Kaposi's sarcoma	Phase II
Neupogen™ Granulocyte Colony Stimulating Factor	Amgen (Thousand Oaks, CA)	AIDS, in combination w/Retrovir	Phase II
rCD4 Recombinant Soluble Human CD4	Genentech (S. San Francisco, CA)	AIDS, ARC	Phase I
Receptin™ Recombinant Soluble Human CD4	Biogen (Cambridge, MA)	AIDS, ARC	Phase I

Vaccines

MANUFACTURER	INDICATION	U.S. DEVELOPMENT STATUS
Biocine (Ciba-Geigy/Chiron) (Emeryville, CA)	AIDS	preclinical research phase
Biotech Research Labs (Rockville, MD)	AIDS	research phase
HIVAC-1e Bristol-Myers/Oncogen (New York, NY)	AIDS	Phase I
Genentech (S. San Francisco, CA)	AIDS	early research phase
Institut Merieux (Lyon, France) Cambridge Bioscience (Worcester, MA)	AIDS	early research phase
VaxSyn® HIV-1 (gp160) MicroGeneSys (West Haven, CT)	AIDS	Phase I as vaccine
	AIDS	Phase I as therapeutic
VaxSyn® HIV–1 (p24) MicroGeneSys (West Haven, CT)	AIDS	IND submitted as vaccine
	AIDS	IND submitted as therapeutic
Otisville BioPharm, Inc. (Otisville, NY)	AIDS	early research phase
Repligen (Cambridge, MA) Merck (Rahway, NJ)	AIDS	animal studies
Viral Technologies (CEL-SCI, Alpha 1 Biomedicals) (Washington, DC)	AIDS	IND submitted
Wistar Institute (Philadelphia, PA)	AIDS	early research phase

Diagnostics

The rapid development and distribution of HIV antibody tests remains one of the most significant medical technology achievements in the fight against AIDS. The tests enable physicians to detect evidence of infection in humans and provide a way to help reduce the risk of transmitting HIV through blood and blood products. The success story of AIDS diagnostics continues as new versions improve detection and analysis capabilities.

23 companies are involved with 46 diagnostics that have been developed or are in development, including 13 new products in our current survey. Most of these tests are for detecting or confirming the presence of HIV antibodies or antigens in the blood. Three are targeted for detection of immune dysfunction in people who have tested positive for the HIV virus.

PMA will no longer list each diagnostic in its quarterly AIDS survey.

Among the companies most active in diagnostic development are:

Company	No. of Diagnostics
Electro-Nucleonics	6
DuPont	4
Genetic Systems/ Bristol-Myers	4
Abbott	3
MicroGeneSys	3
Organon Teknika	3
Thermascan	3

Immuno-modulators

DRUG NAME	MANUFACTURER	INDICATION	U.S. DEVELOPMENT STATUS
Roferon–A Interferon Alfa 2a	Hoffmann-La Roche (Nutley, NJ)	Kaposi's sarcoma	NDA approved
		AIDS, ARC, in combination w/Retrovir	Phase II
SK&F106528 Soluble T4	Smith, Kline & French Laboratories (Philadelphia, PA)	HIV infection	Phase I
Timunox™ Thymopentin	Immunobiology Research Institute (Annandale, NJ)	HIV infection	Phase II
Tumor Necrosis Factor; TNF	Genentech (S. San Francisco, CA)	ARC, in combination w/gamma interferon	Phase I

Anti-infectives

DRUG NAME	MANUFACTURER	INDICATION	U.S. DEVELOPMENT STATUS
Clindamycin with Primaquine	Upjohn (Kalamazoo, MI)	PCP	Phase I/II
Diflucan Fluconazole	Pfizer (New York, NY)	cryptococcal meningitis, candidiasis	Phase III
Mycostatin® Pastille Nystatin Pastille	Squibb Corp. (Princeton, NJ)	prevention of oral candidiasis	Phase III
Ornidyl Eflornithine	Merrell Dow (Cincinnati, OH)	PCP	Phase II (Orphan Drug)
Pentam® 300 Pentamidine Isethionate (IM&IV)	LyphoMed (Rosemont, IL)	PCP treatment	NDA approved for IM & IV use only
Pentam® 300 (aerosol)	LyphoMed (Rosemont, IL)	PCP prophylaxis	Treatment IND (Orphan Drug)
		PCP treatment	Phase III
Piritrexim	Burroughs Wellcome (Rsch. Triangle Park, NC)	PCP treatment	Phase I/II
Pneumopent™ Pentamidine Isethionate for inhalation	Fisons Corporation (Bedford, MA)	PCP prophylaxis	Phase III
Spiramycin	Rhone-Poulenc Pharmaceuticals (Princeton, NJ)	cryptosporidial diarrhea	Phase II
Sporanox® Intraconazole– R51211	Janssen Pharmaceutica (Piscataway, NJ)	histoplasmosis; cryptococcal meningitis	Phase III
Trimetrexate*	Warner-Lambert (Morris Plains, NJ)	PCP	Treatment IND

Other

DRUG NAME	MANUFACTURER	INDICATION	U.S. DEVELOPMENT STATUS
EPREX™ Recombinant Human Erythropoietin	Ortho Pharmaceutical Corp. (Raritan, NJ)	severe anemia assoc. w/AIDS and Retrovir therapy	Phase II/III
Megace® Megestrol Acetate	Bristol-Myers (New York, NY)	treatment of anorexia and cachexia associated with AIDS	Phase III
Vivonex® P.E.N. Total Enteral Nutrition	Norwich Eaton Pharmaceuticals (Norwich, NY)	diarrhea and malabsorption related to AIDS & ARC	uncontrolled human descriptive clinical studies

*Company-sponsored clinical trials have ceased.

The Drug Approval Process

The U.S. system of new drug approvals is perhaps the most rigorous in the world. Here is how a drug is tested and approved.

Preclinical Testing. The promising agent is first subjected to extensive laboratory and animal testing to determine answers to two key questions: Is the compound biologically active? Is it safe? If the answers to both appear to be affirmative, the drug sponsor is ready to test in humans. This stage generally lasts from one to two years.

Investigational New Drug. Before human tests can start, the drug sponsor must file an Investigational New Drug (IND) application with the Food and Drug Administration (FDA), showing the results of all animal testing and how the drug is made. The IND becomes effective if FDA does not disapprove the application in 30 days.

Human Testing (Clinical). There are three phases of human testing, each involving larger numbers of people than the one before.

Phase I. Safety Studies and Pharmacological Profiling: This phase determines the drug's pharmacological actions, its safe dosage range, how it is absorbed, distributed, metabolized and excreted, and the duration of its action. These tests involve a small number of normal healthy subjects (not patients). Phase I clinical testing can usually be conducted in less than one year.

Phase II. Pilot Efficacy Studies: This phase consists of controlled studies in approximately 200 to 300 volunteer patients to assess the drug's effectiveness. Simultaneous animal and human studies continue to determine the drug's safety. Phase II clinical testing may require about two years to complete.

Phase III. Extensive Clinical Trials: Here the testing moves to larger numbers of volunteer patients, usually 1,000 to 3,000, in clinics and hospitals. The drug is administered by practicing physicians to those suffering from the condition the drug is intended to treat. These studies must confirm earlier efficacy studies and identify low-incidence adverse reactions. Phase III clinical trials last about three years.

New Drug Application (NDA). Following completion of Phase III, the drug sponsor must file an NDA with the FDA, containing all the information the sponsor has gathered. NDAs typically run into thousands of pages. The information submitted must include the chemical structure of the drug, scientific rationale and purpose, animal and laboratory studies, results of all tests in humans, formulation and production details, and proposed labeling. On average, the NDA review and approval process by FDA takes two to three years.

Approval. Once an NDA is approved, the company is required to periodically submit reports to FDA, including adverse reaction data and production, quality control and distribution records. For some drugs, FDA requires affirmative post-marketing monitoring, or additional studies to evaluate the long-term effects. NOTE: In October 1988, the Food and Drug Administration (FDA) announced an Interim Rule to speed the approval of drugs for life-threatening and other serious diseases by having FDA work more closely with pharmaceutical companies in expediting preclinical research and development and in designing, monitoring and evaluating clinical trials. Under the plan, if a drug shows sufficient promise after Phases I and II, Phase III would be eliminated. (President Bush's Cancer Panel is also undertaking a review of the FDA approval process for cancer and AIDS drugs.)

GLOSSARY

AIDS—Acquired Immune Deficiency Syndrome.

anorexia—Prolonged loss of appetite that leads to significant weight loss.

antibody—An immunoglobulin molecule produced by plasma cells in response to stimulation by antigen. Antibodies provide a defense mechanism against foreign proteins by binding to them, which in turn counteracts the effects of antigens and therefore protects the body.

antigen—A foreign protein that can cause an immune response by stimulating the production of antibodies in the body.

ARC—AIDS-related complex.

cachexia—Profound and marked state of general ill health and malnutrition.

candidiasis—A fungal infection, usually of the moist cutaneous areas of the body, including the skin, mouth, esophagus and respiratory tract.

CMV—Cytomegalovirus. An opportunistic infection that can cause blindness and be fatal in AIDS patients. ("Sight-threatening" refers to the later stage of CMV that is considered to be an immediate threat to a patient's vision. "Peripheral CMV retinitis" refers to the early stages of the disease, which can become sight-threatening if left untreated.)

cryptococcal meningitis—A fungal infection that affects the three membranes (meninges) surrounding the brain and spinal cord. Symptoms include severe headache, vertigo, nausea, anorexia, sight disorders and mental deterioration.

cryptosporidial diarrhea—Caused by a parasite and characterized by chronic, profuse, watery diarrhea, accompanied by fever, marked weight loss and enlarged lymph nodes.

enteral nutrition—A nutrient substance prepared to be absorbed through the small intestines rather than the stomach.

histoplasmosis—A disease caused by a fungal infection that can affect all the organs of the body. Symptoms usually include fever, shortness of breath, cough, weight loss and physical exhaustion.

HIV—Human Immunodeficiency Virus, the virus that causes AIDS.

IM—Intramuscular.

IND—Investigational New Drug.

IV—Intravenous.

Kaposi's sarcoma—A rare malignant skin tumor that occurs in some AIDS patients. It can be accompanied by fever, enlarged lymph nodes and gastro-intestinal problems.

LAS—Lymphadenopathy Syndrome, or persistently enlarged lymph nodes, which often occur in the early stages of AIDS without any other symptoms.

malabsorption—Faulty absorption of nutrients from the intestines.

Orphan drug—Indicated for rare diseases.

PCP—*Pneumocystis carinii* pneumonia. A severe lung infection found in nearly 80 percent of all AIDS patients at some time during the course of the disease and a major cause of death.

PGL—Persistent generalized abnormal enlargement of the lymph nodes (lymphadenopathy).

Phase I—Safety testing and pharmacological profiling in humans.

Phase II—Effectiveness testing in humans.

Phase III—Extensive clinical trials in humans.

prophylaxis—Treatment intended to preserve health and prevent the spread of disease.

seropositive—Positive blood test for evidence of an infectious disease, such as HIV infection.

H. ROBERT MALINOWSKY

H. Robert Malinowsky is Professor, Bibliographer of Science
and Technology, at the Library of the University of Illinois,
Chicago. He is the editor of *Science and Technology Annual
Reference Review* and *The International Directory of Gay
and Lesbian Periodicals*, also published by the Oryx Press.

GERALD PERRY

Gerald Perry is Reference Librarian and User Education
Coordinator at the Library of Rush University, Chicago, IL.